HEALTH
QUOTIENT

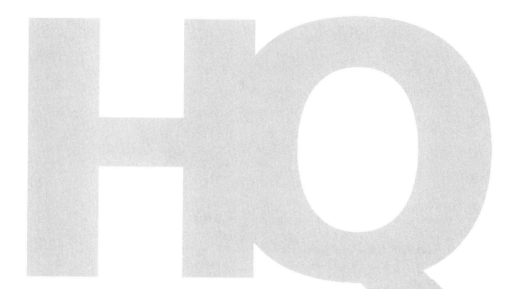

HEALTH QUOTIENT

AN INTELLIGENT APPROACH TO PERSONAL HEALTH

WAH JUN TZE,
CM, MD, FRCPC

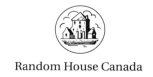

Random House Canada

Canadian Cataloguing in Publication Data

Tze, Wah Jun
  HQ: an intelligent approach to personal health

ISBN 0-679-31055-X

1. Health.   2. Holistic medicine.   I. Title.

RA776.T93 2000   613   C99-933058-6

Pages 296 – 98 constitute an extension of this copyright page.

Cover design: Scott Gibbs
Interior design: Susan Thomas/Digital Zone

Printed and bound in the United States of America

Visit Random House of Canada Limited's Web site: www.randomhouse.ca

10 9 8 7 6 5 4 3 2 1

This book is dedicated to my devoted wife, Theresa, our healthy children, Deirdra and Dennis, and grandchildren, Julia and Jon.

CONTENTS

FOREWORD

The world needs a higher HQ—or Health Quotient—as we move into a new century. That, in essence, is the message of this profoundly important book by Dr. Wah Jun Tze, who has employed his knowledge and experience of Western and Eastern medicine, the sciences and the healing arts of medicine to arrive at a crucial conclusion: we must develop a health model based on wellness, taking the best from both medical worlds, if we are to have effective health systems on this planet. We must take the best of the old, of the new, of the East and of the West. And we all, as individuals, must take more responsibility for our own health—or, more specifically, wellness. Self-care rather than physician-centred care could radically alter the general health of our societies.

In China, the country with a population of more than 1.2 billion, people have enjoyed reasonably good health despite very limited resources. Millions of people are living healthier and longer than ever before. This situation is possible partly because of the underlying importance of centuries-old, traditional Chinese medicine, which emphasizes wellness, gives equal weight to mind and body, and treats the whole person rather than a specific ailment or symptom. In Canada and sister countries, meanwhile, there have been incredible medical and scientific advances that have helped to extend life expectancy and to reduce suffering. But our medical system is stretched to the limit as more and more people, understandably, wish to take advantage of new procedures, drugs and cures.

What's needed, as Dr. Tze shows here, is an integration of all the best philosophies. We must, wherever we live, take advantage of our body's natural healing power and practise a healthy lifestyle. We must remember the important role of the mind in health and health care. We must address not life expectancy alone but also health expectancy and the quality of our lives. More important, we must continually promote scientific and technical advances.

We'd like to commend Dr. Tze for his vision on the future of our health care and everyone's wellness. And we urge you, as you read this book, to regard the concept of HQ with serious thought. The higher your HQ, the better you can control your own health. If HQ were to become a household idea around the globe, we would all be a lot healthier—and happier.

The world really does need a better HQ for the new millennium!

Chen Mingzhang, MD
Minister of Health, China

Hedy Fry, MD
Minister of Multiculturalism, Canada

HQ—THE HEALTH QUOTIENT

Welcome to the world of HQ—a quiet revolution in health! HQ stands for "health quotient." It represents your health intelligence and a radically new approach to your health.

Good health is your most prized possession, worth more than millions of dollars in the bank. You have to save, plan carefully and work hard to have healthy finances, but think of how little time you devote to a healthy mind and body. You take them for granted—until things go wrong.

In this book I aim to give you a hands-on, easy-to-use way of assessing your personal HQ, and the knowledge and resources to improve it. You will create a personal health profile, a blueprint of yourself, and an action plan that could dramatically change your life and your health for the better. Once you understand your HQ and how to use it, you will have the means to live a longer and healthier life, and, more importantly, the quality of your life will be much higher, whatever your age, whatever your medical condition.

Your HQ—like your IQ (intelligence quotient) and your emotional intelligence—is one of your personal characteristics, part of what makes you tick, something that distinguishes you from the next person. But HQ characteristics, unlike those that make up your IQ, are not preordained at birth. Your HQ can be improved by education, knowledge, willpower and emotional intelligence. Once improved, it can give you the power to live a healthier, more satisfying life. It will enable you to make wise, often crucial choices affecting your life and your health. It could mean deciding to go for a walk every day, changing your diet, discovering a new technique to cope with stress or taking up a new sport. But it's more, much more, than that.

Over and above simply taking good care of yourself, to have a high HQ you need to take on the responsibility for your whole health—to practise "self-care." HQ focuses on wellness. This, in essence, means achieving your best level of health and well-being through self-care. That idea will pop up a lot in this book. It means taking charge of your personal health destiny and not leaving everything up to "the experts." In today's medical practice we rely far too heavily on drugs, surgery and certain procedures. Self-care is an important alternative. There is no healing force on earth that is stronger or more universally accessible than your ability to care for yourself through healthful living, personal beliefs and acceptance of your body's innate power to heal itself.

Self-care requires knowledge, which is the core of a strong HQ. The more you know, the better able you will be to make intelligent choices about your health. Through this book I will help you to be more fully aware of modern medical practices, non-mainstream medicine, the mind/body connection, disease prevention, drugs and herbs, types of exercise and stress-relieving techniques, and I will tell you how to have access to a wealth of other information in order to build your personal health action plan.

HQ is a holistic, integrative, evidence-based, all-embracing concept of health, based on the most current evidence and health knowledge. It defines health as not merely the absence of disease but also the state of your wellness. Emotions and your general mental state, your environment and your living situation can all have a direct bearing on your health. Good health in the HQ sense involves all the physical, mental, emotional, spiritual, environmental and social aspects of your existence, and includes a good quality of life.

The HQ concept emphasizes the link between mind and body as a basic part of good health care. A healthy mind—one that is less stressed, calmer, more serene—means a healthier person altogether. Traditional Chinese medicine has for thousands of years believed that stress and emotion can have a direct impact on our physiological makeup, a theory that has been accepted by Westerners only relatively recently. Use of such techniques as mindfulness meditation, hatha yoga and qigong for maintaining health and conquering illness has been common for centuries. Lowering stress through these and other relaxation techniques has been found to help cure a range of ailments and symptoms, from insomnia to infertility.

How does our spiritual and emotional well-being affect our health? It has become increasingly apparent that those who are spiritually fulfilled are often the healthiest among us. According to Daniel Goleman, having a high emotional intelligence, which includes "self-awareness and impulse control, persistence, zeal and motivation, empathy and social deftness," has a positive influence on the three big problems of our age: anxiety, anger and depression.

HQ embraces the best of all health worlds. No one medical system can address all the facets of health care. In the West our doctors are too often trained to identify and treat the symptoms rather than the underlying causes. Our

Western system knows how to use surgery and drugs effectively, but it doesn't have a holistic framework for viewing all the aspects of your life—physical, psychological and social. Our doctors don't comfort you or teach you peace of mind. We have tended to separate the mind from the body. In most parts of Asia, however, doctors have been taught to deal with each person as a unique individual, spending time with patients, getting to know them, understanding how they feel. Even in mainstream medicine some doctors are finding that they can help patients undergoing surgery by preparing them mentally, relaxing their apprehensions and talking to them during operations.

Practitioners of contemporary complementary medicine, such as naturopathy, also believe in the importance of natural healing and the healing power of various natural products and approaches. Again, we are beginning to appreciate the powerful capacity of the human body to heal itself without medical and drug intervention. Healing is a function of our bodies, and it happens continuously.

What can we learn from ancient Chinese medicine today? And what about the ancient Ayurvedic medical system, or North American Native healing, or some of the age-old practices of Africa? Can we combine the best of the old with the best of what's now being discovered? Traditional Chinese medicine's four major components—acupuncture, herbal medicine, food cures and manipulation therapy—are now gaining a wider appreciation in the West. Special exercises like Tai Chi are increasingly seen as having substantial health benefits.

I am not only a Western-trained clinician, pediatrician, academician and scientist but I have also been exposed to the best practices of the East, particularly in China, and have had experience in the field of international health. With my unique background I will help you to sort out the best elements of all these different systems and practices. I am convinced that we can build a healthier, more fulfilled population around the world by bringing together the potential and the best of these medical worlds. In fact, my vision for the future is to create a new HQ health culture, in which people take charge of their personal health in this globally integrated health world.

It's not only time for a change, it's high time.

In spite of all the amazing advances of the twentieth century, our current way of providing health care is in disarray. Our conventional health-care systems are under siege, understaffed and strained to their financial limits. Long lineups for heart surgery have become common and, in some cases, have led to tragedies. In developing countries, poverty and lack of accessible primary health care cause millions of premature deaths and disabilities each year.

Despite all the medical miracles and the daily breakthroughs in our understanding of genetics and health, mainstream medicine is still incapable of dealing effectively with some of the most common chronic diseases and conditions. Cancer, heart disease, diabetes and AIDS continue to claim too many victims around the globe.

Too many of us, older people especially, continue to lead less than adequate lives. As we move into a new millennium, our society in some ways seems sicker than ever. Our physical environment is deteriorating rapidly. More people are living in heavily polluted and crowded cities. More illnesses have environmental origins. Social and stress-related diseases are running rampant in the industrialized nations. The changes in our habits have caused an increase in the prevalence of sexually transmitted diseases, such as HIV/AIDS, and lifestyle-related chronic diseases. Migrating populations mean that diseases move from place to place, from country to country. What are the effects of these conditions on all of us? What are we to do about the growing problem of resurgent and new antibiotic-resistant infections, which we have created by our widespread use and abuse of drugs?

And our affluence has made us fat! Modern society is largely—please forgive the expression—obese. Food is a form of medicine, yet too many of us treat it as a convenience product. It is the fuel for our lives, but many people are more careful about what they put in their cars than what they put into their stomachs.

Against this backdrop, we are unsure how to steer our delivery of health care. The system can no longer cope, and people are demanding changes. The traditional ways aren't working for us, and as a society we are hungry for more HQ health knowledge. The growing number of health resource centres, wellness centres, natural food stores and fitness centres in recent years shows that we are not only ready for, but indeed insisting upon, taking greater responsibility for our personal health and well-being. Our enthusiasm has generated a bewildering array of choices. And thanks to modern technology, we're also in the midst of an information explosion, as sources on the World Wide Web churn out a never-ending stream of health news and advice. Who and what to believe?

That's where your HQ and this book come in. I want to shift your perception of health treatment so that wellness, health maintenance and disease prevention become paramount. My goal is to equip you to sort through the maze of global medical information for credible data and reliable facts, so that you can make your own health decisions. I want to help you learn what is vital for health care and gain the knowledge required to make wise health choices.

At last you have a book that tells the whole story. *HQ* is different from the scores of other health-help books available in bookstores and on library shelves because it suggests a radical new philosophy of health care, one that is not limited to one disease, one kind of medicine, one type of procedure or one way of thinking. I don't want to be the conventional "expert" doctor who simply tells you what to do. My aim is to give you better control of your health by helping you consider the wider sphere—ancient remedies as well as high-tech advances, conventional Western approaches but also the mind/body connection, complementary medicine and the spiritual dimension.

The HQ concept is a wellness ideal through which self-care, a healthy lifestyle, and holistic and integrative approaches to health care, based on the most up-to-date health knowledge, will evolve into a new health culture. This will enable people from all walks of life and from different parts of the world to live longer, healthier and happier lives.

You are different from every other person and have your own health needs. Through HQ, I want to empower you to take control of your own health with confidence, determination and a good understanding of self-care. Don't worry: gaining a high HQ doesn't require you to pore over a pile of medical dictionaries, academic texts and studies. This health enhancement book is enough to help get you started on your way to better health. Use it as a reference and a guide.

Section I tells you what to aim for, how to measure your health and how to assess your results. The goal of the HQ Profile is to help you build a higher HQ and increase your health expectancy with a good quality of life. Section II shows you how to promote your wellness and your HQ throughout the journey of life, from the womb to old age, taking into account your genetic endowment and your environment. In this section I have also devoted two chapters to the mind/body connection and another to the way in which lifestyle can affect your health. In section III I discuss the health options currently available to you and the HQ approach to dealing with illness and disease. Section IV gives you an opportunity to put all your HQ awareness to work and create your own personal health plan. Wondering where to go from there? The last part also suggests resources for further reading. The epilogue contains my vision of a new model of health care: the HQ health culture.

Congratulations! By picking up this book, you have already taken a step towards a healthier life. Stick with it and it will lead you ultimately to the peak of your personal health. Good luck on your way.

SECTION 1

THE HQ PROFILE
AND YOUR HEALTH

CHAPTER 1

THE HQ PROFILE

A Framework for Better Health

"How are you?" Think how many times a day we respond to that universal greeting; but do we tell the truth when we reply? Do we even know the truth?

In this section I will guide you through an all-encompassing health questionnaire that I have devised, and by analyzing your results you will have a complete health profile—the foundation stone of your new HQ awareness. This measurement approach will not only enable you to answer that vital question regarding your health, but it will also give you the means to achieve a happy, optimistic answer. It will show you how to set health goals and enable you to develop a unique personal health plan to reach those goals. It will help you make the best use of available health-care resources and professionals. And at regular intervals you can check back to see how you're doing and whether to readjust your health plan. It's your body and you're the boss.

You don't have to be a health expert to lead a healthy life. Better health and wellness are for everyone, regardless of economic status, cultural background, personal habits, environment or any other individual circumstances. All it takes is a commitment.

Health measurement: letting you in on a well-kept secret

The HQ questionnaire was created by combining the best of Eastern and Western health knowledge, traditional wisdom and the most up-to-date medical advances. It also takes advantage of recent progress in the development of credible and scientific measurements of health status and quality of life. After taking the test and carefully considering the results, along with absorbing the information in the rest of this book, you will have in your hands a new and dynamic tool with which to care for your health. This profile will enable you to make the wisest choices for your personal health and wellness.

That's the beauty of the HQ Profile: it evolves from an extensive, easily understood and affordable gauge of general health and quality of life that can be self-administered by almost anyone. In spite of all the various treatment and preventive health-care methods currently available, most people have never before had the means to assess their own health status and plan a course of action to improve it. In my research and review of the tools available to help people measure their personal health status, I discovered two valuable tests: the World Health Organization's "Quality of Life-100" (WHOQOL-100) and "Short-Form-36" (SF-36) questionnaires. I also found that they are a well-kept secret. Few people have access to this information, nor has it been popularized in any way.

The questionnaire in this book is a synthesis of the two quality-of-life measurements and my own background, experience and observations—all brought together in my vision of a new concept of health. Besides adapting well-established health and measurement systems, I have garnered useful material from my many consultations with experts in various fields. My own credentials cover the spectrum of Western and complementary medicine. I have been exposed extensively to Chinese traditional medicine during more than one hundred trips to China over the past fifteen years. I serve on the editorial boards of a number of scientific and clinical journals and have published numerous scientific articles. While performing ongoing medical research as a full-time professor specializing in the field of pediatric endocrinology and diabetes, I have also founded an institute and other centres for complementary and alternative medicine within conventional medical establishments.

In short, I have immersed myself in the best of the West and the East, the new and the old. And I've tried to use that experience to create the best health measurement plan. My hope is that it will serve as a clear road map and a compass, guiding you on your journey to better health through the confusing and often uncharted territories of our current health care environment. Limited funding, demographic changes brought about by the aging population, the prevalence of many new diseases and changing disease patterns have all led to frustrations and bewilderment even among health professionals. Both developing and industrialized countries are faced with many of the same kinds of challenges and financial dilemmas. In current health care worldwide, a small segment of the population consumes most of the resources, leaving health-care providers and other consumers scrambling to make do with what is left. All these changes and growing demands call for a different perception, a more global approach to health and health-care systems.

The HQ Profile is based on my new vision of a health culture where the focus is on wellness and self-care rather than on illness and reliance upon others or upon a system. This new culture will feature individuals who are knowledgeable about their health and know how to go about improving it on their own, with some guidance and information from experts.

So what is optimal health and wellness?

Without a doubt, health is the most important aspect of your life. Optimal health is a requirement for enjoyable everyday living. It should be your number-one goal, on a day-to-day basis, throughout your life. Unfortunately, many people die prematurely or struggle with poor health, disability or disease. Some don't seek medical advice or obtain treatment when they need it, or don't get the help they need even when they look for it; others simply do not know that many diseases, injuries and illnesses are preventable. Why put up with being sick if you don't have to?

Good health depends on a combination of things: the personal and genetic traits you have inherited, the environment in which you live and work, the care you have received from health-care providers and hospitals, and your personal habits and lifestyle choices. All of these affect health. Many of us fail to see that there are actions we can take ourselves to look and feel healthy. There are serious risks stemming from your personal habits—your lifestyle—that you can control. Health experts now say that lifestyle is one of the most important factors affecting health and quality of life. They believe that many lifestyle choices can have as much impact on your health as the decision of whether or not to smoke. In fact, it is estimated that the risks associated with seven of the ten leading causes of death could be reduced through common-sense changes in lifestyle. Your HQ Profile will show you how.

Health today is far more than the absence of disease and disability. In addition to complete physical, mental and social well-being, health also means achieving a satisfying life. You yourself can add quality to your life. Positive attitudes and awareness, combined with healthy social practices and environment, make a dramatic difference. You have the opportunity to change once you recognize that the combination of your habits, emotional and psychological state, social situation, personality and character affects your health and how you feel every day.

Simply put, for optimal health, knowledge is the key. To be your healthiest, you must identify and realize your health goals. It may well be that to do this you will have to change or find ways to cope with your personal situation. Of course, there are always some factors beyond your control, such as the social practices of the prevailing culture or environmental conditions like air quality.

It takes the community and government to effect those changes. But health-conscious people demand changes, and the actions of each individual do make a difference.

Once you have the information from your health profile, as well as the knowledge and resources that enable you to change, you can improve your health, your well-being and indeed your whole quality of life. "Quality of life"—what does this often-used phrase really mean? There are as many answers to this question as there are people, for we each define quality of life according to our personal values and the expectations of the culture in which we live. It is so much more than mere life expectancy; it's the broad picture, made up of all the brush strokes of our lives—physical health, psychological state, level of independence, social relationships, personal beliefs and the effects of the surrounding world. How good that quality is depends on how satisfied we are with the individual picture we've created. As the artists, we should be trying constantly to paint more meaningfulness and happiness into our pictures.

Many health-care professionals, too, are starting to look beyond diseases, disabilities and symptoms. They are becoming sensitive to the whole picture by helping their patients face their health challenges in the context of their overall quality of life. As a result, both professionals and patients tend to make wiser and more cost-effective choices in the use of health-care resources.

Everyone can benefit from optimal health, but like the ripple in the pond, these benefits often go far beyond the individual to society at large, across borders and even across time, to future generations. Designed to help individuals find or keep good health, the HQ Profile is a tool we can easily share. Who wouldn't want to see loved ones, family, friends and co-workers enjoying better health too? Wellness is contagious; when we see a fit, healthy person, we may be inspired to change. Co-workers can go walking and jogging at lunchtime or play sports together. Businesses will benefit from a healthier workforce, and society will benefit as a whole. People focused on wellness instead of illness spend far less time and money going for medical help, and that leaves costly health-care resources for the people who really need them. As parents, when you set an example of leading a healthier, fitter and more fulfilling life, your children will benefit directly and create their own good health habits. Eventually, as your children grow into adults, the new approach to health will be so much a part of their lives that the new health culture will become a reality.

Taking charge of your personal health

Taking care of yourself means far more than simply avoiding the pitfalls of life. Self-care starts with your ability to view personal health from a holistic— "whole story"—standpoint. It includes identifying self-care resources; choosing and establishing a good rapport with health-care providers; being willing to participate in making health decisions when choices arise; having the determination to practise disease prevention; and using the health-care system in an appropriate way when coping with illness. More than that, practising self-care means improving, where necessary, your living conditions and your lifestyle; making wise use of self-care products and technology; using mind and body health-enhancing techniques such as yoga or Tai Chi; and taking into account how your personal attitudes and beliefs affect your health. In self-care you also need to make an active effort to seek out and digest good health information and resources. For instance, the Internet, CD-ROMs, TV programs and seminars all offer information about self-care. Of course, you have to be careful about the reliability and accuracy of the information.

In today's medical practices there is an overreliance on drugs by both doctors and health-care consumers. One sad result is the increasing number of cases of antibiotic-resistant infections. There has also been overuse of surgery; as a consequence, health-care costs have risen unnecessarily. Medical science and technology, which have so much to be proud of, have encouraged people to hand over responsibility for their personal health to "the experts" and to expect quick fixes for their problems. People practising self-care are familiar with appropriate actions when it comes to disease, symptoms and injury prevention, and are able to cope with minor illnesses. They know when to manage themselves and when it is appropriate to get help. An ability to take an active, well-informed and hands-on role is crucial to becoming healthier and eventually reaching the goal of peak health.

A new health culture can be realized by marrying the familiar scientific, technological approach to the concept of self-care. Scientific research to develop high technology is important and necessary. However, I believe it should be continually directed at specific vital areas, such as acute, traumatic and emergency situations, and at the field of genetic molecular science. The results of such researches will continue to improve life expectancy and repair ailing bodies. The ultimate goal of self-care is a complete about-face from our current practices in order to decrease demand on the health-care system. Disease treatment and expensive high-tech procedures would decline. Such a radical shift in philosophy from high-tech medical care to self-care will also need to be backed up by a major shift of priorities in government health-care funding.

The HQ Profile is the tool you'll need to identify and assess your health requirements so that you can make wise choices for improving your health. Your personal health profile has long-term, ongoing benefits in that it can be used regularly and indefinitely to examine your health status. At any point you can go back to it for another look at your personal health, to target areas that need improvement. This gives you a meaningful way to zero in on your existing health weaknesses in order to face future health challenges. Your profile will provide you with understandable and unbiased information at your fingertips. You will have a unique way to get the clear, whole health picture instead of bits and pieces of information, which may be part of a product pitch or slanted to support a particular point of view.

Approaching health as a dynamic and changeable condition where you, the individual, have a great deal of control can be both motivating and exciting. Such a drastic mental shift is bound to lead to better outcomes in your personal general health and in the future of society's health-care system. If you make the commitment, you will be able to answer that daily question very honestly and very optimistically: "I'm very well, thank you."

The HQ Profile Questionnaire: Measuring Your Health

The HQ Profile encompasses a broad spectrum and measures both your current health situation and the way it can be changed, when necessary, with positive health action. It will provide a clear picture of your current baseline of general health. Although the questions are designed to apply to the widest possible segment of society, some of them may not be applicable to persons with chronic diseases or disabilities. These people can still take the test, but they may need further guidance from their doctors or other health professionals.

All of us want good health, but many of us do not know how to be as healthy as we could be. Good health is not a matter of luck or fate; you have to work at it. The minutes you take to complete this survey may actually help you add years to your life! How? Well, to start, you will be able to identify aspects of your way of life that are risky to your health. This information can help you begin to pinpoint the dangers and rework them into a new, healthy lifestyle. If you do, it's really possible that you will feel better, look better and live longer. Remember, this is not a pass–fail exam. Its purpose is simply to tell you what you need to do to stay healthy or become healthier.

Now, let's take a look at the questionnaire and its categories in more detail.

Each question is a statement. You will be asked to select one of seven words or phrases that expresses most accurately how you relate to the statement or how you would complete it. The test has five major components: Self-care, Knowledge of Health, Lifestyle, The Mind and Life Skills. Each of these areas has four sections, for a total of twenty sections. In turn, each section has five questions, making a total of one hundred questions. Honest and thoughtful answers to the questions will clearly identify risks in your current lifestyle and habits. Then you can read the rest of this book for guidelines and other sources of information about how to eliminate or minimize the dangers. Three months later you can take the test again and judge your own improvements.

Techies take note: if you like, your total scores can be easily graphed to show your health profile, and each section can be graphed separately, facilitating regular checkups. If you want to be really high-tech, you can add to your graph your Initial Score, or Previous Score, and Current Score, allowing you to assess your progress, regression or shortcomings over a period of time. Please refer to the examples in figures 1 to 3 (pages 41 to 44).

I will describe the categories for you in more detail:

I.   **Self-care** identifies your approach to health and wellness, how you manage disease and illness, your awareness of your physical and emotional state, and whether you have a positive personality. This category examines your ability to take a holistic view of personal health. Self-care means taking control of your health—and your life. This involves knowing what to do if you are facing minor illnesses, acute and infectious diseases, chronic diseases, lifestyle-related diseases, surgery or a trip to the hospital. It also means understanding how to improve your surroundings, for example by avoiding second-hand smoke or other pollutants. Self-care presents you with a wide range of opportunities: you can practise self-care with useful supplements, such as vitamins, minerals, antioxidants and tonics; you can use your mind to diminish stressful situations and learn relaxation strategies; development of your inner beliefs can promote healing and wellness; and you can, if necessary, alter some personal characteristics to improve your health, such as bettering your self-discipline, sharpening your curiosity, and firing up your self-motivation and perseverance.

II. **Knowledge of Health** includes your understanding of health itself, the health-care system and health maintenance issues. It also looks at your awareness of risks and the tools needed for monitoring your health. Health knowledge is based on all the information affecting your personal well-being. Much of this knowledge is readily available and not difficult to understand. Through HQ it can be widely disseminated so that everyone in every community has the chance to make it part of a basic health plan. Do you think you're already health-conscious? Check out this list and see if there are any areas you may have overlooked:

- concepts of health and illness
- modern medicine
- diagnostic technology
- unconventional practices (i.e., ancient traditional medicine)
- mind/body health techniques (i.e., relaxation)
- integrated and holistic medicine
- disease/injury prevention
- food, nutrition, diet, drugs and herbs
- nutritional supplements (i.e., vitamins, minerals, antioxidants and tonics)
- risk factors of the major illnesses
- disease transmission
- self-care
- emotional intelligence
- acquaintance with the HQ Profile
- importance of various types of exercise
- quality-of-life measurement
- laboratory data (e.g., cholesterol profile, blood sugar, cancer screening and mammography)
- Internet do-it-yourself study of health and medicine

III. **Lifestyle** zeroes in on your habits, such as smoking, taking drugs or consuming alcohol, as well as your diet, nutrition and eating habits. Exercise, fitness and daily living are also covered. An assessment of these habits—both healthy and unhealthy—gives key information on your personal well-being. Whole health wellness, described more fully in section II of this book, involves a wide range of habits, from smoking, alcohol intake, addiction and substance abuse to some not often thought about from a health perspective, such as interests and hobbies. Other habits include spirituality practice, stress reduction and use of relaxation techniques, sleep patterns and rest, eating preferences, energy levels and exposure to environmental hazards.

IV. The Mind   examines your mental, psychological and emotional states, your personal beliefs and your stress level. That powerful instrument, the mind, is not always used effectively. Most people are competent and skilful in everyday life, but how well they use their intelligence depends on their education and the values of the society they live in. Still, you can make the right choices if you are given good information and the chance to use it. Emotional intelligence comprises your self-awareness, motivation, impulse control, empathy, zeal, persistence, social deftness and effective management of potentially harmful emotions, such as depression, anxiety, anger and stress. Your mind also involves your personal beliefs, mindfulness, techniques for the management of stress and the development of emotional literacy. You can use your mind to control positive and negative feelings, build self-esteem, influence body image and appearance, and upgrade thinking, memorizing and concentrating.

V. Life Skills   explores your home and work environment, social care, social support, personal habits, relationships and core life skills. You need life skills to deal effectively with the demands and challenges of daily living— to make appropriate decisions, solve problems and communicate. You must have them to earn a living and to do something as complex as setting up, running or managing a business. Life skills help you to take proper care of yourself and enable you to stand firm when others propose risky or dangerous activities. You are not born with a set of life skills; they are learned, and can be taught and improved upon. This may give hope to people who find themselves living in situations where physical or emotional abuse, poor mental health, teen and unwanted pregnancies, substance abuse and sexually transmitted diseases are common.

Completing the questionnaire

1.   Complete one section at a time by circling the number corresponding to the answer that best describes you. Try to be objective and truthful.
2.   Then add the numbers you have circled for each question to determine your total section score. Thirty is the highest number that can be scored.
3.   Fill in the score line at the end of each section, then divide this score by three to give you a score out of ten. Write this "total actual score" on the line below.
4.   Don't add up all your scores. You will study your results using the individual scores for each section.

CATEGORY I: SELF-CARE

SECTION 1
Approach to Health and Wellness

This section asks you whether you see attending to health and wellness as a holistic undertaking involving all aspects of taking care of yourself. The statements aim to demonstrate whether you know about actions you can take towards self-care, such as using various health-care options, and about techniques, foods and other resources that can benefit wellness. They also seek to determine your feelings about the connection between your physical condition and the mind, emotions and soul in the search for total health.

1.1   Self-care is important to optimal health.

Strongly disagree	Disagree	Disagree slightly	Neither agree nor disagree	Agree slightly	Agree	Strongly agree
0	1	2	3	4	5	6

1.2   When practising self-care, I am willing to try new and emerging approaches/techniques to maintain my good health.

Never	Almost never	Seldom	Sometimes	Usually	Almost always	Always
0	1	2	3	4	5	6

1.3   I use self-care to prevent the development of diseases related to an unhealthy lifestyle.

Never	Almost never	Seldom	Sometimes	Usually	Almost always	Always
0	1	2	3	4	5	6

1.4   I practise self-relaxation and stress-reduction techniques.

Never	Almost never	Seldom	Sometimes	Often	Regularly	Daily
0	1	2	3	4	5	6

1.5   I control my weight, do self-examination and am alert for the early signs of illness as disease-prevention measures.

Never	Almost never	Seldom	Sometimes	Usually	Almost always	Always
0	1	2	3	4	5	6

APPROACH TO HEALTH AND WELLNESS SCORE: _____

DIVIDE BY 3 FOR TOTAL ACTUAL SCORE: _____

SECTION 2
Approach to Managing Disease and Illness

This section examines your ability to make choices from the various health-care options. Can you, for example, monitor your condition with health tools and search out appropriate helpers and techniques? These statements probe how comfortable you are in managing personal health-care needs that might possibly save you from surgery or a trip to the hospital.

2.1   I actively participate in decision making when dealing with my own health-care needs.

Never	Almost never	Seldom	Sometimes	Usually	Almost always	Always
0	1	2	3	4	5	6

2.2   I feel comfortable caring for myself when I have minor illnesses and infections.

Never	Almost never	Seldom	Sometimes	Usually	Almost always	Always
0	1	2	3	4	5	6

2.3   When I consider my health-care providers, I feel:

Very dissatisfied	Dissatisfied	Mildly dissatisfied	Neither satisfied nor dissatisfied	Mildly satisfied	Satisfied	Very satisfied
0	1	2	3	4	5	6

2.4   The role of the mind is important in the development of disease.

Strongly disagree	Disagree	Disagree slightly	Neither agree nor disagree	Agree slightly	Agree	Strongly agree
0	1	2	3	4	5	6

2.5   When I consider my ability to choose approaches from the different health-care options, I feel:

Very dissatisfied	Dissatisfied	Mildly dissatisfied	Neither satisfied nor dissatisfied	Mildly satisfied	Satisfied	Very satisfied
0	1	2	3	4	5	6

APPROACH TO MANAGING DISEASE AND ILLNESS SCORE: _____

DIVIDE BY 3 FOR TOTAL ACTUAL SCORE: _____

SECTION 3
Awareness of Physical and Emotional State

This section reviews your quality of life by checking your general levels of mobility, pain, discomfort, energy and vitality. These statements identify whether any of these conditions are a problem for you and, if so, assess how much they distress you and interfere with your life.

3.1   I enjoy good health.

Never	Almost never	Seldom	Sometimes	Usually	Almost always	Always
0	1	2	3	4	5	6

3.2   When I consider my energy level, I feel:

Very dissatisfied	Dissatisfied	Mildly dissatisfied	Neither satisfied nor dissatisfied	Mildly satisfied	Satisfied	Very satisfied
0	1	2	3	4	5	6

3.3   I feel free of pain and discomfort.

Never	Almost never	Seldom	Sometimes	Usually	Almost always	Always
0	1	2	3	4	5	6

3.4   I am able to identify the significance of physical symptoms.

Never	Almost never	Seldom	Sometimes	Usually	Almost always	Always
0	1	2	3	4	5	6

3.5   I am able to appreciate the signs of stress and emotional difficulties.

Never	Almost never	Seldom	Sometimes	Usually	Almost always	Always
0	1	2	3	4	5	6

AWARENESS OF PHYSICAL AND EMOTIONAL STATE SCORE: _____

DIVIDE BY 3 FOR TOTAL ACTUAL SCORE: _____

SECTION 4
Positive Personality

This section evaluates whether you feel happy, relaxed and contented. Your views of your perceptions of life and of your ability to solve problems will reveal your likelihood of having a positive personality, which adds to the quality of your life.

4.1   I get things accomplished well before deadlines.

Never	Almost never	Seldom	Sometimes	Usually	Almost always	Always
0	1	2	3	4	5	6

4.2   I am able to prioritize my work.

Never	Almost never	Seldom	Sometimes	Usually	Almost always	Always
0	1	2	3	4	5	6

4.3   I feel relaxed, happy and optimistic about my relationships.

Strongly disagree	Disagree	Disagree slightly	Neither agree nor disagree	Agree slightly	Agree	Strongly agree
0	1	2	3	4	5	6

4.4   I look at problems logically.

Strongly disagree	Disagree	Disagree slightly	Neither agree nor disagree	Agree slightly	Agree	Strongly agree
0	1	2	3	4	5	6

4.5   I am happy with my life.

Never	Almost never	Seldom	Sometimes	Usually	Almost always	Always
0	1	2	3	4	5	6

POSITIVE PERSONALITY SCORE: _____

DIVIDE BY 3 FOR TOTAL ACTUAL SCORE: _____

CATEGORY II: KNOWLEDGE OF HEALTH

SECTION 1
Knowledge of Health

This section seeks to determine whether you understand the many characteristics of health and how they can affect your personal well-being. The statements cover the spectrum from wellness to sickness.

1.1 I would rate my understanding of illness as:

Very poor	Poor	Rather poor	Average	Rather good	Good	Very good
0	1	2	3	4	5	6

1.2 I am satisfied that I have enough health knowledge to assess my health.

Strongly disagree	Disagree	Disagree slightly	Neither agree nor disagree	Agree slightly	Agree	Strongly agree
0	1	2	3	4	5	6

1.3 As far as overall health is concerned, having a healthy mind is:

Irrelevant	Not at all important	Slightly important	Important	Very important	Extremely important	Essential
0	1	2	3	4	5	6

1.4 Regular exercise, well-balanced meals, time for myself, and a happy medium between work and play are important to my lifestyle.

Strongly disagree	Disagree	Disagree slightly	Neither agree nor disagree	Agree slightly	Agree	Strongly agree
0	1	2	3	4	5	6

1.5 Health is more than mere freedom from disease.

Strongly disagree	Disagree	Disagree slightly	Neither agree nor disagree	Agree slightly	Agree	Strongly agree
0	1	2	3	4	5	6

KNOWLEDGE OF HEALTH SCORE: _____

DIVIDE BY 3 FOR TOTAL ACTUAL SCORE: _____

SECTION 2
Knowledge of the Health-care System

This section focuses on how you see the familiar Western health-care system and on your aware-ness of the alternative health-care options that are available to you. Besides calling on the conven-tional doctor, you should know about other types of care. These statements try to pinpoint your knowledge of the availability and importance of these alternatives.

2.1   I would rate my understanding of how the current health-care system works as:

Very poor	Poor	Rather poor	Average	Rather good	Good	Very good
0	1	2	3	4	5	6

2.2   I make appropriate use of the health-care system.

Strongly disagree	Disagree	Disagree slightly	Neither agree nor disagree	Agree slightly	Agree	Strongly agree
0	1	2	3	4	5	6

2.3   My level of awareness of the various health-care options is:

Very poor	Poor	Rather poor	Average	Rather good	Good	Very good
0	1	2	3	4	5	6

2.4   When I consider my ability to choose appropriate health-care providers, I feel:

Not at all confident	A little confident	Somewhat confident	Moderately confident	Quite confident	Very confident	Extremely confident
0	1	2	3	4	5	6

2.5   I intend to find out more about health-care alternatives and want to use them.

Strongly disagree	Disagree	Disagree slightly	Neither agree nor disagree	Agree slightly	Agree	Strongly agree
0	1	2	3	4	5	6

KNOWLEDGE OF THE HEALTH-CARE SYSTEM SCORE: _____

DIVIDE BY 3 FOR TOTAL ACTUAL SCORE: _____

SECTION 3
Knowledge of Health Maintenance Issues

This section explores your awareness and use of health maintenance information, the key to achieving wellness. The statements gauge your knowledge of the fundamental lifestyle patterns and habits and the factors that can threaten your chances of having good health.

3.1   Using an integrated and holistic approach to maintaining my health, I try to inform myself about recent developments in particular areas of medicine.

Never	Almost never	Seldom	Sometimes	Usually	Almost always	Always
0	1	2	3	4	5	6

3.2   I make careful use of health information resources.

Never	Almost never	Seldom	Sometimes	Usually	Almost always	Always
0	1	2	3	4	5	6

3.3   I keep myself updated about new techniques/approaches to health and wellness.

Never	Almost never	Seldom	Sometimes	Usually	Almost always	Always
0	1	2	3	4	5	6

3.4   I can tell when my behaviour or lifestyle is having a major impact on my health.

Never	Almost never	Seldom	Sometimes	Usually	Almost always	Always
0	1	2	3	4	5	6

3.5   I keep up to date on screening methods for disease.

Never	Almost never	Seldom	Sometimes	Usually	Almost always	Always
0	1	2	3	4	5	6

KNOWLEDGE OF HEALTH MAINTENANCE ISSUES SCORE: ____

DIVIDE BY 3 FOR TOTAL ACTUAL SCORE: _____

SECTION 4
Knowledge of Risk Factors and Tools for Health Monitoring

This section looks into your familiarity with the risk factors that can lead to serious illness or disease. You are queried about your awareness of illnesses caused by certain "health" foods, medications and environmental conditions. Your knowledge of methods for monitoring health is also rated.

4.1   I am aware of many risk factors for major diseases and conditions.

Strongly disagree	Disagree	Disagree slightly	Neither agree nor disagree	Agree slightly	Agree	Strongly agree
0	1	2	3	4	5	6

4.2   I am familiar with the potential hazards of some over-the-counter drugs and health-food products.

Strongly disagree	Disagree	Disagree slightly	Neither agree nor disagree	Agree slightly	Agree	Strongly agree
0	1	2	3	4	5	6

4.3   I receive a physical checkup including screening for risk factors.

Never	Rarely	Occasionally	Not regularly	Somewhat regularly	Very regularly	Routinely
0	1	2	3	4	5	6

4.4   I make a point of using good health information in monitoring my health.

Never	Almost never	Seldom	Sometimes	Usually	Almost always	Always
0	1	2	3	4	5	6

4.5   My knowledge about health hazards related to various environments is:

Nil	Almost nil	Weak	Moderate	Quite good	Very good	Extensive
0	1	2	3	4	5	6

**KNOWLEDGE OF RISK FACTORS AND TOOLS FOR
HEALTH MONITORING SCORE:** _____

DIVIDE BY 3 FOR TOTAL ACTUAL SCORE: _____

CATEGORY III: LIFESTYLE

SECTION 1
Smoking, Drugs and Alcohol

This section investigates your habits with respect to smoking, alcohol consumption, and taking medication and other drugs. It also inquires into your knowledge of the hazards of these substances.

1.1   I avoid smoking cigarettes, cigars or a pipe, or ingesting tobacco in another form.

Never	Almost never	Seldom	Sometimes	Usually	Almost always	Always
0	1	2	3	4	5	6

1.2   I avoid being near second-hand smoke.

Never	Almost never	Seldom	Sometimes	Usually	Almost always	Always
0	1	2	3	4	5	6

1.3   My daily intake of alcohol is:

A great deal	Quite a bit	Several drinks	A moderate amount	A little	Almost nil	Nil
0	1	2	3	4	5	6

1.4   I avoid using excessive alcohol or illegal drugs as a way of handling stressful situations in my life.

Never	Almost never	Seldom	Sometimes	Usually	Almost always	Always
0	1	2	3	4	5	6

1.5   I pay attention to the label directions when using prescribed and over-the-counter drugs.

Never	Almost never	Seldom	Sometimes	Usually	Almost always	Always
0	1	2	3	4	5	6

SMOKING, DRUGS AND ALCOHOL SCORE: _____

DIVIDE BY 3 FOR TOTAL ACTUAL SCORE: _____

SECTION 2
Diet, Nutrition and Eating Habits

Since being overweight increases your risk for some diseases, this section examines your eating habits, including what you eat and the regularity of your meals. It also queries your knowledge of foods that are "bad" for you and of the importance of vitamins.

2.1 I eat a variety of foods.

Never	Almost never	Seldom	Sometimes	Usually	Almost always	Always
0	1	2	3	4	5	6

2.2 I take care about what I eat.

Never	Almost never	Seldom	Sometimes	Usually	Almost always	Always
0	1	2	3	4	5	6

2.3 Vitamins are important.

Strongly disagree	Disagree	Disagree slightly	Neither agree nor disagree	Agree slightly	Agree	Strongly agree
0	1	2	3	4	5	6

2.4 I eat at regular intervals.

Never	Almost never	Seldom	Sometimes	Usually	Almost always	Always
0	1	2	3	4	5	6

2.5 I am conscious of my caloric intake.

Never	Almost never	Seldom	Sometimes	Usually	Almost always	Always
0	1	2	3	4	5	6

DIET, NUTRITION AND EATING HABITS SCORE: _____

DIVIDE BY 3 FOR TOTAL ACTUAL SCORE: _____

SECTION 3
Exercise and Fitness

Everyone can gain a health benefit from exercise of some kind. Exercise keeps your heart healthy and eliminates excess weight. This section measures your current state of physical fitness, your body weight and how you feel about the frequency and nature of your exercise.

3.1   I am conscious of my body weight.

Never	Almost never	Seldom	Sometimes	Usually	Almost always	Always
0	1	2	3	4	5	6

3.2   Moderate physical activity, including walking, is important to health.

Strongly disagree	Disagree	Disagree slightly	Neither agree nor disagree	Agree slightly	Agree	Strongly agree
0	1	2	3	4	5	6

3.3   I am aware of rigorous exercises that can enhance my muscle tone and heart function.

Not at all	Hardly at all	Somewhat	Neither aware nor unaware	Slightly aware	Aware	Strongly aware
0	1	2	3	4	5	6

3.4   I take part in family or team activities that can increase my level of fitness.

Never	Almost never	Seldom	Sometimes	Quite frequently	Very often	Regularly
0	1	2	3	4	5	6

3.5   I think that my physical activities or exercise are enough to keep up my desired level of fitness.

Strongly disagree	Disagree	Disagree slightly	Neither agree nor disagree	Agree slightly	Agree	Strongly agree
0	1	2	3	4	5	6

EXERCISE AND FITNESS SCORE: _____

DIVIDE BY 3 FOR TOTAL ACTUAL SCORE: _____

SECTION 4
Daily Living

This section rates your opinion of your ability to perform the usual activities of daily living, including caring for yourself and handling daily responsibilities.

4.1   I am able to cope with the stress generated by my usual daily work and activities.

Never	Almost never	Seldom	Sometimes	Usually	Almost always	Always
0	1	2	3	4	5	6

4.2   When I consider my ability to perform routine activities on a daily basis, I feel:

Very dissatisfied	Dissatisfied	Mildly dissatisfied	Neither satisfied nor dissatisfied	Mildly satisfied	Satisfied	Very satisfied
0	1	2	3	4	5	6

4.3   When I consider my ability to work or perform meaningful tasks, I feel:

Very dissatisfied	Dissatisfied	Mildly dissatisfied	Neither satisfied nor dissatisfied	Mildly satisfied	Satisfied	Very satisfied
0	1	2	3	4	5	6

4.4   When I consider my sex life, I feel:

Very dissatisfied	Dissatisfied	Mildly dissatisfied	Neither satisfied nor dissatisfied	Mildly satisfied	Satisfied	Very satisfied
0	1	2	3	4	5	6

4.5   I feel I am living in a safe and secure environment.

Never	Almost never	Seldom	Sometimes	Usually	Almost always	Always
0	1	2	3	4	5	6

DAILY LIVING SCORE: _____

DIVIDE BY 3 FOR TOTAL ACTUAL SCORE: _____

CATEGORY IV: THE MIND

SECTION 1
Mental and Psychological State

This section explores your feelings about yourself—your outlook and your self-esteem—and how these feelings are reflected in your social group.

1.1   I have positive feelings and am optimistic about life and the future.

Never	Almost never	Seldom	Sometimes	Usually	Almost always	Always
0	1	2	3	4	5	6

1.2   When I consider my mind's capacity to think positively, enjoy learning and reasoning, and concentrate well, I feel:

Very dissatisfied	Dissatisfied	Mildly dissatisfied	Neither satisfied nor dissatisfied	Mildly satisfied	Satisfied	Very satisfied
0	1	2	3	4	5	6

1.3   My self-esteem is important to my health and happiness.

Strongly disagree	Disagree	Disagree slightly	Neither agree nor disagree	Agree slightly	Agree	Strongly agree
0	1	2	3	4	5	6

1.4   When I consider my bodily image and my general appearance, I feel:

Very dissatisfied	Dissatisfied	Mildly dissatisfied	Neither satisfied nor dissatisfied	Mildly satisfied	Satisfied	Very satisfied
0	1	2	3	4	5	6

1.5   When I consider my overall psychological state, such as my motivation, empathy and zeal about life, I feel:

Very dissatisfied	Dissatisfied	Mildly dissatisfied	Neither satisfied nor dissatisfied	Mildly satisfied	Satisfied	Very satisfied
0	1	2	3	4	5	6

MENTAL AND PSYCHOLOGICAL STATE SCORE: _____

DIVIDE BY 3 FOR TOTAL ACTUAL SCORE: _____

SECTION 2
Emotional State

This section deals with your awareness of your emotional makeup, including both your ability to recognize triggers for toxic emotions and your level of satisfaction in how you manage stressful situations. You will also assess how well you get along with others.

2.1   I am aware when my emotional reactions disturb my normal equilibrium.

Never	Almost never	Seldom	Sometimes	Usually	Almost always	Always
0	1	2	3	4	5	6

2.2   Some emotions—anger, anxiety, depression—can interfere with optimal health.

Strongly disagree	Disagree	Disagree slightly	Neither agree nor disagree	Agree slightly	Agree	Strongly agree
0	1	2	3	4	5	6

2.3   I can manage stressful situations and be resourceful when confronted with stresses.

Never	Almost never	Seldom	Sometimes	Usually	Almost always	Always
0	1	2	3	4	5	6

2.4   I enjoy social interactions.

Never	Almost never	Seldom	Sometimes	Usually	Almost always	Always
0	1	2	3	4	5	6

2.5   To maintain good physical health, emotional control is:

Of no importance at all	Of minor importance	Rather unimportant	Neither important nor unimportant	Somewhat important	Very important	Extremely important
0	1	2	3	4	5	6

EMOTIONAL STATE SCORE: _____

DIVIDE BY 3 FOR TOTAL ACTUAL SCORE: _____

SECTION 3
Personal Beliefs

This section inquires into your personal beliefs and how they affect your quality of life, helping you cope with difficulties and unexpected hardships and answering your spiritual and personal questions. These statements are appropriate both for people of mainstream religious beliefs and for those with personal and spiritual beliefs that do not fit into any particular religious orientation.

3.1   My personal beliefs give increased meaning to my life.

Not at all	Very little	Slightly	Moderately	Quite a bit	A great deal	Completely
0	1	2	3	4	5	6

3.2   My personal beliefs help me to deal with difficulties in my life.

Never	Almost never	Seldom	Sometimes	Usually	Almost always	Always
0	1	2	3	4	5	6

3.3   I feel that my personal beliefs can increase my level of satisfaction and happiness.

Not at all	Very little	Slightly	Moderately	Quite a bit	A great deal	Remarkably
0	1	2	3	4	5	6

3.4   My personal beliefs have an impact on my health—for example, by helping me to deal with illness, sadness, despair and hopelessness, and by assisting me in maintaining a healthy lifestyle.

Strongly disagree	Disagree	Disagree slightly	Neither agree nor disagree	Agree slightly	Agree	Strongly agree
0	1	2	3	4	5	6

3.5   My personal and spiritual beliefs give me a general sense of well-being.

Never	Almost never	Seldom	Sometimes	Usually	Almost always	Always
0	1	2	3	4	5	6

PERSONAL BELIEFS SCORE: _____

DIVIDE BY 3 FOR TOTAL ACTUAL SCORE: _____

SECTION 4
Stress

This section addresses an issue that most people have to consider daily: how to deal with stress. These statements focus on how you manage or avoid stressful situations.

4.1   The word(s) that best describes/describe my feelings about my job is/are:

Dislike strongly	Dislike	Dislike slightly	Neither like nor dislike	Like somewhat	Like	Like strongly
0	1	2	3	4	5	6

4.2   I can relax and freely express my feelings.

Never	Almost never	Seldom	Sometimes	Usually	Almost always	Always
0	1	2	3	4	5	6

4.3   I recognize the warning signs when a situation is likely to be stressful for me.

Never	Almost never	Seldom	Sometimes	Usually	Almost always	Always
0	1	2	3	4	5	6

4.4   When I need help or wish to discuss personal matters, I have friends and relatives on whom I can call.

Never	Almost never	Seldom	Sometimes	Usually	Almost always	Always
0	1	2	3	4	5	6

4.5   I can effectively manage stress:

Never	Almost never	Seldom	Sometimes	Usually	Almost always	Always
0	1	2	3	4	5	6

STRESS SCORE: _____

DIVIDE BY 3 FOR TOTAL ACTUAL SCORE: _____

CATEGORY V: LIFE SKILLS

SECTION 1
Core Life Skills

Core life skills are the mental and social abilities that enable you to deal with the demands and challenges of everyday life. This section tests your awareness of these life skills and your ability to use them.

1.1 The skills I have acquired in decision making and problem solving with regard to health issues are:

Nil	Negligible	Few	Average	Quite a few	Numerous	Sufficient for my needs
0	1	2	3	4	5	6

1.2 I use creative thinking to solve my problems.

Never	Almost never	Seldom	Sometimes	Usually	Almost always	Always
0	1	2	3	4	5	6

1.3 When I consider my communication and interpersonal skills, I feel:

Very dissatisfied	Dissatisfied	Mildly dissatisfied	Neither satisfied nor dissatisfied	Mildly satisfied	Satisfied	Very satisfied
0	1	2	3	4	5	6

1.4 I have trained myself to be emotionally aware and empathetic.

Not at all	Hardly at all	Slightly	Somewhat	Quite a bit	A lot	Completely
0	1	2	3	4	5	6

1.5 I am capable of coping with emotions and stress.

Never	Almost never	Seldom	Sometimes	Usually	Almost always	Always
0	1	2	3	4	5	6

CORE LIFE SKILLS SCORE: _____

DIVIDE BY 3 FOR TOTAL ACTUAL SCORE: _____

SECTION 2
Environment and Working

This section looks at your physical and social environments and asks about your work. "Work" includes an occupation that may or may not pay, volunteer service, full-time study, care of the family and duties in the household.

2.1 I do a good job of balancing work demands and the need to spend time with friends and family.

Never	Almost never	Seldom	Sometimes	Usually	Almost always	Always
0	1	2	3	4	5	6

2.2 My financial resources enable me to enjoy life to the fullest.

Never	Almost never	Seldom	Sometimes	Usually	Almost always	Always
0	1	2	3	4	5	6

2.3 When I consider the work I do, I feel:

Very dissatisfied	Dissatisfied	Mildly dissatisfied	Neither satisfied nor dissatisfied	Mildly satisfied	Satisfied	Very satisfied
0	1	2	3	4	5	6

2.4 I work in a comfortable environment where I am able to express myself, interact with others, and accomplish my daily tasks and activities.

Strongly disagree	Disagree	Disagree slightly	Neither agree nor disagree	Agree slightly	Agree	Strongly agree
0	1	2	3	4	5	6

2.5 I am currently living in a healthful, acceptably clean environment.

Strongly disagree	Disagree	Disagree slightly	Neither agree nor disagree	Agree slightly	Agree	Strongly agree
0	1	2	3	4	5	6

ENVIRONMENT AND WORKING SCORE: ____

DIVIDE BY 3 FOR TOTAL ACTUAL SCORE: _____

SECTION 3
Social Care, Support and Behaviour

This section attempts to discover how satisfied you are with your ability to deal with social pressures and demanding social situations, and to receive pleasure and support from your social network.

3.1 In terms of good planning and preparation, I run my life:

Very poorly	Poorly	Sometimes poorly	Neither well nor poorly	Fairly well	Well	Very well
0	1	2	3	4	5	6

3.2 I can withstand peer pressure, such as the pressure to take drugs or to drink alcohol to excess.

Never	Almost never	Seldom	Sometimes	Usually	Almost always	Always
0	1	2	3	4	5	6

3.3 I enjoy and participate in social and leisure activities.

Never	Almost never	Seldom	Sometimes	Often	Very often	Continually
0	1	2	3	4	5	6

3.4 When I consider my ability to get access to social support, I feel:

Very dissatisfied	Dissatisfied	Mildly dissatisfied	Neither satisfied nor dissatisfied	Mildly satisfied	Satisfied	Very satisfied
0	1	2	3	4	5	6

3.5 I make an effort to avoid being socially isolated.

Never	Almost never	Seldom	Sometimes	Usually	Almost always	Always
0	1	2	3	4	5	6

SOCIAL CARE, SUPPORT AND BEHAVIOUR SCORE: ____

DIVIDE BY 3 FOR TOTAL ACTUAL SCORE: _____

SECTION 4
Personal Relationships

This section will question your personal satisfaction with the companionship, friendship, love and support you receive from and give to the people who matter most in your life.

4.1 I have feelings of loneliness.

Always	Almost always	Frequently	Sometimes	Seldom	Almost never	Never
0	1	2	3	4	5	6

4.2 When I consider my relationships with family members, I feel:

Very unhappy	Unhappy	Mildly unhappy	Neither happy nor unhappy	Mildly happy	Happy	Very happy
0	1	2	3	4	5	6

4.3 When I consider my relationships outside the family, I feel:

Very unhappy	Unhappy	Mildly unhappy	Neither happy nor unhappy	Mildly happy	Happy	Very happy
0	1	2	3	4	5	6

4.4 When I consider my actions in giving support to or providing for others, I feel:

Very dissatisfied	Dissatisfied	Mildly dissatisfied	Neither satisfied nor dissatisfied	Mildly satisfied	Satisfied	Very satisfied
0	1	2	3	4	5	6

4.5 When I consider the support I get from family, friends and others, I feel:

Very dissatisfied	Dissatisfied	Mildly dissatisfied	Neither satisfied nor dissatisfied	Mildly satisfied	Satisfied	Very satisfied
0	1	2	3	4	5	6

PERSONAL RELATIONSHIPS SCORE: _____

DIVIDE BY 3 FOR TOTAL ACTUAL SCORE: _____

The results: what your scores mean to you

Scores of 9 and 10   Excellent! Your answers show that you are aware of the importance of this area to your health. Not only that, but you are putting your knowledge to work by practising good HQ—health intelligence. As long as you continue to do so, this area should not pose a serious health risk. It's likely that you are setting an example for your family and friends to follow. Since you scored very high on this part of the test, you can concentrate on other areas, where your scores may indicate room for improvement.

Scores of 6 to 8   Your HQ score shows that your health practices in this area are good, but you obviously could do better. Look again at the items you answered with "Seldom," "Dissatisfied," "Poor," "Never," "Very Dissatisfied" or "Very Poor." What can you do to improve your score? Even a small change can often help your quest for better health.

Scores of 3 to 5   Your HQ health risks are showing! Would you like to have more information about the dangers you are facing and why it is important for you to change? Perhaps you need help in deciding how to make the desired changes successfully? Either way, you will need commitment and effort.

Scores of 0 to 2   It is clear that you were concerned enough about your health to take the test, but your poor HQ score shows that you may be taking serious and unnecessary risks. This is your red flag. Perhaps you are still unaware of the risks and what to do about them. The information you need to help you to initiate personal actions to improve your health is at hand. Study the following sections of this book, and I will show you how to make important changes— before it is too late.

Graphing your HQ scores

A profile of category scores can be graphically represented, showing the positive and negative aspects of your health status and quality of life. Your scores can be modified by your actions and commitment, so a graphic presentation of the data provides an easy-to-read guide for progress towards better health.

Figure 1 is a simple snapshot of John's scores in all sections of the questionnaire.

FIG. 1: HQ PROFILE OF JOHN

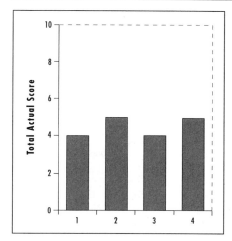

CATEGORY I: SELF-CARE
1. Approach to Health and Wellness
2. Approach to Managing Disease and Illness
3. Awareness of Physical and Emotional State
4. Positive Personality

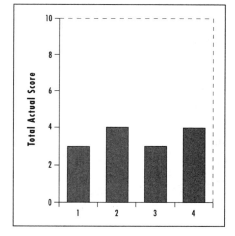

CATEGORY II: KNOWLEDGE OF HEALTH
1. Knowledge of Health
2. Knowledge of the Health-care System
3. Knowledge of Health Maintenance Issues
4. Knowledge of Risk Factors and Tools for Health Monitoring

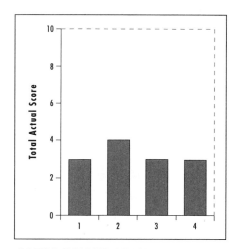

CATEGORY III: LIFESTYLE
1. Smoking, Drugs and Alcohol
2. Diet, Nutrition and Eating Habits
3. Exercise and Fitness
4. Daily Living

FIG. 1: HQ PROFILE OF JOHN (continued)

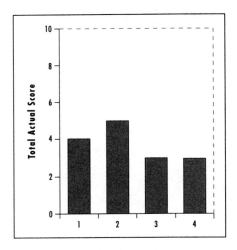

CATEGORY IV: THE MIND

1. Mental and Psychological State
2. Emotional State
3. Personal Beliefs
4. Stress

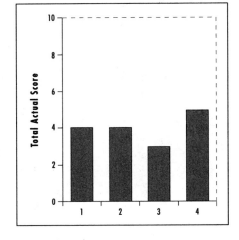

CATEGORY V: LIFE SKILLS

1. Core Life Skills
2. Environment and Working
3. Social Care, Support and Behaviour
4. Personal Relationships

In figure 2, John has averaged his scores for the four sections in each category. You can see how his overall performance varied in each category between three time periods: first, the baseline; second, at the end of period 1 (three months, for instance); then after period 2 (perhaps six months). As you can see, John is improving in all areas.

FIG. 2: HQ PROFILE OF JOHN OVER TIME

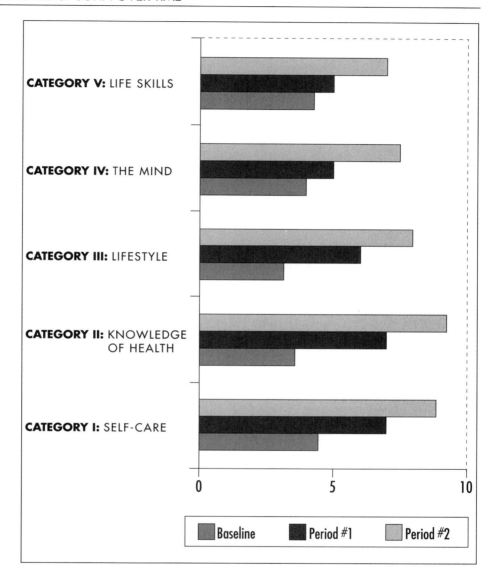

In figure 3, however, we see how Tom has slipped back in the third time period. That's quite possible, after the initial push for improvement. If this happens to you, don't despair: simply look at the areas of slippage and commit yourself to doing better.

FIG. 3: HQ PROFILE OF TOM

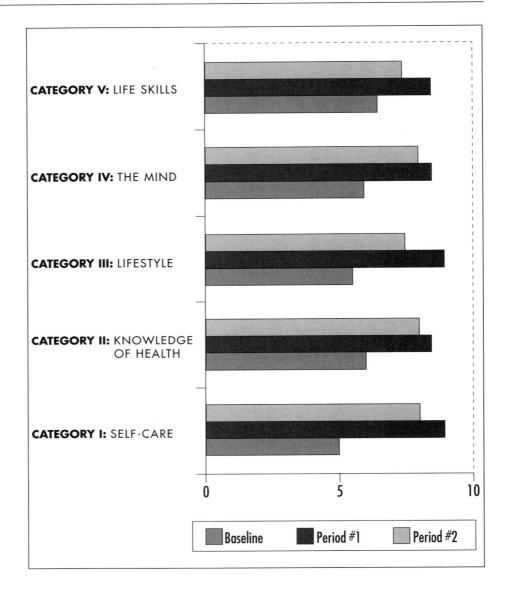

Putting Your HQ Profile to Work

Congratulations! You've taken the questionnaire and the results you have in your hands outline your personal Health Profile. Now, what can you do with it?

Can you do better? Yes, yes, yes! That's what the HQ Profile is for. The whole point of answering this questionnaire is to give you the basis for playing an active part in managing your own health. But it's more than a New Year's resolution: you will need to make an ongoing commitment and a real effort towards bettering your health.

A personal strategy

Now is your chance to improve your knowledge of health, make lifestyle changes, and take a long, hard look at your diet and nutrition, and at your emotional, personal and social situation. Completing the questionnaire has pinpointed your danger zones—those areas that, if left unattended, could bring on disease, suffering or early death. So now you need to:

- find out more about health issues;
- create a healthier lifestyle for yourself by discontinuing bad habits, getting more exercise, and working on unhealthy activities and attitudes;
- understand what you need in your diet and in terms of overall nutrition;
- put stress in its place by working on your coping techniques and making any changes you can to reduce stress in your environment; and
- realize that you often have to make healthful social changes too.

A baker's dozen of common problems and ideas to consider

1. **Avoid smoking.** This is the single most preventable cause of illness and early death. It is especially risky for pregnant women and their unborn babies. Don't start! People who stop smoking reduce their risk of getting heart disease and cancer. If it seems too hard or even impossible to stop completely, you should try the shorter-term goal of cutting back the number of cigarettes you smoke. Never give up trying!

2. **Drink sensibly.** Most people are careful not to drink too much and are capable of handling the mood- and behaviour-changing effects of alcohol. Recent evidence suggests that moderate drinking can actually benefit your health. Nevertheless, regular excessive use of alcohol can lead to cirrhosis of the liver, a leading cause of death. Warnings about the potentially lethal effects of drinking and driving, though well publicized, are still too often unheeded.

3.   **Take care with drugs**—prescription, over-the-counter or "recreational." Today's increased use of drugs, both legal and illegal, is one of society's most serious health risks. Even some drugs prescribed by a doctor can be dangerous in combination with alcohol or driving. Excessive use of tranquilizers or pep pills can cause physical and mental health problems. Use—regular or just experimental—of illicit drugs such as heroin and cocaine can cause all kinds of health damage and even death.

4.   **Eat sensibly.** Overweight people are at greater than average risk for diabetes, gall bladder disease and high blood pressure. Good eating habits include controlling excessive intake of calories and fat (especially saturated fats), cholesterol, sugar and salt. Snacks play a major part in the North American lifestyle, and eating smart snacks, such as fruits and vegetables, instead of high-fat, salty or junk foods can make a huge improvement in nutrition.

5.   **Exercise regularly.** Almost everyone can benefit from exercise, and just about everyone is able to exercise in some way or another. It's always wise to check with a doctor if in doubt. Even a modest commitment of thirty minutes of accumulated moderate exercise daily will help you have a healthier heart, lose extra weight, tone up sagging muscles and sleep better.

6.   **Manage your stress.** Stress is a normal part of life, and everyone is bound to face stressful situations from time to time, whether it's good stress, such as getting a promotion, or the bad kind, such as losing someone you love. The important thing is how you deal with it. Properly handled, stress doesn't have to be a problem. Talking over your worries with someone you trust can often help. Even on busy days it is important to find a few minutes in which to slow down, relax and practise relaxation techniques. It's also wise to learn the difference between the things worth fighting about and those that don't really matter. You will run into major problems if you respond to your stress in unhealthy ways, such as erratic, fast driving, excessive eating or drinking, or sinking into prolonged anger or grief.

7.   **Be safety-conscious.** Think safety first at home, work, school or play, and out on the highway. Buckle seat belts and obey traffic rules. Keep poisons and weapons out of reach of children, and post emergency numbers by your telephone. Take some first-aid training so that, when the unexpected happens, you will be ready for it.

8.   **Improve your life skills.** Coping effectively with the demands and challenges of everyday life is not always easy. Everyone gets frustrated sometimes, but knowing how to avoid or deal with disappointments,

problems, demands and pressures can make things easier. Improving your life skills—your ability to solve problems, make decisions, think critically and creatively, communicate effectively, cope with your emotions and interact successfully with people—will go a long way in helping you through difficult and challenging situations.

9. **Balance work and play.** Finding a balance between work and leisure can be a difficult task for many people. Employees and even the self-employed often find that the demands and expectations being laid on them keep growing. Wages do not always keep up with inflation; job losses and downsizing are a constant threat; and the government spends less now on social services and unemployment benefits than it used to. Many people find themselves working harder and longer to feel more secure in their jobs. There are only so many hours in the day, however, and as a result families and personal lives are suffering. People too often find that they don't have enough time to spend with their families and friends. Fitness and exercise also take a back seat. You must have a reasonable balance between work and play if you want optimal health and happiness.

10. **Care for yourself when possible.** You probably have more control over your own health than you realize. From a preventive point of view, breast self-examination, blood pressure monitoring, immunization, wearing your seat belt or bike helmet, eating properly, exercising and getting enough sleep and rest are all ways of helping to maintain health and prevent disease or unnecessary injury. Remember, an ounce of prevention is worth a pound of cure. If you have care needs that you can't comfortably provide for yourself, seek the help and advice of health experts. There are many people, organizations, agencies and associations that can help you find the most appropriate health-care provider for your particular needs. Take a look at the suggested resources listed in section IV of this book.

11. **Become more knowledgeable about your health.** The best way to take responsibility for your own health is to be knowledgeable about health factors, circumstances surrounding diseases, risk of diseases and so on. Besides knowing the dangers involved and the best ways to avoid these problems, you should be aware of what to do if you find you need care or treatment for a disease or want to talk about symptoms. Your doctor is a valuable source for medical advice, although he or she may not always have the time to give you the extensive information that can be found elsewhere. The Internet, books, journals, television documentaries, seminars

and alternative medical sources are always available, but remember to be critical and cautious when researching or reading information that has not been sanctioned by health experts. Medical professionals are aware of the need for resource centres designed for and made available to those who want to know more about their health and how to take better care of themselves. At present, branches of the public health system provide a great deal of information on immunization, communicable diseases, water and environmental safety, sexually transmitted diseases and some other matters. These agencies, however, are often not equipped to speak about other health issues, complementary health-care systems, the various health-care providers in the community, or different approaches to managing illness and maintaining good health. As the sources of information evolve, we hope that there will soon be resource centres to provide a broader range of information for those seeking it.

12.   **Pay attention to your friendships and interpersonal relationships.** Family, friends, co-workers and others may sometimes thwart your good intentions and feel like thorns in your flesh. If you find this is true of all your relationships, perhaps you need to ask yourself why you are unable to keep up happy or healthy relationships with others. Do you feel positive about yourself? Are you motivated to meet people and engage in conversation? Are you able to feel empathy towards others? Are you willing to both listen and share your own feelings when the occasion arises? Do you feel accepted, worthwhile and valued? All these factors enable you to interact and socialize more easily with people. Friendships can bring you much contentment and satisfaction. Currently, there is a great deal of literature on the theme of interpersonal relationships.

13.   **Encourage your beliefs and faith.** Spirituality is an important but inadequately understood component of health. Some research studies show that people who have strong spiritual beliefs, from whatever faith or spiritual ideal, have a more positive outlook on life, tend to heal more quickly, and worry less than others about the outcome of illnesses. Those with strong personal beliefs generally have a high level of satisfaction and happiness in life, and feel that they can readily deal with illness, sadness, despair and hopelessness.

Your lifelong health journey

A life that is as enjoyable and healthful as possible is not just something to have when you are young: it should be yours for the rest of your life. You make the choices.

- Commit yourself to reaching high HQ Profile scores.
- Encourage your good habits and discard the bad ones.
- Take your health seriously and work steadily towards a healthy lifestyle.
- Be on "health watch." Study regularly and learn as much as you can about health and healthy living.

Often the best way to set off on this health journey is to ask yourself some questions. Am I really doing all I can to be as healthy as possible? What steps can I take to feel better? Am I willing to begin now? Once you are convinced that having the best possible health is a priority in your life, this book will give you the fundamental principles of good health and all the basic information you need to change your habits and develop a whole new healthful lifestyle. The diagram on the next page shows you how this can work.

Most important of all, don't become overwhelmed! If many areas of your health are showing low scores, don't try to remedy everything at once. It may be better to pick an area where you know you are likely to succeed and tackle it first. When you have that one beaten, you can choose the next one.

This is a long-term, ongoing project, and you should not be discouraged if you have already tried to change poor health habits without success. It may be that you needed more support, or perhaps there were influences at work that you weren't aware of at the time. Recognizing these influences is the first step to changing them and their effect on your life. Your challenges will be different from everybody else's, and you will have to resolve them in your own way. When you run into a brick wall, find new solutions, even if it means going for outside help.

Remember: step one is to take the time to complete the questionnaire carefully, thoughtfully and thoroughly. On your own, you can review your results. You may feel delighted, reassured, shocked or something in between by your scores and overall performance. Then it's up to you to make the necessary health changes. As you re-test yourself every month or two, you should begin to see positive changes reflected in your new scores. Hopefully, you will also feel the difference in your general health and quality of life.

It's the long-term, big picture that counts. The real value in creating your health profile is the opportunity it provides for regular testing, clear and useful feedback, and the chance to take appropriate action over time. The profile is not meant for people looking for a quick fix to their health problems. Instead, it has been designed as a "total health program" for people who care enough to commit to the best personal health now and in the future.

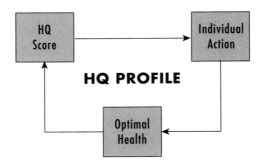

Positive actions taken through the HQ Profile impact positively upon the HQ (health intelligence) score and result in Optimal Health.

As we've said before, making a commitment to your health is the first step in actually becoming a healthier person. Take the time you need to study this test, analyze the results and make yourself aware of the many things you can do to improve your health. This isn't someone else's responsibility. Are you ready to set out on the road to better health? Are you ready to accept responsibility for your own health and for achieving better health? Good! Then you're ready to move on to the next part of this book, which gives you the information you need for remodelling your life the healthy way. As you turn the pages, a bright new future of dynamic health possibilities will open up before your eyes. By the time you reach section IV, you will be HQ aware and more than ready to create the personal action plan that will change your life. Read on, and remember: it's your life and your health!

A Summing-up

The HQ Profile is a practical and easy-to-understand approach to achieving optimal health. Everyone today is looking for a way to be healthier, live longer and enjoy a better life. To many people, however, the road to this ideal seems full of complications and obstacles but short on guideposts and supports. Frankly, it appears unreachable for most people, but only because they haven't had an easy or thorough option for understanding and utilizing their abilities to control and guide their own health.

The focus for a long time has been on increasing life expectancy. For thousands of years, merely finding food, shelter and the basic necessities of life consumed all the time and energy of most people. Only in the last century have we dared to think that life could be easier, and only in the last couple of generations have we expected a lot more from life, including satisfaction and happiness. The quest for "a better life" is now a global phenomenon. People in almost any village anywhere in the world, however poor and undereducated, know that there are antibiotics, immunizations, work opportunities, social prospects and all sorts of other supports that hold out the prospect of a better life. The result has been the emergence of new thinking about health. In addition to the length of life, we are now considering its quality—those values that make life more satisfying. The new term for this shift in priorities is "health expectancy," meaning all the things that make possible good health, meaningfulness and happiness in life.

In North America, people are becoming ever more conscious of health and sickness, and this trend promises to continue in the future. This kind of thinking has the potential to create a new health culture. The focus on wellness, preventive medicine and alternative therapies has evolved from the greater amount and changing kind of information available through the Internet, globalization, the explosion of media communications and multicultural diversity.

Society's enthusiasm for an improved quality of life will require some people to accept more responsibility for maintaining their good health, others to improve their less than optimal health. This self-care begins when you recognize that your individual actions are the most important elements in achieving wellness and optimal health. In accepting responsibility for your own wellness, you must pay attention to proper diet and exercise, stress management, good lifestyle habits, and thoughtful use of technologies, products and services. Focused upon action, self-care requires from you an active interest and prudent and direct moves in dealing with illness and disease. The need for this and the way to accomplish it are clear.

Medical science has indeed increased life expectancy and lessened people's suffering. Overall, society has benefited greatly from these advancements. But while these successes have dominated our thinking about health-care delivery, wellness, and mind and body interaction, the "art" of healing and quality-of-life issues have been partially ignored. Your increasing knowledge of self-care, lifestyle and other issues shown in the HQ Profile will reacquaint and enrich you with the notion of caring for your total needs—in other words, provide a more holistic and integrative approach.

This HQ Profile has been designed with the majority of society in mind, and it stems from the philosophical position that good health care aims not merely at adding days to life but also at adding quality to that life. The profile should be used as a tool to assist you in assessing and reassessing your health status. Its usefulness requires a commitment to active involvement in the management of your own health. Over time, it can produce positive changes in health status and quality of life—effects that can be attained only through your own dedication and action. If you have been conditioned to rely on the existing health-care system, deciding to make use of the HQ Profile will be a new and perhaps somewhat daunting experience. It will help you realize, however, that health maintenance, wellness and disease prevention are largely under your own control and require your particular attention and action.

The HQ Profile questionnaire is designed to provide specific information for each respondent. It is correlated directly to your current state of health, which can be changed by learning, willpower, emotional intelligence and action, all based on personal commitment. The self-administered questionnaire is intended to be completed at frequent intervals, so that you can review changes in your health status. You should complete the questionnaire before reading the rest of this book, returning to it later with a concentration on the areas that need attention. Then, after reviewing this chapter, you can create a plan of action to alter behaviours, lifestyle habits, relationships and so forth. Every two to six months thereafter, you should complete the questionnaire again; your score should be higher, indicating a positive change in your overall health status.

Answering the questions in the HQ Profile questionnaire will enable you to see clearly the aspects of your present lifestyle and behaviour that are risky to your health. The results will show what steps need to be taken to eliminate or minimize the risks or weaknesses identified. This provides the basis for beginning to change habits and lifestyles in a more positive and healthful direction.

To improve your quality of life and health expectancy, you must first be convinced that it needs to be done. When you have the commitment to improve your health and quality of life, you can go into action by devoting twenty minutes to completing and scoring the HQ Profile questionnaire. Following a regime of ongoing self-care actions aimed at health improvement, based on the test outcomes, will certainly guarantee better health for you.

HIGHLIGHTS OF CREATING YOUR HQ PROFILE

- The HQ Profile is a practical and easy-to-understand tool for everyone to use in a personal effort to be as healthy as it is possible to be. For too long it has been a well-kept secret.

- It is no longer good enough simply to focus on life expectancy. Today, there is a quest for a better quality of life, with good health, meaningfulness and happiness and it is global.

- The explosion of health information that has resulted from new technology and rapid communications has created the need for a new health culture, where informed people will take greater responsibility for managing their health.

- The wave of self-care is just reaching the shore. In essence, it requires you to take hands-on action and personal responsibility for your wellness and for responding to illness and disease.

- Good self-care requires knowledge of health, lifestyle and other issues revealed in your HQ Profile. This knowledge will give you a wider and more holistic basis on which to care for your total needs.

- For many people, conditioned to rely solely on the existing health-care system, this may seem to be a radical change. However, it can be both exhilarating and empowering to take control of your personal health destiny. Your success depends largely on your personal commitment and willingness to take action.

SECTION II

HQ AND PROMOTING YOUR WELLNESS

Now that you've read the first part of this book and crafted your health profile, let's build on that framework to raise your HQ and take you to a new level of health and wellness.

Most of the knowledge you need already exists. For the most part it is neither highly technical nor complicated. Most people could easily put it into practice. It does require you to make a strong personal commitment to understanding what health is and the obstacles in the way of becoming healthier or simply staying in good health. You're off to a good start because you picked out this book and, from the assessments you've made in section I, you already know your "health-self" a lot better. Now you're ready to move on.

It's important to remember that health is not static; it is a dynamic process. Your health balance is likely to break down as your conditions change. The information in this section is geared to helping you construct a whole lifestyle for healthy living. More than simply enhancing and protecting your present health, I want you to live a long life in the best possible health until the end of your days—extended health expectancy.

My seven golden rules for good health are the following: have good personal habits; prevent disease and injury; develop life skills; acquire the most valid and appropriate health knowledge; adapt to your psychosocial environment; understand and deal with your health in a holistic manner; and achieve a balance between what's going on around you and your internal healing resources. See the diagram on the next page, which shows how these aspects of your life can interrelate to affect your health.

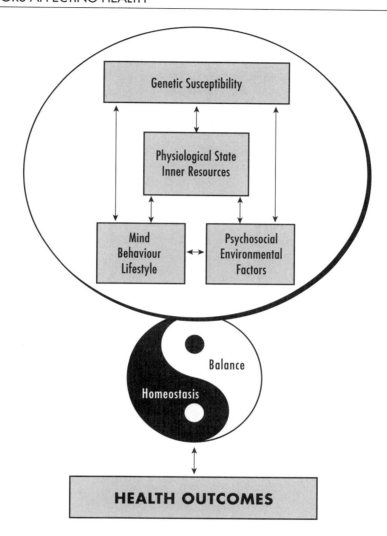

This figure shows the many variables of your life that work together to create your overall state of health. A combination of genetic predisposition, your interaction with your social set-up (such as your social, cultural, ethnic and occupational surroundings) and changes in your habits will alter the internal balance, or homeostasis, and thus affect your health and wellness.

Prevention and wellness are always better than treatment, as Chinese traditional medicine has long shown, but how can you make them happen? How can you maintain health and wellness? Here, HQ plays a critical role.

To answer these questions and to provide information on improving health and staying healthy, this section gives you four chapters. Chapter 2, Your Genetic Endowment and Your Environment, looks at genetic susceptibility, environmental hazards and social conditions as factors in health and illness. Chapter 3, The Healthy Mind, describes the mounting scientific evidence for a strong linkage between mind and body and the mind's impact on physical health, providing insight into this fast-growing, fascinating field of medicine. Chapter 4, Lifestyle and Health, discusses the way we live—our diet, nutrition, exercise and habits—as well as the basic need for a good quality of life. In this chapter I propose a new, healthy HQ eating culture and emphasize the need for physical action to maintain good health. Chapter 5, HQ and Life's Journey, deals with the two issues during each period of the life cycle that are considered to have the most crucial influence on an individual's health, wellness, happiness and longevity.

CHAPTER 2

YOUR GENETIC ENDOWMENT AND YOUR ENVIRONMENT

Two of the most important influences on your health are genetics and the environment. They represent the background of your health picture. The more you know about both, about how they affect your health and how they interact, the healthier you can become.

Genes and Their Role in Human Health

We are in the midst of a genetic revolution in preventing and combatting disease. The Genome Project, which aims to map every part of the human genetic makeup, has potentially mind-boggling implications. Scientists are daily unlocking more of the genetic codes that govern our life and our health. They have even isolated a gene for immortality.

I describe this project in more detail in chapter 6, which looks at the advances in modern medicine. In years to come it seems highly possible that humans will have the ability to reprogram their genetic makeup. In the meantime, there is no reason to shrug and say, "Oh, it's genetic—there is nothing I can do about it." As you will see, by staying on top of your HQ, you have the means to fight and possibly even conquer your genetic predisposition to illness or health problems.

DNA and the genetic code: your blueprint for life

The blueprint for life is programmed into all genetic material. The genetic portrait of just one human being would fill at least a million typed pages. It is amazing that a cell, often not more than one-hundredth of a millimetre in diameter, can store vast quantities of the genetic information that is so vital to heredity and human life.

We now know that DNA (deoxyribonucleic acid) is the carrier of our hereditary characteristics. Most of us are also familiar, through news reports, with the importance of DNA in police investigations. DNA is our individual identity, who we are. It is based on two strands of material twisted around one another, forming a double helix—the gene. Each code word carried can be read by components inside the cell and translated into one of the twenty amino acids that build proteins. Proteins are different sequences of amino acids and the cell's most important tools. In a practical way, they maintain all the reactions needed for supporting life.

Genetics, aging and longevity

It's a common misconception that life expectancy is somehow programmed before birth, in our genetic makeup. Many members of a family may share similar characteristics as they grow old, but this shouldn't be interpreted as evidence that genes play the only role in the aging process. You won't necessarily live the same length of time as your parents or grandparents. Although some factors that promote long life are genetic, it is essential to distinguish family habits, traditions and experiences from genes. Often, family similarities are more closely related to common lifestyle conditions, such as diet and exercise, than to a genetic predisposition to be overweight or underweight. If your father is overweight, you don't necessarily have to be. Take a look at your parents' food preferences and physical activities, and decide whether they are appropriate for you. Moreover, accumulated damage to genes from a lifetime of exposure to environmental pollutants probably underlies some of the changes associated with aging.

Regardless of the genes you inherited as a fetus, you can play an important role in how successfully you age. Much of what you can do depends upon the balance between your genetic influence and the effects of the environment in which you go through life's journey.

Negatively, genes may strongly influence a predisposition to diseases or conditions that shorten life; for example, high cholesterol levels may run in families and can eventually lead to heart disease. But that's only half the story. Where there are strong family histories related to these diseases, environment and lifestyle still have a substantial influence on determining whether or not you will develop the disease or disorder. Exercise, a healthy diet and lifestyle, medications and other approaches are known to delay or completely prevent the emergence of some diseases popularly called hereditary. It is estimated that the effect of these positive influences may outweigh the negative genetic predisposition.

In short, no more excuses! You don't necessarily have to have the same diseases your parents suffered from, if—and it's a big if—you take action. A higher HQ can help minimize or prevent all kinds of so-called genetic problems and extend your health expectancy.

Genetic impact lessens as you get older. In the senior years, heredity has proven to be less important than environment and lifestyle when it comes to keeping up high mental and physical abilities. Where and how you live have the most substantial impact upon age-related changes and quality of life. While certain personality traits can be inherited, your vitality and social skills are more significant for living a long and happy life.

The genetic basis of diseases

People suffering from genetic diseases are victims of a genetic accident. Mutation is an essential fact of life, since it is through "mistakes" in gene replication that genetic variants arise. When we know which genes are present in both healthy and diseased tissues, it is possible to identify both the proteins required for the normal function of tissues and the distorted ones involved in specific diseases. This information allows us to develop new diagnostic tests for various illnesses and new drugs to alter the activity of affected genes or proteins.

Molecular genetics has greatly increased our understanding of the development processes of diseases in which there is a single gene defect, such as cystic fibrosis. Discovering the relevant gene and its function not only helps us understand the development of the disease but also offers an opportunity for possible gene-therapy treatment. Disorders that are caused by several genes, such as diabetes, may soon yield their secrets to the same approach. For instance, an obesity-promoting gene has been identified—clear evidence that genetics does indeed play a role in the development of obesity among some people.

Recent advances have shown that an inherited tendency plays an important role not merely in well-recognized congenital defects or hereditary diseases but also in common diseases that occur in later life, such as coronary heart disease, high blood pressure, diabetes, some cancers and some common mental disorders. We must recognize that genetic predisposition can lead to the premature onset of these diseases. Alzheimer's disease, for instance, the most common form of senile dementia, can run in families and can be linked to at least four different genes. Genetic technology may soon be used to identify people with genetic risk factors for these conditions. The potential for genetically preventing and treating diseases is enormous. As major efforts continue to investigate and develop appropriate preventive strategies and therapies, we need to take a hard look at the implications. At the moment, we have not come to terms as a society with the ethical and social implications of genetic testing.

Hereditary diseases and birth defects

In a typical developed society, congenital and genetic disorders are the most common cause of death in infants, after prenatal factors, and of death in children aged one to four, after accidents. The important thing to know is that many of them can be avoided, and we can take certain actions. Although not all the causes of birth defects are known, some can be prevented by using the knowledge we have already acquired and by taking advantage of the recent research breakthroughs. There is much that women can do to increase their chances of having a healthy baby. For example, they can ensure that they have adequate nutrition throughout the childbearing years (e.g., by eating foods rich in vitamins, folic acid and iodine). They can avoid sexually transmitted diseases. They need to be vaccinated against rubella (German measles) and hepatitis. Women should seek answers to their questions early in their pregnancy from qualified health workers, make a point of getting early and adequate prenatal care, and strictly avoid alcohol, tobacco and certain medicines (thalidomide is an obvious example).

Genes and chronic diseases

Genetic potential may well lead to the premature onset of some common diseases of adult life, such as cancer, heart disease, diabetes, high blood pressure and mental disorders. Let's look at some of them.

Cancer It is not yet certain whether most cancers are hereditary, but a genetic predisposition may be involved in as many as 10 to 25 percent of breast and colon cancer cases. Numerous genes are being identified that may affect susceptibility to cancer development. This in turn has led to a general improvement in the diagnosis and treatment of cancer. For example, a DNA screening test for breast cancer is now available. Advice on the prevention of cancers could eventually be offered to families with different types of cancer risks.

Heart disease Until recently, it was generally believed that environmental factors alone caused coronary heart disease. Lately, however, studies of family histories have uncovered some genetic risk. Mapping the human genome will make the genetic predisposition to heart disease much easier to understand. High blood pressure and high blood cholesterol levels, major risk factors in heart disease, are both genetically influenced. You can counter this with a combination of risk detection, lifestyle counselling, behaviour changes and drug treatment. I believe this could significantly reduce the incidence of heart attacks to the much lower levels of two or three generations ago.

Diabetes About 85 percent of diabetes cases in developed countries are the non-insulin-dependent form of the disease (Type 2 diabetes), which has a strong tendency to run in families. Again, diet, exercise and weight control can delay or help to prevent the onset of this problem. Evidence for a genetic element in insulin-dependent diabetes mellitus (Type 1 diabetes) has emerged from studies showing a higher occurrence in identical twins (25 to 30 percent) than in non-identical twins (5 to 10 percent).

Mental disorders Evidence from studies of families and twins demonstrates genetic predisposition to some common mental diseases. The recent discovery of several genes whose malfunctioning leads to Alzheimer's provides the pharmaceutical industry with important molecular targets for drug development. Only through the discovery of these kinds of genes can biomedical research stop this difficult and debilitating cause of human senility. Research may eventually lead also to the development of drugs that will be useful in preventing or delaying the onset of the disease.

Genes and addictions

Genetic traits may cause some individuals to feel a different effect from alcohol than is typical, or may make them more susceptible to dependence. The identification of a genetic marker, a measurable genetic characteristic, could have a major impact on dealing with alcoholism and might even predict the likelihood that an individual may suffer various physical consequences, such as cirrhosis of the liver. Genetic traits affect the onset and persistence of tobacco dependence in much the same way that they create alcohol dependence. Genes are also suspect in substance abuse and dependency.

Your Environment and Your Health

Now that we've looked at the enormous importance of genes, let's go on to the critical issue of the environment—your living conditions—and how your HQ can be improved with an understanding of the role the environment plays in your health. When I refer to environment, I mean both your physical surroundings and your psychosocial atmosphere, which is made up of your economic status, degree of social isolation, and the availability of networks for social affiliation and support. In other words, it may not be so widely recognized, but who your friends are and how much money you make will definitely affect your health. Other fringe psychosocial factors can be ethnicity, culture, occupation and social stress. Heart disease, for example, has been linked to economic status, age, ethnicity, psychological stress, job stress and lack of social resources. But more of that later; at this point, I want to blow the whistle on pollution.

Environmental health hazards in daily living occur everywhere. In the open, car emissions and second-hand tobacco smoke can lead to cancer, some pollutants can exacerbate or create asthmatic conditions, sun and UV light exposure can cause skin cancer and cataracts, and a host of other pollutants can cause or contribute to ill health. You are subjected to these hazards simply by being outdoors, in both rural and urban areas, or in open-air workplaces.

What may surprise you is that when you move inside and shut the front door, the situation doesn't get any better. In fact, recent studies have shown that the worst environmental pollution occurs inside the home. It's a jungle in there! Of course, nobody wants to live in a plastic-wrapped environment or a sanitized bubble, but we don't have to sit back helplessly sucking in toxins until it's too late. Micro-organisms, dust particles and dust mites can invade the home or a building's ventilation system, causing problems from headaches to legionnaires' disease. These hazards need to be detected and corrected early in order to protect the health of the family or of office employees.

Toxic pollutants in daily life

Significant advances have been made in techniques for assessing exposure to toxic substances. Highly sensitive analytical instruments and pollution monitoring devices have recently been developed. These devices are portable and simple to use, and the more we use them, the better able we'll be to keep a sharp eye on the poisons out there.

Already these devices have been used in large-scale field studies to assess people who have been exposed to potentially dangerous toxic substances or chemicals. These studies have produced amazing information about the concentration of environmental hazards and how they cause sickness. For example, Wayne R. Ott and John W. Roberts conducted a study in 1980 to assess human exposure to toxic substances. Over three thousand candidates, "a carefully chosen slice of the population meant to be representative of most North Americans living in urban or suburban areas" were studied for the prevalence of volatile organic compounds, carbon monoxide, pesticides or dangerous particles in their daily surroundings. The majority of the investigations used monitoring instruments that showed which pollutants existed close by and in what concentration, and that were small and light enough for people to carry as they went about their regular activities. The disturbing results of the study were published in *Scientific American*: "… most citizens were very likely to have the greatest contact with potentially toxic pollutants not outside but inside the places they usually consider to be essentially unpolluted, such as homes, offices and automobiles…. The chief sources appeared to be ordinary consumer products, such as air fresheners and cleaning compounds, and various building materials." Everyday substances found in any household, such as moth repellents, pesticides, solvents, deodorizers, cleansers, dry-cleaned clothes, dusty carpets, paint, particle-board, adhesives, and fumes from cooking and heating, can act as pollutants. The good news is that you can choose to get rid of most of them.

Common household toxins

The pollutants found indoors include biological contaminants and toxic pollutants common to every kitchen, bathroom or garage. Here's what to beware of: volatile organic compounds found in paints, resins, cleaning agents, kitchen and bathroom cleansers, air fresheners and building materials; human-made mineral fibres such as fibreglass insulation, construction dirt and paper dust; and biological contaminants, including bacteria, fungi, moulds, viruses, pollens and dust mites. Perchloroethylene, which is commonly used to dry clean clothes is known to cause cancer in laboratory animals. Paradichlorobenzene, which is found in moth-repellent cakes or crystals, toilet disinfectants and deodorizers is also known to cause cancer in laboratory animals.

Carbon monoxide poisoning is not uncommon. It interferes with the oxygen supplied to the body by the blood, and excessive amounts cause death. Generally people are more commonly exposed to carbon monoxide indoors than outdoors, particularly in the garage. Better ventilation can help lower exposure.

Lately, there has been considerable concern about the danger from fine particles, which can penetrate the lungs. Smoking, cooking, burning candles and burning firewood can all lead to production of these particles. A connection between a high concentration of fine particles found indoors and premature death has actually been documented.

Researchers have demonstrated that indoor air can contain a concentration of pesticides at least five times higher than outside air. These poisons can be traced to dirt carried on people's shoes or the careless spraying of pesticides directly on indoor surfaces. Toxic organic chemicals called polycyclic aromatic hydrocarbons (PAH) are often deposited on carpets by shoes. PAH has been shown to cause cancer in animals and may also induce cancer in humans.

Indoor pesticides and PAH may cause as many as three thousand cases of cancer each year in the United States alone.

Small children are at high risk from second-hand tobacco smoke and toxic house dust as well as from all the above pollutants because they are likely to play on floors and carpets and regularly put their hands in their mouths. Because of their smaller size, children take in relatively more pollutants than adults. The Ott–Roberts study found that "for small children, house dust is a major source of exposure to cadmium, lead and other heavy metals, as well as polychlorinated biphenyls and other persistent organic pollutants. Carpets are most trouble-some because they act as deep reservoirs for these toxic compounds (as well as for dangerous bacteria and asthma-inducing allergens, such as animal dander, dust mites and mould." Obviously, floors, carpets and doormats must be kept clean to reduce pollutants in the house.

Avoiding tracking dust indoors and using an effective vacuum cleaner, can actually reduce the amount of toxic substances in carpets to about a tenth of the original level. You can further reduce household pollutants by limiting the use of latex gloves, deodorizers and cleansers.

We need much better public education in this area. There has to be a greater awareness that toxic pollutants in the home and workplace cause illness.

Resulting health problems

In recent years, problems associated with indoor environments have become a huge health issue. Clinical symptoms and illnesses have increasingly been attributed to non-industrial indoor conditions. It's now clear that the familiar home environment is more threatening to our health than industrial pollu-tion. The Ott–Roberts study looked at benzene, for instance, a chemical known to cause leukemia in people who are exposed to it in high concentrations over a long period of time. The study showed that "45 percent of the total exposure of the U.S. population to benzene comes from smoking (or breathing smoke exhaled by others), 36 percent from inhaling gasoline fumes or from using various familiar products (such as glues), and 16 percent from home sources (such as paints and gasoline stored in basements or attached garages)."

Building-related illnesses Certain agents found indoors can lead to serious illness. Exposure to moulds, spores, allergenic chemicals and other people's illnesses can cause such conditions as rhinitis, asthma, hypersensitivity pneu-monitis and sinusitis, conjunctivitis and laryngopharyngitis. Several infectious diseases, such as legionnaires' disease, viral infections and tuberculosis, are known to spread under particular indoor conditions. Not only respiratory disorders but also certain skin disorders, such as allergic and irritant dermatitis and urticaria, are associated with specific indoor agents, including allergens and fibreglass, which is a common and potent irritant. Buildings can contain other agents that cause long-term risk if there is a prolonged exposure to them; these include radon, asbestos and tobacco smoke in the air.

Sick-building syndrome (SBS) The term "sick-building syndrome" has emerged in recent years. People who work or live in such buildings complain of upper-respiratory irritation symptoms, headaches, fatigue, visual disturbances and even outbreaks of hideous rashes. SBS first gained attention after the development in the 1970s of more energy-efficient buildings that depended on mechanical ventilation systems to circulate fresh air and control temperature and humidity. Greater use of synthetic building materials, a greater proportion of the population working in office settings, and an increase in work stress may also be factors contributing to SBS.

Effects of outdoor environmental pollutants on health

Fine-particle air pollution is the most dangerous outdoor air pollutant. Airborne particles come from a variety of sources and can be either natural or created by human activities. Human-created pollutants such as cigarette smoke, wood smoke, motor vehicle emissions and industrial processes are the most common. These particles, smaller than ten microns in diameter, are also called fine particulate matter, or PM-10. They can be inhaled and deposited in people's lungs, and they are incredibly harmful. In a number of studies it has been estimated that every time the PM-10 concentration rises by ten micrograms per cubic metre in the air, there is a 1 percent rise in the daily mortality within the exposed population (Dockely et al., 1993).

Although sunlight is essential to maintaining life on our planet, it is also the main source of ultraviolet (UV) radiation on earth. It is now well known that excessive exposure to UV radiation can lead to skin cancer. UV radiation is, in fact, one of the most significant carcinogens in our outdoor physical environment. Three types of skin cancer have been linked to UV radiation, and one of them, malignant melanoma, is frequently fatal. UV radiation exposure can also cause cataracts and premature aging of the skin as well as having an adverse effect on the body's immune system. Suntanning may still be fashionable, but it's a health hazard. Intelligent self-care indicates that it is very important for you to protect yourself and your family from excessive UV exposure.

While advancing civilization, humans have been the chief culprits in polluting the atmosphere. We've heard much in recent years about the depletion of

COMMON SOURCES OF OUTDOOR POLLUTION
_____

- Entrapped outdoor sources: factory chimney exhaust, motor vehicle exhaust and industrial waste discharge.

- Environmental physical factors: warming and humidity machinery, noise and lighting, radon, nuclear waste and UV radiation.

- Contaminants generated by human activity: carbon dioxide, perfume, wood smoke, gas-leak waste, fuel combustion products, environmental tobacco smoke, cleaning agents, pesticides and building materials.

the ozone layer through the use of chlorofluorocarbons (CFCs). This has resulted in an increase in the intensity of UV radiation at the earth's surface.

Are you susceptible to environment-related cancer?

Most cancers result from the interaction of genetic predisposition with the environment. Although genetics by themselves are thought to explain only about 5 percent of all cancers, *genetic susceptibility* is still the most significant factor in cancer development. Despite recent advances in genetic technology, it's still too early to offer testing to either high-risk families or the general population as part of routine general medical practice, although it is predicted that this will be coming within the next decade.

We have seen that individual genetic susceptibility together with environmental factors such as smoking, diet and pollutants are to blame for most human cancers. New scientific evidence indicates that, even leaving aside the predisposing genetic traits, some groups—certain ethnic populations, the very young, women, and people with poor health and nutritional status—may be at higher risk from certain environmental exposures. These are now called *acquired susceptibility* factors.

Whether you consider yourself to be at risk or not, eat your greens! Epidemiological studies have shown that fruits and vegetables rich in antioxidants and other micronutrients have a protective effect against various cancers, including those of the lung, esophagus, mouth, larynx, cervix and breast. These micronutrients may act through a variety of mechanisms to block DNA damage and mutation and the carcinogens carried by oxygen radicals, PAH and other chemicals. Recent studies indicate that heavy smokers with low concentrations of certain micronutrients, such as vitamin E and specific minerals, take in more carcinogens than do others when they are exposed to the same environment.

A new vision for environmental health research

Kenneth Olden, director of the National Institute of Environmental Health and Safety (NIEHS) in the United States, has proposed a new "vision" for environmental health research. It encompasses an environmental genome project, a survey of exposures to chemicals, the development of speedier chemical screening methods and a study of chemical mixtures. This is a departure from the conventional approach to environmental research and takes advantage of the advances in technology, molecular biology and the human genome project. Essentially, Olden is suggesting that we put environmental factors at the very top of our health-care research. I think this makes a lot of sense. It's about time we opened our eyes to what's really going on around us.

The Social Environment and Your Health

Environment in the broadest sense includes variables in our psychological, social, cultural, ethnic and occupational surroundings. Over the past few decades, studies have been enormously successful in identifying the risk factors of major diseases. Most of this research has focused on diet, cholesterol levels, exercise and lifestyle, and behaviour. Social conditions, however, also play an important role in human health and illness. Low economic status and lack of social support have been proven to contribute to the causes of disease. Society cannot afford to ignore this.

Many aspects of our social and economic worlds influence our health. Good health is underpinned by a strong economy, physical safety, a stable income, meaningful work, positive conditions in our schools and workplaces, supportive family and friends, quality care in early childhood, and social justice. These social and economic factors do not in themselves create health, but they do provide opportunities to achieve better health. Economic status, race and ethnicity also play a role in wellness.

Your health correlates to your position in society: the better off are usually healthier. People of lower economic status tend to die earlier from all causes and have higher rates of heart disease, diabetes, high blood pressure, chronic bronchitis and tuberculosis than those who are more advantaged. However, this relationship between lower economic status and health is not the result of poverty alone. Poor nutrition, inadequate hygiene and lack of access to medical care are also negative factors. Such personal habits as smoking, lack of physical activity, excess weight and alcohol consumption are closely tied to both economic status and overall health results. Obviously, the personal and social characteristics of individuals are also important influences on the state of health. In the United States, the effect of personal habits can be seen in the degree to which all economic segments of the population have benefited from the decline in mortality from heart disease during the past thirty years.

Unemployment also contributes to poor health. The unemployed have significantly more psychological distress, anxiety, depression, disability days, health problems, hospitalizations and family problems than the employed (D'Arcy, 1986). However, work is not always the answer.

Work stress and the work environment

Work stress happens when the job we have to do overwhelms us. Work-related anxiety is a common source of stress for many people. Job strain also occurs when an employee holds a job that offers little opportunity for control or independent decision making. In studies involving white men, a greater incidence of heart disease, stroke and high blood pressure is seen where there is job strain. Men employed in responsible jobs that offer few rewards for good work are at increased risk for heart attacks. Individuals who are constantly struggling against a demanding and non-supportive work environment are at increased risk for developing high blood pressure.

Social isolation

Social isolation and lack of social support can increase vulnerability to disease. Social isolation is the condition describing someone with few intimate relationships or social contacts. It is often measured by whether or not a person lives alone and how many organizations, such as clubs or churches, he or she belongs to. Lack of social support describes a condition of having few friends or family members who can provide emotional or tangible support in times of trouble. Data from large-scale studies show that socially isolated people are more likely to die prematurely from all causes when compared with their more socially integrated counterparts.

By now you have probably seen yourself "at risk" somewhere in this chapter. Indeed, you have to be extremely vigilant to be safe even in your own home. But don't be discouraged by the health dangers that may seem to lurk at every turn. Instead, look at them positively, as potential ways to improve your health. Often it's the small daily changes that make the most difference to your long-term health. For example, encourage your family and friends to remove their shoes and leave them by the door as they come into your home. And do you really need all those toxic cleaning agents? Sometimes organic, non-toxic cleansers—and elbow grease—do the jobs just as well. When you pick up your dry cleaning, hang it outside in the fresh air if possible, to dissipate some of the chemical fumes before bringing it into your home. Even better, purchase clothing that does not need dry cleaning and the harsh chemicals that process involves. These are just a few suggestions. Your HQ wisdom will no doubt enable you to come up with many more.

GENES AND ENVIRONMENT—A SUMMARY OF WHAT YOU CAN DO

- Take a clear and realistic look at your family health background. How much of your family's health problems can be blamed on a genetic factor? Or are they the result of family traditions and lifestyles? Discover what you can do to break or change the patterns leading to ill health.

- Where you see patterns of illness, there is much you can do to counteract or conquer genetic predisposition to disease. Become aware so that you can make wise choices to increase your chances of beating the odds. Recognize that lifestyle and environment become more important than genetics as you get older.

- Keep abreast of the exciting new developments in the Genome Project and be prepared to play your part as society wrestles with the ethical dilemmas it will create.

- Understand the role genetics and the environment play in the development of chronic diseases such as cancer, heart disease, diabetes and mental disorders, and in the development of addictions to drugs and alcohol.

- Become the master/mistress of your own house. Be aware that indoor pollution is just as bad as, if not worse than, outdoor hazards. Open your cupboards and be prepared to make intelligent choices about the everyday products you use.

- How healthy is your workplace? Is it time to get it tested so that you don't become a victim of sick-building syndrome?

- Slap on the sunscreen and get out of the sun. There is no arguing with the statistics: ultraviolet radiation does cause skin cancer and cataracts.

- Should you be extra careful? Some people are particularly susceptible to the dangers in the environment. Assess your surroundings and use your HQ knowledge to find out if you are one of them.

- Pay attention to your whole environment, including your home and workplace surroundings. Deal wisely with work-related stress or the anxiety caused by unemployment.

- Finally, make lots of friends and build a strong network of social support. Be prepared to lean on your friends and your social network when you become ill. They will help in your healing!

CHAPTER 3

THE HEALTHY MIND

The mind and the body are one. Sounds obvious, doesn't it? Yet for centuries, despite mounting evidence that a healthy mind really means a whole healthy body, doctors have treated the two as separate entities. It's only in the past quarter-century that we have begun to look seriously at the interconnection between mind and body.

I will help you understand how your mind can help your body get healthy and stay healthy. Furthermore, by learning to control your mind, you can even prevent illness and disease from occurring. There is, without question, a tangible and real link between mind and body. Stress, for instance, plays a part in everyone's life. Sometimes stress can bring on terrible illness. But stress does not necessarily have to be a bad thing. If stress is well managed and you pay attention to all your emotions, you are setting yourself up for a longer and healthier life.

Your mind is crucial to your HQ. The key is to deal effectively with potentially damaging emotions, such as anger, depression and anxiety. A healthy mind means that you develop a strong emotional intelligence and have a good level of self-esteem; accept your body image; enjoy a reasonable ability to think, learn, memorize and concentrate; experience a broad range of positive emotions; and are able to sense what other people are feeling. Using your mind, you are capable of creatively solving your problems, dealing with stress and bad feelings, and making intelligent decisions regarding your health.

Feeling skeptical? You don't have to take my word for this. Let's take a look at the mounting body of evidence, proof positive of the vital health link between mind and body.

The Mind/Body Connection

Advances in the last two decades have led to greater understanding of the mind/body connection. Much of the information I am presenting here comes from medical pioneers Herbert Benson of Harvard University and Daniel Goleman, a psychologist, writer for *The New York Times* and best-selling author of *Emotional Intelligence*, which has popularized the link between mind and body.

The strong connection between the mental and the physical has been a principle in the philosophy of traditional Chinese medicine (TCM) for centuries. TCM recognizes that disturbance of the mind causes internal disease. Seven primary emotions are thought to affect health and well-being: joy, anger, anxiety, sorrow, thought, fear and shock. These seven emotions are responsible for internal damage and are causes of disease. Each of them can disturb the body's balance, resulting in the development of diseases, particularly if the emotion is strongly or frequently expressed. Each emotion is related to a specific organ. For instance, joy affects the heart, anger is related to the liver, anxiety and sorrow to the lungs, thought to the spleen, fear and shock to the kidneys.

In other systems of medicine, too, the mind's power to affect the body has been recognized for centuries. In the placebo effect, the power of healing stems from a patient's positive attitude. If you think the doctor is curing you, even if he or she has merely given you a pill made of sugar, there's a good chance you will be cured by the power of positive thought. In spite of all the advances in medical science and technology, surgery and drugs, doctors still use the placebo technique. It works! The effectiveness of placebo healing is real. Study after study has shown that in virtually any disease, roughly a third of the symptoms improve when patients are given a placebo treatment with no pharmacological content whatsoever.

Using powerful imaging technology, neuroscientists have demonstrated what goes on in the brain during an emotional reaction. These neuroscientific findings help to explain how brain activity in response to an emotional reaction, such as a feeling of stress, influences bodily functions. Here's some supporting evidence of the mind/body connection.

The mind and your immune system

A relatively recent branch of neuroscience is psychoneuroimmunology (PNI). This long word has huge implications. In this new realm, scientists have produced strong evidence for a direct connection between emotions and the immune system.

Research has revealed a direct, measurable link between what you think and feel and what goes on inside your body. To the astonishment of many immunologists, it turns out that our thoughts and feelings are acted upon by the brain chemicals that also regulate our body's defences. Dr. Candace Pert has demonstrated that neuropeptides—chemicals within the brain associated with feelings of anger, sadness, love or hate—are also present in the immune system, including the spleen, the lymph glands and the thymus gland.

Dr. James Gordon, head of the Center for Mind/Body Medicine, states: "The fact that there are the same receptors, the same peptides whether they are in a brain cell or a lymph cell or an endocrine cell indicates that major parts of our body are in continuing and ongoing communication with one another." It has also been shown that emotions have a powerful effect on the autonomic nervous system, which is essential for the proper functioning of the immune system.

Another link between emotions and the immune system is the hormones that are released under stress. The catecholamines, cortisol, prolactin, and the natural opiates beta-endorphin and enkephalin are all released during stress arousal. Each has an influence on immune cells. The relationships are complex, but the main effect is that the immune cells are hampered in their functioning, so that an attack of stress suppresses immune resistance in the body's defence mechanism, at least temporarily. If the stress is ongoing, constant and intense, that suppression may become long-lasting and bring on physical illness.

We are finding out more all the time. Scientists are discovering other connections between the brain and the cardiovascular and immune systems. It is becoming obvious that if your psychological distress affects your immune system, you are more likely to get sick.

A buffer against disease

There is a good side to all this. You may actually be able to create a buffer zone against disease by dealing positively with worry, anxiety, hostility, anger, pessimism and depression. A Stanford University study showed that women with terminal breast cancer who were in support groups survived twice as long as those who were not supported.

A growing body of research now bears out the use of meditation, relaxation training and support groups in preventing and dealing with illness. There is little risk, at any rate, while the potential benefits can be quite high. It has been shown that by reducing the effects of stress and improving your emotional state, you can lessen your chances of getting sick and even prevent everyday nuisances such as flu and the common cold.

It helps to be an optimist!

Where your health is concerned, it helps to be upbeat. A positive attitude does make a difference. Numerous studies have linked characteristics such as optimism, hope and a sense of control with greater physical well-being. Healthy optimism is not an unrealistic attitude but one that embodies the belief that people can be active players in their own lives. Pessimism, on the other hand, breeds passiveness and a sense of defeat—what psychologists call "learned helplessness"—which is often linked to poor health.

In the largest study of its kind, researchers at the University of Pennsylvania showed that pessimists aged twenty-five were less healthy than optimists aged between forty and sixty. How does this happen? Attitudes probably influence health in a number of ways. Some studies suggest that the immune system may play a mediating role. Others point to interpersonal reasons, such as social support, or to behaviour patterns, such as eating well and exercising regularly. Most likely, all of these factors are involved. Although questions remain about these links, health professionals are already exploring ways to change people's attitudes and thus enhance their health. One important tool may be mind therapy; originally designed to counteract depression, it has now been found to boost optimism as well.

What can you do? Well, it is possible for you to change negative attitudes, but the key to success may be to deal with other problem areas of your life while you work on becoming more upbeat. This will give you a sense of control, which is essential to your health.

Another Q!

Are you ready for another Q? You've heard about IQ, EQ and HQ. Now let me tell you about AQ! This stands for Adversity Quotient, and it refers to your basic human need for some control or mastery over your life. Paul Stoltz, who devised the concept, puts forward some essential ideas for understanding how human motivation, effectiveness and performance are the building blocks for good health and happiness. He picks out these elements:

> *Helplessness:* This negative emotion adds to depression.
> *Optimism and Pessimism:* Optimists live longer than pessimists.
> *Hardiness:* Fortitude enables you to withstand adversity.
> *Resilience:* The better you can bounce back, the healthier you are.

Hardiness and resilience are predictors of overall performance and health. There is a direct link between your response to adversity and your mental and physical health. Hardiness can influence your immune functions, recovery from surgery and vulnerability to life-threatening diseases.

A pampered upbringing may prove to be a disadvantage in the long run. Research shows that those who face and overcome adversity as children appear to fare better later in life than those with more serene childhoods. The survivors of difficult early years enjoy stronger marriages and better health. Beware the silver spoon: it may not gleam so brightly as the years go by!

Another study, at Duke University, demonstrated the importance of a good AQ in recovery from major surgery. The death rate among those who perceived the effects of surgery as severe and long-lasting was more than double that among those who regarded the hardship as more limited and fleeting. Follow-up research at the Montreal Heart Institute discovered that among 222 heart patients, those who responded to the adversity with depression and anxiety had double to triple the death rate of those who remained upbeat.

Your friends will help you to live longer

I've touched upon this already, but it is such a valuable idea that it bears repeating: acquire friends and live longer. Men and women with few social ties are significantly more likely to become ill and die prematurely than people who are socially involved with a rich network of family and friends. Strong social networks are linked to better health. Go join that club!

HQ wellness and your spirituality

Historically, spirituality has been known to be a great healer of both mind and body. Well-documented records show that religion and medicine traditionally work side by side to heal the sick. In the distant past, religious and healing rites were often conducted by the same person, the priest. As medical science advanced, the business of healing began to separate from religion. Now we're coming full circle. Amid the resurgence of "spirituality," there is increasing evidence of a correlation between good health and positive spiritual and religious practices. Over two hundred studies have been conducted to assess "the faith factor" in health and healing. Three individuals—Dale A. Matthews, Harold G. Koenig and David B. Larson—are tireless in promoting and engaging in research on the link between spiritual and religious practices on the one hand and physical health and healing on the other.

More research is being undertaken in this field in response to the increasing interest in spirituality and religious beliefs. Most religions, faiths and personal creeds are based on the experience of a power, a life force, an energy, whatever name is applied to it. From a health point of view, the difference doesn't seem to matter. Whatever term is used, the outcome is the same: people who believe in something usually have fewer health problems.

Churchgoing can be good for more than just your soul. Researchers have demonstrated that people who belong to religious communities live longer. Not only that, but during a measured time period, those who regularly attended religious services were less likely to die. Among people recovering from open-heart surgery, those who attended religious services regularly during the six-month post-operative period were less likely to die than those who did not attend services.

And there's more. Mind/body medicine pioneer Herbert Benson suggests that people who are seriously involved in religion smoke and drink less heavily and generally tend to practise healthier lifestyles. He also suggests that historically there have been additional stress protection and enhanced well-being in the religious communities, possibly resulting from "a coherent world view, an amplified sense of belonging, more stable marriages, and the rest and meditation associated with frequent prayer" (Benson and Stuart, 1993).

Indeed, prayer and meditation have a measurable physical result. When you engage in a repetitive prayer and passively disregard intrusive thoughts, you can elicit a relaxation response that provokes a set of physiological responses. There is decreased metabolism, heart rate and rate of breathing, and the brain waves are distinctly shorter. These changes are directly opposite to those induced by stress. The result can be an effective therapy against a number of diseases, such as high blood pressure, many forms of chronic pain, insomnia, infertility, premenstrual syndrome, anxiety, and mild and moderate depression. Clearly, prayer and meditation are both therapeutic, and your spirituality and personal beliefs may well lead to better health.

Coping with Stress

Stress seems to be the byword for our age. The person next to us at the office is stressed. The shopper surrounded by bags on the bus is stressed. Those drivers on the freeway, road-raging their anger at you and everyone else, are stressed. Even our kids are stressed, worrying about exams and their future in an uncertain world.

What is stress? It is a psychological and physical state brought on when demands are too much for you, when you just can't take it any more. There are two forms of stress: short-term (or acute) and long-term (or chronic). Many people can handle short-term stress. It could be an exam, an appearance on stage, a speech, an interview. Usually you get through it. On the other hand, long-term stress may cause real damage to your immune system and health. It can lead to higher blood pressure, and in the worst-case scenario it can make you more susceptible to severe illness, such as cancer and heart disease.

Stress seems to be everywhere, particularly in the workplace, where an increasing number of absences are stress-related. "Stress leave" is a relatively new part of the labour vocabulary. We are even beginning to see the emergence of stress consultants in the workplace. One of these, Eli Bay of Toronto, says that 80 percent of people who live in North American cities have Type A, competitive personalities. Type A personalities produce 400 percent more stress hormones than Type B, or more relaxed, personalities.

How do you fight stress in the workplace? There are many ways, but these—from Gilman Haldane Consulting in Vancouver—are helpful:

- Spend time with friends and family at least three times a week.
- Don't be afraid to ask for support when you're overwhelmed or under pressure. That's a sign of health, not weakness.
- If you have spiritual beliefs, increase or maintain your involvement in this aspect of your life.
- Use stress-reduction methods, such as exercise, nutrition, hobbies and relaxation techniques like meditation or yoga.

Effects of stress

Not surprisingly, understanding stress and treating it are increasingly important in conventional medicine. Between 60 and 90 percent of all medical visits in the United States are for stress-related disorders. The three major components of stress are physiological, behavioural and psychological. Let's take a look at what is happening to you in each case.

Physiologically, stress begins when a threat is perceived. Your unconscious response to a stressful event occurs before you think about reacting to it. For example, when you have been insulted, your blood pressure goes up long before you have decided how to respond. This innate physiological response to stress is often referred to as an "emergency reaction," similar to the kind that prepares an animal for fight or flight. Responding in this way may have been a necessary part of our evolution, but in modern life it can lead to serious consequences. Growing evidence shows that stress hormones are the villains in a wide variety of illnesses. For example, changes triggered by stress may affect the heart in these and other ways:

- Blood pressure is elevated in both healthy individuals and people with borderline high blood pressure and may induce a spasm or sudden constriction of the arteries of the heart.
- Under extreme, acute stress, the brain's control over the heart rate may be disrupted, leading to abnormal heart rates and even sudden death in patients with coronary heart disease.
- Stress hormones may indirectly increase the blood's tendency to clot, which can block the supply of blood to the heart muscle and lead to a heart attack.

Behaviourally, stress has a direct influence on how we handle our responsibilities in life. Even a little stress will compromise the performance of our daily tasks. For jobs that are solely dependent on physical exertion, such as building a brick wall or mending a leaky tap, stress may be quite a nuisance. Tasks that call for fine motor skills or that involve intense concentration may well be endangered by even a small amount of stress. Nobody wants to see a bus driver, an airline pilot, a truck driver or a brain surgeon undergoing even minor stress.

And what is a typical result? We see it every day. As stress increases, so do smoking, alcohol abuse, drug abuse, poor food choices and even violence. What about you? Perhaps you are a victim of stress without realizing it. Look at yourself in the mirror. Nicotine-stained fingers? Too much junk food? Too much anger? The odds are that you've got too much stress in your life.

Psychologically, as a result of the mind's conditioning, we get caught up in patterns of thinking that create and exacerbate stress. Generally, when we feel stressed, it is because we are dwelling on the past or worrying about the future, wanting something we don't have or having something we don't want. These mental tendencies lead to anxiety, fear, guilt, anger, dissatisfaction and confusion, which stimulate the sympathetic nervous system and produce physical distress. The physical symptoms of anxiety then magnify the disturbing mental and emotional patterns. Once we get caught up in this anxiety cycle, we are riding on the stress merry-go-round and feel out of control. The creative potential of our mind is overridden by worries, obsessions and fears as we go round and round in stress-bound circles.

Fortunately, even when these vicious circles have become extreme, it is possible to reverse them by shifting the mind's focus. It takes a positive focus to bring the mind up to the present and move beyond negative thoughts.

Relaxation methods, meditation and other mind/body techniques are some ways of coping with stress. What an enormous relief it is when the mind becomes calm and absorbed in a positive focus. I'm not saying that reconditioning the mind is going to be easy. Sometimes when you are trying to soothe your anxiety-filled mind, it feels instead like a drunken monkey stung by bees. Yet with determination it is possible to draw away from this stress-induced tyranny and become quiet, serene and sure of yourself once more.

The following goals will help motivate you to practise stress management:

1. I want to be more energetic and less prone to fatigue.
2. I want to think more clearly and logically.
3. I wish to look and feel better.
4. I hope to experience greater self-confidence and relief by knowing that I can control my stress.
5. I want to be happier about my work, my life and my family.
6. I want to be better able to keep myself calm and to handle emotional problems.
7. I want to enjoy wellness and better health.
8. I would like to have fewer physical and psychological symptoms and complaints.
9. I want to reduce the likelihood that I will develop lifestyle-related diseases.
10. I want to achieve higher HQ Profile scores.

Some relaxation techniques

The relaxation response One of the ways I often recommend to combat stress is the relaxation response technique. It's one of the most helpful of the self-care antistress devices. Herbert Benson discovered it through the study of meditation. It's a little like chanting a mantra. The physiological changes it triggers represent a natural relaxation that is the opposite of the fight-or-flight response to stress. In this respect it resembles other relaxation techniques. I would like to see this type of relaxation strategy used much more widely to help people, and especially young people, counter the stress in their lives. Too many young people seek relief from stress and anxiety through alcohol, smoking and drug use; others who cannot cope with the stress of modern life become violent or commit suicide. Fortunately, the strategy is slowly starting to catch on. Stress management courses, based on relaxation, are now being offered in many high schools in the United States.

So, how do you induce a relaxed frame of mind?

There are several relaxation techniques. Here is one standard set of instructions used at the Mind/Body Medical Institute in the United States.

1. Pick a focus word or short phrase that's firmly rooted in your personal belief system. For example, an individual who does not follow a particular established religion might choose a neutral word like "one" or "peace" or "love." A Christian person desiring to use a prayer might pick the opening words of Psalm 23, "The Lord is my shepherd," while a Jewish person could choose "shalom."
2. Sit quietly in a comfortable position.
3. Close your eyes.
4. Relax your muscles.
5. Breathe slowly and naturally, silently repeating your focus word or phrase as you exhale.
6. Throughout, assume a passive attitude. Don't worry about how well you're doing. When other thoughts come to mind, simply say to yourself, "Oh well," and gently return to the repetition.
7. Continue for ten to twenty minutes. You may open your eyes to check the time, but do not use an alarm. When you finish, sit quietly for a minute or so, at first with your eyes closed and later with your eyes open. Then remain sitting for one or two minutes.
8. Practise the technique once or twice a day.

You can also do this relaxing technique during exercise, such as walking or jogging. Follow these steps provided by the Mind/Body Medical Institute:

1. Get into sufficiently good condition that you can jog or walk without becoming excessively short of breath.
2. Do warm-up exercises before you jog or walk.
3. As you exercise, keep your eyes fully open, but attend to your breathing. After you fall into a regular pattern of breathing, focus in particular on its in-and-out rhythm. As you breathe in, say to yourself silently, "in"; when you exhale, say "out." In effect, the words *in* and *out* become your mental devices or focus words in the same way that personal focus words or phrases are used with other relaxation response settings. If this in/out rhythm is uncomfortable for you, you may focus on something else. For example, you can become aware of your feet hitting the ground, silently repeating, "One, two, one, two" or "Left, right, left, right." There is, of course, equal merit in focusing on a faith-oriented word or phrase during this exercise.

4. Remember to maintain a passive attitude, simply disregarding disruptive thoughts. When they occur, think to yourself, "Oh well," and return to repeating your focus word or phrase.
5. After you finish walking or jogging, return to your normal after-exercise routine.

Practising qigong or Tai Chi are also excellent and enjoyable ways to elicit the relaxation response. I have included a description of qigong in appendix 8 at the end of this book, and Tai Chi techniques are described on page 110.

Mindfulness meditation The second major mind/body technique for coping with stress is mindfulness meditation. It offers a unique way to deal with stress, pain and chronic illness. Mindfulness meditation can induce deep states of relaxation. In this technique you don't ignore distracting thoughts, sensations or physical discomfort; instead, you focus on them. This form of meditation practice, which is perhaps 2,500 years old, stems primarily from the Buddhist tradition. It was developed as a means of cultivating greater awareness and wisdom, with the aim of helping people live each moment of their lives—even the painful ones—as fully as possible. Jon Kabat-Zinn has made a major contribution by disseminating knowledge about this important mind/body technique.

Mindfulness meditation focuses your attention on one object and brings your mind back to this focal point when it inevitably wanders. This practice of observing thoughts, feelings and sensations can help you achieve a calmer and broader perspective on them, one that sees and understands the mind and its activities more clearly. Mindfulness can be practised anywhere, in any situation, but it is important to practise on a regular basis to deepen insight and self-understanding, and to lessen your tendency to react automatically to stressful events or circumstances. Many of those who practise mindfulness find that it deeply enhances their mental and physical well-being.

Some tips for coping with daily anxiety and stress The following is a modified list of recommendations suggested by the Mind/Body Medical Institute for management of stress:

- Recognize your own signs and symptoms of stress.
- Identify and reduce the sources of your stress.
- Don't be afraid to say no.
- Organize your work priorities and get ahead of deadlines.
- Try to solve job problems with co-workers.

- Ask for support from your family and friends when you need it.
- Learn stress-coping techniques.
- Practise relaxation and meditation as part of your daily routine.
- Improve your emotional intelligence.
- Avoid situations in which you feel you may lose control.
- Practise a healthy lifestyle.
- Eat a well-balanced, healthy diet.
- Exercise regularly.
- Allow adequate time for sleep and rest.
- Find time for relaxation.
- Don't rely on cigarettes, alcohol or drugs to deal with stress.
- Practise a "Stop–Breathe–Reflect–Choose" approach to stressful situations.

Emotional Intelligence and Health*

Emotional intelligence has become an increasingly popular concept over the past decade. At the same time there has been mounting scientific and clinical evidence that emotion plays an important role in health and illness. Anger, anxiety, depression or even feelings of sadness are all potentially toxic emotions that can profoundly affect your health.

"Emotional intelligence" refers to the capacity for recognizing our own feelings and those of others, for motivating ourselves, and for good management of emotions within ourselves and in our relationships. Peter Salovey, a Yale psychologist, expanded the definition of emotional intelligence into five basic emotional and social competencies:

Self-awareness—knowing what we are feeling at the moment and using the resulting preferences to guide our decision making; having a realistic assessment of our abilities and a well-grounded sense of self-confidence

Self-regulation—handling our emotions so that they facilitate rather than interfere with the task at hand; being conscientious and delaying gratification to pursue goals; recovering well from emotional distress

---

* Most of the information in this section comes from Daniel Goleman's book *Emotional Intelligence*.

Motivation—using our deepest preferences to move and guide us towards our goals, to help us take initiative and strive to improve, and to encourage us to persevere in the face of setbacks and frustrations

Empathy—sensing what other people are feeling, being able to take their perspective and cultivating rapport with a broad variety of people

Social skills—handling emotions in relationships well; accurately reading social situations and networks; interacting smoothly; using these skills to persuade, lead, negotiate and settle disputes with the aim of promoting co-operation and teamwork

A study of people who had experienced chronic anxiety, long periods of sadness and pessimism, unremitting tension or hostility, or relentless cynicism or suspicion found that they had double the normal risk of disease. Their resulting illnesses ranged from simple headaches to asthma, arthritis, peptic ulcers and heart disease (Friedman and Booth-Kewley, 1987). Dr. Goleman suggests that the health consequences of such negative emotions are just as bad as those from smoking or high cholesterol levels.

Chronic anxiety, agitation and distress will make you vulnerable to many diseases, not least the common cold. At a specialized colds research unit in England, volunteers were systematically exposed to cold viruses. Of those people undergoing a little stress, 27 percent came down with a cold; among those experiencing high stress, 47 percent contracted the virus.

Anger can even affect life expectancy. Anger appears to do the most harm to the heart. A study of two thousand factory workers found that chronically angry people were one and a half times more likely to die over a twenty-five-year period than those who were seldom angry. Another study, begun in the mid-1950s, involved a group of medical students who were tested and classified according to their levels of hostility. When they were tracked down twenty years later, it was found that those with high hostility scores were five to seven times more likely to have died prematurely than those with low scores. Most of the deaths among those who were angry occurred before age fifty. The conclusion: the angry seem likely to die young.

Depression impedes medical recovery and increases the risk of death. Depression generally means a feeling of sadness, self-pity or hopelessness. It is more likely to interfere with the recovery process than with the course of the disease. At the Mount Sinai School of Medicine in New York City, psychiatrists evaluated levels of depression in elderly people who came to the hospital with a broken hip. Those who were not depressed were three times more likely to walk again than those who were depressed. Depression also poses a medical risk for heart-attack survivors. At the University of Montreal, among patients treated for a first heart attack, those who were seriously depressed afterward were five times more likely to die than were patients with comparable heart disease but no depression.

Now for the good news: emotional intelligence is not fixed; it can be nurtured and strengthened. Ease your mind and work on those positive emotions, such as optimism and equanimity, and on a healthful state of calmness. Optimism, a sense of control, and social interaction work together to give you a healthy advantage. They can keep you from becoming depressed when you must deal with the bad things that happen in your life, and they will help you remain upbeat in the face of setbacks. In one study, started in the 1940s, students at Harvard University were classified as pessimists or optimists based on essays they had written explaining events in their lives. About thirty years later, the health histories of these same students were examined. Starting in their forties, the pessimists had more serious diseases and health problems than the optimists.

To achieve a state of calmness or equanimity, people have to learn some relaxation techniques. Many individuals use meditation to good effect. As we've related, calming practices can gently ease the body into a state of relaxation and healthy equanimity.

There are many instances where positive feelings, such as a sense of control, have led to greater health. For example, some Yale University psychologists persuaded the administrators of one nursing home to let a group of elderly people have more control over what they ate and when they received visitors. They also gave everyone in this group a plant to nurture. A year later, the group that had been given more control and autonomy had half as many deaths as the group with less sense of control.

Your friends and your social network may prove to be your lifeline. A classic study conducted by Stanford University divided women with advanced cases of breast cancer into two groups. One group of patients was given the usual medical treatment. The other group had the same treatment but also met for group therapy once a week for a year. They talked about their feelings concerning the cancer and what it meant for their families. They became very close as a group, with a lot of love being generated in the meetings. They also learned a self-hypnotic technique for pain control. After ten years, the death rate was twice as high in the group that had not received therapy.

In another study, University of California researchers interviewed five thousand people, house to house, in a big city. After nine years, the people who had very few friends were twice as likely to have died as those who had many friends. Clearly, human connections help. A new strategy in the medical community is to create support groups, where people who are ill meet with others with the same disease for emotional support.

There is no doubt about the medical value of positive relationships; the healing power of close ties and high-quality relationships is well documented. Closely allied with this is the healing power of emotional support. Beneficial medical effects come from voicing the most troubling thoughts. Confession has also been shown to produce a positive effect on health, as well as decreasing the number of visits to health centres and days missed at the workplace.

Medicine's blind spot

It must be said that patients' emotional needs are largely unmet by today's system of mainstream medicine. I see many ways in which medicine can expand its view of health to encompass the emotional realities of illness. Patients could routinely be offered fuller information to enable them to make the necessary decisions about their own medical care; they would then be more like partners with their physicians. Another approach is needed to prepare people for surgery: teach them to be effective questioners of their physicians, teach them relaxation techniques and answer their questions well in advance of surgery. Also, it makes sense to tell people several days ahead of surgery precisely what they are likely to experience during their recovery. The result would be patients recovering from surgery an average of two to three days sooner than before.

Relaxation training can help patients deal with some of the distress their symptoms bring as well as with the emotions that may be triggering or worsening their symptoms. Relaxation and yoga are at the core of an innovative and effective program for treating coronary heart disease without surgery developed by Dean Ornish, the well-known cardiologist. Many patients can benefit measurably when their psychological needs are attended to along with their purely medical ones.

Emotional care represents an opportunity too often lost in today's medical practice; it is medicine's blind spot. There is added medical value when a patient has an empathetic physician or nurse with the time to listen and counsel. This is what is meant by "relationship-centred care." Medical schools should teach and assess emotional intelligence, self-awareness, and the arts of empathy and listening.

From a practical point of view, treating patients' emotional distress can save money. It prevents or delays the onset of sickness, and it can help patients heal more quickly. Such care also leaves patients feeling more satisfied with their physicians and with the health-care system. An editorial in the *Journal of the American Medical Association* comments on a report that depressed patients who have been treated for heart attacks are five times more likely to die than non-depressed patients. It states: "The clear demonstration that psychological factors like depression and social isolation distinguish the coronary heart disease patients at highest risk means it would be unethical not to start trying to treat these factors." Medical care that neglects how people feel as they battle chronic or severe disease is no longer good enough.

Think about it. If we help people to manage their feelings of anger, anxiety, depression, pessimism and loneliness, it will serve as disease prevention. The potential medical payoffs are as great as getting heavy smokers to quit. I would love to see a broad-based public health effort designed to impart to children as many basic emotional intelligence skills as possible, enabling them to develop healthy minds and good habits to last a lifetime. Furthermore, I believe that it would be useful for people reaching retirement age to learn emotion-management skills. Populations at risk—the very poor, single working mothers, residents of high-crime neighbourhoods—all live under extraordinary pressure. How much better off they might be medically if they had help in handling the emotional toll of their stresses.

All this is simple and sound common sense, but I fear that it has become lost somewhere in our headlong rush towards the latest pills and medical techniques. I sincerely believe, however, that it makes HQ sense. Care and compassion are a vital part of good medicine.

A SUMMARY OF THE LINK BETWEEN MIND, BODY AND YOUR HEALTH

- The mind/body connection has been a fundamental principle of traditional Chinese medicine for centuries. While not officially acknowledged, mainstream medical techniques in the Western world routinely use the placebo effect because it works.

- Neuroscientists have clearly demonstrated that emotional reactions have a direct influence on the physical body.

- The proven link between emotions and the immune system means that you can create a buffer zone against disease by using techniques such as relaxation and meditation. It's inexpensive and easy.

- Bolster your health by practising an upbeat, positive attitude and working on ways to have a sense of active control over your life. You are responsible for your emotional intelligence and for maintaining physical health through mind management.

- Be aware of your "adversity quotient" and how you respond to the difficulties or hardships that you face in life. Don't pamper or overprotect your children: learning how to face up to life's dilemmas will prepare them better for later life.

- Get friends, join clubs and make plenty of connections with the people around you. Your strong social networks will help to keep you healthy.

- Pay attention to the spiritual dimension of your life. Prayer and meditation will serve to soothe your soul, calm your mind and make you healthier.

- Jump off that stress merry-go-round, slow down, and move steadily and thoughtfully to a calmer, more confident state of mind.

- Yes, the angry do die young. Understand the importance of dealing positively with your emotions. Nurture and strengthen your emotional health.

- Research relaxation techniques to find the one that works best for you, whether it is yoga, mindfulness meditation, Tai Chi or qigong. This is a way to improve your health without worrying about side effects or complications. Why not start now?

CHAPTER 4

LIFESTYLE AND HEALTH

What is lifestyle and why is it one of the most important parts of a high HQ? The dictionary defines lifestyle as "the way in which an individual lives, as to habits, values, friendships, etc.," but in contemporary society it often takes on a frothy, almost frivolous meaning. Today's newspapers put lifestyle on the back pages, behind the hard news and insight sections. I believe, however, that your lifestyle is vital to your health. Habits and attitudes are known to have a direct effect on health and wellness, especially in the area of chronic diseases. I want to show you how your own actions are the best way to ensure a long, satisfying and healthy life. This is at the core of the HQ idea—how you live, your lifestyle—and is inextricably tied to your health. Remember, it's your life and your health. You can take charge!

So, what kind of lifestyle do you lead? Arnold Mitchell in *The Nine American Lifestyles* (1983) described a group of lifestyles that typifies the North American culture. He provides a comprehensive look at the values, beliefs, drives, needs and social trends that shape us as individuals and help to form what our lives will be like down the road. The nine types are Survivor and Sustainer (need-driven lifestyles); Belonger, Emulator and Achiever (outer-directed lifestyles); I-Am-Me, Experiential and Socially Conscious (inner-directed lifestyles); and Integrated (a combination of inner-directed and outer-directed lifestyles). Mitchell concludes that the Integrated lifestyle is the best one for good health and happiness.

This is good as far as it goes, but I want to add to Mitchell's guide. A healthy HQ lifestyle means making healthy habits, personal beliefs and sound behaviour part of an integrated lifestyle, within accepted social and cultural values.

Unfortunately, in spite of the damning weight of evidence linking chronic diseases to smoking, a physically sedentary life, poor diet, excessive eating, alcohol dependence and stress, these habits seem deeply rooted in our society and culture. Also, we seem to be hurtling along the fast-food track to disaster. The Western lifestyle, in particular, boasts a diet rich in calories and animal fat but poor in fresh fruit, vegetables and fibre. This type of diet is often associated with cancers of the breast, colon-rectum and prostate as well as with circulatory diseases and diabetes. There is growing alarm at the global spread of this style of eating, which will eventually lead to an increase in disease in many developing and newly industrialized countries. Ironically, as you will see later on in this chapter, the traditional diet of Asian countries, with its emphasis on vegetables instead of meat, is now seen to be one of the healthiest. That's the one that should be catching on!

What's needed is a general cultural shift towards a more sensible, life-enhancing way of being that includes adequate physical activity, proper diet, and stress and environmental management. This will not only safeguard human health from the potentially adverse effects of biological, chemical and physical factors but also improve the quality of life. Only then can something be done to change global disease patterns and reduce health-care costs.

It's never too early to start the promotion of healthy lifestyles—at home and in the classroom. Parents or teachers who encourage their youngsters to eat more fruit and vegetables, to exercise, to avoid smoking and, eventually, to drink alcohol only moderately are launching them on a hopeful, healthful life.

I'm not saying this is going to be easy. Unhealthy habits are often deeply entrenched, and not everyone has strong willpower. That said, people have to make healthy living a priority both individually and collectively. A healthy population costs society less in economic terms, and makes for a happier, more productive community. As a society we need to encourage people to work towards this goal by developing their personal skills, creating supportive environments, strengthening community action, building healthy public policy, and bringing about a healthy and caring population.

Eat Right for Your Health

Why put bad fuel into your body? Better to treat yourself like a sleek, expensive automobile, one that needs pampering every day. Good food and nutrition do far more than simply provide your body with the necessary energy to live, breathe, work and function. They also help you achieve a better outlook on life and maintain satisfactory body composition, which is made up of lean body mass, bone and fat. People with sound nutritional knowledge who have appropriate body mass and strong self-esteem are well equipped to avoid eating disorders and other weight-related diseases.

Researchers tell us that what we eat affects our long-term risk of heart disease, cancer, diabetes and other illnesses. Food may actually be the most powerful drug you will ever take. This is ancient wisdom. As Hippocrates, the father of medicine, once said, "Let your food be your medicine and let your medicine be your food."

Are you enjoying the good life?

In the past, society ate more healthily in many ways. Foods were grown without the use of chemical fertilizers and pesticides, were often harvested by the families that consumed them and were prepared in simple ways. Over the years there has been a cultural shift in the kinds of foods we eat and the ways in which they are cooked. During the past three decades, because of time pressures and, yes, lifestyle changes, more and more people have begun to eat fast foods and prepared foods. Compared with our ancestors, today's affluent populations consume twice the amount of fat, a much higher ratio of saturated to unsaturated fatty acids, a third of the fibre, many empty calories like those in soft drinks, much more sugar and sodium, fewer complex carbohydrates and relatively small amounts of micronutrients. Worldwide, this diet has been accompanied by a major increase in coronary heart disease, strokes, various cancers, diabetes and other chronic diseases. So much for the good life! It's time to fight back.

Nutrition: it doesn't have to taste bad!

Although most of us derive great pleasure from eating, we are often uncomfortably aware that what we should be eating and what we are actually eating are two entirely different things. I am happy to tell you that when you put more thought into the selection and preparation of a nutritious diet, healthy foods can be delicious. Eating can be both one of life's great pleasures and a way to promote optimal health. Most people who switch to a healthier diet feel better, have more energy and have a better ability to concentrate. Some believe that they look better, too.

For people in developed countries, the problem with food is not how to obtain enough of it but how to choose from among the great variety of foods available. In the past decades North Americans have shown a propensity for consuming too much animal fat, which contains a high percentage of saturated fat and cholesterol. This kind of eating results in a rise in both the total blood cholesterol level and the low-density lipoprotein (LDL), or "bad cholesterol," creating a major risk factor for coronary artery disease. A high-fat diet has also been associated with an increased risk of cancer of the breast, colon and prostate. While fats may hurt you, eating fruits and vegetables may actually protect you from disease. Recent data show that a diet rich in fruits and vegetables can reduce blood pressure levels in a matter of weeks, particularly when combined with low-fat dairy foods and a reduced intake of saturated and total fats.

North Americans do not generally eat enough vegetables, fruits, whole-grain products and legumes, all good foods that are rich in fibre, vitamins and minerals while being low in fat. In the world of high HQ, these foods should not be thought of as "side dishes" but should form the major part of our diets. Think for a moment about that radical approach: instead of building your meal around a steak or a chicken, build it around a vegetable or fruit, with meat on the side. Try this and you'll be amazed at the difference in your health after only a week. There are signs that this way of eating is catching on. In the United States between 1970 and 1994, for instance, fruit and vegetable consumption per person increased by 22 and 19 percent respectively.

Ancient Asian secrets of good eating

Yes, eating Chinese-style is good for your health. It turns out that the traditional diets and lifestyles of many regional cultures in Asia are extremely good for you. A proven formula has been developed to promote a long, healthy life. Even better news is that the prescription is rooted in the kinds of foods and active lifestyles that have traditionally characterized Asia.

One of the biggest and most comprehensive medical studies ever conducted on diet and health shows that the vegetables and grains embraced by many rural Chinese for centuries are precisely the ones that best suit humans. The long-term study, conducted jointly by Cornell University in the United States, Oxford University in England and the Beijing-based Chinese Academy of Preventative Medicine, set out to examine the eating habits and illnesses of 6,500 rural Chinese. The results challenge conventional thinking with the finding that obesity is also a function of the quality of one's diet, not just its quantity. This conclusion is based on the discovery that, in a study adjusted for height, Chinese consume 20 percent fewer calories than Americans do, but Americans are 25 percent fatter. On average, Chinese people eat just one-third of the fat that Americans consume, one-tenth of the animal protein and three times as much fibre. Their diet contributes to lower incidences of heart disease, diabetes and cancer. The finding has led to an Asian Food Pyramid (see the diagram on the next page). As you can see, the Asian model puts more emphasis on vegetables and far less on meat.

THE ASIAN FOOD PYRAMID

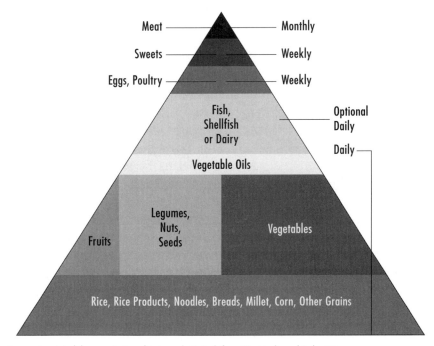

Meat —————— Monthly

Sweets —————— Weekly

Eggs, Poultry —————— Weekly

Fish, Shellfish or Dairy — Optional Daily

Vegetable Oils — Daily

Legumes, Nuts, Seeds

Fruits

Vegetables

Rice, Rice Products, Noodles, Breads, Millet, Corn, Other Grains

Source: Reprinted, by permission of Asiaweek Limited, from Tim Healy and Helen Wong, "The Road to Fit and Trim," *Asiaweek*, August 21, 1998:58–59.

This study found one especially surprising consequence of a mostly vegetarian lifestyle: a low incidence of osteoporosis, or brittle bone disease. Although the Asian diet contains relatively little calcium, a low intake of animal fat is believed to make the difference. Researchers now believe that an animal-based diet actually draws calcium out of the bones.

The cloud over all this good news is that, in recent years, the average Asian diet has become more Western—and less healthy. Asians have increased their fat intake from 10 or 15 percent of total energy consumed to 25 or 30 percent. This will probably be to the detriment of their health. In fact, there is already a dramatic increase in the prevalence of diabetes among the Chinese population.

Other dietary recommendations

Canada's Food Guide to Healthy Eating is also a good tool for helping people understand what makes up a healthy diet. The guide consists of the following four food groups and the daily amounts you should eat:

GROUP 1	2	3	4
Bread, cereal, rice and pasta	Vegetables and fruits	Milk, yogurt and cheese	Meat, poultry, fish, dry beans, eggs and nuts
5 to 12 servings	5 to 10 servings	2 to 4 servings	2 to 3 servings

Legumes The great nutritional value provided by beans and lentils makes them a major component of a healthy diet and an ideal replacement for meats. They are rich in protein, iron, fibre and many vitamins and minerals, besides being low in fat and cholesterol-free. Try to use beans and lentils in soups, salads, chili and sandwich fillings.

Soybeans are an incredibly versatile nutrient. Research has linked soy or soy's components to major health issues, including prevention of cancer and benefits in heart disease, diabetes and kidney disease. There are over twelve thousand soy-based products on the market today, with more to come. The more common soy products are whole soybeans, tofu, soy milk, tempeh, meat analogues, soy flour, natto, miso, soy sauce, okara and soy oil. Adding more soy to your diet can reduce the risk of disease.

Cholesterol There are two types of cholesterol: blood cholesterol and dietary cholesterol. Blood cholesterol, which occurs naturally in the body, is manufactured mainly by the liver. Again, there are two types: high-density (HDL) and low-density (LDL). HDL-cholesterol is often referred to as the good cholesterol, since it gathers up excess cholesterol in the bloodstream and carries it back to the liver to be excreted. The level of HDL in your blood is mainly influenced by exercise, weight, smoking and genetics. LDL-cholesterol is commonly called the bad cholesterol because excess levels build up on your artery walls. The fat portion of your diet can play an important role in controlling LDL levels. Foods high in fat, especially saturated fat, increase LDL-cholesterol levels. It is desirable to have low LDL and high HDL levels.

Dietary cholesterol is found only in foods of animal origin, primarily egg yolks, shrimp, prawns, liver, dairy products and meat. We now know that dietary cholesterol doesn't affect blood cholesterol nearly as much as dietary fat. If you're concerned about your blood cholesterol level, pay more attention to the total fat content in your diet, and particularly saturated fat, than to dietary cholesterol. When you cut back on fat, you automatically reduce your cholesterol intake! To learn more about fat you should become familiar with the information in appendix 6.

Glycemic index (GI) The glycemic index is a method of ranking foods according to their effect on your blood sugar level. This effect is clearly influenced by the form in which we eat our food, such as whether we use whole grain or refined flour, the size of the chunks of food we swallow, even the methods of processing, cooking and preparing the foods. Add to that the biologic nature of the starch (complex carbohydrates) we consume and you will discover a whole new food science to contemplate! Low glycemic index levels are better because high glycemic index foods cause a greater increase in the blood sugar level, requiring more insulin to be released by the pancreas to bring the level back to normal. Insulin plays a key role in your body's metabolism. It is not only able to lower the blood sugar level, but it also promotes the formation of fat and protein and the elevation of cholesterol levels. As well, insulin inhibits the breakdown of body fat. A prolonged and chronic high blood insulin level is undesirable and will lead to harmful metabolic changes. This could be deadly for people with diabetes, obesity or coronary heart disease. Understanding and using this concept has proven to be more valuable for people such as diabetics than the standard dietary advice of lowering fat and increasing fibre content.

Low-index foods are filling and, if eaten before prolonged strenuous exercise, can increase endurance. "Carbo-loading" has become a familiar catchphrase with distance runners. Research is still going on in this area to provide information that is simple and practical to follow. Take a look at appendix 5 to find out the glycemic index of some common foods and how to substitute low-index for high-index foods.

Dietary fibre Fibre became a food fad for a while when people began to realize the valuable role it played in overall health. Fibre is the non-digestible portion of a plant, and it has several jobs to do in maintaining your health. It helps to prevent diverticulitis and constipation, bowel conditions that are much less common among people with a high-fibre diet. A high-fibre, low-fat diet may help to prevent colon cancer. Fibre can also fill you up quickly. Try starting your lunch and dinner with a large salad or a serving of raw vegetables and plenty of water, especially when you're trying to lose weight.

A certain type of fibre can help to lower serum cholesterol and bring about better blood-sugar control in diabetics. This water-soluble fibre is found in oat bran, oatmeal, legumes, barley, apples, figs and carrots. In fact, most fruits and vegetables have both water-soluble and insoluble fibre. Insoluble fibre too is a very important food, since it helps to maintain good digestion and may help to protect against colon cancer. It is easily available from whole wheat bread and a variety of fruits and vegetables.

To increase dietary fibre, choose a diet with plenty of fruits and vegetables, whole grain breads and cereals, beans, lentils and peas. Adults should take in 20 to 35 grams of fibre daily.

Sugar Is refined sugar a dietary villain? Yes. Although simple sugar does not seem to cause illnesses, it does contribute to tooth decay, overweight, obesity and risk factors for diseases. The rising consumption of sugar in the past several decades is considered to be a major factor in the increasing prevalence of obesity and diabetes. It also makes sense that when you fill up with candies and desserts, you usually do so at the expense of healthier foods. Sugary foods are often fatty, too, like ice cream. Candy bars and soft drinks provide a hefty dose of refined sugar. Total elimination of refined sugar is desirable, but in any event it should form only a very small part of any diet.

Salt Several large population studies have shown that there is a definite link between excessive salt consumption and high blood pressure. Many people with hypertension can lower their blood pressure by reducing sodium intake. The U.S. Dietary Guideline Advisory Committee recommends a salt intake of less than six grams (one teaspoon) per day, and a more rigorous restriction may be recommended for hypertensive individuals.

Phytochemicals and phytoestrogens These are the good guys—a kind of plant chemical (phytochemical) found in withered plants, soybeans, fruits, vegetables and flaxseed, which appear to have a physiological effect resembling that of the hormone estrogen in humans. Studies suggest that consumption of a phytoestrogen-rich diet, as seen in traditional Asian societies, is associated with a lower risk of breast and prostate cancer as well as a lowered incidence of cardiovascular disease. Cruciferous vegetables, including broccoli, cabbage, cauliflower and Brussels sprouts, contain phytochemicals that appear to be powerful cancer fighters. Even garlic and onions can help, by lowering your cholesterol.

More studies are required to establish the protective role of phytoestrogens in the onset or development of cancer. Post-menopausal women who have the greatest breast cancer risk are being encouraged to increase their phytoestrogen intake. Research in vegetables, legumes and fruits has uncovered a wide range of natural plant chemical compounds that are thought to play a protective role against cancer, heart disease and other chronic illnesses in conjunction with vitamins, minerals and other nutrients. Again, good foods are nature's medicine.

Now ponder a Chinese dietary puzzle

The rate of cardiovascular disease in mainland China is about one-fifth that in the developed world. To try and find out the reasons for this, researchers used ultrasonography to measure reactivity of the artery in healthy people from Sydney, Australia, and from a village in southern China. Young people in both countries had similarly healthy arteries. Among the elderly, however, the Australians were far more likely to show signs of artery abnormality than their Chinese counterparts (Woo et al., 1997).

Arteries don't inevitably break down with age, and cardiovascular disease is not purely genetic. So it appears there is something in the Chinese environment that is protecting people from the age-related decline in arteries that we see in the developed world. Somewhat surprisingly, the difference was not explained by varying cholesterol values: these were similar in elderly Chinese and Australian people. Nevertheless, diet may be the answer, as the Chinese consume large quantities of antioxidant flavonoids found, for example, in green tea and soybean products. Flavonoids may help protect arteries from damage.

Vegetarian diet   A carefully chosen vegetarian diet can indeed help to lessen the risk of heart disease and other illnesses because it is lower in fat and cholesterol and higher in fibre. Vegetarian diets are made up of fruits, vegetables, grains, legumes, nuts and seeds. Eggs and dairy products may or may not be included. Vegetarian diets are generally classified as follows:

Lacto-ovo-vegetarian	— excludes meat, poultry and fish but includes dairy products and eggs
Lacto-vegetarian	— excludes meat, poultry, fish and eggs but includes dairy products
Vegan	— a strict vegetarian diet; all animal products, dairy products and eggs are excluded

A carefully chosen vegetarian diet will be nutritionally adequate. Taking in enough protein is usually not a problem. Many plant foods, particularly legumes, contain plentiful protein. The body can produce complete proteins if a good variety of plant proteins are consumed over the course of a day. Extra attention, however, must be paid to some micronutrients. I don't recommend this diet for rapidly growing young children or for seniors.

A person following a strict vegan diet will need vitamin D and calcium supplements. In addition, vitamin B-12 should be increased by either eating a fortified breakfast cereal or taking a supplement.

Supplements   These are the subject of much debate, but I believe that supplements are necessary even with a good diet. Studies continue to show health benefits from certain nutrients, vitamins and mineral supplements. You should be cautious, however, when taking supplements. Generally, a multivitamin and mineral supplement in one-a-day form is recommended. And keep in mind that supplements should never be viewed as replacing a good diet.

Supplements of the micronutrients enhance the immune system, act as antioxidants, and reduce levels of cholesterol and homocysteine, an amino acid in the blood. Abnormal elevation of the homocysteine level has been found to be a major risk factor for heart attack, cardiovascular disease and stroke. Some supplements are known to protect people against cancer, heart disease and other chronic diseases. Their protective qualities are particularly useful among the elderly, children and pregnant women.

An important recommendation: pregnant women need to take 400 micrograms (0.4 milligrams) of folic acid daily. Recent studies have shown that women who have adequate folic acid intake can reduce the risk of having a baby with brain damage. Many multivitamin supplements contain an adequate amount of folic acid. Good food sources for this B vitamin are green vegetables, such as spinach, broccoli, kale and romaine lettuce, oranges and orange juice, grapefruit juice, cantaloupe, legumes, nuts and seeds, fortified breakfast cereals and wheat germ. Commercially available folic acid is a synthetic and heat-stable compound, approximately twice as potent biologically as the folate that occurs naturally in foods such as dark green leafy vegetables, seeds, fruits, liver and kidneys.

Why is folic acid so important? Mothers who take folic acid during their pregnancy have healthier babies. The United States Public Health Service recommends that all women who could become pregnant consume 400 micrograms of folic acid each day. Women consuming an average diet containing 200 micrograms of food-derived folate plus 400 micrograms of supplemental folic acid in a multivitamin or fortified cereal could achieve full protection against congenital neural tube defect.

A recent report suggests that folic acid can benefit everyone. Since the mid-1970s, 25 percent of American adults have consumed a daily multivitamin containing 400 micrograms of folic acid. An editorial in the *New England Journal of Medicine* (1998) has recommended that adults should take 400 micrograms of folic acid supplement while continuing to consume a healthy diet with more vegetables, fruits and whole grains. Blood homocysteine is a sensitive indicator of folate deficiency. Inadequate intake of folate or a lower level of folate will lead to increases in the blood homocysteine level. Men with abnormally high homocysteine levels have a threefold greater risk for heart attack than those with lower levels of homocysteine.

In adults, daily folic acid intake of 400 micrograms appears to play a major role in the prevention of coronary artery disease, stroke, peripheral vascular disease and certain cancers, such as colon, gastric and throat cancer. Adequate folic acid intake allows the body's normal defence and repair mechanisms to function. A long-term study of ninety thousand women recently published in the *Annals of Internal Medicine* found that women who took folic acid supplements for at least fifteen years decreased their risk of colon cancer by about 75 percent.

Another study, of men this time, at the University of Arizona found substantial reductions in the incidence of prostate cancer among men who had taken selenium supplements.

Antioxidants   Over the past few years, "antioxidant" has become a common buzzword among the health-conscious public. You or your friends may have started taking antioxidant nutrients like vitamins E and C, beta-carotene and selenium in an attempt to beat cancer, heart disease and natural aging. Another term frequently batted about these days is "free radicals." The idea is that antioxidants act as protective agents that block the dangerous action of free radicals.

Free radicals are atoms or groups of atoms. They are normally present in the body in small numbers as by-products of normal metabolism. A diet that is high in fat can increase free radical activity because oxidation occurs more readily in fat molecules than it does in carbohydrate or protein molecules. Exposure to radiation, whether from the sun or from medical procedures, or exposure to environmental pollutants such as tobacco smoke and automobile exhaust, can lead to the production of free radicals in the body. Excessive free radical formation could cause damage to DNA, mutate genes and produce abnormal proteins, thus weakening the immune system.

Free radicals are normally kept in check by the action of antioxidants, the free-radical scavengers that occur naturally in the body. Antioxidants can be obtained from food sources such as sprouted grains and fresh fruits and vegetables that contain a large amount of micronutrients rich in antioxidant activity. Therefore, a high intake of foods with antioxidant nutrients appears to be effective against chronic diseases and the aging process. You can also minimize free-radical damage by taking supplements of key nutrients with high antioxidant activity. This is further scientific evidence that eating a diet rich in vegetables and fruits will help to maintain health and protect against diseases.

A recent book, *The Antioxidant Miracle*, by Lester Packer, a professor of the Department of Molecular and Cell Biology at the University of California at Berkeley, puts the power of antioxidants succinctly. Suppose, Packer states, there was a pill that could keep your heart strong, your mind sharp and your body youthful "well into your seventies, eighties, nineties and beyond." And what if that pill could extend your life and improve your sex life as well as preventing cancer and keeping your skin wrinkle-free? Packer, a mainstream scientist, suggests that people might consider him a weird futurist. Yet, he points out, antioxidants—which he has studied for most of his seventy years—have incredible power. According to him, the most important antioxidants are vitamins C and E, lipoic acid and Glutathione coenzyme Q10. Vitamin E is considered to be nature's master antioxidant.

Eating patterns

We have been emphasizing that a healthy diet and good eating habits can lead to a longer, healthier and happier life. You should also know how your eating patterns—the process of eating, digesting and absorbing food—can affect your body. You need to know how often to eat, which foods provide the best nutritive value, and the amounts of food required for the best health. The most important thing to keep in mind is that even a few small changes can make a big difference. Healthy eating does not always require a major change in the way you eat or entertain or shop for groceries. Just eating less fried food, for example, can make a huge difference.

Your habits can have a profound impact on your health. A regular eating pattern with three small balanced meals and two snacks is a very good physiological approach to maintaining the normal body's metabolic status. Eating is an enjoyable aspect of life and deserves your full concentration. Selecting the right amount and kind of food can help you considerably. Alcohol in moderation is also believed to be beneficial in providing protection against some chronic diseases. Green tea is believed to be effective in preventing heart disease, stroke and certain cancers. Regularity in eating also seems to be important to health and longevity.

One of the great challenges to healthy eating may be altering your familiar mindset and practices with regard to food selection, preparation, presentation and consumption. Although well-balanced meals and optimal nutritional details have already been discussed, I am really suggesting a whole new strategy that shifts the focus from meat to vegetable/grain/fruit/legume dishes without requiring a complete abandonment of meat products.

Traditional meals for many North Americans and other cultures have centred on meat as the main course. Vegetables and other foods have generally been regarded as "accompaniments" or "side dishes." In fact, meat has historically been a status symbol among the well-to-do, the food-proud, chefs and culinary experts. Meat is also the focus of many cultural and familial traditions and therefore holds a special place in our minds. Today, however, it's time to view meat and the part it plays in our diets in a different light.

Our perceptions of meat are moulded not only by traditions in the home and within various cultures but also by advertisements and what is made available at restaurants and in the marketplace. Most restaurants feature only meats on their specials-of-the-day menu. Furthermore, restaurants usually arrange their selections in chicken, beef, pork or fish categories. This encourages society to think about meat first and everything else second.

Eating out, eating right

Shifting our attitudes towards food so that the culture emphasizes healthy eating, with an emphasis on vegetables, grains, fruits and legumes and without compromising variety, will have significant ramifications for the restaurant industry. Imagine a menu that categorizes dishes based on whether they feature dark green vegetables, root vegetables, beans or tofu. Then, various meats could be included as side dishes, or perhaps grilled and served on top of the vegetable dish. Beef and broccoli may become broccoli and beef; pork and beans would be known as beans with pork. This type of cooking has been practised and popularized for a thousand years in China.

A rethink in home cooking, too

Familiarizing people with a menu centred on vegetables rather than meat can be a first step towards encouraging a new way of thinking about food selection, preparation and consumption at home. Meat can still be offered for its flavour, texture, protein and other nutritive value, but it should be played down in importance, to reduce the amount of animal, saturated and hydrogenated fats we consume.

A more vegetable-centred diet doesn't mean exclusive vegetarianism but a better balance among the items on our basic list, including meats. Eating can be even more enjoyable and varied, and a new emphasis on preparation and cooking methods can provide fun and a chance for the family to participate. A new approach to combining the foods in the food pyramid will give you the chance to create a new cuisine for your family. It is an excellent opportunity to amend existing recipes or develop new ones that are healthful and exciting. Cultural tastes and traditions can still be attended to, and particular dietary needs met.

Some suggested menu ideas

Let's look at how this change might work. Here's a different way of thinking about mealtimes, with some new suggestions for the preparation of various courses. A word of caution: it's tempting to overindulge at special occasions, parties or picnics. You can avoid this by planning ahead and choosing a simple food-and-drink menu. Many people also find that weekly menu plans make shopping more efficient and economical and meals more nutritious.

1. *Appetizers*   These can feature meatless soups and salads centred on vegetables, fruits, and nuts or grains. Many chilled vegetable or fruit soups are very tasty and provide valuable nutrients; grilled and/or marinated vegetables or seafood can make delicious hot or cold hors d'oeuvres. Soups plus side-dish or main-course salads will often make a meal. Watch carefully when you select salad dressings: most of the popular dressings contain high amounts of calories and fat.
2. *Main Course*   This can be built around vegetables such as beans and peas, colourful stir-fried or steamed vegetables, and casseroles and chili dishes that emphasize vegetables over meat. Fish, tofu dishes and mixed-grain entrees with vegetables and tasty accompanying sauces make nutritious and filling main courses. Eggs, rice and pasta can easily be used to create nutritious and exciting main-course dishes that maintain unique cultural flavours and other distinctions. Try to avoid fried foods.
3. *Side Dishes*   Small amounts of meat or meat-with-vegetable dishes can be introduced here as an accompaniment to the main course; meats that are lean (10 percent animal fat or less) and cooked by grilling or baking are best. Remember to cook with the less-saturated fats and oils, such as olive and canola.

4. *Food Staples.* Whole grain products make up a necessary part of an everyday balanced diet and should be included in meals throughout the day. This diverse category includes hot and cold cereals, whole wheat bread, rice, noodles, pasta, and grains such as millet, barley and oats. Rice is eaten every day by half the world's population and comes in many varieties, providing a base that offers endless opportunities for adding flavours. All grains make an attractive bed on which to serve a main course. Remember to add oat bran to baked products and substitute oat flour for all-purpose flour whenever possible.

5. *Dessert* Substituting fruit for sugary desserts gives you more nutrition without compromising flavour. Fresh fruits, fruit compotes, poached fruits and dried fruit stews all provide natural sweetness and flavour. Puddings, mousses and sorbets can provide a light, low-calorie end to a meal. Top fruit desserts with yogurt instead of whipped cream.

6. *Fresh Juice* is more than just a delicious drink; it provides us with some of the nutrients and micronutrients (vitamins and minerals) that help us to cope with stresses and strains. There are many special drink recipes available that are suggested as health cures. Since almost all fresh fruit and vegetable juices are good for your health, the best juice recipes are the ones you like the most. Keep in mind that pulp is a good source of fibre.

7. *Green Tea* Yes, it really is as good as they say! Coffee is entrenched in our culture, but from a health point of view, green tea or juices should be the beverages of choice. Green tea, with its antioxidant properties, has been found to have an anti-cancer effect. For fluid intake you should drink water instead of soft drinks,which have a high sugar content.

8. *Wine* Go ahead and pour yourself a glass with my blessing. Since modest amounts of alcohol in the form of red wine have been found to protect against cancer and heart disease, there is no reason why you shouldn't enjoy one glass of wine with a meal.

Your total food experience

Selecting, preparing and cooking foods more nutritiously requires thinking about food in a new way. Your total "food experience" can be made even more exciting if you employ a new style of cooking, such as steaming or boiling, rather than frying, and learn new food preparation techniques, like carving or chopping and slicing, that will enhance the presentation of the meal. Changing the way you view food does not necessarily mean that it can't be an important and enjoyable part of your life. Instead, you can learn to savour other aspects of the food experience that help keep you healthy and fulfilled.

HOW TO EAT RIGHT FOR A HEALTHY LIFE

- Food is the most powerful drug you will ever take, so give yourself the best you can. Good food choices are the key to healthy eating, and they can be delicious. You should choose food that reflects good variety and provides a well-balanced diet. Ideally, foods should be organically grown and fresh. Avoid fast foods, junk foods and overprocessed foods.

- Put meat in its place, at the side of the plate, and move the vegetables, fruits and whole grain products from the side to become front and centre in your diet. Check out the Asian Food Pyramid (page 94), and remember that the rule of thumb is to choose lots of whole grain foods; fruits, vegetables and legumes; fewer dairy products, fish, eggs and nuts; and minimal amounts of meat and poultry. Soybeans and legumes are great protein substitutes.

- Be aware of good and bad cholesterols and the glycemic index. Aim for a combination of foods that are high in fibre but low in fat, saturated fat, salt and cholesterol, have a low glycemic index and contain negligible refined sugar.

- Find out about nature's medicines, such as the potential benefits of flavonoids, and about which foods provide important phytochemicals and phytoestrogens.

- Know both the value and the dangers of taking supplements. Generally, you should consider daily micronutrient supplements in the form of a multivitamin. Excessive supplementation in the form of macrovitamins, however, is not recommended. Although taking supplements should never replace a good diet, I recommend choosing a supplement that contains:
  - antioxidants (vitamins E and C, beta carotene, selenium), which neutralize free radicals and are effective against chronic diseases and the aging process;
  - folic acid, which is required in a pregnant woman's nutrition to prevent brain and spinal cord malformations in the fetus, and which decreases the homocysteine level, a risk factor for heart disease; and
  - vitamin D and calcium, which are important for post-menopausal women and for seniors, and are required by vegans.

- Eating should be a pleasure. Try a new philosophy of healthy eating by using the suggestions in my menu ideas. Most problems with food and eating can be addressed by using meat merely as an enhancement to the meal rather than as the focal point, by emphasizing the role of vegetables and by substituting fruit for sugary desserts.

Instead of reaching for the tried-and-true gratification of a large slice of meat, you can get equal satisfaction through your new style of cuisine. I would like to see a gradual but major change in our food and eating habits—to the HQ way. We can all be a lot smarter in the ways we choose, prepare, cook and present our foods. Even traditional or cultural meals can be adapted to be health smart. Who knows—this may bring a whole new culinary world to your dinner table. So fire up the stove, set the table, light the candles and bon appétit!

Exercise, Stay Young

The more active you are, the longer you'll live; for most of us, it's as easy as that. Regular aerobic exercise and physical activity are keys to preventing sudden death and lowering the possibility of sickness or death from heart disease. Regular exercise makes the heart stronger and more efficient. Exercise is a protective factor and also serves to lessen the impact of other potent dangers, such as high blood pressure, high cholesterol and obesity. Physical activity can alter the course of diabetes, mood disturbances, osteoporosis, arthritis and heart attack (Matheson et al., 1989). Couch potatoes, please sit up and take notice: a sedentary lifestyle puts you at major risk for death from heart disease and other chronic diseases.

A study by the Framingham Heart Studies shows that active men live longer than sedentary ones. The scientist Steven N. Blair reported that men who maintain or improve adequate physical fitness are less likely to die from all causes than men who are persistently unfit. Physicians should encourage men who are out of shape to improve their fitness by starting a physical activity program (Blair et al., 1995).

What exercise can do for you

Regular exercise is essential for top physical functioning of the human body. You'll benefit both physically and psychologically. Regular exercise improves digestion and elimination, increases endurance and energy levels, promotes lean body mass while burning fat, and lowers overall blood cholesterol while raising the proportion of good to bad cholesterol. It can be a great way to relax, and it can help you deal effectively with the stress of daily life, which contributes to so many illnesses.

Physical changes occur during aerobic exercise. There is a decrease in resting heart rate, a decrease in resting blood pressure and a decrease in body fat. Aerobic exercise also produces an increase in maximal output from the heart and an increase in maximal oxygen consumption. All important—and significant to your health!

Researchers have found that exercise can decrease anxiety and depression and improve your self-image. It also elevates your mood and makes you feel good. So, get out there and walk, run or jog. Any exercise, however limited, will be beneficial as long as you do it regularly. According to a 1996 report by the Aerobics Centre Longitudinal Study, published in the *Journal of the American Medical Association*, low fitness levels may pose as great a risk to health as smoking, and a greater risk than high cholesterol, high blood pressure or obesity. It was reported that smokers who are moderately physically fit but have high blood pressure and high cholesterol live longer than non-smokers who are healthy but sedentary. The statistics are in and there is no debate about it: an active and fit way of life will improve your health and lower your risk of early death.

Eating less and exercising more will help you to lose extra weight and keep it off. Research consistently shows that regular physical activity, combined with healthy eating habits, is the most efficient and healthful way to control your weight, whether you are trying to lose weight or maintain it. When you eat more calories than you need to perform your day's activities, your body stores the extra calories and you gain weight. Everything you eat contains calories, and everything you do uses calories, including walking, sleeping, breathing and digesting food. Balancing the calories you use through all activities with the calories you eat will help you achieve your desired body weight. Any type of physical activity you choose to do—strenuous ones such as running or aerobic exercise, or more moderate ones like walking or household work—will increase the number of calories your body uses.

Regular physical activity can help to protect you from the following health problems:

- **Heart disease and stroke** Exercise strengthens your heart muscle, lowers your blood pressure, raises your high-density lipoprotein levels and lowers low-density lipoprotein levels, improves blood flow and increases your heart's working capacity. A recent study published in *The Lancet* (October 1998) showed that exercise could not only reduce the risk of stroke but also help stroke survivors recover motor skills. In a thirteen-year study of more than eleven thousand men, those who took moderate exercise (a brisk one-hour's walk five days a week) had a 46 percent lower stroke risk than those who did little or no exercise.

- **High blood pressure**   Regular exercise has been proven to reduce high blood pressure levels. It also reduces body fat, which is associated with high blood pressure.
- **Non-insulin-dependent diabetes**   A focus on fitness will lead to weight loss, which can help to prevent or control this type of diabetes.
- **Obesity**   Physical exercise helps to reduce body fat by building or preserving muscle mass and improving the body's ability to use calories. When combined with proper nutrition, it can help control weight and prevent obesity, a major risk factor for many diseases.
- **Back pain**   By increasing muscle strength and endurance and improving flexibility and posture, regular exercise helps to prevent back pain.
- **Osteoporosis**   Regular weight-bearing exercise promotes bone formation and may prevent many forms of bone loss that come with aging.

In summary, weight management through exercise can improve your physical appearance, muscle strength, flexibility, cardiovascular efficiency and endurance, and make you less vulnerable to the development of diseases by enhancing your immune system.

Psychologically, too, you can benefit from regular exercise. It acts as a buffer against stress and may thus help protect the cardiovascular and immune systems from the consequences of stressful events. Frequent exercise is an effective treatment for anxiety and has proven to be as effective as psychotherapy in treating mild or moderate depression. Exercise seems to lighten your spirits both through its physical effects on the nervous system and through its direct psychological effects on the mind. For instance, studies have found that regular exercise can improve your mood and the way you feel about yourself. It distracts you from everyday concerns and gives you time to relax and reflect. Any form of enjoyable exercise can give you a psychological lift and help counteract the effects of stress in your life. Most people who exercise say that they feel better, think better of themselves and have a more positive outlook on life. They feel better not only physically but mentally and emotionally as well.

Besides helping to reduce stress and induce a relaxation response, you may realize some of the following specific benefits from recreational exercise:

- increased cardiovascular efficiency
- increased fat utilization (weight control)

- improved aging/longevity
- increased bone density (prevention of osteoporosis and possible fractures)
- increased high-density lipoprotein (HDL), or good cholesterol, and decreased triglycerides
- decreased hypertension
- decreased platelet aggregability (blood clots)
- enhanced glucose tolerance and increased insulin sensitivity
- decreased sensitivity of the heart muscle to stress hormones
- decreased upper-respiratory infections (URI)
- cancer prevention

How to go about exercise planning

At this point, you are probably thinking, "That's all very well, but how do I fit more exercise into my already busy daily routine?" Or perhaps you feel that you are simply not able to do strenuous and vigorous exercise. Remember, though, that you don't have to run a marathon to make this work for you. Moderate and cumulative exercise is good enough to help your health.

The first step in starting an exercise regime is to learn what kinds of exercise are right for you. For instance, think about exercises of varying type, frequency, intensity and duration, and identify what you would enjoy. There are therapeutic exercises that can target a particular health problem you may have. Recreational activities can provide both aerobic and non-aerobic exercise as well as skill development, if you are hoping to achieve other benefits as well.

For a recreational exercise program to be part of your life, it has to be:

- an enjoyable program suited to your personality
- varied, so that you don't become bored with it
- an activity that you can realistically and comfortably pursue
- capable of becoming a part of your lifestyle
- open to participation from family or friends
- easy to begin
- clearly beneficial to your physical and psychological well-being
- an improvement in your quality of life
- an activity that gives you a sense of satisfaction with your health

Each kind of exercise produces different physiological effects. To obtain the best benefits the key is to choose an exercise that is enjoyable and that fits your personality. The list of possibilities is enormous. There's yoga (see page 190), Tai Chi (see below), qigong (see page 215), weight training, aerobic training and all kinds of options that you may not have considered before.

Motivation is the main problem. If you know that you are not easily motivated, make sure that you try an activity that is relatively easy to fit into your daily life and one that you think you will enjoy—even a walk to the store instead of a trip by car!

How about trying Tai Chi?

Tai Chi, a slow, graceful and precise series of circular and supple movements inspired by stylized combat, originated in ancient China. All vital functions of the human body are stimulated. Tai Chi's flowing movements and "energy meditations" have the therapeutic effect of slowing down the pace of your life, reducing stress and improving energy. Tai Chi relaxes the mind and the body, slows activities of the nervous system, benefits the heart and blood circulation, improves digestion, loosens stiff joints, tones up muscles and refreshes the skin. It re-establishes balance both physically and mentally, encouraging your body and mind to return to a rested state. The regular practice of Tai Chi improves health and vitality, and promotes a supple body, the harmonious development of physique, better posture, and a mind free of the annoyance of everyday jitters.

Tai Chi is well known as a way to achieve relaxation and tranquility. As a physical exercise system, Tai Chi utilizes the principles of non-exertion and internal energy exercise. It teaches the art of fluid movements and gentle, relaxing exercise to develop and strengthen the whole body, gradually and evenly. At the same time it has the capacity to rejuvenate the body, increase resistance to disease and illness, and improve physical fitness. As a healing art, Tai Chi is widely used by the Chinese to alleviate, or in some cases cure, insomnia, arthritis, rheumatism, anemia, chronic indigestion, listlessness, mental strain, depression and nervous breakdown. Thus, the benefits of Tai Chi are physical, mental, emotional and spiritual.

There are five essential principles in the practice of the art of Tai Chi: relaxation, concentration, meditation, harmony and breathing. The five essential qualities of Tai Chi movement are slowness, lightness, clarity, balance and calmness. During Tai Chi exercise the mind is focused on the mental imagery of each movement, with continuous abdominal breathing. It is a good and enjoyable way to elicit relaxation.

Recent studies have shown that people aged seventy and over who took part in a fifteen-week Tai Chi program reduced their risk of falling by 47.5

percent (Wolf et al., 1996). Tai Chi exercises have also proven effective in improving balance and strength among older people (Wolfson et al., 1996), and have been found to lower blood pressure.

Tai Chi is a reminder that relatively "low-tech" approaches should not be overlooked in the search for ways to prevent disability and maintain physical performance in later life. It is an inexpensive approach to helping the elderly avoid unnecessary frailty and potentially debilitating falls. This low-intensity exercise can be done easily at home alone or in public parks with friends, once they have been given the proper training.

How much exercise is enough?

The answer depends on each person, but there are goals to aim for. In 1995 the Center for Disease Control and Prevention and the American College of Sports Medicine jointly reviewed the evidence related to physical activity. They concluded that every adult should accumulate thirty minutes or more of moderately intense physical activity on most, if not all, days of the week. The thirty minutes could be accumulated intermittently and could include routine activities such as yard work, housework and walking the dog, or recreational activities like playing with children, dancing and sports, as well as traditional exercise regimes. Less intense activities should be done more often, or for longer periods of time, or both. Adults exercising at this level, comparable to a brisk, two-mile walk, will easily burn about two hundred calories a day. Over time these add up to a huge health benefit.

The new *Physical Activity Guide* (1998) of the Canadian Society for Exercise Physiology aims to help lethargic Canadians get up and go. It claims that you can improve your fitness and your heart by doing light activity for ten-minute periods, adding them up for an hour's worth each day. Light walking, easy gardening and stretching are all acceptable; you don't have to go for gruelling workouts to improve your health. Accumulating sixty minutes of gentle exercise every day will help you stay healthy or improve your health. This goal can be reached by building physical activities into your daily routine. The guide indicates that it's easy to achieve six ten-minute periods of activity in a day, helping reduce risk of premature death, heart disease, diabetes, high blood pressure, and even depression and stress. As you progress to more demanding activities like jogging or aerobics, you can cut down to thirty minutes of exercise, four times a week, according to the guide.

If you have been inactive for a while, you may want to begin slowly, with easy exercise like walking or swimming at a comfortable pace. As you build up your strength over time, you will become steadily fitter without straining your body.

Once you are in better shape, you can graduate to more vigorous and demanding activities.

Moderate-intensity activities include some of the things you may already be doing on a daily or weekly basis, such as gardening and housework. You can do these in short spurts—ten minutes here, eight minutes there. Alone, each action does not have a great effect on your health, but if you regularly accumulate thirty minutes or more of activity over the course of the day, you can reap substantial health rewards.

To become more active throughout your day, take advantage of any chance to get up and move around. The point is not to make physical activity an unwelcome chore but to make the most of the opportunities you have to be active.

Aerobic activity is a great kind of moderate-intensity exercise. Aerobic exercise is an extended activity that makes you breathe hard while using the large muscle groups at a regular, even pace. It helps make your heart stronger and more efficient. Aerobics also use more calories than other activities.

To get the best health benefits from an aerobic workout you should exercise at a level strenuous enough to raise your heart rate to your target zone. Your target heart-rate zone is 50 to 75 percent of your maximum heart rate (the fastest your heart can beat). To find your target zone, look for the category closest to your age in the chart below and read across the line. For example, if you are thirty-five years old, your target heart-rate zone is 93 to 138 beats per minute.

TARGET HEART RATE DURING AEROBIC EXERCISE	
Age	**Heartbeats per minute**
20–30 years	98 to 146
31–40 years	93 to 138
41–50 years	88 to 131
51–60 years	83 to 123
61+ years	78 to 116

To see if you are exercising within your target heart-rate zone, count the number of pulse beats at your wrist. Your heart should be beating within your target heart-rate zone. If your heart is beating faster than your target heart rate, you are exercising too hard and should slow down. If your heart is beating slower than your target heart rate, you should exercise a little harder. When you begin your exercise program, aim for the lower part of your target

TIPS FOR A SAFE AND SUCCESSFUL PHYSICAL ACTIVITY PROGRAM

- Make sure that you are in good health when you begin. Follow a gradual approach to exercise to get the greatest benefits with the fewest risks. If you have not been exercising, start slowly, and as you become fitter, gradually increase the duration and the pace of your activity.

- Regular exercise can make physical activity a part of your lifestyle. Be sure to choose activities that are safe and comfortable, and that offer you pleasure and enjoyment, so that you will stay with your exercise routine. Exercising must be convenient and offer variety, so that you will want to stick with it and do it almost every day. It would be advisable to invite friends and/or family into your activities, so that you can encourage one another to persevere.

- Choose activities that you enjoy and that fit your personality. For example, if you like team sports or group activities, pick something like soccer or aerobics. If you prefer more individual activities, get into swimming, biking or walking.

- Exercise regularly. For the best health benefits it is important to exercise as consistently as possible. Make sure your activities will fit into your schedule.

- Exercise at a comfortable pace. For example, while jogging or walking briskly, you should be able to hold a conversation. If you feel uncomfortable within ten minutes of beginning your exercise, you are working too hard.

- Maximize your safety and comfort. Wear shoes that fit and clothes that move with you, and always exercise in a safe location.

- Vary your activities. Choose several so that you won't get bored with any one thing.

- Challenge yourself. Set short-term as well as long-term goals, and celebrate every success, no matter how small.

zone (50 percent). As you get into better shape, slowly build up to the higher part of your target zone (75 percent). If exercising within your target zone seems too hard, work at a pace that is comfortable for you. You will find that, with time, your body will get used to the exercise demands and you can slowly increase to your target zone.

Stretching and muscle-strengthening exercises, such as weight training, could also be a part of your physical activity program. In addition to burning calories, these exercises strengthen your muscles and bones and help prevent fractures.

Unhealthy Habits, Unhealthy Living

Tobacco use, alcohol dependency and substance abuse are all bad for you. How bad? Read on.

Smoking

There is overwhelming evidence to prove that smoking is extremely detrimental to your health and well-being. You need to know the truth. I am going to look at some plain statistics, facts and information, collected over decades, to show the devastation that smoking causes. I will also give you some ideas to help you stop smoking. If you don't smoke, well done; you can skip this section. If you do, stub out that cigarette and take note.

Tobacco smoke is a major cause of premature death and mortality. The estimates show just how destructive the tobacco epidemic has been in developed countries over the last half of the twentieth century. Between 1950 and 2000, about 62 million people died in these countries from tobacco use, most (52 million) of them men, with the majority (38 million) dying in middle age (thirty-five to sixty-nine years). On average, those killed by tobacco in this age group lost more than twenty years of life expectancy. Currently, smoking causes 30 percent of all cancer deaths in the United States, making tobacco smoke the single most lethal carcinogen in that country today. Few researchers doubt that repeatedly exposing parts of the body to the chemicals in tobacco smoke may eventually bring about the cellular changes that can lead to cancer. Studies also demonstrate that one in four deaths among males is attributable to smoking. Smoking now causes about a third of all male deaths in middle age, plus about a fifth of those in old age. Smoking is the cause of about half of all male cancer deaths in middle age and about a third of male cancers in old age. Indeed, analysis of the statistics shows that smoking accounts for virtually all the differences in cancer trends between men and women, and between countries. When the effects of smoking are removed, cancer trends are remarkably similar, at least in middle age, for men and women, and for different countries. This finding reinforces the need to sound the alarm bells even louder. National cancer control agencies should be blasting tobacco as public enemy number one in their fight against the disease.

The epidemic has not yet reached its peak among women in any country. Female deaths from smoking have become common in only a few countries (most notably the United States, the United Kingdom, Denmark, Hungary and Ireland), but the death toll will rise in other countries where many young women now smoke. Already in the United States, smoking is the cause of a third of all female deaths in middle age, and overall about 225,000 American women die each year from tobacco use. The mortality rate of females from tobacco use is expected to exceed that of males within about a decade.

Smoking, mainly of cigarettes, causes cancer of the lung, and there is strong evidence for its association with cancers of the upper respiratory tract, esophagus, bladder and pancreas, and probably of the stomach, liver, kidney and colon as well. Whether smoking will result in cancer depends on several things, including the number of cigarettes smoked, the cigarettes' tar content and, most important, the duration of the habit. Youngsters who take up smoking dramatically increase their risk. These dangers vary from one type of cancer to another. Passive smoking, or inhalation of tobacco smoke in the surrounding air, also causes lung cancer and other diseases associated with smoking.

Smokers harm others

Environmental tobacco smoke, or second-hand smoke, causes lung cancer and other diseases in individuals exposed to it. Second-hand smoke is also known to make your family's allergies and asthma worse. When one or both parents smoke, there is some correlation to sudden infant death syndrome, and to higher rates of middle ear infection and respiratory illnesses, such as bronchitis, colds and pneumonia, in children. Pregnant women who smoke cause the deaths of about 5,600 babies and 115,000 miscarriages in the United States every year.

Passive smoking is the breathing of side-stream smoke or of smoke exhaled by the smoker. It poses health risks to the non-smoker similar to those threatening the smoker. It contains particles of smaller diameter and is therefore more likely to be deposited deep in the lungs. The U.S. Environmental Protection Agency has classified environmental tobacco smoke as a Group A carcinogen. A non-smoker living with a smoker gains a 30 percent higher risk of death from heart disease or heart attack. Lung cancer risk also skyrockets in this situation.

TOBACCO AND YOUR HEALTH: THE FACTS

To help you appreciate the magnitude of the health hazard from cigarette smoking, here are some facts from *Tobacco or Health*, a publication of the World Health Organization and UNICEF:

- Tobacco is the leading cause of preventable death.

- Tobacco kills three times more people than alcohol, AIDS, illicit drugs, car accidents, murder and suicide *combined*.

- There are 1.1 billion smokers worldwide; the number of women who smoke is increasing in many countries.

- Each year, 6,000 billion cigarettes are smoked.

- About 3 million smoking-related deaths occur annually, with about one-third of them in developing countries.

- Cigarettes currently cause just under 20 percent of all deaths in developed countries.

- Smoking rates have declined among adults in developed countries; however, the tobacco industry has been quick to shift its attention to other markets, and smoking prevalence has increased in many developing countries.

The harmful health consequences of smoking

Nicotine is the main active ingredient of tobacco, but it is only a small component of cigarette smoke, which contains more than 4,700 chemical compounds, including forty-three cancer-causing substances. Toxins in cigarette smoke have broken down the DNA in cultured human lung cells. In some cases these carcinogens greatly accelerated the mutation rate in dividing cells, which in turn can lead to cancer development.

Unfortunately for the smoker, no threshold level of exposure to the toxins has been found. What is clear is that every year of cigarette smoking vastly increases the risk of developing several fatal conditions. In addition to being responsible for more than 85 percent of lung cancers, smoking is associated with cancers of the mouth, pharynx, larynx, esophagus, stomach, pancreas, uterus, cervix, kidney, urethra, bladder and colon. Smoking also increases the risk of cardiovascular disease, including stroke, sudden death, heart attack, peripheral vascular disease and aortic aneurysm. Ingredients of cigarette smoke damage the inner lining of the blood vessels, which can lead to the development of atherosclerosis. The toxins can also stimulate elements that close the passages in coronary arteries, resulting in the formation of clots and triggering spasms. Furthermore, cigarette smoking is the leading cause of such pulmonary illnesses as pneumonia, emphysema, bronchitis and influenza.

The health consequences of smoking among women are of special concern because of the damaging effect on their babies and young children. Smoking reduces fertility, spurs the rate of spontaneous abortions and still-births, can cause excessive bleeding during pregnancy, and results in lower birth weights in infants. Moreover, children of smokers do not grow as large or attain the same educational standard as unexposed children. Smoking is a significant cause of cardiovascular diseases and strokes in women. A final grim statistic: lung cancer has now surpassed breast cancer as the primary cause of death from cancer among women.

The elderly also face special harm from smoking. Among persons older than sixty-five, the rates of death among those who continue to smoke are twice those among people who have never smoked. Smoking is associated with a variety of age-related ailments as well, such as cataracts, delayed healing of broken bones, gum disease, predisposition to ulcer disease, high blood pressure, brain hemorrhages and even skin wrinkles.

What can giving up smoking do for you?

There is much to be gained by those who kick the habit. The immediate and long-term benefits of quitting are dramatic. After a year of not smoking, mortality from heart disease drops halfway back to that of a non-smoker; after five years it drops to the rate of non-smokers. Your risk of lung cancer after giving up smoking is cut in half in five years; by ten years it drops almost to the rate of non-smokers. Smokers who quit before age fifty halve their risk of dying in the next fifteen years compared with smokers who do not quit by that age. Smokers who quit in their mid-sixties also significantly reduce their risk for heart disease, stroke and smoking-related cancers. Such gains make sense, however, only if smokers quit in time, before they show any signs of tobacco's lethal effects.

Prevention of smoking

It's not all doom and gloom. The dramatic decline in some smoking rates in North America over the past thirty-five years is one of the great success stories. Prevention programs in schools, mass-media communications, train-ing for health-care providers—as well as research on the effects of nicotine—have all helped.

Nevertheless, still more effective primary prevention efforts are needed. The key to cutting tobacco use is to persuade people never to take up the habit in the first place. More than half of all high-school students who smoke are dependent on nicotine, and almost 90 percent have withdrawal symp-toms when they try to quit smoking. These are good reasons to concentrate on prevention among children of elementary and middle-school ages.

Intervention: taking positive action to promote changes in behaviour

Although most smokers who quit do so on their own, smokers who participate in an intensive group plan to stop smoking have higher rates of success. The primary focus of stop-smoking programs is prevention of relapse. Nicotine replacement therapy (by gum or transdermal patch) has helped prevent many from relapsing and has nearly doubled the success rates. Nicotine gum as a sole intervention may be no better than a placebo, but if it works, that's great.

Who stops smoking?

People who are most likely to succeed in quitting are on average older, have higher incomes and educations, are less dependent on nicotine, and have suffered acute health problems because of their level of smoking. Often they are highly confident of their ability to succeed. Clearly, they are more than ready to try to quit.

Anti-smoking strategies

The risk of relapse is high soon after smokers quit, so this has to be a major focus of all antismoking programs. People who relapse soon after they quit may be responding to the effects of nicotine withdrawal. Those who relapse after a long period without smoking are more likely to have given way to psychological stress, concerns about weight gain and failure to cope with old temptations associated with smoking.

Many of the successful stop-smoking programs attempt to prevent relapse by taking these problems into account. They use social support and mind and behaviour strategies, and they also pay attention to weight, stress manage-ment and exercise. Quitting groups that meet often and use many strategies typically produce a success rate of one year without smoking among 20 to 25 percent of the participants. Only 5 percent or fewer of the smokers who receive no help are estimated to succeed in stopping.

Alcohol

Alcohol poisoning is so prevalent in our society that it is hard to keep up with the statistics. It is thought possible that as many as 120 million people worldwide are afflicted with alcohol dependence syndrome. Alcoholic beverages have been estimated to contribute to about 3 percent of total cancer deaths in the developed world.

Alcohol dependence and abuse are responsible for at least 100,000 deaths annually in the United States, where medical care, lost productivity and other social costs from alcoholism amount to $200 billion every year. Fifty percent of the higher risk of mortality among alcoholics is the result of cardiovascular disease. Up to one-quarter of all cases of high blood pressure are associated with alcohol and heavy drinking in both men and women, regardless of age or weight. High levels of alcohol consumption also increase the risk of fatal and non-fatal strokes, arrhythmias, sudden cardiac death, heart disease and cardiomyopathies.

High doses of alcohol produce short-term increases in blood pressure and heart rate, and even impairment of the heart function and sudden cardiac death. Long-term excessive use of alcohol is associated with depressed cardiac output, abnormal contraction of the heart muscle and irregular heart rate. In addition, excessive alcohol has many other harmful effects. It has been linked to several forms of cancer, and it causes cirrhosis of the liver. Use of alcohol accounts for more than 10 percent of the high blood pressure observed in men. In addition, high intake of alcohol sometimes leads to more damaging behaviour such as increased hostility and depression. Alcohol consumption and tobacco smoking in combination are believed to cause cancer in the upper respiratory and gastrointestinal tracts, as well as breast cancer. Besides being coupled with smoking, the overuse of alcohol is often accompanied by a poor diet. Abuse of other drugs, too, is common among individuals who misuse alcohol. Unhappily, as we are all too well aware, alcohol is implicated in a range of social problems, including automobile accidents, crime, violence, marital breakdown and major losses in work productivity.

A family history of alcohol dependence is a multi-faceted risk. Indeed, the social and psychological frustrations of living with at least one alcoholic parent probably contribute to future alcohol abuse by the children. As interaction between parent and child breaks down, the children start drinking as well, and as teenagers they inevitably get into trouble. Children who use alcohol and drugs usually begin during early adolescence, and the habit is reinforced by substance use among their peers.

The benefits of moderate drinking

The news about alcohol is not all bad. Moderate drinking—about one or two alcoholic drinks a day—seems to cut down on death from heart disease. Alcohol actually helps to prevent the formation of blood clots, which are a major cause of stroke and heart attack. People who drink wine and beer in moderation tend to live longer than heavy drinkers and—here's the irony—even longer than those who do not drink at all! This phenomenon has become known as the "French paradox," because the French traditionally have low rates of heart disease despite a diet relatively high in saturated animal fats. French people drink wine in the same way that Americans and some Canadians consume soft drinks. Numerous studies show that alcohol consumed in moderation also helps to prevent the deterioration of the arteries, called atherosclerosis, which is the underlying cause of most heart attacks. Phenolic flavonoid, an antioxidant that occurs in red wine, may play a protective role in this.

A Harvard University study of 89,000 middle-aged women found that those who drank three to nine drinks a week were 40 percent less likely to develop heart disease than non-drinkers. A ten-year study of nearly 130,000 men and women found that people who usually consumed one or two drinks a day were 30 percent less likely to die from coronary heart disease than people who abstained from alcohol altogether. According to the American Heart Association, moderate alcohol consumption was linked to an increase in protective HDL-cholesterol and reduction in coronary heart disease. Another positive side effect, however, is that alcohol appears to provide some relief from mental anxiety and frustration. These effects may vary, depending on the amount of alcohol consumed and the time that has passed since it was consumed.

For women, one drink a day is considered moderate and has a biological effect similar to that of two drinks a day in men. But alcohol is still a no for pregnant women; they should not drink at all, since alcohol can affect the fetus.

The wisdom of cutting back

Of course, many of the detrimental effects of alcohol abuse can be reduced or reversed by stopping alcohol intake. Ending alcohol abuse and getting treatment can reduce cardiovascular illness and risk of early death significantly. For example, abstinence reduces the risk of death for patients with diseased heart muscle and can make important reductions in blood pressure levels in some individuals. Counselling has sometimes been used effectively for treating problem drinking. As with smoking, it's critical to maintain abstinence after someone has initially stopped drinking.

Many alcoholics actually need to address several drug-abuse problems. These complications make it difficult to help these patients. Recently, counselling has focused on changing specific habits associated with alcohol use. There may be other conditions, such as heart or behaviour problems, that have to be treated at the same time as the alcohol abuse.

A SUMMARY OF ADVICE ON DRINKING ALCOHOL

- Clearly, for many reasons, heavy alcohol consumption should be avoided. Alcohol is addictive.

- If alcohol is consumed at all, it should be limited to less than two drinks a day for men and one drink for women (none for pregnant women because of detrimental effects on the fetus and breast-feeding).

- Binge drinking is extremely harmful.

- Consume no alcohol if you are taking medications. Hundreds of medications interact with alcohol, many causing serious damage.

- If you achieve on your own a level of confidence and motivation sufficient to succeed in quitting drinking, you may not require any professional intervention.

- Controlling drinking by reducing the strength of the drink, alternating alcoholic with non-alcoholic beverages, and eating at the same time as drinking are good strategies.

Drug abuse

Globally, the production and trafficking of illicit drugs has increased dramatically over the last twenty years. Moreover, the worldwide trend among persons dependent on drugs is towards the use of multiple psychoactive substances. People move from one substance to another and use drugs in various combinations. Amphetamines are increasingly used in every region of the world, and one, methamphetamine, sometimes known as ice, poses a significant public health threat at this time. Amphetamines often have a longer-lasting effect than cocaine. Because they increase endurance, delay sleep and give a sense of added energy or euphoria, some of them have become an established part of the all-night parties of youth culture in many countries. They are also used by some groups of workers, such as long-distance truck drivers and others who work very long hours or feel the need for greater alertness.

It is likely that the public health consequences of drug use, particularly intoxication, poisoning and overdoses, will increase as the new combinations of substances are used. In many countries drug injection is becoming increasingly common, which leads to the sharing of needles and the risk of spreading HIV/AIDS, hepatitis B and C, and other blood-borne infections.

Addiction is as much a disorder of the brain as any other form of mental illness. Scientists are more and more convinced that dopamine, a chemical that transmits pleasure signals, is the villain in a wide range of addictions. Recently, a fascinating story published in *Nature*, one of the most prestigious scientific journals, reported findings suggesting that dopamine, more than a mere transmitter of the feel-good sensation, is actually a master molecule of addiction. It's the surge of dopamine in an addict's brain that triggers a "high," and there is mounting evidence that it is to blame in a whole range of addictions, from hard drugs to marijuana, alcohol, nicotine and caffeine.

The dopamine hypothesis raises hope that more effective therapies can be found. In the meantime, we are all too familiar with the devastation that drug abuse can cause.

The way ahead

There must be more efforts to educate young people about the dangers of addiction. Many other problems arise when young people misuse drugs, problems that are also related to smoking. There is clear evidence that tobacco is all too often the gateway through which young people pass on their way to the use of other drugs. In North American countries and some others, this can happen at a very young age. In the United States, it has been estimated that daily cigarette smokers aged twelve to seventeen are 14 times more likely to have binged on alcohol, 32 times more likely to be frequent cocaine users and 114 times more likely to be frequent marijuana users, compared to their peers who do not smoke tobacco. So, if we can convince our youngsters not to smoke, they will be far less likely to embark on other forms of substance abuse. This is a war that must be fought on many battlegrounds. Programs to keep people from starting, highlighting the grave dangers of illicit drug use and alcohol abuse, are the front line. They are crucial to the future well-being of all young people.

If you are struggling with an addiction, take heart from the *Nature* report that addictions can be reversed with learning. Many victims of the vicious circle of drug addiction do succeed in stopping on their own. Others can benefit from self-help groups or professional treatment. A great many drug users successfully change their habit by using all sorts of strategies, ranging from psychotherapy to twelve-step programs. These can and do help. Cognitive therapy, which supplies people with coping skills, appears to hold particular promise. In recent years, acupuncture treatment for narcotic addiction has achieved some degree of success.

For people who have had substance addictions for some time, the first step in the healing process may be to seek help from a qualified counsellor or support group, such as Alcoholics Anonymous or Narcotics Anonymous. The first impulse of everyone dealing with an addiction is to think it can be handled alone, using willpower and forgoing any outside help. Unfortunately, this thought process is part of the classic pattern of addiction and simply becomes part of the problem. Most people find that to heal an addictive pattern permanently, they need help and support from others who have experience of the problem. Society does care; don't hesitate to ask for help.

IT'S TIME TO BANISH THOSE UNHEALTHY HABITS

- Tobacco, public enemy number one, is a major cause of mortality and premature death, responsible for 30 percent of cancer deaths in the United States. Women are now beginning to outsmoke men, with alarming results.

- Second-hand smoke also causes diseases. Smoking at home affects all family members, often causing asthma and allergy problems. A pregnant woman who smokes will adversely affect her unborn baby.

- Tobacco is indeed "the smoking gun." It is one of the main causes of heart and lung disease. Among seniors especially, it also leads to many other illnesses and problems.

- Find out how to quit. Society has many resources to help you. Use self-help groups and expert assistance if necessary. Be aware of the dangers of relapse, which is all too common.

- Excessive alcohol intake leads to deaths from accident, cirrhosis, suicide and homicide. The cost of the health consequences of alcohol abuse is $200 billion a year in the United States. They include high blood pressure, some cancers and damaging social behaviour.

- Alcohol is not all bad. In fact, there is evidence that people who drink in moderation live longer than those who do not drink at all. It may be the result of that flavonoid phenomenon again! A reasonable alcohol intake is two drinks a day for men, one for women and none for pregnant women, as alcohol clearly affects the fetus and development of the unborn child.

- It may be that dopamine—a chemical found in the brain—is the master villain behind all kinds of addictions. There is ongoing research in the hope that effective therapies may be developed for addicts. In the meantime, don't hesitate to ask for help.

CHAPTER 5

HQ AND LIFE'S JOURNEY

Good health starts in the womb and continues until very old age. Health, through HQ, is vital to your lifelong journey. I'll help you understand and initiate sound health practices not only for yourself but also for your children and other family members.

In the industrialized countries we are already seeing people live to a great age in numbers that would have been unimaginable a hundred years ago. Since 1950, every decade has seen an increase in life expectancy. There are two main reasons for this: first, a reduction in deaths in infancy and childhood, and second, and more recently, a decline in deaths among middle-aged and elderly people. Nowadays, babies and children benefit from better care from their mothers, the availability of clean water, better food, and the control or eradication of infectious diseases with immunization and antibiotics. Preventable injuries now pose a greater danger to young children and adolescents than do diseases. The mortality rate for middle-aged and older populations is also going down because people are taking better care of themselves. In addition, science and medicine, through technological and pharmaceutical advances, have helped millions live longer through control of chronic and formerly fatal diseases and disorders.

Life is a continuum. It encompasses growth, development, maturing and aging. Across this sequence of events, which spans all human life, there are ongoing changes. The early stages are characterized by rapid growth and development. A normal, healthy infant, child or adolescent grows and develops at a genetically predetermined rate, but the rate can be hindered or accelerated for all kinds of reasons, such as an unbalanced diet or poor nutrition. Growth and development taper off as we move into early adulthood. After growth ceases and maturity is complete, the process of cell turnover becomes static; old cells die and only some are replaced. Eventually we see aging, which in essence is the slowing down of physiological functions in the course of advancing years. This process is governed by genetics, race and gender, but it is also influenced by the events of our youth, such as early nurturing, social surroundings, physical activity, diet, habits and accompanying disease conditions. Let's start at the beginning.

Child-bearing Women

The first few months of life—inside the womb—are critical to future development. Fetal organs begin to form within three days of the first missed menstrual period, often before women even suspect that they are pregnant, and formation is complete by the fifty-sixth day after conception. That's why all women of child-bearing age should try to be healthy and careful about eating habits and lifestyle, especially if they are planning to have children. In the first three months of pregnancy, when the fertilized egg increases 2.5 million times in mass, the danger of harm to the developing child is far greater than during the rest of the pregnancy.

A great deal of new information has been gathered recently about the relationship between lifestyle habits before pregnancy and future problems such as miscarriage, birth defects, low birth weight and premature birth. As a result, there is now a movement to encourage all women of child-bearing age to take extra care of themselves, even before conception.

Of special concern are women who have been using the birth-control pill and those with poor eating habits. Both of these groups may be deficient in folic acid and vitamin B, which help to prevent severe birth defects of the spinal cord and brain, such as neural tube defects and anencephaly. As a preventive measure against these birth defects, adequate folic acid and vitamin B must be taken before conception. Congenital neural tube defects affect ten to twenty out of every thousand babies. The main sources of folic acid in a typical North American diet are dark green leafy vegetables and some fruits. I have talked about this already, but I can't emphasize enough how important it is that women of child-bearing age think about taking a daily vitamin supplement that supplies 400 micrograms of folate, the biologically active form of folic acid.

Embryo and fetal development

A mother's prenatal condition is key to the successful intrauterine growth, development and birth of her baby. Eating for two means eating well. The best possible nutrition is needed for the different stages of development of the baby's organs and systems. As stated above, the most vulnerable period in the growth and development of a fetus is the first three months of gestation. During this time it is essential that the growing embryo gets enough nutrients to avoid birth defects. The healthier you are, the healthier your baby will be. It's extremely important that pregnant women not use tobacco, alcohol or drugs and protect the growing baby from exposure to harmful substances. Mothers-to-be will give their babies the best start in life by making wise health choices and participating in prenatal care.

The remaining seven months of gestation are a period of rapid fetal growth and development. Again, good food, in both quantity and quality, is essential for the fetus's health and normal weight gain. During the last three months the fetus gains more than two-thirds of its full-term birth weight. If the mother's nutrition is poor and inadequate, it may result in premature birth and low birth weight, which could endanger the health of the newborn.

Care during pregnancy

It's important for the pregnant woman to be calm and relaxed throughout her pregnancy. A study at the University of Kentucky found that stressed moms have stressed babies. Women with "wanted" babies, high self-esteem and ample social support had the calmest fetuses. Heart rates of fetuses with stressed mothers were significantly higher, and the study suggested that women with high stress hormone levels were also more likely to deliver premature babies. Meditation or relaxation exercises can help stressed pregnant women lower their blood pressure.

It's true that genetics play a large part in the growth and health of the embryo and fetus. For some babies, genetic inheritance adds to their risk of disease and affects their future health prospects. Nonetheless, many of these risks can be minimized if women maintain a healthy lifestyle and carefully consider the following preventive measures:

- *Screening of all pregnant women at high risk for Down's syndrome or other birth defects*   It has been well established that pregnant women at high risk are those over thirty-five, or who have already had a child with a serious birth defect, or who have a family history of birth defects. Down's syndrome, a form of mental retardation, is the most common and best known of all the chromosomal disorders. About one child in eight hundred is born with Down's syndrome, and it occurs most often in infants of mothers over age thirty-five.

- *Encouraging rubella immunization*   for all women to prevent congenital rubella syndrome. This syndrome, which may include multiple birth defects and mental retardation, occurs in about 25 percent of infants born to women who acquire rubella (German measles) during the first three months of pregnancy. Rubella can be prevented through immunization.
- *Avoiding fetal alcohol syndrome (FAS),*   which is recognized as perhaps the major cause of mental retardation and growth retardation. Since FAS is directly related to alcohol consumption during pregnancy, it is entirely preventable. No lower limit of safe alcohol consumption in pregnancy has been firmly established, and until that limit is determined, pregnant women should consume no alcohol, particularly in the first three months of pregnancy.
- *Encouraging folic acid as a daily supplement*   for all women who become pregnant. The recommendation includes 400 micrograms of folic acid for most women and 4 milligrams for women who have already had a child with a neural tube defect. Make sure you're eating those leafy vegetables and legumes during pregnancy, too; they may be some of the most valuable foods you will ever consume.

The Critical Period: Newborn to Three Years

Your new baby has a whole lot of growing to do. The first thirty days after birth are a vital time of adjustment. Energy and nutrient requirements have to be high to maintain the baby's basal metabolism and to support growth. During infancy, the first year of life, your baby has a threefold increase in body weight. In this period of high nutritional demand, your baby needs two to three times as many nutrients as adults do. In response, nature has designed a great gift for mothers to give to their newborn children: breast-feeding.

Breast milk is free, healthful and the perfect fast food. It is also the most nutritious and hygienic food available for newborns and small babies. Breast milk is absolutely the best. Here are seven reasons why:

1. *It's the perfect food for infants.*   Breast milk provides an infant's total nutrient requirement for the first four to six months of life. When combined with appropriate weaning foods, it is an invaluable source of nourishment until past the second birthday. It prevents malnutrition, allowing the child to develop fully.

2. *It serves as the first immunization.*   Born into a world full of germs and infections, a newborn has colostrum (the mother's first milk) as its strongest defence. Colostrum, produced by the mother in the first few days after birth, provides the baby's first immunization. Breast milk contains antibodies and live cells that protect infants from bacterial and viral sources of disease. This protection works both before and during the time when the baby acquires active immunity through vaccination.

3. *It bonds mother and child.*   Although bonding between mother and child is continuous, the first hours of a baby's life are a critical part of the process. Mother and baby imprint their feel, smell and visual image on each other, which has a positive, lifelong effect on their mutual relationship. The baby's instinct for protection and nurturing at this time is remarkably strong. In natural childbirth it is the newborn who initiates breast-feeding. Research shows that breast-feeding raises intelligence by 8.3 points. Now that's a Health Quotient target!

4. *It prevents diarrhea and other diseases.*   Infants up to two months old who are not breast-fed are twice as likely to have diarrhea, and their chances of dying from its effects are up to twenty-five times greater. A protein called mucin in human milk has been found to suppress the reproduction of a rotavirus, a major cause of infant diarrhea. Breast-feeding also reduces the risk of gastrointestinal, respiratory, middle ear and other infections. It also helps to prevent sudden infant death syndrome (SIDS).

5. *It helps in birth spacing.*   Frequent suckling from the time of birth maintains high levels of progesterone in the mother's body, which inhibits ovulation and therefore pregnancy. Exclusive breast-feeding offers 98 percent protection against pregnancy during the first six months after birth. Increasing the interval between births helps both maternal health and child health and development. This cannot, however, be considered an absolute form of contraception.

6. *It saves some mothers' lives.*   When suckling starts within the first hour after birth, the placenta is expelled faster and the risk of after-birth bleeding, which can kill the mother, is reduced. Breast-feeding also substantially reduces the mother's risk of developing breast cancer or ovarian cancer in later years.

7. *Breast-feeding also saves money.*   This is not small change! Breast milk is readily available and convenient. Breast-feeding is an economic benefit for families, hospitals, communities and countries.

A child's developing brain

It seems unbelievable, but that tiny newborn snuggled in your arms has trillions of brain cells waiting to be programmed. From birth, a baby's brain cells proliferate wildly, making connections that may shape a lifetime of events. The many and varied experiences of the young child help to form the brain's circuitry for music, math, language and emotion. In this respect the first three years of life are critical.

When a baby comes into the world, some of the brain cells have already been hard-wired by the genes in the fertilized egg into the circuits that command breathing or control heartbeat, regulate body temperature or produce reflexes. But trillions and trillions more have pure and infinite potential as unprogrammed circuits. If these brain cells are used, they become integrated into the circuitry of the brain by connecting to other brain cells; if they are not used, they may die. It is the experiences of infancy and early childhood that determine which of these neurons are used. These experiences determine whether the child grows up to be intelligent or dull, fearful or self-assured, articulate or tongue-tied.

It's generally believed that there are two broad stages of brain wiring: an early period, when experience is not required, and a later one, when it is. Once wired, there are limits to the brain's ability to re-create itself. Time limits, called "critical periods," refer to the windows of opportunity that nature flings open before birth, and then slams shut, one by one, with every year that passes.

The first years last forever

The positive emotional, physical and intellectual experiences that a baby has in the early years are equally necessary for the growth of a healthy brain. The brain is the part of the body that allows us to feel joy or despair, to respond to others in a loving or angry way, to use reason or simply to react. These capacities don't magically appear; they result from the interplay between heredity and childhood experiences.

At birth, the parts of the brain that handle thinking and remembering as well as emotional and social behaviour are very much underdeveloped. The fact that the brain matures in the world, rather than in the womb, means that young children are deeply affected by what happens to them in the early months. Relationships with parents and other important caregivers, the sights, sounds, smells and feelings they are exposed to, and the challenges they face influence far more than their moods; these experiences actually affect the way a child's brain becomes "wired." In other words, early experiences help to determine brain structure, thus shaping the way a person learns, thinks and behaves for the rest of his or her life.

It is evident, then, that everyone who cares for young children, including parents, family, friends, teachers and child-care providers, can make a difference. Essential to all of these efforts is a child's basic health and safety. The following ten guidelines, adapted from suggestions by the Canadian Institute of Child Health in Ottawa, can help parents and other caregivers raise healthy, happy children and confident, competent learners.

1. *Be warm, loving and responsive.* When children receive warm, responsive care, they are more likely to feel safe and secure with the adults who take care of them. Researchers call these strong relationships "secure attachments," and they are the basis of all the child's future relationships. We have always known that children thrive when they feel secure; now we know that children's early attachments actually affect the way their brains work and grow.

    If I just love my child, is that enough? Not exactly. It is the *expression* of your love—touching, rocking, talking, smiling and singing—that affects how your young child's brain is wired and helps to shape later learning and behaviour. Babies experience relationships through their senses: they see the way you look into their eyes and the expressions on your face; they hear you cooing, singing, talking and reading; they feel you holding or rocking them; and they take in your familiar smells. Touch is especially important; holding and stroking stimulates the brain to release important hormones necessary for growth.

2. *Respond to your child's cues and clues.* Infants can't use words to communicate their moods, preferences or needs, but they send many signals to the adults who care for them. Among the cues and clues they send are the sounds they make and eye contact. Children become securely attached when parents and caregivers try to read these signals and respond with sensitivity. They begin to be sure that when they smile, someone will smile back; that when they are upset, someone will comfort them; that when they are hungry, someone will feed them. Parents who pay close attention to their children's cues for stimulation as well as for quiet times help them form secure attachments.

    But won't my newborn get spoiled with all this attention? You might think so, but studies show that newborns who are quickly and warmly responded to when crying typically learn to cry much less and sleep more at night. After all, newborns have just come from a warm, snug place where they could hear and feel the rhythmic beating of their mother's heart, and where they were never hungry or cold. Before birth, everything was regulated. After birth, when the baby is hungry, uncomfortable or upset in his or her new environment, the brain's stress-response systems turn on and release stress hormones. The baby expresses distress by crying. When the caregiver responds and provides food or warmth or comfort, the baby tends to be calmed. The stress-response systems in the brain are then turned off, and the infant's brain begins to create a self-soothing network of brain cells. You cannot spoil a newborn baby by responding to its needs.

3.   *Talk, read and sing to your child.* Making up stories about daily events, singing songs about the people and places they know, describing what is happening during daily routines—all of these "conversations" give your child a solid basis for later learning.

   Why talk or read to infants before they can talk? It may seem that very young children can't take in what you're saying, but in important ways they do. Infants don't yet grasp the meaning of words, but it is through these early "conversations" that language capacity grows. When babies hear you say words over and over, the parts of the brain that handle speech and language develop. The more language they hear in these conversations, the more those parts of the brain will grow and develop. Talking, singing and reading to your child are not only important for brain development but a wonderful opportunity for closeness with your child.

   You can read picture books and stories to very young children, even to infants. By about six months, infants show their excitement by widening their eyes and moving their arms and legs when looking at a book with pictures of babies or other familiar things. Studies find that the way you read to children makes a difference. Read stories in a way that encourages older babies and toddlers to participate—by answering your questions, by pointing at what they see in a picture book, by telling you what they think will happen next in the story, and by repeating the rhymes and refrains. Telling the same stories and singing the same songs over and over may feel boring to you, but not to children. They learn through repetition, and that doesn't apply only to language.

4.   *Establish routines and rituals.* One toddler knows it is nap time because his mom sings a song and closes the curtains, as she always does. Another toddler knows it is nearly time for her dad to pick her up because her child-care provider gives her juice and crackers. Daily routines and rituals associated with pleasurable feelings are reassuring for children, as caregivers have long known.

   Repeated positive experiences, which form strong connections between neurons in the brain, provide children with a sense of security.

They also help children learn what to expect from their environment and how to understand the world around them. Children who have safe and predictable interactions with others have also been found to do better in school later on.

5. *Encourage safe exploration and play.* In the first months of life the parents will be the child's whole world. Interactions between parent and child form the basis of all subsequent learning. As infants grow and are able to crawl and walk, they begin to explore the world beyond their caregivers. Parents should encourage this exploration and be receptive when the child needs to return to them for security.

    Play is equally important as a learning experience. While many of us think of learning as simply acquiring facts, children actually learn through playing. Just watch a toddler at play, and it is easy to see how much he or she is learning.

6. *Make TV watching selective.* Television by itself can't teach an infant language, and it can't teach him or her how to communicate. Studies show that children who learn best in school have families who limit the amount of time they spend in front of the TV and are selective as to the kinds of shows they watch. Very young children are still learning the difference between what is real and what is pretend. Some TV images strike them as delightful, but other images can be confusing or even frightening.

    Be selective and involved in your children's TV habits. Don't use TV as a babysitter. Whenever possible, sit and watch programs with your child, and talk about what you are viewing.

7. *Use discipline as an opportunity to teach.* As children grow, they become capable of even more exploration, discovery and experimentation. In the process, they often experience a lot of confusion and frustration. At times their feelings can become very intense. As children explore their ever-expanding world, they need limits and consistent, loving adult supervision. Studies reveal that the way in which adults provide discipline, which really means teaching, is crucial to their children's later development.

    How can I discipline my young child? Don't expect young children to do what you say all the time. Young children are normally impulsive and will hit, yell or fall apart at times, because their feelings of frustration and anger exceed their ability to control themselves. Helping them learn self-control is a long-term process. It is also normal for children to test a rule by breaking it. When you respond in a supportive, consistent way, you are helping your child to feel safe in the world.

- Communicate to your child what needs to be done at that moment: "I know you're having fun at the park, but it's time to get ready to go now."
- Redirect your child's attention or activity by using neutral or positive language: "It's not OK to draw on the wall, but here is some paper you can use."
- Say no while maintaining love: "I love you, but I don't love what you're doing."
- Give the reason for your rule: "Don't run with scissors; you might fall and hurt yourself."
- Acknowledge children's feelings, but set limits: "I know you're angry, but no biting."
- Help children see how their actions affect others: "Your sister is upset because you pinched her. How would you feel if she hurt you?"
- Help children see how they can use words to communicate their feelings: "Tell your brother you don't like it when he hits you."
- Acknowledge positive behaviour: "You did a good job picking up your stuffed animals. Thank you."

NEVER HIT OR SHAKE YOUR CHILD. Brain research has shown that these forms of "discipline" can have long-term negative effects. Discipline is about learning, and the only things a child can learn from this dangerously harsh punishment are fear, humiliation and rage. If you hit or shake your child, he or she is far more likely to come to feel that violence is an acceptable way of reacting. Take time out for yourself. Count to ten, or call a friend or relative for support. Do not harshly criticize and shame the child. Direct your comments to their behaviour, not to who they are as people.

Disciplining your children will inevitably cause moments of disconnection when they will feel upset by your disapproval. It is important for you as parents to repair this ruptured connection so your child will continue to feel loved and supported. If you feel you have overreacted or disciplined your child inappropriately, you can say that you made a mistake and are sorry.

8. *Recognize that each child is unique.* Children have different temperaments: one child is outgoing while her brother is more bashful and slow to warm up. Children also grow at different rates. Their ideas and feelings about themselves reflect, in large measure, your attitude towards them.

How can I help my children feel good about themselves? When children master the challenges of everyday life, they feel good about themselves, particularly when you acknowledge their accomplishments with specific praise: "You climbed those stairs all by yourself." When children receive concrete praise, they begin to see the connection between their actions and your response. Parents who are sensitive to their particular child's cues and clues will have children with positive self-esteem.

9. *Choose quality child care and stay involved.* Choosing a child-care provider is one of the most important decisions families make. Research shows that high-quality child care and early education can boost children's learning and social skills when they enter school. However, it is often difficult to decide which programs are good enough.

    What should we look for in a child-care setting? To make a good choice, visit child-care providers and observe how they respond to and interact with the babies and children in their care. Seek a provider who responds warmly and responsively to the baby's needs. Select someone who cares about children, is eager to learn about their development, will give children individual attention, and will engage them in creative play and exploration. Find a setting that is clean and safe. Make sure there are enough caregivers that your child can get individualized attention. Carefully check the provider's references.

    After choosing your child-care provider, stay involved. Drop in unannounced occasionally so you can see what your child's world is like during the day. Ask for frequent "progress reports." And don't be afraid to offer constructive suggestions to improve your child's experience. Studies show that children who achieve well in school have families who stay involved in their care and education.

10. *Take care of yourself.* In the final analysis, parents and caregivers need care too. Taking care of our children is the most important, the most wonderful and often the most challenging job in our society. Because you provide the primary environment for infants and young children, your health and welfare are extremely important. When you are exhausted, preoccupied, irritable, depressed or overwhelmed, you will probably have a harder time meeting the needs of young children.

    When you feel overwhelmed, take care of yourself. Reach out and get some help. Family, friends, neighbours, pediatricians, child-care providers and others can assist you in fostering your child's healthy development and school-readiness. Bear in mind that there are many ways to reach this goal.

Childhood to Adolescence

They're growing up. Maturation and education are the two key issues of childhood. This is a period during which habits are formed—particularly eating habits—and behaviours are moulded. Early childhood experiences have a major influence on your child's ability to lead a full, rewarding life as an adult. The childhood years are also a crucial time for the development of emotional intelligence, as Daniel Goleman clearly spells out in his book *Emotional Intelligence*.

As we know, the human brain is by no means fully formed at birth; it continues to shape itself throughout life. Children are born with many more brain cells than their mature brain will retain. The brain cells actually lose the connections that are less used and form strong connections with the circuits that are used most often. Experience, especially in childhood, impacts the structure and function of the mature brain.

It is interesting that, of all species, humans take the longest to achieve fully mature brains. The sensory areas mature during early childhood and the limbic system by puberty, while the frontal lobes continue to develop into late adolescence. Anatomically, the limbic system of the brain is considered to be the seat of the emotions and is responsible for learning and remembering; the frontal lobes are the seat of emotional self-control, understanding and artful response; and the neocortex, the top layer, is considered to be the thinking brain.

Emotional habits and patterns that are repeated over and over again during childhood and the teenage years will aid in the development of the neuronal connections, the brain circuitry. The opportunity for encouraging emotional abilities begins during the earliest years and continues throughout the school years. Childhood is therefore a crucial time for shaping lifelong emotional intelligence. There are several key periods throughout childhood for acquiring this intelligence. Each period represents a window of opportunity for helping the child absorb beneficial emotional habits. If these chances are missed, the good habits are much harder to develop later in life. Severe stress during this time can impair the brain's ability to learn.

A child's readiness for school depends upon the most basic of all knowledge: how to learn. A report from the National Center for Clinical Infant Programs lists seven key ingredients of this crucial capacity, all related to emotional intelligence; these are confidence, curiosity, intention, self-control, relatedness, capacity to communicate and co-operativeness. Whether or not a child arrives at school on the first day of kindergarten with these capabilities depends largely on the environment and kind of care that parents, caregivers or preschool teachers have provided.

The Adolescent Years

You know you're there when all the food in your fridge magically disappears overnight!

Yes, adolescence is a period of incredibly rapid growth. The total nutritional requirement of adolescents is greater than that of adults except during pregnancy and lactation periods. Relax. Teenagers who keep raiding the refrigerator are simply trying to keep pace with growth. The challenge for us as parents is to keep them away from junk food. Meeting the nutritional needs of adolescents is complicated because, at this stage in life, elements of their physiological, psychological and social development may endanger good food habits. Teenagers are the most likely group to fall victim to poor eating habits.

We have all watched teenagers grow and develop. In the process they must also learn life skills. Many of them are strongly influenced by peer pressure and social pressure, so it's not surprising that emotions and psychological well-being affect their health.

The hazards of being a teenager

This is no joke. Teenagers belong to the only age group in society that has not seen a reduction in overall mortality in the past four decades. Most teenage deaths in North America result from traffic accidents, and though teenagers make up only 12 percent of drivers, they account for 38 percent of accidents. The most common age of death in a traffic accident is eighteen years. The second most common cause of teenage death is suicide; the third is homicide. Teenagers may die as a result of drug misuse, sexually transmitted diseases, depression and suicide, violence, teenage pregnancy and running away from home.

Worldwide, there are 100 million teenagers living in unfavourable conditions. In North America, between 30 and 40 percent of teenagers on the streets are substance abusers, and a third say they have attempted suicide. Teenagers are strongly affected by social pressure: how they see themselves and how they want others to see them. It is largely because of pressure that the number of young female smokers has actually increased over the past ten years. Tobacco ads encourage and condition young people to think that, if they smoke, they will become more attractive, sexy, strong, adventurous and worldly.

Teenagers will be the next group to experience an epidemic of deaths from AIDS. Among teenage girls on the streets, prostitution has almost doubled since 1980; among teenage boys on the streets, it has more than doubled during the same time period. The percentage of adolescents having sexual intercourse increased during the 1980s, and rates of curable sexually transmitted diseases rose dramatically among some groups of adolescents. It's a scary world out there, and the important thing is to be aware and to be there for your teens. Your timely and appropriate support or intervention may enable young people to become responsible members of society rather than victims of adverse circumstances.

A word about life skills

Good health and happiness are affected by the way you meet the demands and challenges of daily living, through your ability to make appropriate decisions, solve problems and communicate. From a more practical point of view, life skills are necessary if you are to gain a livelihood. Life skills involve concepts such as knowing how to care for yourself properly, and how to assert yourself in instances where peers or others propose risky or dangerous activities.

Life skills are psychosocial competencies, and they can be modified or learned. They have real and practical implications, especially for people who find themselves in situations of physical or emotional abuse, or suffering from depression, low self-esteem or poor mental health. Life skills are the best defence for people living in an environment where teen or unwanted pregnancies, substance abuse or sexually transmitted diseases are prevalent. They help in problem solving and decision making, critical and creative thinking, communication and interpersonal skills, self-awareness and empathy, coping with stress and other damaging emotions, and social adjustment.

Don't underestimate the importance of life skills. Your ability to deal with life issues affects your health. Family, occupation, financial resources, education, sexual behaviour, social support, cultural considerations, community involvement, social adaptability, personal relationships, and participation in and opportunities for recreation and leisure activities all influence and affect your health and well-being. Understanding how to manage and deal with these elements through life-skills training can make all the difference to your life and your health.

The Adult Years

Congratulations! You made it through all the trials and tribulations of adolescence. Your life is on track, you're gaining confidence and things are humming along nicely. Watch out: you are busy with many things, but this is not the time to neglect your health needs. As you move through the adult years, the clinical signs of the slow, insidious process of chronic disease can begin to appear. For adults, achieving and maintaining a healthy lifestyle will make all the difference to reducing the risk of developing chronic disease. In fact, this period of your life is absolutely critical in the run-up to healthy aging, living longer and improving health expectancy. To maintain your best health as an adult, you will have to cope successfully with social pressure and stress, social adjustment, career development and assumption of family responsibilities.

The main issues relating to health in the adult years were addressed in detail in chapter 4. Overweight and obesity are major clinical conditions that are products of the twentieth century. These are directly related to an unhealthy lifestyle, with inappropriate eating and sedentary habits. The prevalence of these conditions has reached epidemic proportions and is one of the most serious health problems of our time. The trend is happening not only in industrialized countries but also in developing countries, as the Western lifestyle and culture increase in influence. Ironically, economic improvement has not always been a blessing to some of these countries, as it has caused a general decline in the fitness levels of their populations. Obesity is clearly documented as a serious health hazard and a major risk factor for many diseases, particularly the development of diabetes. It has contributed to disability and premature death.

Control your weight, avoid obesity

Prevention of obesity is one of the greatest public-health challenges in developed countries. One-third of the American adult population is currently overweight: 35 percent of women and 31 percent of men aged twenty and older. Among children and adolescents, 25 percent are considered overweight. Obesity is a particular problem among minorities, especially minority women. It also occurs disproportionately among individuals of low economic status.

Your physical appearance is often an accurate means of determining whether you are overweight or obese. More scientifically, overweight and obesity are determined by the body mass index (BMI) measurement, which takes into account height and weight to estimate total body fat. It is calculated according to the following formula:

$$\text{BMI} = \frac{703 \times \text{weight in pounds}}{(\text{height in inches})^2}$$

A BMI score exceeding 27 for women and 28 for men is rated as overweight, and over 30 for women and 31 for men is considered to be obese. The National Center for Health Statistics recently adjusted the definition of overweight to include adults with an index reading of 25 to 26. Statistics Canada estimates that slightly under half of all adult Canadians (46 percent) are either overweight or obese.

These statistics are of importance because excess weight is associated with high blood pressure, high blood cholesterol, diabetes, heart disease, osteoporosis and even cancer. Overweight people increase their risk of dying from heart disease and are more likely to experience breathing problems, particularly sleep apnea. There are also negative psychological and social impacts from being fat. It's unfair, but statistics show that overweight people are less likely to be hired for a job or to get married than their slimmer peers.

Obesity is also one of the main problems in Type 2 diabetes. Formerly called non-insulin-dependent diabetes or adult diabetes, the Type 2 form usually arises because of insulin resistance, in which the body fails to use insulin properly. This is a major concern for the nearly 157 million North Americans who have this type of the disease. Type 2 diabetes occurs most commonly in people who are over forty-five and overweight.

Research shows that it makes a big difference where extra fat is accumulated. Independent of overall obesity, the distribution of body fat relates directly to heart disease and death from all causes. A more central distribution of body fat, defined as a higher ratio of waist to hip circumference, is associated with increased rates of high blood pressure, high blood insulin, glucose intolerance, increased triglycerides in the blood, heart attack, angina, stroke and death. It is interesting to note that genetic factors are connected with distribution of body fat.

A large belly is not to be shrugged off lightly. The increased health risks that accompany excessive girth are attributed to obesity within the abdominal cavity. Dr. Bruce Breeder of the University of Saskatchewan studied 10,054 men and women aged eighteen to seventy-four and found that a person's girth is the single best predictor of heart disease risk. Those over age forty with a waist circumference (WC) between thirty-six and forty inches, or ninety and one hundred centimetres, had a considerable heart disease risk. Individuals with a WC of forty inches (one hundred centimetres) or more have double the normal risk of high blood pressure and diabetes. Research also demonstrates that stress, lack of activity and smoking are associated with visceral fat. Many studies show that even a modest weight loss can lower blood pressure, decrease bad cholesterol levels while increasing good ones, improve insulin sensitivity and the blood sugar level, and cut down on sleep apnea.

Causes of obesity

Obesity results from an imbalance between intake of calories and output of energy. Low levels of physical activity and intake of excess calories and dietary fat are major causes of obesity. High-fat diets, in particular, are to blame for obesity, perhaps because they are more palatable than other diets. In addition, fat is high in calories that are consumed more easily and stored in the body more efficiently than the excess calories from other nutrient sources, such as complex carbohydrates.

Although research has shown that genetic predisposition plays a major role for some obese people, there is clearly a difference between people who have gained weight because of overeating or a poor diet and those who are overweight for genetic reasons. New findings show that the body's fat cells release into the bloodstream a hormone known as leptin, which by its level in the blood signals the brain to stop gaining fat reserves. There is a possibility that in some obese people the signalling mechanism is defective for genetic reasons. So far, scientists have learned only that the body indeed has a fat control system, but there is hope that one day it will become possible to correct defects in the leptin mechanism.

Apart from our tendency to consume too many calories, other familiar reasons for weight gain are inactivity, pregnancy and giving up smoking. Studies indicate that large weight gains are most likely to occur in both men and women between the ages of twenty-five and thirty-four, when there is a general decline in physical activity. Women continue to gain weight as they age, averaging almost one pound a year during menopause. Men and women both tend to gain weight when they stop smoking, and the effect is particularly pronounced in women. Anecdotal evidence suggests that weight gain is also associated with stress. Nevertheless, there is overwhelming evidence that environment and diet are chiefly to blame for people getting too fat.

How to combat obesity

It's a formidable challenge. Intervention is usually aimed either at preventing people from becoming overweight or at treating people who already have a weight problem. There is no simple solution. Attempts to prevent obesity that are targeted at groups of people in communities, work sites and schools have been found to have little effect for individuals. Personal action seems to have a greater chance of success. While attempting to diet, it is important for us to understand how natural metabolism functions. Research has shown that the body burns calories more slowly than normal after weight is lost and faster than normal when weight is gained. Metabolism is adjusted by making the muscles more or less efficient in burning calories.

Some success has been reported in treating weight problems in children eight to twelve years old. Treatment of overweight adults, however, has been far less successful. Typical programs that combine diet, exercise and behaviour training to manage eating habits result in an average weight loss of about nine kilograms over twenty weeks. True success, however, means keeping the weight off, and that is a greater challenge. The success rate is improved by greater contact between patient and therapist, emphasis on both diet and exercise, use of certain strategies such as self-monitoring, and a well-structured plan to prevent relapse. Even when weight loss is modest, the results are beneficial to an individual's blood pressure levels and lower the risk of heart disease. These benefits remain for as long as the weight is kept off. Don't be discouraged by the yo-yo phenomenon. Previous concerns about the potentially bad effects of weight cycling (repeated weight loss followed by weight gain) appear to have been disproved. Most studies now show that weight cycling per se does not cause problems.

Growing recognition that some drugs may have serious adverse side effects has dampened enthusiasm for using drug treatments to help people lose weight. Now, drugs tend to be recommended only for the very obese. They may be more effective when combined with diet, exercise and behaviour changes. Although drugs are not the solution for obesity, new findings show that drugs may help in some cases. Recently, the largest and longest study ever conducted of an obesity medication has found that a new drug, orlistat, can help obese people shed weight and keep it off (Davidson et al., 1999). Orlistat, with the brand name Xenical, blocks an enzyme that is needed to digest fat, and it is found to have no serious side effects. The drug is in the final stage of approval by the U.S. Food and Drug Administration. Other promising research on treatment of obesity involves leptin, the anti-obesity hormone first discovered in mice, which is made by fat cells and circulates in the body. It is believed to have a role in food intake and body-weight regulation. In laboratory studies, mice genetically deficient in leptin became obese; when given extra leptin, they grew thinner.

In a recent study, leptin and placebo injections were given to fifty-three lean people and seventy who were moderately obese. All participants were placed on a weight-reduction diet. At the end of six months, the leptin injections proved to have been effective in causing weight loss without significant adverse effects (Greenberg, 1998).

SOME PRACTICAL TIPS FOR LOSING WEIGHT

Physical activity must be given top priority. Exercise as a way of burning calories is the most important part of any weight-reduction program.

Reducing fat intake in the diet is essential. For weight loss, fat intake must be substantially lower than 30 percent of the total calorie intake, even with a low-calorie diet. In order to reduce fat intake, you need to cut back on or eliminate added fats and hidden fats. These are found in muffins, hot dogs, ice cream, nuts, pie, doughnuts, luncheon meats and fried foods. A diet with plentiful grains, fruits, vegetables and soybean products is a great alternative.

Alcohol, like fat, is very high in calories. People trying to lose weight should reduce their alcohol intake.

Eat at regular intervals. It is far better to eat small, frequent meals or snacks than to fast or skip meals in an attempt to lose weight.

Availability of food must be monitored. Often, individuals overeat simply because the food is available. They need to take control of their environment rather than let their environment control them.

Emotional stresses are often associated with overeating. Emotions such as loneliness, frustration, boredom, anger and depression can all trigger overeating. We are familiar with the term "comfort food." It does seem that food can comfort people when they are stressed and give them a sense of satisfaction.

Eating habits, including your surroundings, may need to change for weight loss. It is important to make eating an enjoyable experience, to eat at regular intervals in a pleasant setting, and to focus on the food without other distractions.

The Senior Years

Fitter, more active retirees are making a mockery of the classic rocking-chair image of old age. Clearly, the senior years are not a time to become passive about your health. Active aging involves every dimension of our lives: physical, mental, social and spiritual. Successful aging is determined not so much by genetic inheritance as by your lifestyle, choices in diet, exercise, pursuit of mental challenges, ability to look after yourself and involvement with other people. There is much the individual can do to remain active and healthy in later life.

The process of natural aging

Elderly people who are functioning well may still be at risk for disease or disability as their aging organs gradually lose strength with the years. The elderly become more vulnerable to chronic diseases as these organs decline.

In medical terms, human aging is characterized by the progressive diminishing of the homeostatic reserve of every organ system. In most people this decline begins in their thirties, long before they notice that anything has changed. While the decline is almost always gradual and progressive, its rate and extent depend on the individual. Much depends on diet, environment and personal habits, as well as personal genetics. All of these things will determine your life expectancy. You can achieve a good HQ even in old age, but obviously, a whole life well lived will usually mean a longer, happier life in old age. The MacArthur Foundation's report (Rowe and Kahn, 1998) lists three characteristics of a healthy old age: low risk of disease and disease-related disability, high mental and physical function, and an active engagement with life.

So, your good habits are still essential. Avoid smoking, high blood pressure and poor eating habits, and carry on an active lifestyle to lessen the likelihood of premature sickness and death. It's also important to keep alert and stimulated with hobbies and activities, both intellectual and physical; this will keep you in good spirits and good health. Successful aging is largely determined not by genetic inheritance but by such lifestyle choices. Social interactions are important at all stages of life, but particularly among older people because lack of mobility and other problems may make a vigorous social life difficult.

Natural aging and your vulnerability

Health professionals tend to stereotype older people into two groups, the "diseased" and the "normal." Many people placed in the "normal" group are in fact very vulnerable to disease, but they may not yet have reached some arbitrary diagnostic threshold of disease—and these diagnoses can often be arbitrary. By calling people who are on the borderline of disease "normal," we underestimate their vulnerability, and they remain unknowingly on the verge of developing illness.

It's true, of course, that modest increases in blood pressure and blood sugar levels and decreases in bone density are common among "normal" elderly people. We tend to view anything called normal as harmless, carrying with it no risk. This is a mistake, because these small changes may increase the likelihood of disease. The first step in rationalizing these conditions is to stop underestimating the power of lifestyle factors such as diet, exercise and stopping smoking; these can make a dramatic difference to your chances of getting sick and to the quality of life in your senior years. Traditionally, doctors have focused on treating the "diseased" and disabled, but I believe that so-called normal people on the borderline also deserve to be treated. Their blood pressure and blood sugar level should be controlled, their weight brought into a healthy range, and so on. Eventually, I would like to see society shifting its view of the aging process from one of inevitable decline to one of sustained success! Being "OK for your age" is not good enough.

Too many in the "normal" group have already experienced disturbing physiological changes, such as the small increases in systolic blood pressure, abdominal fat and blood sugar noted earlier. If you show these signs, you are not OK for your age. These changes, along with faster declines in the functioning of the immune system, lungs, kidneys and other organs, set the stage for the development of disease. Many people characterized as "normal" suffer, often silently, from the syndrome of unnatural aging, a condition associated with significant risk of disease. If they are stressed, too, it compounds their risks.

The average healthy eighty-year-old non-smoker has only about two-thirds of the lung function of young adult counterparts, and an immune system that is impaired as well. The difference between young and old in these instances is purely related to the consequences of natural aging. To illustrate this, take the case of an eighty-year-old grandfather who has developed pneumonia. His initial symptoms may be the same as those of his young adult grandchild with the same diagnosis. However, even if he too is given the appropriate antibiotic, the course of his illness might be much more severe because there has been a decline in his recuperative power.

Consider, too, the risks of high blood sugar and high insulin levels, known as the "pseudo-diabetes of aging." This is a common and worrisome feature of natural aging. It can adversely affect health, whether or not the person actually develops full-blown diabetes. Both high sugar and high insulin levels increase the risk of coronary heart disease. Increasing levels of blood sugar within the range previously considered "normal" are dangerous. The higher the level of blood sugar, the greater the risk of both stroke and heart attack.

You, not your genes, are in charge!

A recent study of natural aging looked at middle-aged and older men at risk for heart disease. It compared the effects of a nine-month diet-induced weight loss to the effects of a constant-weight aerobic exercise program. At the start the participants were obese and had modest increases in their blood pressure, blood sugar and insulin; all had a blood lipid profile, including cholesterol levels, typical for the development of vascular disease. The low-calorie diet significantly reduced weight, blood sugar, insulin levels, blood pressure and levels of bad cholesterol in the blood; the good cholesterol increased. In sum, the diet improved or reversed every single risk factor. While the older weight-loss subjects lost less weight than the middle-aged subjects and had more modest improvements in their blood sugar levels, they made equal progress in the reductions of all other risk factors. In general, the weight-loss intervention had greater effects than the constant-weight aerobic exercise program, thus highlighting an important approach to natural aging.

Another important study of high systolic blood pressure showed that after an average of 4.5 years of standard treatment that effectively lowered blood pressure, the incidence of strokes was 36 percent lower and the incidence of heart attacks was 27 percent lower in the treatment group. Even participants over eighty years of age achieved the health benefits of blood pressure reduction, regardless of race or gender. These results confirm our belief that it is possible to change the susceptibilities common to the usual aging syndrome. Even more importantly, the results highlight the value of finding out whether you are at risk and of learning aggressive prevention strategies if you are in this segment of the older population.

To a much greater degree than we realized, we are responsible for our own health in old age. This is true whether people are in their seventies, eighties or nineties. They can end up sick, demented and sexless, or vigorous, sharp and lusty, depending upon how they have lived their lives. According to John W. Rowe, director of the MacArthur Foundation Consortium on Successful Aging, "Only about 30 percent of the characteristics of aging are genetically based; the remaining 70 percent are not." The MacArthur Foundation research team further discovered that staying active, both physically and socially, contributes to successful aging. "People are largely responsible for their own old age," it points out bluntly. Genetics plays the greatest role in

NATURAL AGING: THE FACTS

So, what exactly happens to your body during the process of natural aging? Data from the Baltimore Longitudinal Study of Aging outline these general changes:

Heart The heart grows slightly larger with age. Maximal oxygen consumption during exercise declines in men by about 10 percent with each decade of adult life and in women by about 7.5 percent. Cardiac output remains basically the same, even with increased efficiency of the heart.

Lungs Maximum vital capacity declines by about 40 percent between twenty and seventy years of age.

Brain The brain loses neurons but increases connections between cell synapses, and regrows branchlike extensions called dendrites and axons, which transmit brain messages.

Kidneys The kidneys lose efficiency in extracting wastes from the blood at the same time as there is a decline in bladder capacity. Inability to retain urine occurs if tissues waste away.

Body fat The body redistributes fat from under the skin to deeper parts of the body. Women tend to store fat in their hips and thighs, whereas men store fat in the abdominal area.

Muscles Muscle mass decreases by about 22 percent for women and 23 percent for men between thirty and seventy years of age.

Sight Loss of visual sharpness and difficulty in focusing begin in the forties. Susceptibility to glare and difficulty seeing in the dark increase with aging.

Hearing Hearing declines more quickly in men than in women, with a particular decline in the ability to hear higher frequencies.

Personality Personality is consistent unless it is altered by a disease process.

Just as no two people are alike, everyone will age at a different rate. And the gap widens as people get older. As health professionals, we must fight the tendency to overgeneralize about the health and abilities of older people.

health characteristics early in life, "but by age eighty, for many characteristics, there is hardly any genetic influence left."

Studies have shown that the serious losses in physical and mental functioning commonly attributed to age are not inevitable, nor are they impossible to change. As we have seen, a background that leads to successful aging includes regular physical activity, continued social connections, resilience (the ability to bounce back readily after suffering a loss) and self-efficacy (a feeling of control over one's life). People have the power to counteract negative forces as they age by putting their lives and their well-being under their own control. I believe that society has a crucial role to play in helping older people achieve this goal.

Older people who have more emotional support have a better self-image, which in turn is related to the better working of their mind and body. Verbal intelligence doesn't necessarily decline with age; it can actually increase. Older people should not be discouraged from doing what they think they can do. Keep going and stay involved with life—it's good for you. Researchers have clearly demonstrated that people who continue to be productive after they retire are more likely to have a successful old age.

Nutrition as we age

Many older people eat poorly, for a variety of reasons. Long-term bad habits, poverty, dental problems or a lack of knowledge can all play a part. Healthy older people need to be aware that, while the general guidelines for healthy eating still apply, there are some specific age-related changes. As we get older, the body requires less energy—because of a decline in physical activity and loss of lean body mass. Nevertheless, it is just as important to keep up the nutrient requirements in old age. This often means taking supplements.

Many individuals who are sixty-five or over are not eating enough protein, fibre, calcium, zinc, vitamins B, A, D and E, selenium and carotenoids. Deficiencies in one or more of these can increase the risk of suffering a heart attack or stroke, developing cancer or osteoporosis, or contracting a serious infectious illness like pneumonia. Jeffrey Blumberg, a nutrition researcher at Tufts University, maintains that, because there are such widespread dietary deficiencies among older Americans, recommending micronutrient supplements for older people is justified.

Dietary suggestions

Calories Over time, aging men and women progressively lose muscle mass, which means that living and functioning normally requires fewer calories. The so-called basal metabolic rate, that is, the energy we use to perform basic body functions, drops significantly by the age of seventy-five. Add to that the fact that older people are less physically active and the result is a substantial decline in the caloric needs of older adults. Older people should make a point of eating a wide variety of foods containing calories adequate for their needs.

Water balance Several causes conspire to put older people at a relatively high risk for dehydration. Two of these are a diminished capacity to conserve water through the kidneys and a significantly reduced sensation of thirst. This is particularly troublesome in the face of acute illnesses with fever, such as common colds and flu, which make dehydration worse. In fact, dehydration increases the danger of complications related to influenza in older people. Older people should consume about one and a half to two quarts of fluid daily.

Fat Aging people should follow the general rule of thumb that no more than 30 percent of total daily calories should come from fat. They do have one less thing to worry about: since cholesterol does not appear to carry as much risk for the elderly as it does for younger adults, it doesn't seem necessary to limit foods containing cholesterol.

Carbohydrates Dietary carbohydrates should supply 55 to 60 percent of daily calories. The emphasis should be on complex carbohydrates, which contain soluble fibre and are found in some fruits, peas, beans and lentils. These can help reduce the occurrence of constipation and other gastrointestinal problems. Dietary fibre also reduces blood fat and sugar levels and may be important in preventing heart disease.

Protein Older people may need more protein than younger people. At least 12 percent of total caloric intake should come from protein. A chronic shortage of dietary protein may reduce the body's ability to fight disease and heal wounds and may accelerate loss of lean muscle tissue. Less expensive sources of protein that may also be easier for seniors to eat include beans, peas, lentils and soybean products.

Supplements for seniors

While it is always best to improve health by eating more nutritious foods, this tactic is not always practical for older people. As people age, shortfalls can result from social isolation, limited mobility and dexterity, tight budgets, chronic illness, dentures and digestive difficulties. Older people need fewer calories, so they must get more nutrients from less food.

Older North Americans are often found to be deficient in folate, vitamins B_{12} and D, and calcium. A low intake of folate, vitamin B, and vegetables like spinach, okra, asparagus and dried beans and peas can result in a high blood level of homocysteine, which raises the risk of heart disease and stroke. I recommend that older people take about 400 micrograms of folate daily, found in one multivitamin.

Seniors are less able to absorb vitamin B_{12} from foods and may do better by taking a supplement, which is more readily absorbed. Vitamin D shortages in older people result from the skin's diminished ability to form vitamin D from sunlight and also because they probably spend less time outdoors. A larger calcium intake—up to 1,500 milligrams a day for older men and women—is necessary to reduce bone loss and resulting fractures. The elderly may also need a small increase in zinc, which aids immune function and healing of wounds. Also recommended is a daily dose of 100 to 400 international units of vitamin E, which acts as a potent antioxidant that may counter cataracts, macular degeneration, atherosclerosis, carcinogenic assaults on cells, and premature aging of cells throughout the body.

Hormones

Can hormones prevent aging? The National Institute of Aging (NIA) in the United States points out that, while our hormone levels decrease as a normal part of aging, pills, shots or medicated skin patches can all help increase the body's hormone levels. But can they prevent aging? There is no scientific evidence available to support any specific claim. And while some supplements can help people with genuine deficiencies, they can also cause harmful side effects. The right balance of hormones helps us stay healthy, the NIA points out, while an imbalance might be dangerous. Speak to your doctor before venturing into the world of hormone supplements—and don't take any supplement as an anti-aging remedy.

A SUCCESSFUL LIFE'S JOURNEY

Many stages throughout life present windows of opportunity for bringing about healthy development. Once you become aware of them, you will be able to seize the moments as they arise. The following chart summarizes these unique chances to make the most healthful choices for optimum behavioural, physical, intellectual and emotional development at each stage of the human lifespan.

STAGES OF LIFE	OBJECTIVES	APPROACHES
Intrauterine	Healthy beginning/ healthy foundation	Achieve optimal maternal health to ensure normal fetal growth and development
Birth to 3 years	Good brain	Provide parental love, stimulation and good parenting; practise breast-feeding
Childhood	Emotional intelligence and healthy habits	Capture opportunity to provide good schooling and health education; develop healthy habits and emotional intelligence
Adolescence	Coping with turbulent period of life	Provide training in life skills to deal with stress and social pressures
Adulthood	Avoid lifestyle-related disease and premature death	Engage in healthy lifestyle and achievement of social adjustment; control weight and avoid obesity
Old age	Healthy aging and longevity	Manage natural aging process; care for adequate nutritional needs and take supplements if necessary; remain active

TEN GOLDEN RULES FOR A SUCCESSFUL AND LONG LIFE'S JOURNEY

Less meat, more vegetables

Less sugar, more fruit

Less worry, more sleep

Less greed, more charity

Less riding, more walking

Less salt, more vinegar

Less food, more chewing

Less complaining, more laughter

Less clothing, more bathing

Less talk, more action

SECTION III

HQ AND THE FUTURE OF HEALTH CARE

You are now familiar with the importance of taking personal responsibility for your wellness, health maintenance and disease prevention. This section will help you go farther on your HQ journey.

Achieving a long, happy and healthy life based on personal efforts—the HQ goal—means keeping up with the latest developments in health, taking advantage of the advances in communications and medical technologies, and remaining actively involved in the decisions about your own health care. I'll help you to wade through the morass of information to understand what is important and why.

How can you achieve full recovery and optimal quality of life when you are sick? How can you promote self-healing and deal with the root cause of an illness? How important is self-care? You must be armed with all the information before you can make wise health decisions. I take a detailed look at some lifestyle-related chronic illnesses and show you how you can attack them in a radical and effective manner.

What is the future of health care in the new millennium? You'll find information about new research and technologies that will have a great effect on the way we'll live tomorrow. These pave the way for future medical miracles. As we are living in an age of information, complex scientific and clinical information will be translated into understandable description and practical, everyday language. I'll also suggest how holistic and integrated approaches to health care will be acceptable and accessible.

In this section we look at what modern medicine has achieved and what it is capable of achieving in the future. In chapter 6 we consider whether mainstream Western medicine is sufficient, or whether we should start seriously to consider integrating other systems of health care with it, such as mind/body medicine, spirituality and complementary medicine, as described in chapters 7 and 8.

Once you've read this, you will have a wider appreciation of mainstream medicine, mind/body medicine, traditional medicine and the modern-day alternatives that I call contemporary complementary medicines. You'll learn of their unique roles in helping you to achieve better health. This will lead you ultimately to the climax of your journey to better health: HQ medicine, or how to manage your personal health care with intelligence. Described in chapter 9, this is the integration of all these systems and my vision of health care for the twenty-first century, which includes the exciting developments in computer-based medicine.

The incredible and unprecedented developments in the past one hundred years have set the stage. I believe that, armed with HQ wisdom, we are now poised to be part of a quiet but dramatic revolution in health care around the globe. Join in—you don't want to be left sitting on the sidelines when it comes to your health!

CHAPTER 6

MAINSTREAM MEDICINE

The advances in mainstream—or conventional—medicine have been staggering over the course of the twentieth century. We have moved at lightning speed from the Dark Ages of medicine into an exciting world of innovations barely conceivable forty years ago. We're beginning to talk seriously about gene therapy and putting artificial hearts into humans. Who's to say we won't see all this before too long? We have already seen life conceived in a test tube. We are already in the future of mainstream medicine, where just about anything seems possible. Yet, as we are making giant leaps forward, we slip backward at the same time.

After giving you a general overview of the progress and advances achieved, I will take a good hard look at the current status of mainstream medicine and its major battles against chronic, new and resurgent infectious diseases. I will finish on the bright side, giving you an exciting glimpse of the future and a positive assessment by the World Health Organization (WHO). First, though, take a moment to reflect and cast your mind back to the early days of medicine at the beginning of this century.

Progress in Modern Medicine

Who could have imagined on that September morning in 1928, when British bacteriologist Alexander Fleming returned from vacation to find a blob of mouldy fungus on one of his culture plates, that this would lead to penicillin—arguably the most important medical find of this century? The birth of antibiotics—the magic bullet—dramatically altered the course of both clinical and medical research. An alliance of governments, university laboratories and the private sector became the driving force behind the subsequent advances in medical science and medicine that have ranged from the molecular level of genetic engineering to major-organ transplantation. Look, and marvel, at the following summary of some of the most important milestones in modern medicine, beginning with Fleming's 1928 discovery.

A CENTURY OF SCIENTIFIC ACHIEVEMENT

1928   British bacteriologist Alexander Fleming discovers penicillin, the first antibiotic.

1953   Geneticists James Watson and Francis Crick show DNA's double-helix structure.

1954   Dr. Joseph Murray, a surgeon, performs the world's first kidney transplant.

1955   Public-health officials begin inoculating children with Dr. Jonas Salk's polio vaccine.

1972   British engineers invent the computer-assisted tomography (CAT) scanner, which assembles thousands of X-ray images into a highly detailed picture of the brain.

1978   Louise Brown, the world's first test-tube baby, is born in England.

1979   The World Health Organization announces that smallpox has been eradicated.

1981   Acquired immune deficiency syndrome, or AIDS, is first described in the United States, and HIV is subsequently confirmed as the cause of the syndrome.

1982   The U.S. Food and Drug Administration approves the first drug developed with genetic engineering, or recombinant DNA technology: a form of human insulin.

1985   Kary B. Mullis develops the Polymerase Chain Reaction (PCR) method for mass copying of DNA.

1999   An international team of scientists deciphers the genetic code of a human chromosome.

2000   Francis Collins and Craig Venter announce the sequencing of the human genome.

There's no question about the remarkable progress of mainstream medicine over the past several decades. This branch of medicine has made historic and formidable contributions towards longevity and the reduction of pain and suffering. It has brought about such widely varied innovations as lifesaving antibiotic treatments, new anaesthetics, childhood vaccination, public-health initiatives, computer-assisted diagnosis, magnetic resonance imaging and other important technologies. Meanwhile, we have seen the eradication of many diseases and disabilities, the successful transplantation of various human organs, and logical and reasoned explanations for many processes of health and illness. Mainstream medicine has also initiated crucial research into the genetic backgrounds of health and illness. At the same time, it has sought to highlight the associated ethical, moral and social dilemmas that will continue to challenge us in the future. Researchers and physicians in the mainstream are tackling many new health challenges: HIV and AIDS, cancer and a host of other chronic diseases. Some have been able to embrace therapies and approaches that have been proven to work but for which there may not always be a scientific explanation.

Mainstream medicine has established a bona fide and fully accepted role in bringing typically Western-style medicine to other parts of the globe and is keeping up a high standard of education and information to health professionals. Research, evaluation and peer review have always been its touchstones and promise to be so well into the future.

Around the globe, more people than ever before now have access to at least minimum health care and to safe water supplies and sanitation facilities. Most of the world's children are now immunized against the six major diseases of childhood. We have made spectacular progress in reducing death among children under five in the last few decades: there were 91 million such deaths in 1955, but only about 10 million in 1997. Overall, average global life expectancy at birth in 1955 was just forty-eight years; in 1995 it was sixty-five years. It's getting better all the time.

In the developing countries, we are steadily winning the battle against the infectious diseases, such as poliomyelitis, leprosy and guinea-worm disease, that have afflicted hundreds of millions of people. Smallpox has been eradicated. In the industrialized world, prevention programs, education and improved treatment have resulted in declines in disability from heart disease and some cancers. Progress in medical research, treatment, care and rehabilitation, and technology is happening every day.

Most exciting is the advance in molecular genetics. This is the most profoundly important development in medicine as we enter a new century. Analyzing how genes work in health and illness has yielded deep insight into the origin and progression of diseases. The understanding of molecular genetics has created unprecedented opportunities to discover important drugs, to develop vaccines and diagnostic tests, and to provide treatment.

The Human Genome Project

The fifteen-year-long international Human Genome Project, begun in 1990 and funded by various governments, has been conducted in a number of international centres, including university and government laboratories in the United States, the Sanger Centre of England, and at facilities in Germany and Japan. It was targeted to be complete in the year 2005. But on June 26, 2000, five years ahead of schedule, Dr. Francis Collins, director of the Genome Project at the U.S. National Institutes of Health, joined by Dr. Craig Venter, president of Celera Genomics, announced the successful sequencing of the entire human genome, spelling out the 3.1 billion chemical letters that make up the human DNA.

This project is the most important scientific endeavour ever undertaken by the human race. That may sound overblown, but this project can literally change the whole fabric of health care in the twenty-first century. It has the potential to be more important than any other medical undertaking in history. Why? Because it will help us understand the genetic basis of diseases so that we can develop more effective screening and treatment methods. This research will eventually lead to the identification of every gene that is linked to susceptibility or resistance to diseases.

The project is divided into two phases. Phase one, now essentially complete, involved the creation of a detailed map of the human genome. The second phase involves defining the DNA sequence of all 50,000 human genes and it is already far advanced in some particularly interesting parts of the genome. The new knowledge gained in both phases of the project will change all our current thinking about the progress and treatment of disease. The implications are huge.

The gene maps enable scientists to pinpoint a faulty gene's precise location on a specific chromosome. This will be a crucial weapon in the battle against diseases. The resulting information will help patients adopt treatments and lifestyles that could head off genetic or genetically related diseases before they occur. Although a flawed gene cannot be repaired by making lifestyle changes, we can affect the way it develops by taking early preventive measures. The Human Genome Project will thus allow preventive medicine and prediction of disease to be part of everyday medical practice.

The project will provide enormous commercial opportunities for the pharmaceutical and biotechnology industries, which have been quick to recognize the potential for new treatments. The completion of the project should make the search for "disease" genes much quicker and will increase still further the importance of gene-based ways of dealing with diseases. Information and technologies derived from genomic research are already beginning to revolutionize the study of disease.

In the not too distant future, DNA testing will be an everyday tool for health care. It is anticipated that in another fifteen or twenty years every physician will be having to decide each day whether he or she needs the kind of information available only from DNA testing and will then counsel patients about the results of those tests. Imagine a physician discussing with a patient the results of a blood test to determine the patient's genetic profile. The test reveals that the patient's risk for colon cancer is four times the average, and the risk for diabetes is twice the norm. After discussing the implications of the results, the physician, the patient and the nurse design a preventive medicine program to maximize the patient's chances of staying well—avoiding cancer and diabetes altogether. We're not too far away from this scenario. I've talked much about genetic predisposition in this book and how, by understanding our vulnerabilities and health threats, we can work towards a healthier future.

Indeed, the future is now. Testing for breast and colon cancer susceptibility is becoming feasible for those with a family history of these conditions. A National Institutes of Health Consensus Development Conference in the United States has advocated offering DNA-based testing to couples contemplating a pregnancy to determine if either partner carries the gene responsible for cystic fibrosis.

The physicians of the future will need sound education in the broad field of genetics, as well as counselling and genetic diagnosis abilities, and access to gene therapy and genetic specialists. To ensure that health professionals are prepared to practise in this new era, health leaders must work together to make genetics education a priority. It will also be essential to develop an Internet-based communication and information hub pertaining to genetic medicine for both physicians and lay people.

Francis Collins recently wrote of the importance of gene therapy in medicine: "The new technology of gene therapy symbolizes a revolutionary landmark in medicine. It can potentially cure or affect the treatment for a vast majority of diseases. Almost every illness arises in part or as a whole from one or more abnormal genes." Until recently there was no way to isolate and characterize the bad genes; they were known only by their consequences in the form of diagnosed disease. Now, specific faulty genes are implicated in virtually every major human disease, including cardiovascular disease, diabetes, cancer and asthma. Every week or so a new disease gene is discovered.

A single defective gene causes more than four thousand conditions, among them Severe Combined Immunodeficiency and cystic fibrosis. Many other chronic diseases, such as cancer, heart disease, arthritis and senility, are caused by one or more impaired genes involved in the body's defences. These defences include not only the immune system but also the body's mechanisms for maintaining itself. For example, liver cells manufacture proteins that help clear cholesterol from the blood. If there is an imperfection in the gene for this protein, the result may lead to high cholesterol levels, atherosclerosis (hardening of the arteries) and heart disease.

Physicians can apply gene therapy in one of two ways. In the first method, a healthy copy of a gene is inserted into the patient's cells in order to compensate for a defective gene. There are several methods for transporting genetic material into the diseased host cells; viruses are one of the known carriers. Cells with defective genes are removed from the patient and normal copies of the affected DNA are introduced into them before they are returned to the body. The second approach is somatic-cell gene therapy. In this procedure, carriers bearing corrective genes are introduced directly into the tissue where the genes are needed.

Gene therapy should ultimately become simpler and less costly to apply. Sometime in this century, gene therapy is expected to be no longer limited to genetic diseases but used regularly and routinely in treating a wide range of illnesses. Future use will allow doctors to treat many diseases by injecting the required genes directly into the bloodstream. The genes will be contained in viral carriers that seek out targeted cells, such as tumour cells. When the carriers reach their targets, they will unload their genetic material, which will then produce a helpful protein, able to kill a malignant cell.

In the world to come, it will probably be routine to diagnose and repair a faulty gene in a fetus. Ideally, this should pose no more of a threat than removing impurities from the water supply.

Five percent of the Human Genome Project budget is allocated to the ethical, legal and social questions that may arise from genetic diagnosis and gene therapy. In terms of the ethical debate, I hope that HQ wisdom will prevail. I believe that genetic diseases are random tragedies that we should do everything in our power to prevent. A potential mother, who is likely to be the one most involved with the upbringing of her child, should have the authority to make the decision regarding the outcome of her pregnancy. We cannot, however, ignore the challenges this scientific breakthrough creates. We are already in the midst of medical ethical dilemmas. DNA samples are now almost routinely tested for the presence of specific mutant genes. These tests may warn of an impending disease with no available cure. What should be done? Should the potential victims be told? Do they even want to know? There is also growing alarm that genetic heritage may be vulnerable to unwanted prying. We have to face up to these bioethical and social implications of genetic testing. I take the stand that working intelligently and wisely to see that good genes, not bad ones, dominate as many lives as possible is a sensible and moral way to proceed.

Advances in neuroscience: understanding the brain

The last ten years have produced more knowledge about the brain and how it develops and functions than the work of all the previous centuries. We are beginning to unlock the secrets of the mind.

In the past, investigations of the brain relied heavily on animal studies. Research on humans concentrated primarily on case studies of people with neurological disorders. Autopsies were also an important source of knowledge. Today, animal studies and autopsies continue to be important research tools, but with the help of new technologies, scientists have the means to study the brains of living people with methods that are designed to be non-invasive. Magnetic Resonance Imaging (MRI), a technological breakthrough, has given neuroscientists a far more detailed view of the brain than was previously possible; a related technology, known as functional MRI, offers new insights into how the brain works.

The PET (Positron Emission Tomography) scan is perhaps the most notable advance in brain imaging in recent years. It allows scientists not only to observe brain structure in great detail, but also to record and measure with considerable precision the activity levels of various parts of the brain. The PET scan does far more than simply help us to diagnose illness. These images have let us see how normal brains develop in the early years of life and, with other technologies, have made it possible to study and get a glimpse of the brain's intricate circuitry and how it evolves. The knowledge gained has far-reaching consequences. It has taught us better ways to nurture children and give them the stimulation and care they require for future health (as discussed in chapter 5). Scientists also now understand far more about brain chemistry and the effects of various environmental factors. At the same time they have gained insight into the nature of a dysfunctioning brain.

Advances in medical technology

It's hard to keep up! All these successes in medical technology contribute to human health, health care, disease prevention and progress in the medical sciences. I have chosen to highlight three more of them: recombinant DNA technology, imaging technology and computer-aided diagnosis.

Recombinant DNA technology The techniques of biotechnology are being applied in many industries and research fields, leading to products and processes that contribute to a cleaner environment, improved diagnosis and treatment of diseases, more vigorous food crops and alternatives to petroleum as a source of energy. One of the best examples of biotechnology's usefulness is the production of insulin. Scientists take the gene for insulin production in humans and paste it into the DNA of *Escherichia coli*, a bacterium that inhabits the human digestive tract. The bacterial cells divide very rapidly, making billions of copies of themselves, and each bacterium carries in its DNA a faithful replica of the human gene for insulin production. As a result, an unlimited amount of pure human insulin can be produced. This technology not only produces a better, less allergenic and more effective human insulin for the treatment of millions of diabetics around the world, but it also renders obsolete the old technology, in which insulin was extracted from animal (pig and cow) pancreata. The world need no longer worry about a short supply of animal pancreata. The use of human insulin in human diabetics since 1982 has eliminated the initial concern about potential risks.

Other benefits of biotechnology, such as production of vaccines and drugs, may play an essential role in the fight against infectious diseases. The new and better vaccines may dramatically reduce the annual toll of up to 13 million deaths from childhood diseases in developing countries. These benefits are also likely to far outweigh any potential risks.

In 1997, eminent scientists, experts in medicine, and representatives of various concerned organizations and industries from around the world met at the World Health Organization in Geneva to examine issues related to biotechnology and their relevance to diseases such as cholera, tuberculosis, malaria and AIDS. They recommended public information and drew up a series of safety and ethical considerations to assist health regulators, particularly those in developing countries.

The new DNA technologies open doors to more powerful weapons against disease. The greatest global impact of DNA technology is likely to be in the field of vaccine development. The first such vaccine, a recombinant-derived hepatitis B vaccine, has already been successfully developed using genetically altered yeast, and has gained widespread international use. Vaccines against bacterial and parasitic diseases, as well as new drugs, are likely to be developed in the near future by recombinant technology. The drug discovery process has been radically changed by biotechnology. More than two hundred products are at present in clinical trials for a wide range of diseases and disorders, including osteoporosis, rheumatoid arthritis, Alzheimer's disease and cancer. We have seen only the tip of the iceberg. The best is yet to come.

Progress in imaging technology In 1972, British engineers invented the computerized tomography (CAT) scanner, which assembled thousands of X-ray images into a highly detailed picture of the brain. Later models were able to scan the entire body. Since then the technology has advanced rapidly to become even more sophisticated.

With the improvements in medical imaging technology, radiologists are now able to make pictures of the internal human body with clarity and great detail. Advances in radiology and ultrasound techniques have helped to achieve amazing accuracy in diagnosing, preventing and treating disease. Imaging technology can also guide more direct explorations, usually by surgery, and examination of biopsies. Advanced techniques such as positron emission tomography (PET) and magnetic resonance imaging (MRI) can study physiological function of the organs. The most recent advance in medical imaging methods (technically known as single-photon emission computed tomography, or SPECT) can produce 3-D images of the workings of the body.

Ultrasound is a procedure that produces computerized images of internal body parts based on the echoes produced by sound waves. Ultrasound is a simple, safe, non-invasive technique widely used for diagnosing various diseases. Used for the past two decades during pregnancy, it provides a good opportunity for early diagnosis and treatment of diseases of the fetus. (Of course, moms and dads have also been delighted to see their children before they're born!) More recently, high-resolution ultrasound recordings have allowed scientists to study fetal behaviour and document early brain development during the prenatal period.

I've already mentioned MRI and PET scans, but I'd like to tell you more about these safer, less invasive ways of studying the human body and the brain. MRI exposes the body to a magnetic field and measures the energy. Computers then translate these data into detailed images. A development of this technique, called functional MRI, can zero in on various parts of the body, including very specific regions of the brain, to see how they operate. It can give an amazingly detailed picture of what happens when a person speaks, solves a problem or undertakes various tasks, such as squeezing a hand.

The PET scan differs from the MRI in that it not only shows the brain's structure and function but also reveals how the brain uses energy. To perform a PET scan, scientists play a trick on the brain. They inject a tracer chemical, a compound containing an isotope that gives off particles called positrons. This compound closely resembles glucose, the brain's chief energy source. As a result, the brain is "tricked" into taking up the tracer chemical and trying to use it to provide energy for its various activities. In addition to measuring the brain's activity level, PET scans can be used to record and measure blood flow to various parts of the brain, oxygen utilization, protein synthesis, and the release and binding of neurotransmitters, specialized brain chemicals that transmit information from one brain cell to another.

Computer-aided diagnosis Of course, nowadays, the mighty computer is just as much a part of mainstream medicine as it is of everyday life. The hardware and software improve by leaps and bounds as fast as you're reading this sentence. Three-dimensional multimodal display and computer-aided diagnosis, for example, are two of the latest developments for detecting and treating cancer.

Besides letting physicians see more clearly inside the body, computer-aided techniques help them to interpret the images they see. Computers can complement the radiologist's eye. The availability of high-quality digitizers and fast computers makes it possible to process medical images in minutes. For example, the interpretation of mammograms is a repetitive task that requires attention to very minute details, but out of every thousand sets of mammograms taken for screening purposes, only about five will actually contain images of cancerous lesions. Computer-aided diagnosis may direct radiologists' attention to the suspect regions and thus prevent oversights. There is also widespread, routine use of computer technology to replace the filmed imaging techniques.

Other medical advances Other exciting advances in the past two decades include greater safety and efficacy in drugs, anaesthetics and surgical techniques; more effective chemotherapy; improved reproductive technologies; progress in radiology; and vastly improved radioisotope methods for accurate diagnosis and treatment. The expanding pharmaceutical industry has benefited from many of the scientific discoveries over the years, and now produces a variety of effective drugs and medicines for treatment of diseases as well as vaccines for disease prevention.

The progress of the behavioural sciences, through health education and promotion, has heightened public awareness about the important roles of lifestyle and environment. In recent years tobacco smoking has significantly decreased in the industrialized countries. More and more people have started to pay attention to their unhealthy lifestyles and habits. Successful public-health programs, including clean water and sanitation, immunization, micronutrient supplements, rehydration fluid for acute diarrhea, and early treatment of acute respiratory diseases, have dramatically reduced infant and child mortality in both developed and developing countries. Prenatal and obstetric care and education for better maternal health have improved maternal and infant mortality rates. Improvements in the emergency care and treatment of trauma are also major successes of modern medicine.

So where does all this take us? Let's make a cool, HQ-style appraisal of where we stand in modern medicine.

The Current Status of Mainstream Medical Practice

As we enter a new millennium, we have learned one overwhelming medical lesson: we are no longer powerless when it comes to our health. We live in an age of medical miracles. Millions of people around the world are living longer and healthier lives thanks to the combined energies of scientists, physicians, public and private institutions, the pharmaceutical industry and, particularly, active health consumers themselves. Disease, disability and discomfort have been dramatically reduced through medical advances in recent years. A little Aspirin tablet can help relieve a headache—or prevent a heart attack. A new heart can save a life. The production of insulin through biotechnology, and other innovations, are helping millions of diabetics live normal, active lives. There are even signs that the war against AIDS is making favourable progress.

The 1998 health report of the World Health Organization rated longer life expectancy, reduced suffering and improved quality of life as major achievements in mainstream medicine. The death rate from heart attacks has been dropping over the past three decades. Treatments for certain childhood cancers, leukemia, Hodgkin's disease and several other malignancies have improved markedly. Quality of life for people in their seventies and older has greatly improved, aided by such innovations as artificial joints, lens implants and a wide assortment of pharmacological health aids.

Together, vaccines, antibiotics, new drug treatments, sophisticated surgical procedures and biotechnology have given us greater confidence than ever before that we can conquer or combat many of the health problems that confront us. At the beginning of the twentieth century there was no penicillin, no insulin, no heart or brain surgery. Today, medical science is recording breakthroughs every day. The progress in molecular genetics and the Human Genome Project offer breathtaking possibilities for the medicine of the future. Technology is making it easier for us to detect diseases; hi-tech scanners and imaging are enabling us to make more intelligent and accurate diagnoses. Our ability to look at the anatomical and biochemical makeup of the body has been greatly enhanced. Remarkable imaging technologies have helped to advance neuroscience—the science of the nervous system—and to demonstrate how the brain functions in different emotional states. Scientific support for a strong tie between the mind and the body continues to grow. At the same time, complementary health-care approaches are getting attention and a higher level of research.

With the eradication of smallpox and the near-eradication of polio through the global immunization program, is it any wonder that people feel they can live a more satisfactory and healthy life than at any previous stage in human history?

Yet among the triumphs there is still tragedy and despair. Cancer, heart disease, diabetes and AIDS continue to claim too many victims around the globe. There has been an increase in the number of illnesses with environmental origins. Recently, the proliferation of antibiotic-resistant infections has been alarming. Social and stress-related diseases are running rampant in the industrialized nations of the world. Too many of us, older people especially, continue to live poor-quality, less than adequate lives.

Despite the miracles, mainstream conventional medicine is incapable of dealing effectively with the chronic diseases and conditions. Our conventional health-care systems face the dilemma of increasing demands for medical care and shrinking budgets. Our newspapers daily chronicle stories of people waiting too long for medical help, which in some tragic instances comes too late. In developing countries, poverty and lack of accessible primary health care cause millions of premature deaths and disabilities.

In a few decades the ancient art of healing has been eclipsed by the magic bullet of the antibiotic era and the seemingly endless vistas of the molecular age. Many new fields of medicine and medical disciplines have developed, resulting in an even closer intimacy between science and clinical medicine. The remarkable progress of medicine in the past few decades may herald even more marvellous advances, perhaps now unimaginable, but any amount of miracle making does not preclude the need for attention to the art of healing and humane medicine.

Quality of life for the growing number of elderly people may be much better, but their longevity has created a need for ways to deal more adequately with chronic diseases, degenerative diseases and the common problems of natural aging. The wide prevalence of Alzheimer's disease, for example, has only recently gained attention. Now, intensive efforts are underway to identify its causes, improve diagnosis and find possible treatments. The advances of modern medicine are simultaneously up against other challenges: the dehumanizing effect of supertechnology, ethical dilemmas resulting from biomedicine's enhanced ability to prolong life, and an assembly-line style of care that strains the doctor–patient relationship.

We need a whole new blueprint for health care, one in which the patient will take greater control of his or her destiny. It is a wellness model that we can use to address the desire for health expectancy in a time of rising costs for health care. Furthermore, our health-care services should be drawing the best from all health-care systems and taking a holistic approach to health and illness that acknowledges the interaction of mind and body.

The whole idea of HQ is to make you aware of the potential of all medical systems. But it will also make you aware of their limitations. There are many limits to what mainstream Western medicine can currently provide to patients around the world. Science and technology are roaring along, but it's the art of practising medicine that often lags behind in the conventional medical world. We have yet to see effective, patient-based management of chronic diseases, a focus upon wellness, a recognition that mind and body are intertwined, and well-balanced doctor–patient relationships.

The battle against chronic diseases

It is these non-infectious (non-communicable) chronic diseases, particularly cancer, heart diseases, diabetes, arthritis and mental disorders—including dementia—that now pose the greatest threats to health in developed countries. These are diseases that tend to strike later in life, so that, as life expectancy increases, we can expect them to become more prevalent. Chronic diseases are responsible for more than 24 million deaths a year, or almost half the global total. The most common chronic diseases are the circulatory diseases, including heart disease and stroke, cancer and lung disease. In 1997, of a global total of 52.2 million deaths, 17.3 million were due to infectious and parasitic diseases, 15.3 million to circulatory diseases, 6.2 million to cancer, and 2.9 million to respiratory diseases, mainly lung disease. Already, the outlook for most individuals in the developing world is that, if they manage to survive the infectious diseases, they will succumb in later life to the chronic ones.

In the history of medicine and public health we have been successful in curing many infectious diseases. However, chronic diseases, with a few exceptions, have not lent themselves so easily to cure. They do not spread from person to person. Every case of chronic disease is a personal disaster for people who, depending on circumstances, may or may not have access to treatment or support. If the majority of chronic diseases cannot be cured, the emphasis must be on preventing their premature onset and delaying their development in later life. This also involves lessening the suffering caused by the disease and providing a supportive social environment to care for those who become disabled. So far, modern medicine hasn't done a very good job.

As I have already said, the development of chronic diseases is seldom, if ever, the result of a single cause. In addition to genetic susceptibility, many lifestyle habits, such as smoking, heavy drinking, inappropriate diet and inadequate physical activity, are known to increase the risks. Let me say this one more time: as a well-informed person with a high HQ, you have the means to lower your risks for chronic disease, because lifestyle is mostly within your personal control. I strongly believe that promoting a healthier lifestyle should be a top priority of ongoing health-care practices. However, despite some improvements in recent years, we still have a long way to go—a very long way. HQ would help.

One of the major deficiencies of our mainstream health-care system is its failure to pay effective attention to the health-related quality of life in chronic diseases. Your health status is much more than the biological progress of a disease; it's also your own sense of well-being and ability to perform in the multiple roles that define a normal life. Your health encompasses a broad range of consequences, from simple matters of mobility and self-care to the fulfillment of family and social responsibilities. This is all about patient-centred care and, although modern medicine does not yet give it due weight, I believe it plays a major part in your overall medical situation.

In recent years, there has been significant progress in measuring quality of life, as I mentioned in the first part of this book. This has to be taken into account when deciding how to treat certain chronic diseases. One of the aims is to balance the expected benefits of treatment against the disabilities and discomforts that they may cause and the effects on overall quality of life.

Health-related quality of life is a relatively new area of research. Nevertheless, it is likely to assume growing importance as the medical community and the people it serves recognize that the ability to participate in life's major activities is a patient's right, and thus an essential part of medical evaluation and decision making. As you know, your health profile—which I hope you have already filled out at the beginning of this book—is more than just the absence of illness. Quality of life is an essential part of helping you stay healthier and live longer. The medical profession needs to understand more about you than can be gained from the average six-minute visit in your GP's office.

A warning about diabetes mellitus

This chronic disease poses one of the most daunting challenges at the present time. Recent data show that approximately 135 million people worldwide suffer from diabetes mellitus and predict that this number will rise to almost 300 million by the year 2025. The forecast is based on the aging population, unhealthy diets, obesity and sedentary lifestyles. While the rise will be of the order of 45 percent in developed countries, it will be almost 200 percent in developing countries.

Diabetes is likely to become the pre-eminent public-health problem of the twenty-first century. "The incidence of type 2 diabetes rose rapidly by 9 percent per year over the decade ending in 1996," according to a report by Michael P. Stern at the American Diabetes Association's 1998 annual scientific sessions. Apart from the health devastation, there are huge economic implications. It is a particularly costly disease for the health-care system, the affected individual and society as a whole because of its chronic nature, the severity of its complications and the means required to control it.

The war against microbes: old and new infectious diseases

Thanks to the successes of antibiotics, vaccines and public health campaigns, there was, until quite recently, a widespread feeling that the struggle against infectious diseases was almost won. The means of controlling most of them seemed either available or discoverable without undue difficulty. Spectacular progress has indeed been made: smallpox has been eradicated and six other communicable diseases will soon be eliminated. Tragically, with optimism came a false sense of security.

Acquired Immune Deficiency Syndrome, or AIDS, caused by the human immunodeficiency virus (HIV), came along in the 1980s with its associated serious health problems from infections. This has become the great new global health challenge. As yet, there are no effective vaccines for HIV infections, and AIDS has rapidly become an epidemic and a major public-health concern.

Soon after AIDS burst upon the world scene, physicians began to encounter more and more strains of bacteria that did not respond to the antibiotics that had once destroyed them. Four decades of use, overuse and inappropriate use of these drugs have allowed certain forms of microbes with mutated genes to develop and to resist drugs, leaving no viable antibiotic treatment options. People of all ages in recent years have been dying of infectious diseases that once seemed easy to treat.

Re-emerging infectious diseases are infections that were familiar at one time but had fallen to such low levels that they were no longer considered a public-health problem. Of these, malaria and tuberculosis are making a deadly comeback in many parts of the world. At the same time, plague, diphtheria, dengue, meningococcal meningitis, yellow fever and cholera have reappeared as public-health threats in many countries after years of decline. Some of them may subsequently reappear in epidemic proportions. Some scary statistics:

according to the World Health Organization, the leading killers among infectious diseases are acute lung infections (3.7 million), tuberculosis (2.9 million), diarrhea (2.5 million), HIV/AIDS (2.3 million) and malaria (1.5 to 2.7 million).

Other, previously unknown infectious diseases are emerging at an alarming rate. In the last twenty years, more than thirty new and highly infectious diseases have been identified. One of them, the virulent Ebola-type hemorrhagic fever, struck terror in our souls as it dominated the news for weeks. For this and some HIV/AIDS diseases, there is no effective treatment, cure or vaccine.

At the same time, fewer new antibiotics are being produced, in part because of the high costs of development and licensing. As the treatment of communicable diseases becomes less effective, more people will need hospitalization, illnesses will last longer, treatment will cost more, and absenteeism from school and work will increase. So, while substantial progress has been achieved in many areas of science and medicine, other developments are negating or minimizing these achievements.

There are many reasons for the appearance of new diseases and the resurgence of old ones. Among them are the increase in international air travel and the growth of megacities with enormous populations, inadequate supplies of safe water and poor sanitation. The risk of food-borne diseases has also been increased by the globalization of trade and changes in the production, handling and processing of food. Environmental factors, too, can lead to the exposure of humans to diseases previously unknown. For example, man is destroying forests and moving into once remote animal and insect habitats where there are high risks of exposure to disease and often no control over mosquitoes and other carriers of disease.

Meanwhile, in rich and poor countries alike, resources for public health are being reduced as other priorities demand the limited funds. As a result, the rise of new diseases, the re-emergence of known diseases or the development of antibiotic resistance may go unnoticed until it is too late. A striking example is HIV, which was recognized only after it had already infected large numbers of people in many African countries. Early awareness is crucial. Potential epidemics, even those on a global scale, can be prevented or at least minimized if they are detected soon enough.

Another red flag warning: adverse drug reactions

A recent report in the *JAMA* raised the red flag about adverse drug reactions. It revealed an extremely high incidence of serious and fatal drug reactions among patients in U.S. hospitals. And the World Health Organization estimated that, in 1994 in the United States, 106,000 hospital patients died from adverse drug reactions, making this possibly the fourth leading cause of death after heart disease, cancer and stroke in the United States. That's a statistic we haven't often heard about. We shouldn't ignore it: adverse drug reaction is a major problem of Western medicine, and it may well be one of the reasons people turn to other sources, such as complementary or alternative medicine.

A Glimpse of the Future

So, what's on the horizon in the brave new world of mainstream medicine? Let's peek even deeper into our medical future. I have told you much about the new world of genetic technology. The next millennium will also see drugs by design, better vaccines, telemedicine, robotic medicine, microchip implants, pocket-sized medicine, laser therapy, construction of artificial organs and xenograft transplantation. Here's a taste of tomorrow.

Genetic Map The successful sequencing of the entire human genome could transform the world of medicine, ushering in a "genomic era" in which the secrets of human health and disease at the molecular level will be known. The Gene Map will allow scientists to understand individual genetic variability and determine which gene could lead to a predisposition to a particular disease. Within five years, individuals may be able to carry a record of their genetic makeup embedded in the magnetic strip of a smart card. At the same time, drugs that would match an individual's genetic makeup, guaranteeing their effectiveness and wiping out side effects, are expected to be available. Dr. Francis Collins, head of the Human Genome Project, predicts that "within ten years, tests for genetic predisposition to twenty-five major causes of illness and death in North America will be widely available."

Living longer We accept that we're now living longer than our grandparents. We now expect, if we're healthy, to live to 80 or, if we're very lucky, 90. But how about 150 or 200? Researchers are saying that a few small genetic manipulations could allow humans to live twice as long as they do now. Scientists have had astonishing success in recent years in extending the lifespans of laboratory animals such as fruit flies and worms. Researchers suggest that, given adequate funding and a few lucky breaks, they could stretch the human lifespan to unimaginable lengths. The scientists suggest, too, that extending your life would also mean extending your vitality and health; you wouldn't have to creak along for more than a hundred years!

Designer drugs Most drugs on the market today were found either by chance observation or by systematic screening of large numbers of natural and synthetic substances. In many cases, trial and error led to their acceptance as effective therapy. In spite of the relative inefficiency of the traditional scientific approaches, they enabled us to devise treatments for everything from minor aches and pains to life-threatening illnesses. Those traditional methods of drug discovery are now being supplemented by a more direct approach, called structure-based drug design, made possible in part by our improved understanding of the molecular causes of diseases.

The designer drug is created from scratch, aiming for a specific molecular target in the body. A chemical is created that precisely fits the molecular target and can alter its activity. This technique can yield promising drugs more quickly and less expensively. Indeed, because the final products are custom-tailored to their targets, they tend to be more potent, more specific and less toxic than remedies discovered in traditional ways.

This innovative approach to developing drugs has recently spawned many promising drug therapies, including several now used in trials for treating AIDS, cancer and other diseases. Captopril is one designer drug already widely used for the treatment of high blood pressure. Several others, produced by various laboratories, are currently being tested on humans for a host of disorders, including psoriasis, a form of T-cell lymphoma, cancer, AIDS, glaucoma and the common cold. There will be increasing use of this scientific method for drug production among the pharmaceutical industries in the future.

Vaccines The most dramatic and worthwhile changes in the last two decades will have a major impact in our battle against cancer. Leading researchers are hopeful that vaccines against several deadly cancers caused by infections will be developed in the near future. A more distant but very exciting prospect is that advances in molecular biology will produce vaccines against other forms of cancer that are not connected to infections.

There is also hope of better vaccines for the prevention of childhood diseases. New vaccines produced using DNA techniques may eventually replace the generation of vaccines currently in use. A shortcoming of the present vaccines is that they require multiple doses given at intervals of several weeks. Too many people fail to turn up for all the injections, resulting in incomplete immunization. Multiple doses also add to the cost. Biotechnology also offers the possibility of combining several vaccines into one simple product. A single vaccine that will provide protection against several major childhood diseases is an exciting and challenging area of research.

Telemedicine The mainstream medical world of tomorrow may regularly make use of long-distance diagnosis and treatment. Essentially, telemedicine combines medical expertise with telecommunication and computer technologies to send medical services over great distances. We're already beginning to see examples of this in Canada, where a specialist in Vancouver can, via TV, diagnose and suggest treatment for a patient hundreds of miles away in northern British Columbia. Telemedicine has enormous, mind-boggling potential. It can bring quality medical care to almost every part of the world. The key here is the specialist. A heart doctor might not be available for a patient in a town in Africa, but with a television set and a computer, a heart specialist in New York could diagnose a patient and recommend suitable treatment to a local doctor. We'll also find patients talking directly to doctors via modem and TV. Using future computer technology, doctors will be able to make full video visits to their far-off patients and even send them to appropriate Internet sites for more information.

Out of telemedicine grows telediagnosis. Its main purpose is to seek a second opinion from, or to confirm a primary diagnosis by, distant specialists. Telediagnosis can be especially helpful to rural physicians who are a long way from specialists in the main centres. We're entering a golden era. The next decade will see the introduction of national and international telemedicine networks, based on the principle of improving patient care and increasing cost-effectiveness.

A word of caution as we rush to embrace the opportunities that telemedicine brings. There are challenges to be faced, too. How, for instance, can we ensure that long-distance telemedicine is not too impersonal, too clinical, too swift? Telemedicine looks good on paper (or the computer screen), but we must make sure that it really improves health care—and a patient's quality of life—while reducing costs and inconvenience.

Laser therapy From a medical point of view, the laser is a convenient and easy-to-control, highly focused beam of light. The range of clinical applications is enormous. There's the simple carbon dioxide laser, used as a non-contact scalpel. The precision of the dioxide laser makes it suitable for such delicate tasks as reshaping corneas. And there is the "flash lamp pumped dye laser," used to close the small blood vessels of disfiguring port-wine birthmarks. The precision of light delivery and the ability to predict biological reaction to laser therapy are now making it possible to destroy early cancer tissue. More and more often, patients won't go under the knife but under a laser of light.

Robotic medicine   The robot has a future in mainstream medicine. Robot systems are already being tested in various surgeries, such as orthopaedic surgery of the hip or knee. Robotics are used for various keyhole surgery procedures, and two new robotic surgical techniques allow doctors to operate on a beating heart without using a heart-lung machine. These techniques should make coronary bypass surgery safer and less expensive. More recently, microbots have been developed that could one day be used as microsurgical instruments to move single cells or catch bacteria. Several organizations have systematically begun to integrate robotic devices into their laboratory automation schemes. We'll be seeing more automation in the laboratories and operating rooms of the future.

Microchip implants   Conditions such as blindness, kidney failure and nerve damage are common chronic complications of diabetes. Control of the disease with daily insulin shots has been only partially successful. Injection of the insulin hormone once or several times a day helps to bring down the high blood sugar level in diabetic patients, but the appropriate insulin dosage for each patient may vary widely from day to day and even from hour to hour. Often, amounts of insulin cannot be given precisely enough to maintain blood sugar levels in the normal range and thus prevent complications of the disease later in life. That's where the microchip comes in. Innovative research in microchip delivery may someday make insulin injections obsolete. In many diabetics, the disease is caused by the destruction of islet cells (insulin-producing cells) in the pancreas. It is possible to envisage a microchip implant device that would function like the pancreas, constantly monitoring glucose levels and secreting the appropriate amount of insulin in response.

At the Massachusetts Institute of Technology, an implantable, self-contained pharmacy-on-a-chip has been developed that releases controlled pulses of a drug on demand. The device enables the delivery of precise amounts of medication exactly where and when you need them, according to MIT. The plan is to implant the microchip under the skin. Potential applications include local delivery of extremely tiny amounts of potent morphine "analogues" to areas experiencing heavy pain.

Pocket-sized medicine   Miniaturized devices already let doctors take the emergency room with them. They may even encourage the return of the old-fashioned house call. Pocket-sized medicine is based on a miniaturized version of every diagnostic tool needed to assess a patient, along with a full supply of standard emergency-care drugs. Pocket-sized medicine may eventually feature functional electrocardiogram (EKG) machines no bigger than a box of chocolates, blood-sample analyzers no larger than a cellular telephone, and portable ultra-sound machines that fit into a briefcase. It may all seem incredible, but the U.S. Food and Drug Administration has already approved a paperback-sized automatic defibrillator that can shock a stopped heart back into a normal rhythm.

All this new, miniaturized equipment will enable physicians to bring their high-tech tools to their elderly, housebound or disabled patients, thereby improving both the efficiency and the efficacy of patient care. The results will bring radical changes to medical practice.

Construction of artificial organs   Millions of people around the globe suffer organ and tissue loss every year from accidents, birth defects and diseases such as cancer. Over the next three decades, medical science will move beyond the practice of transplantation and into the era of fabrication. The idea is to make organs rather than simply move them. Advances in cell biology and plastics manufacturing have already enabled researchers to construct artificial tissues that look and function like their natural counterparts. In tandem with this, genetic engineering may come up with universal donor cells, which would not provoke rejection of these artificial tissues by the immune system.

Spinning plastic into tissue has given rise to many new strategies in the field of tissue engineering. Development of "plastic tissue" depends upon the manipulation of ultrapure, biodegradable plastics or polymers to create a surface on which cells can be grown. Using computer-aided design and manufacturing methods, researchers shape the plastics into intricate scaffolding that mimics the structure of specific tissues and even organs. During the past several years, human skin grown on these polymer plastics has been grafted onto burn patients and the foot ulcers of diabetic patients, with some success. Eventually, whole organs such as kidneys and livers will be designed, fabricated and transferred to patients. Similarly, engineered structural tissue will replace the plastic and metal prostheses used today to repair damaged bones and joints. These living implants will merge seamlessly with the surrounding tissue, eliminating such problems as infection and loosening at the joint, which plague many users of contemporary prostheses.

The day may not be too far off when tissue engineering will produce complex body parts like hands and arms. The structure of these parts can already be duplicated in polymer scaffolding, and most of the relevant tissue types, such as muscle, bone, cartilage, tendon, ligaments and skin, grow readily in culture.

Xenograft (cross-species) transplantation   There are never enough replacement organs available to meet our needs. Transplantation of organs from animals may help alleviate the shortage. Several approaches under investigation involve breeding animals whose tissues will be accepted in humans and developing antirejection drugs.

Surgeons at Duke University in the United States have successfully transplanted hearts from genetically altered pigs into baboons, proving that the hope for cross-species transplantation is not unrealistic. Someday, xenograft transplantation will become a major clinical approach to organ failure and to prolonging longevity.

Drug delivery

Significant progress has been made in the field of drug delivery. There is increasing use of non-invasive techniques that don't involve the dreaded needle. The drug industry is working on a variety of alternatives, including skin patches and inhalation through the mouth and nose. One example was recently described in a report on the effectiveness of inhaled insulin for treatment of diabetes. Diabetics may soon be spared the discomfort, inconvenience and expense of multiple daily insulin injections.

Alongside this work, scientists are developing a new field, chronobiology, which is concerned with timing. Research in this field has shown that the function and processes of the human body can be predicted over daily, monthly and yearly cycles, and it explains why the symptoms of certain diseases and conditions are worse at particular times of the day, month or year. This leads to chronotherapy, which aims to deliver the right therapy at the right time to optimize medical treatment. Timing treatment according to the body's natural rhythms can make surgery and drug therapy more effective, significantly reduce side effects and even prolong life.

Life in the twenty-first century: the World Health Organization report

All of the foregoing may sound like the stuff of science fiction, so let's get our feet back on the ground by taking a look at the World Health Organization's crystal-ball view of life in the twenty-first century. *World Health Report 1998* gives us an expert assessment of the global health situation, which it uses as a basis for projecting health trends to the year 2025. Examining the entire human lifespan and sifting through data gathered over the past fifty years, the report studies the well-being of infants and children, adolescents and adults, older people and the "older old." The most important pattern now emerging is an unmistakable trend towards healthier, longer life. In many ways, the face of humanity is being rapidly reshaped.

Without question, the world of 2025 will be significantly different from today's world, and almost unrecognizable when compared with 1900. The stunning technological advances of recent years, particularly in global telecommunications, computer networking and the Internet, have made the planet seem smaller than ever before. By 2025 it is likely to seem smaller still, and with continuing population growth it will certainly be much more crowded. Increasing life expectancy and falling fertility rates mean that by 2025 we can expect that:

- worldwide life expectancy, currently sixty-six years, will reach seventy-three years—a 50 percent improvement;
- the total global population, now about 5.8 billion, will increase to about 8 billion;
- the number of people aged over sixty-five will have risen from 390 million in 1997 to 800 million, and from 6.6 percent of the total population to 10 percent; and
- the proportion of young people under twenty years of age will have fallen from 40 percent of the total population in 1997 to 32 percent.

These trends will have profound implications for human health in all age groups. The past few decades have seen the growing impact of poverty and malnutrition on health in some parts of the world, and widening health inequalities between rich and poor almost everywhere. These are only some of the problems on the public-health agenda left unsolved at the end of the twentieth century. The war against ill health in the twenty-first century will have to be fought, as we have seen, against two main enemies: infectious diseases and chronic, non-communicable diseases. Many developing countries will be particularly hard hit because, as heart disease, cancer, diabetes and other "lifestyle" conditions become common, infectious illnesses may remain undefeated. Of this latter group, HIV/AIDS will continue to be the deadliest menace. Experience shows that reduced spending on control of infectious diseases can enable them to return with a vengeance, while globalization, and particularly the expansion of international travel and trade and the transportation of foodstuffs, increases the probability of their global spread.

That said, the weight of past and present evidence shows that humanity has many good reasons to be hopeful about the future. Unprecedented advances in health during the twentieth century—the control and prevention of some diseases, the development of vaccines and medicines, and countless other medical and scientific innovations—have laid the foundations for further dramatic progress in the years ahead. Overall, the World Health Organization report gives us plenty of reason to be optimistic.

THE KEY FEATURES OF MAINSTREAM MEDICINE

- The advent of antibiotics in 1928 set the stage for seventy years of stunning achievements in mainstream medicine. Statistics have clearly shown that people are healthier and living longer than ever before. This is largely the result of the twentieth century's progress in medical science and technology.

- Molecular genetics has advanced so far that diagnosis of viral and bacterial infections has become faster and more accurate; comparisons, verifications and dating of organic materials can be achieved; and the genetic makeup of embryos can be determined.

- Biotechnology and the associated recombinant DNA technology have tremendously expanded our knowledge of how living things grow, reproduce and guard against disease.

- Neuroscience has recently provided some important information about the brain and how it develops. This information assists in understanding the nature of brain dysfunction and the need for various brain stimuli.

- Imaging techniques, including MRI and PET scans, enable doctors to see and understand many anatomical and physiological factors, knowledge that is essential to treating disease most effectively. In addition, these techniques have provided a glimpse of the brain's circuitry and early development.

- The current system of medical practice involves limitations and communication problems for both the doctor and the patient. These are becoming increasingly apparent with the growth of chronic diseases and the lack of focus on quality-of-life issues. Also, antibiotic-resistant infections, the appearance of new diseases and re-emergence of old ones, and frequent adverse reactions to drugs make it abundantly clear that, in spite of stellar achievements so far, mainstream medicine still has a long way to go.

- Finally, it will be prudent to keep an eye on some important health topics and issues in the new century, such as increasing life and health expectancy; falling fertility rates; improvement of women's health; use of current vaccines and development of new ones to eradicate diseases; and advances in communications and computer technology. Of course, we also anticipate continued progress in the fields of genetics, molecular biology, imaging, pharmacology and disease-based research.

CHAPTER 7

MIND/BODY MEDICINE

Without a doubt, mind/body medicine is one of the most powerful tools in health care. It can enhance both self-healing and resistance to disease. For your HQ it is important to know about this medicine and how it arises from the unique relationship between the mind and the body.

Mind/body medicine includes a variety of treatments and strategies, from meditation and relaxation training to biofeedback, imagery, hypnotherapy and social support groups. I believe that mind/body medicine could—and should—be integrated into the mainstream health-care service, not as a substitute but as a valuable accessory. Whereas some people classify this type of medicine as "complementary," it has already, in fact, far greater scientific proof than most therapies that come under that classification. As we have seen in previous chapters, the science behind mind/body medicine has become more solid in recent years. I have already discussed what happens when stress hormones are released into the body, the effects of the mind on the immune system, and the exciting progress in neuroscience that confirms how emotions have a direct impact on the body.

For years, the mind has been used in healing; recall the placebo effect I discussed in chapter 3. Lately, mind/body medicine has attracted growing interest from the mainstream medical community. More and more prestigious medical centres are offering mind/body techniques to their patients and conducting research on the use of this approach. The Mind/Body Medical Institute at Harvard University has been leading the way in research and education and is busy expanding clinical services not only within the institute itself but nationwide. The institute has published an impressive list of research results that provide substantial proof of the undeniable effectiveness of mind/body medicine. Here are some examples:

- Patients with chronic pain reduced their visits to physicians by 36 percent.
- There was a reduction of approximately 50 percent in visits to physicians after a relaxation-response-based treatment, which resulted in significant cost savings.
- Among hypertensive patients, 80 percent had lowered blood pressure and decreased medications; 16 percent were able to discontinue all of their medications.
- Open-heart-surgery patients had significantly fewer post-operative complications.
- All insomnia patients reported improved sleep, and 90 percent reduced or eliminated their use of sleep medication.
- Infertile women reported decreased levels of depression, anxiety and anger, and 35 percent were able to conceive.
- Women with severe post-menopausal syndrome experienced a 57 percent reduction in physical and psychological symptoms.
- Cancer patients had significant decreases in the nausea and vomiting that were expected to accompany therapy.
- Cancer patients lived twice as long, on average, as those who did not participate in mind/body therapies.
- People with HIV disease experienced a significant reduction in HIV-related symptoms and an increase in vigour and hardiness.
- Health-promoting habits (i.e., good nutrition, social supports, self-esteem, health responsibility and exercise) increased after the program was finished and were maintained six months after the program in a follow-up study, which also revealed that 80 percent of patients continued to experience a decrease in their physical symptoms.
- Anxiety and depression lifted for most participants and remained at a normal level six months post-program.
- Women in menopause had fewer incidents of "hot flashes," and experienced lower blood pressure, improved sleep, and decreased depression, anxiety and anger.

Apart from the obvious medical benefits, use of low-tech and inexpensive mind/body techniques can save money—no small matter, given the current financial crisis in medical care. Already, many of these mind- and behaviour-changing methods have earned their place in regular clinical practice. Mind/body therapies have been used along with drugs in treating the major chronic diseases, such as heart disease, cancer, arthritis, and smoking and chemical dependencies, as well as many other diseases and conditions.

Although they are hard to measure, I feel strongly that belief systems, positive emotions and spiritual values have a crucial role to play not only in your personal well-being but also in creating an effective health-care system for the future. This is a key part of my HQ vision—what this book is all about.

The Role of the Mind in Illness

In chapter 3, I discussed at length the effects of stress on your body and how important it is for you to take care of yourself by finding ways to cope with the acute and chronic stresses in your life. It seems that your individual personal characteristics and how you relate to the world around you will play a role in determining whether stress makes you sick or not. So, if you do succumb to sickness, mind/body medicine may well be the answer. Many studies have proved its effectiveness in treating diseases related to stress.

How do you know if you are experiencing negative stress? The following is a list of stress symptoms compiled by University of Miami psychologist Michael Antoni and his colleagues.

- *Cognitive symptoms:* anxious thoughts, fearful anticipation, poor concentration, difficulty with memory
- *Emotional symptoms:* feelings of tension, irritability, restlessness, worries, inability to relax, depression
- *Behaviour symptoms:* avoidance of tasks, sleep problems, difficulty in completing work assignments, fidgeting, tremors, strained face, clenching of fists, crying, changes in drinking, eating or smoking behaviours
- *Physiological symptoms:* stiff or tense muscles, grinding of teeth, sweating, tension headaches, faintness, choking feeling, difficulty in swallowing, stomach ache, nausea, vomiting, looseness of bowels, constipation, frequency and urgency of urination, loss of interest in sex, tiredness, shakiness or tremors, weight loss or gain, awareness of heartbeat
- *Social symptoms:* Some people in stressful times tend to seek out others for companionship; others withdraw under stress. Also, the quality of relationships can change when a person is under stress.

As I mentioned earlier, evidence from a raft of recent human and animal studies clearly shows that stress can suppress the immune function. In most cases these immune system changes may be quite small and probably will not have any severe consequences, particularly if you are otherwise healthy. But if you have recently experienced a major disruption in your life, like a divorce or a move, your health may indeed be affected, especially if age or certain medical conditions have already weakened your immune system. (Appendix 7 shows estimates of the relative amounts of stress associated with different life events.) At the same time, studies indicate that relaxation, group support and other forms of stress management can counteract these effects.

Although research results are promising and are beginning to suggest ways in which we can affect the balance between health and disease, there is much we don't know. This should motivate you to do whatever you can to have a healthy, stress-free mind and avoid making yourself vulnerable to major conditions, such as heart disease, cancer, diabetes, gastrointestinal diseases, asthma, infertility, pain, insomnia and obesity. The latest information suggests that there are things you can do both to improve your chances of staying healthy and to recover from illness. Beyond following the basics, such as getting flu shots, eating sensibly, exercising, getting enough sleep and taking the drug treatments you need, if you feel you are under serious stress, you may want to try one of the many stress reduction programs now available. It could be helpful to talk about how you feel with your family and friends or with a therapist. Whatever you do, don't bottle up your feelings. As I have said, supportive personal relationships appear to help maintain your immune system and your physical health. They also improve the prognosis of your illness and lessen your suffering.

Recently, Branda Penninx, reporting on aging, confirmed for the first time that older people who are chronically depressed have a higher risk of cancer. This could be because depression can suppress the immune system. The author analyzed information about 4,800 men and women over the age of seventy, including those assessed for depression, using a standard test. After accounting for age, sex, smoking and other factors, the depressed people had an 88 percent higher risk for all forms of cancer.

Stress and illness

How does stress relate to specific conditions or diseases? How may the mind affect them? I have discussed these questions already in general terms, but I want to highlight some of the important implications for specific conditions as discussed in the publication *Mind/Body Medicine*, edited by Daniel Goleman and Joel Gurin.

Coronary heart disease Conditions that will increase your likelihood of developing heart disease and dying from it prematurely include a hostile personality, subjection to chronic stress, such as social stress and severe job pressure, and lack of social support. The reason is that these factors increase the body's levels of stress hormones and insulin resistance, which can in turn raise blood pressure and cholesterol levels and cause the formation of clots that lead to blockage in the heart's arteries. Hostile people are also more likely than others to have poor health habits, such as overeating (or eating the wrong foods), smoking and excessive alcohol consumption, problems that may also be more common among socially isolated people.

Cancer Many people have come to believe that the mind and emotions play a significant role in the development of cancer. There is, however, no conclusive evidence that specific emotions, personality types or stressful events predispose a person to cancer. Of course, being able to express your emotions and maintain a fighting spirit will help you face any crisis in life. Social support too has definitely been shown to lengthen survival for cancer patients, probably because it helps people cope more effectively and keep a better attitude.

Chronic pain Pain is one of the symptoms that people complain about the most. In many cases the specific cause remains unknown, and no effective medical treatment exists. Although psychological reasons alone rarely cause persistent pain, they can trigger or worsen attacks of pain and contribute to distress and disability. A healthy mind can improve a patient's outlook and lessen the severity of the pain symptoms.

Diabetes Stress may play a role in triggering diabetes. High levels of stress can affect glucose metabolism and can cause insulin resistance and increase your blood sugar level. Stress and emotional instability can also make diabetes more difficult to control once the disease has developed.

Skin problems There are all kinds of reasons for skin problems, but the skin is undoubtedly highly responsive to emotional changes. Do you break out in a rash when you're worried about paying those bills or when you're all set to go out on a date? Any skin problem may have stress as one of its causes.

Gastrointestinal disorders Stress and other emotions can play a role in various gastrointestinal disorders. These are illnesses for which there is no known physical cause. By far the most common of them is irritable bowel syndrome.

This may have other causes, but people who are psychologically vulnerable may be more likely to develop the condition or to see it worsen. Some evidence shows that illness patterns, often learned in childhood, can also contribute to the problem. It's still a medical mystery why stress affects patients in different ways: it may lead to diarrhea in one and constipation in another. Tension may also play a role in gastrointestinal disorders and in the everyday upsets often experienced by otherwise healthy people. Also, stress can contribute to ulcers, although it is not their primary cause.

Arthritis Arthritic patients' state of mind and ability to cope with day-to-day activities will affect the course of their disease. Attitude will also make a difference in how well they respond to drug therapy.

Asthma Stress and emotions won't cause the disease, but for some people they may precipitate asthma attacks or make them more severe. In general, attacks may worsen during times of emotional turmoil or depression. Episodes of intense emotion, like a fit of anger, can trigger an attack. And in some people with a conditioned response, simply thinking that they have been exposed to something they are allergic to, for example a cat, can bring on a bout of wheezing. Family stress plays a role too: family conflicts have been linked to fatal asthma attacks in adolescents and can trigger non-fatal attacks in many children and adults with the disease.

Infertility and pregnancy The desire to have children has profound meaning and may lead to deep emotional upsets. In particular, the inability to conceive can create enormous stress, which may in turn worsen the problem of infertility. During pregnancy, prolonged emotional stress on the mother can affect her fetus, although the simple stress of working at a demanding job is not necessarily hazardous. In the critical period of labour and delivery, supportive stress-reducing measures, such as the presence of a labour coach or companion, may ease the process and cut down the risk of complications.

Somatization This is the clinical term for malingering—when physical symptoms have no medical cause. Research has shown us that many of the patients in a doctor's waiting room do not really suffer from a medical problem but from emotional distress that they have translated into a physical symptom. Doctors call such patients "somatizers." Often the maladies they complain of are those that are still somewhat mysterious to medical science and cannot be easily diagnosed; these days, they are often environmental allergies and chronic fatigue syndrome. In many cases the complaints are linked to the patient's real physical vulnerabilities. For example, a somatizer who has a history of legitimate allergies may be susceptible to mysterious allergic reactions under stress.

Although these patients do not have a physical illness, their suffering is real; they're not making it up. They often travel from doctor to doctor in search of a cure, but they are rarely helped unless an insightful physician refers them to a psychotherapist. Through therapy, patients can come to understand that their physical symptoms are an expression of their emotional conflicts. They learn to confront their stress and to develop a range of healthier strategies for coping with it. Research shows that offering such patients brief psychotherapy can dramatically cut the number of their visits to doctors and hence the cost of their health care.

Mind/Body Techniques and Treatments

No mind/body intervention is a substitute for the well-documented benefits of conventional standard medical care, but it can complement them. In terms of serious illness or chronic diseases, well-designed programs, such as the ones organized by the Harvard University Mind/Body Medical Institute, can definitely improve quality of life and serve as a reinforcement to mainstream medical treatment. Recent scientific research is vindicating the notion that the right mental attitude, thoughts and emotions can cure illness and minimize physical symptoms. There is a wide range of techniques in addition to the relaxation response exercises and mindfulness meditation discussed earlier. For starters we can consider imagery, biofeedback, hypnosis, yoga, progressive muscle relaxation and autogenic training. These are all health-enhancing and can definitely aid in your recovery from disease.

The relaxation response as therapy

Individuals under stress often experience the fight-or-flight response. In essence, this means you either want to stay and fight the stress or would rather run away and hide from it. As described in chapter 3, the fight-or-flight stress response triggers physical reactions such as increases in blood pressure, heart and respiratory rates, and metabolism. Facing up to your stress in a positive manner is obviously the better way to go. Dr. Herbert Benson has found the relaxation response to be an effective inborn form of stress protection that is the opposite of the fight-or-flight response. Research data has shown that the relaxation response actually reduces the signs and symptoms of many illnesses, especially those arising from cardiovascular disease. This kind of mental workout has proved its worth as an accessory to standard medical treatment. It effectively reduces hypertension, insomnia, anxiety and pain, and in many instances it allows the sufferer to dispense with the use of medication. Apart from reaping the physical rewards, you are able to reach a calmer, more realistic state of mind, which is a forward step towards balance and healing. If you would like to try this technique, please refer back to chapter 3, where I tell you how to go about it.

Mindfulness meditation as therapy

In chapter 3, I talked about the value of mindfulness meditation in deepening your insight and self-understanding and helping you to have a calm reaction to stressful events or circumstances. It can also improve your ability to cope with medical and illness-related emotional challenges. You should realize, however, that this type of meditation is far more than just a medical therapy; it is a way of life. Regular practice can often deeply enhance your mental and physical well-being. I mentioned earlier the ongoing contributions that Dr. Jon Kabat-Zinn at the University of Massachusetts and his colleagues have made in our understanding of mindfulness meditation and health. One of his studies, an eight-week mindfulness training program, improved a range of physical symptoms. It reduced pain, depression and anxiety, enhanced feelings of trust and connectedness, and helped to motivate patients. These benefits have far-reaching effects beyond the actual mindfulness training sessions. More controlled studies are being carried out to investigate whether mindfulness can influence the healing process and help in the treatment of a variety of diseases.

Imagery

Through guided imagery, a patient attempts to stimulate changes in parts of the body usually considered inaccessible to conscious influence. Therapeutic imagery usually consists of a twenty-minute session that begins with a relaxation exercise to help focus attention and centre the mind. Patients concentrate on a predetermined image designed to assist them in controlling a particular symptom. Suggestive imagery is generally considered to be a powerful and effective way to relieve physical symptoms. It is simple and safe. You can do it yourself with the help of a book or videotape, or get the guidance of a therapist. In mind/body medicine, imagery is a valuable way to enhance emotional awareness, provide insight and heal the body.

Most people learn quickly how to relax using imagery. You can then try more complex forms of imagery. In cases of chronic symptoms, you should regularly practise active imagery. Success of the treatment varies with the individual. It also depends on the patient's physical and emotional state at the beginning of the therapy. Imagery is often used in conjunction with hypnosis.

Hypnotherapy

A hypnotic state is a relaxed state of intense, focused concentration where patients become open to suggestions for improving their mental or physical health. These suggestions are made in the form of imagery, utilizing the ability of your mind to experience imagined sensations of sight, hearing, touch, smell and taste. Hypnotherapy can be used for medical and emotional problems as a primary or additional treatment. Pain control is the most common medical use of this therapy, which has also been widely used to change unhealthy habits. There is some preliminary evidence that hypnotic suggestion may influence the human immune system. This technique is especially effective in helping children, probably in part because of children's great power of imagination and their openness to suggestion.

The one drawback of hypnotherapy is that it is by no means a speedy treatment. Since most of the problems to be dealt with, such as poor health habits or chronic physical problems, have evolved over long periods of time, it takes much time and effort to eliminate them.

Hypnosis can be self-taught and self-administered, but it is easier to master with guidance from an expert.

Biofeedback

Biofeedback detects and amplifies signals from your body that you would normally be unable to notice. These very small body signals are transformed into audio and visual form on a computer. The feedback can help guide you to make use of these body signals. It can alleviate physical complaints and generally improve your health by making you aware of your involuntary responses, thus giving you the ability to alter them.

The increase in awareness of bodily processes and vital signs gives many patients the incentive to learn to control them better. Research and experience back up the use of biofeedback procedures and treatments as either primary or complementary treatments for some symptoms and disorders. Biofeedback treatment is non-invasive and carries very low risk. For patients with chronic health problems, such as chronic pain, recurrent headaches and incontinence, biofeedback may help increase their sense of control, heighten their optimism and lessen their feelings of helplessness.

Biofeedback is a form of self-medication. Doctors and therapists can help to evaluate whether biofeedback is working or not. It helps to have a well-qualified therapist, too.

Physical exercise for stress control

I've already devoted many words to the healthful wonders of exercise. As you know, physical activity, whether it is running, jumping, playing tennis, swimming or whatever, can keep you fit and healthy in body and mind. It is just as important in terms of sickness and ill health. I cannot emphasize enough the preventive benefits. Regular physical exercise protects you from stress and may help to strengthen the cardiovascular and immune systems. Frequent exercise is an effective treatment for anxiety and may be as effective as psychotherapy in the treatment of mild or moderate depression.

Yoga

Hatha yoga is the most common form of this technique. It does not require a central mental focus, mantra or prayer. The practice involves focusing on breathing and on a series of physical postures requiring slow movement and concentration. In effect, it is basically a form of mindfulness meditation and thus differs from approaches like transcendental meditation. Yoga also elicits the healthful changes of the relaxation response.

Progressive muscle relaxation

Increased muscle tension is one of the main physical responses to stress. For the progressive muscle relaxation technique, you lie down in a quiet room, cultivate a passive attitude, and are taught how to recognize the sensations of muscle contractions or tension. In this way you learn how the muscles can be released to achieve a deep physical relaxation. This knowledge then enables you to control muscle tension in all kinds of stressful circumstances.

Autogenic training

Autogenic training makes use of a series of brief, repeated phrases designed to focus attention on various parts of the body in order to induce changes. It is termed "autogenic" because the technique helps you to change from within. This technique initiates a reaction to counter the stress-induced fight-or-flight response. The standard exercises concentrate on feelings of heaviness and cultivate a sense of warmth in the limbs as well as a passive focus on breathing. There is a peaceful quality to this exercise. It should be one of passive, not intense, concentration, evoking a spontaneous and tranquil nature.

Transcendental meditation

Transcendental meditation means that the mind transcends the thought impulse and allows itself to settle down to the simplest state of awareness. This state of awareness is known as transcendental consciousness, and it creates a pattern of profound rest and balance in the body's metabolism. During transcendental meditation, metabolism is reduced to a state even lower than that experienced during sleep or eyes-closed rest. In medical terms this slows down your breathing but does not deprive you of oxygen; it also slows your heart rate, decreases your blood pressure and stabilizes your nervous system. It may sound like a contradiction in terms, but during transcendental meditation you are in a state of restful alertness. Regular practice of transcendental meditation would significantly benefit your health as it helps to counteract the effects of stress on the heart and other organs.

Cognitive therapy

In cognitive therapy, patients discuss their thoughts about illness, explore their fears of death, talk about problems they are having with treatments, and try to replace negative thought patterns with more realistic ones. I've suggested earlier that optimistic people are usually a lot happier—and healthier—than pessimists. It seems self-evident, perhaps, but it's an important health issue.

Cognitive therapy, designed to counter depression, apparently boosts optimism as well. It enables patients to look on the bright side, to be more realistic about their circumstances and to be in a better position to deal with dire expectations and the consequences of disease. Success may depend upon the patient's ability to change other aspects of his or her life at the same time. Patients will probably achieve better results from cognitive therapy if they also take part in spiritual practices and work closely with their health-care providers.

Stress-management group programs

Group programs are becoming a common mind/body treatment for chronic illnesses. The stress-management program is an extremely effective way to teach people how to tolerate the psychological burden of their illness. Research data on men infected with the AIDS virus have shown that these groups also reap physical benefits from this management technique.

These programs offer relaxation training to calm the body and mind in times of distress. In addition, there are four specific coping strategies that can assist the participants in dealing with stressful circumstances; these are known as cognitive restructuring, assertiveness training, information or communication strategy, and social support. *Cognitive restructuring* allows you to recognize irrational thought patterns that cause negative emotions, and to replace these negative emotions with rational thinking. *Assertiveness training* empowers you to express your wishes clearly and strongly while still respecting the needs and desires of the people around you. This kind of communication can reduce stress in some situations and improve your relationships with others. *Information strategy* is the sharing of knowledge through discussion of the causes and signs of stress as well as specific illness problems. *Social support* is one of the most important of the group strategies. Members are taught to recognize the many types of support available and how to lean on them when coping with stress. In itself, the group becomes a model of good social support, offering its members a secure place in which they can learn and share.

Active participation

Active participation is a mind/body therapy that helps you to manage the negative thoughts and reactions that might otherwise hinder your medical treatment. It is a positive—indeed, therapeutic—way of putting you in control of what is happening to you. You can often prepare yourself mentally for stressful medical procedures, such as surgery or a CAT scan, by being an active participant. Of course, you need to communicate closely with all the health professionals involved so that you are knowledgeable about the medical care you are receiving; this is one of my important HQ goals. It doesn't detract from the good diagnosis, advice and treatment offered by conventional care, but patient-centred medicine brings the sense of control back to you.

Doctor–patient communication is becoming popular with patients because it makes medical care more equitable and effective. In essence, the doctor is no longer a demigod prescribing treatments. Research has demonstrated that active, assertive patients generally do better than passive ones. An active health approach means knowing how and when to practise self-care and how to communicate effectively with a physician. The truth is that a great many people handle their own medical problems and don't even bother to go to the doctor. As people are becoming more responsible for their own health, physicians are learning to be more attentive to their patients. They are more often willing to have a constructive dialogue with patients during treatment. This positive new trend has great potential for the future of health care, and the HQ approach to health can only speed it along the way.

Outside help with mind/body medicine

Many of the mind/body therapies require you to seek outside, sometimes professional, help. You might need a therapist with special skills, a psychiatrist, or a mental heath professional familiar with the needs of patients who are physically ill. Your assistants might also be non-professionals—friends, family members and fellow patients. Therapy treatments can take place one-to-one, in the form of social support, or in a self-help group.

Sharing is healthy. I've mentioned throughout this book that having a high level of social support produces a positive effect on your health; strong support can also greatly improve the outcome of your illness and your chance of having a full recovery from the disease or its symptoms. Self-help groups allow members to learn more about their common illness, exchange experiences and feelings with fellow patients, and lend each other various kinds of support. Studies have demonstrated the advantages these groups provide: they enhance your sense of control over your life and your ability to deal with the illness. This is especially true for the terminally ill patient, for whom such support provides comfort and emotional nourishment.

These self-help groups can be located through your family physician or hospital, on the Internet, in the Yellow Pages or by talking to other patients. To find out if a particular group works for you, simply attend the first session. It's up to you to decide if you feel comfortable—and supported—in that environment. In health care, this is the medical equivalent of Alcoholics Anonymous: you have a shared problem, and the group can help support you in your darker moments. Support groups have an important place in medical care, improving a patient's quality of life and perhaps even his or her prognosis.

Psychotherapy/psychiatric therapy

Psychotherapy and psychiatric treatments can be very helpful for sick people, even if their illness is physical in origin. For instance, elderly people with hip fractures and patients with HIV infection or cancer may all benefit from this type of treatment. It will have the best results if the source of the emotional problem is well diagnosed, if treatment begins early and if therapists have a close working relationship with the patient's regular doctor.

In cases of chronic illness, psychotherapy allows the patient to cope better with the day-to-day challenges and the stress of the disease. It gives patients a more realistic view of their medical condition, which allows them to make the most of their capacity to take care of themselves. It may well help to motivate them to have regular exercise, select a good diet, stick to their medical regimen and establish a good rapport with the doctors supervising their treatment. Psychotherapy can also help patients deal with frightening and debilitating thoughts, such as rage and betrayal, that may arise as a result of their illness.

Sometimes the feeling of helplessness brought on by an illness is even more crippling than the actual physical impairment of the disease. Psychotherapy and counselling can often help those with severe physical problems to adjust to their situation and live fuller and more productive lives.

The Use of Mind/Body Medicine

The purpose of mind/body medicine is to improve your quality of life, reduce your physical symptoms, enhance the self-healing process, and help you regain a sense of control and well-being. How can you effectively use the mind/body approach in its entirety to combat a specific medical problem? Here are a few suggestions, recommended by Goleman and Gurin in their book *Mind/Body Medicine*.

Cardiovascular disease There are ways to diminish the negative health effects of hostility, low social support and job stress. Hostility can be countered by a commitment to change, by learning to control your reactions and by having better emotional intelligence. Research also shows that support groups can improve the prognosis for heart patients, and it is reasonable to believe that strong social support can help healthy people prevent heart disease.

Cancer Support groups and mind therapies can definitely help cancer patients improve their quality of life. Once the illness is diagnosed, patients and their loved ones often have difficulty coping; some patients may become so depressed or anxious that they are unable to pursue treatment. In such cases, individual or group therapy can make a tremendous difference.

Relaxation, guided imagery, hypnosis, biofeedback, meditation, distraction and other therapies can all help people deal with the side effects of treatment for cancer as well as with pain from the cancer itself. We have only begun to explore cancer's emotional landscape, but we can already offer patients social and psychological treatments to help them deal with the illness. One day, we hope, we will learn to harness the mind to help them fight their disease even more effectively.

Chronic pain People who suffer from chronic pain are likely to feel helpless and hopeless, but they can take an active role in managing their condition. A number of self-management approaches, including biofeedback, exercise, imagery and cognitive strategies, can help people develop a sense of mastery over their pain. You may find it helpful to go to a pain clinic if you have trouble battling pain on your own.

Diabetes There is some evidence, though it is still preliminary, that relaxation techniques may help control the disease in some people with Type 2 diabetes, especially if they are under significant stress. Methods tested to date include biofeedback and progressive muscle relaxation.

Skin problems A variety of mind/body techniques, including simple relaxation training, hypnosis, imagery, psychotherapy and biofeedback, can help relieve skin conditions. Itching and scratching can be relieved, even in severe cases, with a combination of mind and behaviour techniques. Warts are clearly treatable by hypnosis, and herpes may be as well. Researchers are also looking into the use of mind medicine to treat psoriasis and a number of other skin problems.

Gastrointestinal disorders When these disorders are linked to emotions, there are numerous mind/body treatments, particularly psychotherapy, relaxation training and hypnosis, that can help in prevention and treatment. Although biofeedback has been useful in documenting the mind's influence on the gastrointestinal tract, it is generally not a very effective treatment for stress-related symptoms. (It is, however, the treatment of choice for incontinence.) Our understanding of the best treatments will certainly improve as we learn more about the link between the mind and intestinal illness.

Arthritis Self-efficacy—the feeling of confidence that you can cope with the disease—is the key to dealing with arthritis; it gives you that therapeutic sense of control. One self-help-group approach, available nationally to people with arthritis, works by enhancing this sense of control. People who go through this group approach find that they experience less pain and have fewer visits to the doctor.

The ideal approach to arthritis treatment for most people embraces self-efficacy and the whole gamut of medical care. It is a combination of having a supportive physician and other health-care professionals, using appropriate drugs to relieve pain and inflammation, and learning new coping strategies and putting them into practice. By themselves, these tactics are not likely to be effective; together, they can do a great deal to treat rheumatic disease.

Asthma Hypnotherapy can help lessen the effects of asthmatic attacks through post-hypnotic suggestion, and basic relaxation techniques may be effective in some cases. Psychotherapy is often helpful both in defusing the emotions that can trigger attacks and in helping people deal with the emotional consequences of the disease.

Pregnancy and delivery   Emotional support should be incorporated into obstetrical care from the time of conception through the first months of parenthood. In particular, support groups help prospective parents deal with any stress associated with the changes they are experiencing at this important stage of their lives. At the time of delivery, the presence of a labour coach or companion has been shown to make birthing easier and to lower the risk of complications. In addition to the potential health benefits for mother and baby, such support can clearly enhance the quality of life for the new family.

Surgery and other medical procedures   Any invasive medical procedure can provoke anxiety, and undergoing surgery can be extraordinarily stressful. Research indicates that the more you know about what to do and what to expect before, during and after surgery, the more likely it is that the surgery will go smoothly and you will recover rapidly. Few hospitals offer programs to prepare patients to withstand the physical and emotional trauma associated with surgical procedures, but there are steps you can take yourself.

The best approach is to think of yourself as an athlete training for a major event. Enter surgery with specific plans for your part in the event. Learn about the surgery beforehand, and consider giving yourself specific instructions to assist your body in muscle relaxation or to improve blood circulation. You can ask your surgeon well ahead of time what kind of areas you should focus on to help in your recovery. Simple techniques might make all the difference. For example, you can plan ahead to use earplugs or, better yet, a cassette player during surgery to block out any disturbing sounds that you may perceive unconsciously and to provide comforting sounds, music or verbal suggestions.

At every step, work closely with your surgical team. Communicate your needs assertively, but respect their professional judgment as well. Don't be afraid to discuss all aspects of your treatment, from premedication to anaesthesia and post-surgical pain control. An action plan will help to limit the psychological trauma of undergoing surgery and to put you on the road to recovery more quickly.

Mind/body medicine programs

Several mind/body medicine programs are being offered by health organizations, such as the Beth Israel Deaconess Medical Center at Harvard Medical

School. These integrated programs are conducted in group settings, and they combine relaxation response techniques with nutrition, exercise and cognitive therapy. For more details about this one and others, please refer to the resources section at the back of this book.

Outpatient programs

A variety of pioneering multidisciplinary outpatient programs now exist for the treatment of all kinds of symptoms and diseases caused or aggravated by stress. These include cancer, AIDS, heart disease, presurgery, insomnia, chronic pain, infertility and menopause. These programs give patients the opportunity to train in self-care, to use mind/body techniques, and to access specific video and audio tapes about their conditions. These programs also serve to relieve the burden on the existing health-care system by diverting more people to outpatient clinics and decreasing the length of their hospital stay. Hospitals such as Beth Israel Medical Center, the Columbia-Presbyterian Medical Center and Memorial Sloan-Kettering International Center in New York City, are staking their reputations and millions of dollars on the belief that their patients will heal more quickly and less traumatically with the use of support groups, meditation and a variety of relaxation and mind techniques.

A Summing-up

While chapter 3 emphasized the importance of the mind/body connection and its role in maintaining health and wellness, this chapter has highlighted ways in which you can take advantage of mind/body approaches not only to maintain health but also to treat diseases and symptoms. The Office for Alternative Medicine of the National Institutes of Health in the United States includes mind/body medicine within the area of "alternative medicine." I would suggest that mind/body medicine should be much more widely used as a complementary or regular part of mainstream medical care. Although there remains a need for more scientifically based support for mind/body medicine, it has far more substantiation than other forms of complementary medicine. In fact, mind/body medicine deals with many issues that simply make good common sense and impinge on facets of life that affect each and every one of us: the presence of stress and other emotions that can adversely affect optimal physical health. We fully expect that research into the field of mind/body medicine will progress rapidly and that eventually all aspects will be investigated scientifically.

It is indisputable that the mind plays a role in the development of diseases. Stress, for instance, has been shown to cause the development of diseases and the exaggeration of symptoms. Stress adversely affects the body's balance, resulting in a weakening of the body's immune system and healing power. Stress has been shown to cause the release of stress hormones that interfere with normal lipid profiles, blood coagulation and other physiological processes, which, if left unchecked, can cause poor cardiovascular function and other negative physiological as well as psychological effects.

Emotional intelligence is also fundamental to optimal health. Your zeal, persistence and ability to empathize, among other factors, are all important to your ultimate health. Chronic anxiety, anger or depression can have a direct negative influence on your health and are notable features in causing disease and exaggerating symptoms.

The effects of stress and the importance of emotional intelligence should not be underestimated. This chapter has discussed a host of diseases to provide examples of the role the mind plays in the development of disease and the worsening of chronic symptoms. Fortunately, there are mind/body intervention approaches and techniques, from relaxation response to social support groups, that can lessen the effects of disease and symptoms.

There are a number of techniques and methods that can assist you in managing your own health and other approaches that require outside assistance. Through advances in the neurosciences that clearly explain how the brain works during times of stress and emotion, researchers have been able to understand the benefits of relaxation response and meditation. Dr. Herbert Benson has shown that a repetition of words or phrases, combined with a passive attitude, will bring on the relaxation response, the physiological effects of which are the opposite of those induced by stress—a decrease in heart rate, blood pressure and other potentially negative physiological parameters. These results ultimately make you relax and positively affect your health state. Furthermore, Benson clearly describes the benefits of spirituality and religion, and the power of personal beliefs in eliciting the relaxation response and achieving a more relaxed and peaceful state.

Another technique that can be used in a self-care approach is mindfulness meditation, which I described in chapter 3. It involves focusing on the present moment. Although the method is somewhat different than that of the relaxation response, the outcome is similar—tranquility and quietness. Both techniques serve to improve health, prevent illness and the development of disease, alleviate symptoms and improve quality of life.

Clinical programs, notably those developed by the Mind/Body Medical

Institute, incorporate the philosophy and practical approaches of mind/body medicine to improve the health of many people. One of these programs designed to treat chronic pain and diseases is an example of how health professionals can play a role in their patients' quest for better health, improved health expectancy and optimal quality of life. Other techniques beyond self-care approaches that have proven validity include support groups and the services of psychotherapists and psychologists.

Mind/body medicine has established itself as a real, genuinely important aspect of achieving optimal health and wellness, managing chronic pain and suffering, and abating disease and related symptoms. Mind/body medicine has the capacity to prevent or slow disease processes and improve prognosis. Furthermore, if you already have a disease, mind/body medicine can help you cope better and reduce suffering from symptoms related to your disease. Finally, this augmenting approach to managing your health care provides a simple, convenient, safe and inexpensive way to achieve improved health outcomes, either by yourself or with the help of health professionals.

Mind/body medicine cannot be ignored, but neither can it be a replacement for mainstream medicine. In general, mind/body medicine can play an important role in total health-care maintenance and as an adjunct or part of mainstream medicine. This kind of care is starting to make headway in the more standardized approaches to health care and maintenance.

More and more people are looking for medical care that takes into account their thoughts and emotions as well as their overt medical problems. Mind/body medicine offers exciting opportunities for integrating its useful techniques into routine mainstream medicine. HQ is taking mind/body medicine very seriously; in fact, it is a major component of the HQ approach to health care.

THE HIGHLIGHTS OF MIND/BODY MEDICINE

- There is increased evidence and growing awareness of the success of the mind/body approach not only in maintaining health but also in treating diseases and symptoms.

- Indisputably, the mind plays a role in the development of diseases. **Stress can make you sick.** Stress adversely affects the body's balance, resulting in a weakening of the body's immune system and healing power.

- Where do you stand on the stress scale? If you think you might be vulnerable, check yourself against the list of symptoms on page 183. Then measure the impact of life events listed in appendix 7. Perhaps they apply to your situation and you have good reason to be stressed.

- There are many ways to access the power of the mind to counteract the damaging effects of stress and toxic emotions. Some of them are: relaxation response, mindfulness meditation, imagery, hypnotherapy, biofeedback, yoga, muscle relaxation, autogenics, transcendental meditation, cognitive therapy, self-help groups and psychotherapy.

- If you already have a specific illness or disease, such as heart disease, cancer, chronic pain, diabetes or arthritis, mind/body medicine can help you to cope better and reduce the suffering from related symptoms. Find out how the power of your mind can help you to heal and feel better. For example, you can try the technique of approaching surgical procedures as if you were an athlete training for an important event.

- Mind/body medicine cannot be ignored, but neither can it replace conventional medicine. I believe it can play an important role in total health-care maintenance as a valuable adjunct to mainstream medicine. This kind of care is already starting to make headway among the more standardized approaches to health care.

- More and more people are looking for medical care that takes into account their thoughts and emotions as well as their overt medical problems. Mind/body medicine offers exciting opportunities for integrating its useful techniques into routine mainstream medicine. HQ takes mind/body medicine seriously as a major component of the HQ approach to health care.

CHAPTER 8

NON-MAINSTREAM MEDICINE

Twenty years ago, alternative medicine therapies were considered wacko and weird. Now, these non-mainstream therapies, which I prefer to call complementary medicine, are winning new converts every day. Ginseng, herbal remedies, acupuncture, homeopathy, naturopathy and many others are the unconventional health therapies of our age. The array of treatments and ideas can often seem confusing.

What is complementary medicine? Basically, it is medicine without drugs, a more holistic approach that embraces self-healing and encompasses a plethora of therapies not usually taught in conventional medical schools. And we're not calling it "alternative" any more; that word seems a bit too confrontational as more and more people get on board. Gradually it is being replaced by "complementary," which sounds a lot more appropriate in today's more broad-minded world. Although many in mainstream medicine continue to be suspicious or dismissive, millions of people are turning to complementary treatment to replace or supplement modern health care. Ordinary people are flocking to these treatments in droves for a very good reason: in many cases they are benefiting from them.

An elderly woman's chronic pain is relieved by acupuncture; the stressed-out executive is calmed by qigong or meditation; and the child whose persistent skin eczema had defeated conventional treatments is cured when she starts drinking a Chinese herbal concoction. Is it hokum? Or can complementary medicine, in its many guises, produce the miracle cures that its followers believe it can?

Let me say at once that I don't believe all complementary therapies are wonder cures. Most of them are still scientifically untested. But I do believe strongly that standard medical services and complementary therapies can work together to heal people and to help them stay well. I'll go even farther: for the good of all, mainstream and complementary medicine must work together, in an integrated fashion, as we enter the new millennium. My HQ model embraces a much broader health-care world. And you can improve your personal HQ by investigating unconventional therapies. Don't be restricted to mainstream health care, especially if conventional treatment has not worked for you. Take a look at other health-care ideas, such as acupuncture, massage or herbal treatments. Perhaps for you the therapy may simply mean switching to a healthier diet, doing regular exercise or making a health-conscious lifestyle change. Yes, even what you eat is part of complementary care.

The most promising complementary therapies focus on self-healing grounded in healthy living. In spite of the vast arsenal of medical equipment we acquired in the past century, good health often still comes down to sound common sense: eat well, exercise, reduce the amount of fat in your diet, manage your stress, and allow your body to maintain balance and to heal spontaneously, naturally. Many conventional doctors are now adopting some of the complementary ideas, often without being aware of it. Increasingly, the disciplines are overlapping. If you want to have a high HQ, you will need to be fully aware of all the possibilities.

In 1992 the U.S. National Institutes of Health (NIH), the most reputable research institution in the world, created the Office of Alternative Medicine, more recently named the National Center for Complementary and Alternative Medicine. This organization has given complementary medicine a great boost. Operating mainly as a grant agency to stimulate and motivate research into complementary therapies, it has produced reverberations around the globe. In Britain, Prince Charles recently urged mainstream physicians to look seriously at integrating alternative approaches. A group established by the European Commission is also investigating the therapeutic significance of unconventional medicine.

The Office of Alternative Medicine classified complementary therapies into seven categories:

1. Mind/body methods, such as hypnosis, meditation and yoga, that use the mind to enhance health.
2. Diet and nutrition: therapists in this area advocate the use of specific foods, vitamins and minerals to prevent illness and treat disease.
3. Herbal medicine: plants are used as natural medicines and tonics.
4. Manual healing methods, which use the hands to promote healing. Massage, chiropractic and osteopathic manipulation fall into this category.
5. Pharmacological and biological treatments, which use various substances to treat specific medical problems.

6. Bioelectromagnetic therapies: these use electrical currents or magnetic fields for healing. An electric current, for instance, is used to help heal broken bones.
7. Alternative systems of medical practice: medical treatments from other cultures, such as Chinese medicine (acupuncture, for example).

We saw in the last chapter that mind/body treatment is one of the fastest-growing and most fascinating fields of medicine. Relaxation techniques suddenly make a lot of sense. Up to now, however, those techniques haven't routinely been offered by your friendly family doctor. Although there seems to be a heartening increase in research, there is still enormous work to be done. We need to make a full scientific study of the various therapies. This will take time. Even so, I predict that in this century complementary medicine will become part of everybody's mainstream health care. If the twentieth century was a time of incredible scientific breakthroughs, the twenty-first will continue that momentum but take us, medically, in another direction, in which we take more control over our personal health care and engage in self-healing.

Traditional Chinese medicine, natural medicines, herbs, acupuncture, manual healing, complementary treatments—all of these will be front and centre in the health care of people around the world. They have to be; there's no choice. As we've seen, the current Western model of health care is struggling to cope with all the demands on it. Of course, it will continue to march forward scientifically, but I believe that the old-style ways of treating nothing but symptoms and illness will be replaced by holistic and integrative health care. This approach and the encouragement of wellness are the basis of HQ medicine. It is part of my dream for the HQ culture of tomorrow.

In the next few years various complementary techniques will come under microscopic scientific scrutiny. Some of them will be found to be hogwash; others will stun the scientific community as valuable, low-cost, low-tech and extraordinarily effective. I welcome this open-minded scientific research. As health professionals, our job is to identify promising therapies, confirm the ones that work and weed out the ones that don't. The world, as ever, is full of mountebanks and charlatans, and even among the effective treatments there is a lot of work to do. We must discover any potential side effects, fully addressing the important safety issues. We must determine how therapies should be administered—for how long and, where applicable, in what dosage. Are they poisonous in any way? Although many of the therapies have been around for a long time, they have existed on the fringes of society and are largely unregulated.

Even ginseng, the miracle root that Chinese people have been taking for centuries as a tonic and life extender, is only now coming under intense scrutiny. Many studies are looking at the plant's impact on Alzheimer's disease and aging. I anticipate that it won't be long before we understand why this plant has held wonder-drug status for millions of people through the ages and begin to make better use of it in general health care. It may be early days for complementary plant tonics, but we have mounting evidence—not all apocryphal—that many of them can and do work. Perhaps we are doing more than a kindness when we bring grapes to people in hospital: reveratrol, a natural product derived from grapes, has proven to be effective in heart disease and cancer prevention. Dean Ornish, the best-selling author of *Dr. Dean Ornish's Program for Reversing Heart Disease*, has shown that, as an alternative to surgery, heart disease can be treated with lifestyle change, including diet and an exercise program (see pages 241–2). Andrew Weil, author of the best-seller *Spontaneous Healing*, has brought into sharp focus the body's natural healing system. With interest in these therapies and methods growing, the popularity of complementary treatment is burgeoning around the world.

It's a bottom-up, people-driven phenomenon. More and more ordinary folk, dissatisfied with conventional care, are looking for other ways to treat their ailments and attain a better quality of life. Much of the drive for these new "cures" has come from people with chronic or terminal illnesses who feel they are getting inadequate help from their conventional doctors. We've seen, for instance, tens of thousands of people turn to chiropractors to treat chronic lower-back pain. Chiropractors, once regarded as the pariahs of the medical movement, are now well respected as highly trained practitioners able to make a difference in the aching day-to-day lives of people with lower-back pain. The acupuncturist, whether relieving pain or helping drug addicts, is no longer the mysterious Eastern needle man or woman. Now, in the West, acupuncture is accepted as an effective technique in treating pain and other illnesses. Recently, a panel of experts at NIH endorsed acupuncture as an effective treatment and encouraged doctors to integrate it into their mainstream standard health care. Also recently, a new study was announced to find out if acupuncture can aid in the treatment of Vancouver's downtown heroin addicts.

A recent study of another therapy in China suggested that traditional Chinese medicine may even help in preventing breech births through moxibustion, a method that uses the heat generated by burning herbs to stimulate acupuncture points. In this case the method was used to stimulate "acupoint BL 67," which is beside the outer corner of the fifth toenail. It may sound somewhat unusual to a Westerner, but moxibustion is a popular and much-appreciated therapy in China. The study found that the therapy had some impressive results, with the breech problem literally turned around for a large number of pregnant women.

As people flock to different health ideas, governments and the medical establishment have to sit up and pay attention, and now is the time to do it. We are living at a time when ordinary people are more and more health-conscious. Exercise and diet were the buzzwords of the 1990s. People are working out, riding bicycles, jogging and eating carefully. They're using relaxation to lower their stress levels. They're assiduously reading the labels on food packages. How much fat? How much sugar? How many calories? They're looking for answers. Some of these people already have a high HQ because they've awakened to the idea of wellness and have gone out to acquire knowledge on their own. These people often make intelligent choices based on their own research and experience, such as deciding to be cautious about taking a new tonic or remedy. There's a health reformation in progress. You only have to read or listen to the mainstream media to learn daily about new findings connected to complementary medicine. Even some politicians are beginning to wake up to the fact that complementary medicine can't be ignored. The public is urging change, and governments will eventually respond with more research grants and official sanctioning and classification of complementary therapies and natural products. Scientists and doctors will research complementary medicine and develop acceptable ways to measure the results. It's a volatile atmosphere as public demand drives the debate forward at a rapid pace.

While some physicians are cautiously experimenting with complementary therapies, others fear that this type of medicine is garbage, full of snake-oil salesmen and loonies. Although it is quite understandable for highly trained health professionals to be suspicious of miracle cures or strange lotions and potions, I expect that narrow view to change over time. As we learn more about certain treatments and have that information thoroughly scrutinized in vigorous scientific research, those natural suspicions will begin to disappear. There is already an indication that a steadily increasing number of doctors and scientists are becoming more open-minded and less critical, judgmental and resistant. Change always takes time, but gradually these therapies and treatments will seem less "alternative" and more fascinating. The day will come when we will see medical schools teaching not only conventional medicine but also various forms of complementary therapies. In fact, in some places it is already starting to happen: in Germany and the United Kingdom, colleges are teaching herbal medicine and acupuncture.

The complementary medical movement is a worldwide phenomenon. Though most of the traditional therapies originated in Asia, the West has embraced them with gusto. The practice of acupuncture is licensed in many American states. In Australia, traditional Chinese medicine enjoys a stunning popularity. In Britain and North America, natural food stores—which also stock herbs and natural vitamins—have become extremely popular. In France, homeopathic medicines are stocked alongside traditional drugs in pharmacies.

Using complementary or ancient traditional medicine doesn't—and I must stress this—mean turning your back on mainstream medicine. An integrated approach—the HQ approach—uses the best of all worlds. Results of a national study in the United States (published in *JAMA*) concluded that complementary medicine users are finding some health-care alternatives more in line with their own values, beliefs and philosophical orientation towards health and life.

In some countries the use of traditional medicine is not only a matter of medicine but also an expression of culture. In my discussion of traditional medicines I will focus mainly on traditional Chinese medicine (TCM) because it is the one I know extremely well. Also, traditional Chinese medicine stands out as an example of a comprehensive system with proven successes over thousands of years. Nowadays in China, traditional and Western medicines are practised side by side.

Traditional Medicine

Traditional medicine is based on practices and customs developed before the arrival of modern medicine. It is part of the tradition of a country, an indigenous array of healing practices handed down from generation to generation. In some cases these have evolved into a sophisticated theory and system, such as those of traditional Chinese medicine and Ayurvedic medicine. Most of the population in developing countries (more than 80 percent) use complementary medicine as their primary health care, according to the World Health Organization. Many elements of traditional medicine are beneficial, but others are not, and it will be one of the great challenges of the new century to separate the wheat from the chaff. Herbal medicines have existed for many centuries, but only a relatively small number of plant species, perhaps five thousand, have been studied for their possible medical applications. Safety and efficacy data exist for only a much smaller number of plants and their extracts and active ingredients. Regulating the use of plant medicines through effective standards and quality control has become a major concern.

The World Health Organization has long supported the use of traditional medicine. As early as May 1977, the thirtieth World Health Assembly urged "interested governments to give adequate importance to the utilization of their traditional systems of medicine, with appropriate regulations as suited to their national health systems." More recently, this organization has set up studies and collaboration centres in various countries to conduct research and to assess the development of traditional medicine as a viable form of complementary medicine.

Acupuncture is spreading worldwide because it is a cheap, simple and low-tech treatment with few side effects. It has been used routinely in China for thousands of years and spread to other oriental countries long ago. Consumer surveys in the West consistently show positive public attitudes towards this therapy. We are making important advances in our understanding of how it works, particularly for the treatment of acute and chronic pain. There is also research into acupuncture analgesia, which has traditionally been used following surgery.

In China, both traditional Chinese and Western medicines are honoured and used regularly in the health-care system. Medical students at either TCM or Western-oriented medical colleges and universities get the same amount of education and training. Graduates from these two different systems are equally respected and recognized. Each province has a college and a research institute for traditional Chinese medicine. In India, the government provides financial support for research and development of Ayurvedic practices and their increasing use as part of health services.

Such traditional medical systems as these focus on wellness and are directly involved in primary health care. Research institutes and foundations have also been established to study these methods in industrialized countries, for example the Office of Alternative Medicine in the United States. More recent has been the establishment of our own Tzu Chi Institute for Complementary and Alternative Medicine in the Vancouver Hospital and Health Sciences Centre, a major general hospital and one of the best teaching hospitals in Canada.

Traditional Chinese medicine: an introduction

Traditional Chinese medicine has existed for more than five thousand years, with written records dating back more than two thousand years. It is an integral part of Chinese culture. Through centuries of experience, TCM has developed into a whole medical system with a theoretical basis and a variety of different treatment methods. In the past few decades it has grown significantly. Traditional Chinese medicine was founded on natural philosophy instead of natural sciences. Classics such as the *Book of Medicine of the Yellow Emperor*, *The Golden Chest*, *Shang-hang Lun* and *Herbal Materia Medica*, which document the experience and expertise of great masters, are part of this cultural heritage and have influenced TCM professionals over the centuries.

This ancient art of healing is based on the belief that people achieve well-being by harmonizing the mind, body and spirit. It is thought that disease will develop if this state of harmony is disrupted. The biological view of the patient is quite different than in Western medicine. TCM views each human being as unique, while Western medicine believes human beings are biologically similar. For this reason, two people with the same disease will probably not receive exactly the same treatment in TCM. Other aspects of traditional Chinese medicine are not easily measured, unlike in the West, where uniform research standards are easier to meet because it is usual to prescribe the same drug or surgical procedure for patients with the same disease.

TCM doctors focus on certain characteristics of their patient's body and mind as key indicators of health and disease. They can determine where disharmony lies by examining the tongue and pulse and by thoroughly observing and questioning their patients. Where TCM is practised, physicians who treat people after they have become sick are considered to be inferior to those who are mainly involved in preventing disease, which is a critical part of TCM. Priority is usually given to building up health and strengthening the body's natural healing power. This is a striking difference from modern Western practice, where doctors rarely see their healthy clients except for baby care and routine checkups for some adults.

It is said that TCM succeeds in "relieving symptoms" by treating the underlying cause of disease. It can also assist in helping body, mind and spirit achieve a harmonious and balanced state of well-being. As well as freedom from illness, the principle behind TCM is achieving total wellness in all respects—physical, psychological and social. The practice of TCM therefore revolves around sustaining the body's natural balance.

The philosophy of TCM includes the theories of qi (pronounced "chee"), yin-yang and the five elements. *Qi* is vital energy, the basic "particle" that constitutes the cosmos and produces everything in the world through its movement and changes. Human life is believed to be endowed with the qi of nature and to be maintained by qi energy. The various actions and changes of qi, accompanied by energy transformation, are the basis of all of life's activities.

The theory of *yin-yang* is a primitive form of dialectical thinking—the law of the unity of opposites. According to this theory, everything in the world contains two opposite aspects, yin and yang, which are in conflict and at the same time interdependent. Traditional Chinese medicine asserts that the human body is full of opposites and that good health depends on the normal balance of yin-yang. It also requires co-ordination of yin-yang between the human being and the external environment. It is believed that disease occurs when that balance or co-ordination is broken down, so treatment is aimed at restoring the normal equilibrium.

Another key part of TCM is the *five elements*. The five elements refer to wood, fire, earth, metal and water. In the human body, key organs correspond to the five elements: wood to the liver, tendons and eyes; fire to the heart, blood vessels and tongue; earth to the spleen, flesh and mouth; metal to the lungs, skin, hair and nose; and water to the kidneys, bones and ears. Four laws—production, control, attack and resisting control—govern the relationships among the five element areas.

Causes of disharmony leading to disease

In TCM there are thought to be three causes of disharmony: internal, external and miscellaneous. Internal organs influence not only the physical body but also its psychological and spiritual makeup. The major internal causes of disharmony are considered to be psychological in nature and are termed the "seven emotions." These are anger, joy, sadness, grief, pensiveness, fear and fright.

Six external causes of disharmony relate to climatic conditions. Known as the "six pathogenic factors," these are wind, fire and heat, cold, dryness, damp, and summer heat.

The miscellaneous causes of disharmony are the internal and external effects of lifestyle, work, exercise, diet, sexual activity and unforeseen events.

As applied to medicine, all these philosophies emphasize a holistic view, with various parts of the body linked into an integral whole through an ongoing series of relationships. In a nutshell, it's all about checks and balances and making sure the various parts are in harmony.

All these ideas were originally philosophical thoughts, but later they became basic medical theories when they were applied to healing. Later, they were revised on the basis of medical practice. This led, ultimately, to the characteristics of TCM we see today.

Holism is the belief that the human body should always be viewed as an organic entity. In TCM the holistic view governs medicine in a way that can hardly be imagined by many Western-trained medical doctors. For example, pulse taking is believed not only to show changes in the cardiovascular system but also to provide information about almost all the organs and systems. Simply by inspecting the tongue, traditional Chinese practitioners can get information about the organs and all the body systems and where

TCM AT WORK

How does TCM work in a particular medical situation? Just for your interest, here's a table showing how traditional Chinese medicine diagnoses and treats chronic gastritis—inflammation of the stomach—by Dr. Xie Zhufan.

SYNDROME	DIAGNOSTIC CRITERIA	TREATMENT PRINCIPLE WITH HERBAL MEDICINE
Stagnation of qi of the liver and stomach	Distending pain in the epigastrium involving the side and back, accompanied by frequent belching; thin and white tongue coating; stringy, taut pulse	To regulate the flow of qi and pacify the stomach
Heat in the stomach	Severe pain with fullness and distention, distress in the stomach, acid regurgitation, irritability, bitterness in the mouth; reddened tongue with yellow, greasy coating; rapid pulse	To reduce heat and pacify the stomach
Deficiency of the stomach yin	Dull epigastric pain with burning sensation, distress in the stomach, feeling of hunger, reduced food intake, dryness of the mouth; dry and reddened tongue; rapid and thready pulse	To replenish the stomach yin
Deficiency—cold spleen and stomach	Continuous dull pain, aggravated when the stomach is empty and alleviated after meal or by pressure and warmth; watery regurgitation, lassitude, cold limbs, loose stools; pale tongue; deep, thready pulse	To warm and invigorate the spleen and stomach

there may be disease. The ears are viewed as parts of the body that are closely linked to all the internal organs, so these can be treated by pricking or stimulating a certain point of the ear.

In Western medicine we tend to treat the disease or the ailment. In TCM the idea is to treat the person. It's a big difference. When you go for diagnosis and treatment, traditional Chinese doctors will look at your body as a whole. They are observing your five functioning systems, each with a different organ at its core, all linked by meridians. After years of making these observations, traditional Chinese doctors have honed their skills and have a deep understanding of the human body, how all the systems interrelate, the nature of diseases and how to treat them.

The philosophy of Chinese medicine offers many alternative perspectives from which to diagnose and treat the disharmonies revealed by physical and mental complaints. The Eight Principles provide a systematic way to organize a lot of information about a very dynamic energy system—the human body. These Eight Principles are yin and yang, internal and external, cold and hot, and deficiency and excess. In addition, eight grand methods of treatment have been established in TCM as the guiding principles for medical practice. They are treatment by means of inducing perspiration, clearing heat, inducing bowel movements, striking a balance, warming up coldness, tonification, eliminating, and inducing vomiting.

Once you have been diagnosed, there are four main areas of treatment: acupuncture and moxibustion (heat stimulation), herbal medicine, food, and manipulation or exercise therapy. There is an old Chinese saying, "First you use the needle, then fire [moxibustion], and then herbs."

Acupuncture

This three-thousand-year-old Chinese medical treatment is one of the most popular complementary medicine methods, and it is probably the one most familiar to people in the West. Acupuncture therapy is intervention in the body by the use of specialized needles that are inserted into specific anatomic points on the meridian system where pools of qi—energy and electromagnetic charges—are located. It's thought that since the meridian pathways are linked to the internal organs, needle manipulation can unblock qi or blood stagnation as well as expel disease-causing toxins. Acupuncture is used to regulate or correct the flow of qi to restore health.

Throughout Chinese history, acupuncture steadily evolved into a practical and complex system, eventually offering treatments for various medical conditions. The meridian system is very important. The concept and its application have changed very little in the last two thousand years. Acupuncture has been adopted through the centuries by Japan, Korea and France (in the nineteenth century). In the past forty years it has become a well-known and reasonably available treatment in developing and developed countries.

Acupuncture was not introduced to North America until the 1970s, when China resumed political and cultural contacts with the West. In 1972, *New York*

Times columnist James Reston underwent an emergency appendectomy while in China. He later wrote about the successful acupuncture treatment for his post-operative pain. Quietly and significantly, acupuncture is making massive inroads in North America, and it has become an increasingly established health-care practice. An estimated three thousand conventionally trained U.S. physicians have taken courses to incorporate acupuncture into their medical practices. Americans make an estimated 9 to 12 million visits to acupuncturists annually, according to the U.S. Food and Drug Administration.

Research has produced some scientific evidence of how acupuncture works, helping to explain some of the effects of remote stimulation. Acupuncture-induced general analgesia, for example, is explained by the release of beta-endorphins in the brain. A series of controlled studies has revealed the efficacy of acupuncture in the treatment of a variety of conditions, including osteoarthritis.

Acupuncture has been effective in treating nausea caused by pregnancy and cancer chemotherapy drugs, as well as asthma, back pain, painful menstrual cycles, bladder instability, migraine headaches and pain resulting from surgery. It has also been used to induce surgical anaesthesia. Studies have shown positive results when acupuncture is used in chronic pain management and in the management of drug addiction—two common problems where conventional Western medicine has achieved only very limited success. Acupuncture has won the seal of approval from many Western health professionals. A panel of non-federal, non-advocate experts who convened in November 1997 for the National Institutes of Health endorsed acupuncture as an effective way to deal with pain. High-quality studies evaluating acupuncture for the treatment of pain have concluded that it is more than a placebo.

A long list of stories in which acupuncture was used successfully to treat patients with different clinical problems is well documented. For example, the British Journal *Anaesthesia* reported that laser stimulation of acupuncture point P6 reduces post-operative vomiting in children undergoing strabismus surgery. Now, the World Health Organization lists more than forty conditions for which acupuncture may be effective. Other studies have shown that acupuncture significantly reduces the need for drugs or lengthy stays in costly treatment facilities. Although acupuncture alone is usually not sufficient to relieve severe pain, researchers have noted that it works well when combined with lower doses of pain-killing drugs. It also seems to lessen the side effects, such as nausea, that the drugs may produce. In studies of substance abuse treatment, groups that received acupuncture had reduced cravings and improved psychological conditions.

Moxibustion   This ancient Chinese therapeutic technique is used to treat many diseases and symptoms. In moxibustion, the heat generated from burning a specific herb is used to stimulate acupuncture points. This treatment approach has been used routinely in hospitals in China. Extensive documentation and anecdotal evidence of its effectiveness have been recorded in the Chinese medical literature. More recently, a controlled trial by Cardini and Weixin found that moxibustion is helpful in late pregnancy in correcting the problem of a breech presentation.

Herbal medicine

This is the backbone of TCM. Chinese herbs are prescribed according to the body's state of disharmony. Their use in medicine is based upon ancient Chinese knowledge of their nature and capabilities. A TCM physician is familiar with a vast array of herbs and formulas and knows how to use them for various situations.

Herbal remedies have three important properties: flavour, energy and action. There are five flavours, four energies and four movements in Chinese herbs. The five flavours are pungent, sweet, sour, bitter and salty. The four movements are to push upward, to push downward, to float and to sink. The four energies are cold, hot, warm and cool.

The use of herbal medicine has been growing quite rapidly all over the world throughout the past decade. There have been many articles in scientific and medical journals reporting on the effectiveness of herbal medicine in treating disease. For instance, artemisin, an ancient malaria remedy, has been hailed as one of the biggest medical breakthroughs of the century. This so-called magic drug is derived from a native Chinese plant called qing hao. It was first described as a herb that could combat malaria in AD 341. Now, new studies suggest that it can be effective in treating not only malaria but scores of other ailments as well. The artemisinin family of herbs has also been used to treat drug-resistant malaria.

The *Journal of Diabetic Care* reports that ginseng effectively boosted the regular treatment of non-insulin-dependent diabetics. Ginseng therapy elevated people's mood, improved performance and assisted in lowering their blood sugar levels and body weight. The *British Medical Journal* reports that Chinese herbs can be used effectively against eczema. The prominent scientific journal *Science* reported that arsenic trioxide, an ingredient in a traditional Chinese remedy, has been used successfully to treat and cure acute promyelocyte leukemia, a fatal disease. More recently, Alan Bensoussan, head of the Research Unit for Complementary Medicine at the University of Western Sydney, and his colleagues discovered in a scientific trial that a Chinese herbal medicine formulation improves symptoms of irritable bowel syndrome. In fact, every day herbal medicines are found to be useful and effective in treating a host of diseases.

Food therapy

What the Chinese have known for centuries is that ordinary foods contain powerful healing properties. Chinese "dietotherapy" is based on traditional medicine and features food-based medicinal materials. According to TCM, medicine and food are of the same origin; as much of both originate from plants. I have found that the Chinese system of food cures is a fascinating and proven practical approach to health and to coping with the effects of aging and diseases. I urge you to read the booklet *Chinese System of Food Cures— Prevention and Remedies* by Henry C. Lu.

It is believed that the flavours, energies and actions of foods serve to nourish qi and the body's organs on a daily basis. Food, then, is essentially a medicine, not just fuel. The practice of using food as medicine is quite similar to that for herbs, which I have just described. Food cures show results only after a relatively long period, ranging from weeks to a few months or even longer. You may want to continue a cure throughout your life if it has proven beneficial to your health.

Fast food is anathema to practitioners of traditional Chinese medicine. The way we shovel food down as we rush out the door, or "grab a bite" in takeaway restaurants or wherever we are in our too busy modern world, stands in stark contrast to the discipline of a traditional Chinese meal. In order to gain maximum benefit from food, it is considered crucial to eat the right amount at regular times and in a disciplined manner. Begin now to bring greater harmony and health into your life with the most effective, most natural disease-prevention system of all: the foods you eat each day.

Manipulation or massage therapy

Acupressure, also known as Tui Na, is a form of massage therapy used to treat injuries and aid internal organs. It relieves symptoms and treats diseases through acupuncture points and the meridian system. This treatment can be used over general areas of the body to promote qi energy and good blood circulation. It can be employed on its own or with other treatment strategies. For example, acupressure massage is often used before acupuncture treatment.

There are three basic acupressure techniques used by the therapist:

- the calming technique, for a too active qi
  Use the whole palm evenly to gently rub or stroke the area concerned.

- the enhancing technique, for deficient qi
  Apply firm and stationary pressure with the thumb or middle finger to the chosen point.

- the releasing technique, for stagnant or blocked qi
  Apply firm pressure, but then move the pressure by making a small rotation of the thumb around the point, or by pressing in and out on the point.

A simple and straightforward acupressure technique can be used on yourself or on friends and relatives. Tension headaches and travel sickness often respond well to this type of treatment.

Exercise therapy

The practice of exercise techniques and specialized meditation, qigong and Tai Chi (see chapter 4) are believed to create a continuous flow of qi energy and to strengthen the immune system.

Qigong   Part of the ancient healing tradition of Chinese medicine, qigong began to be practised in the fourth century AD. Since then it has been passed down through the generations and has become an integral part of the Chinese culture. It is essentially an exercise for regulating the mind and breathing by helping the qi, the vital energy of the human body, to circulate freely and nourish the internal organs. Qigong also improves quality of life by concentrating on the mind, body and breath. Some of the benefits of qigong exercise are preventing or alleviating diseases, strengthening the constitution, avoiding premature aging and prolonging life.

Generally speaking, there are two types of qigong. One is "quiescent," performed when you are standing, sitting or lying down; it uses special breathing techniques to focus the mind. In the second, "mobile" type, the participant practises a set of movements while keeping a proper balance between mind and emotion, qi and strength. The mobile type usually combines qigong and physical exercise or self-massage.

Qigong is not the same as gymnastics or other modern sports. It can certainly strengthen the tendons, bones and skin and improve appearance, but it has other qualities as well. The exercises that are part of it have been shown to help in the treatment of many different diseases and medical conditions. Medical qigong can be divided into two main categories: internal qigong and external qigong. The patients themselves practise the first kind to preserve and promote their own health. Internally, qigong can enhance the spirit, the qi and the mind. In the second type, a qigong master leads the exercises for treatment of diseases or conditions.

I would like to see qigong as an option in mainstream Western health care. It is suitable for everybody—old and young, men and women, wealthy and poor, strong and weak. Those who persevere in practising the qigong exercises often find themselves feeling younger and stronger than ever before. Eight million people in China now arise early every morning to practise qigong together in parks and even at their worksites. These exercises have been attracting attention from health professionals and intellectuals around the world. See appendix 8 for instructions on practising internal qigong.

Can TCM be part of your self-care?

Yes! There are all kinds of ways you can use some of the elements of Chinese medicine to help you stay healthy. Let me suggest a few:

- *self-assessment:* using a self-reflective exercise, such as Tai Chi, to assess your state of mind and body
- *self-practice:* including meditation, Tai Chi and qigong
- *self-control:* which embraces all the good things in life, like a healthy diet, healthy lifestyles and the use of supplements such as tonics, vitamins, herbal remedies and minerals
- *self-treatment:* in which you learn about and perhaps try healing practices like acupressure and qigong in addition to using food and plant remedies and herbal teas

We need research to bring it all together

Extensive research has been done in China through the institutions of traditional Chinese medicine, but only in the past quarter-century have biomedical scientists in China characterized and identified active agents in much of the traditional medical formulations. I've already talked about the difficulties of measuring the effectiveness of traditional Chinese medical treatment. Still, it is imperative to make the attempt if some of these valuable ancient healing arts are to take their rightful place in modern medicine. It's worth doing, and it's about time the West uncovered the secrets that for centuries have been benefiting millions of Chinese people.

In November 1998, a *JAMA* editorial recommended that research funding for complementary medicine should be directed to investigating the relevant clinical problems in areas where alternative therapies have shown encouraging

COMPARISON OF THE TWO MAJOR MEDICAL SYSTEMS

	WESTERN SCIENTIFIC MEDICINE	TRADITIONAL CHINESE MEDICINE
Attention directed to	Trauma Acute illness Chronic illness Prevention of illness	Wellness Health maintenance Prevention of illness Chronic illness
Philosophy concentrates on	Materialistic explanation, anatomy, physiology, natural science	Non-materialistic explanation, qi (vital energy), yin-yang, five elements, natural philosophy
Principles based on	Evidence	Non-evidence
Intervention focuses on	Physical body Homeostasis of physiological state	Energetic body Flow of energy within the body and between the patient and the cosmos (adaptability); healing through balancing the bodily harmonies
Biological view of patient	Human beings are biologically similar, therefore similar treatment for same disease	Each human being is unique, therefore individualization in treatment for same disease
Clinical approaches	Focus on diagnosis and treatment Symptoms relieved	Unique system of diagnosis: pulse taking, inspection of the tongue, syndrome differentiation Treatment: holistic approach, promotion of healing, treatment of underlying cause
Body/mind interaction	Separation	Strong connection

results. The editorial urged researchers to focus on common medical conditions, especially those that have stymied conventional medicine. Of course, thorough and top-quality research is essential. There is no doubt that from now on these unconventional techniques will be subjected to the new, demanding style of evidence-based medicine that marries systematic clinical experience with painstaking research.

Other traditional medicines

Ayurveda is a traditional, natural system of medicine that has been practised in India for more than five thousand years. Practitioners believe that all disease begins with an imbalance or stress in people's consciousness. Ayurveda takes an integrated approach to preventing and treating illness, through lifestyle changes and the use of natural therapies. There are ten Ayurvedic clinics in North America, including one hospital-based clinic that has served twenty-five thousand patients since 1955.

In India, Ayurvedic practitioners receive state-recognized training in accredited institutions, parallel to that of their conventional physician peers. There is also a growing body of research into the effects of meditative techniques and yoga postures. Published studies have documented a reduction in the risk factors for heart disease, including lower blood pressure levels, reductions in bad cholesterol and better reaction to stress, among people who practise Ayurvedic methods.

Laboratory and clinical studies on Ayurvedic herbal preparations and other therapies have shown them to be useful in preventing and treating certain cancers, treating infectious disease, promoting health and addressing the problems associated with aging.

North American Native peoples have their own medical systems and beliefs. They have developed several rituals and practices, such as sweating and purging, the use of herbal remedies gathered from the surrounding countryside and sometimes traded over long distances, and the healing wisdom of the much-respected holy shaman. These shamanic healers often invoke spiritual powers to aid them in their healing techniques.

There has been little formal research into the techniques, although Native people have much faith in their healing ceremonies and herbal remedies. It's claimed that their approach can cure ailments and diseases such as heart disease, diabetes, thyroid conditions, cancer, skin rashes and asthma.

Latin America also has its community-based practices. These include a folk system of medicine called *curanderismo*, which is actively used in much of Mexico and among some Hispanic U.S. citizens.

Contemporary Complementary Medicine

Contemporary complementary medicine, sometimes referred to as New Age medicine, has become very popular in recent years. Nevertheless, it has quite a way to go before it's accepted by the mainstream. There's still a lot of suspicion. One of the problems is that there are so many "new" complementary therapies out there that it's difficult to separate the good from the bad, the effective from the downright dangerous.

I don't like all complementary therapies, but many of them have real potential, in their entirety or in part. Here you'll really have to do your homework by carefully testing which complementary or natural system works well for you. More reliable information is on its way, thanks to better communication. Again, the Internet is a useful place to search for information.

What is complementary medicine?

A panel at the World Health Organization in 1997 defined complementary medicine as "a broad domain of healing resources that encompasses all health systems, modalities and practices other than those intrinsic to the politically dominant health system of a particular society or culture in a given historical period." In other words, you will find most of these "healing resources" advertised in alternative papers and magazines but not used at your local hospital or clinic. It's a constantly evolving medicine, where the boundaries change from one day to the next. One of the more comprehensive and widely accepted areas of complementary medicine is naturopathy.

Naturopathic medicine: an introduction

This is one of the fastest-growing complementary systems. As you might guess, it is rooted in the natural. In this healing method, natural means are used to empower people to become healthy. It's a comprehensive system for health and illness that draws on the healing wisdom of various health-care systems.

As practised today, naturopathic medicine integrates traditional natural therapeutics—including botanical medicine, clinical nutrition, homeopathy, acupuncture, traditional oriental medicine, hydrotherapy and naturopathic manipulative therapy—with modern medical diagnostic science and standards of care.

Benedict Lust, the founder of naturopathic medicine, put forward his ideas in 1918 in a treatise called "The Principles, Aims, and Program of the Nature Cure System." He wrote: "The natural system for curing disease is based on a return to nature in regulating the diet, breathing, exercising, bathing and the employment of various forces to eliminate the poisonous products in the system and so raise the vitality of the patient to a proper standard of health." Official medicine, he went on to say, has over the years attacked the symptoms of disease without paying attention to its causes. Natural healing aims to get to the root cause of the ailment. These cures avoid the use of medication and thus are styled "a system of drugless healing."

A history of naturopathic medicine

Naturopathic medicine, as a distinct American health-care technique, is almost one hundred years old. Here are some of the milestones:

LATE NINETEENTH CENTURY	founded by Benedict Lust; origin in the Germanic hydrotherapy and nature cure traditions
1900 TO 1917	the formative years; convergence of American dietetic, hygienic, physical culture, spinal manipulation, mental and emotional healing, homeopathic/eclectic and homeopathic systems
1918 TO 1937	the halcyon days; during a period of great public interest and support, diversification of the philosophy and scope of the therapies to encompass botanical, homeopathic and environmental medicine
1938 TO 1970	days of decline; legal and economic suppression as a result of the American infatuation with technology and the emergence of "miracle" drugs and effective modern surgical techniques perfected in two world wars
1971 TO PRESENT	naturopathic medicine re-emerges; reawakening of public awareness about health prevention and concern for the environment; regeneration of public interest through modern, accredited physician-level training

The principles of naturopathic medicine

Seven major concepts provide the bases for naturopathic medicine:

1. *The healing power of nature* Nature acts powerfully through healing mechanisms in the body and mind to maintain and restore health. When

these inherent systems are not working, naturopathic physicians try to restore and support them by using methods, medicines and techniques that are in harmony with the natural processes.

2. *First, do no harm*   Naturopathic physicians prefer non-invasive treatments that minimize the risk of harmful side effects. They are trained to know which patients they can treat by these gentle methods and which should be referred to other health-care practitioners.

3. *Find the cause*   Every illness has an underlying cause, often rooted in the lifestyle, diet or habits of the individual. Naturopathic physicians are trained to locate the source of the problem and help their patient find ways to overcome it.

4. *Treat the whole person*   Health, or lack of it, arises from a complex interaction of your mental, emotional, spiritual, physical, dietary, genetic and environmental situations. Naturopathic physicians treat the whole person, taking everything into account.

5. *Preventive medicine*   The naturopathic approach to health care helps avoid disease altogether and aims to prevent minor illnesses from developing into more serious or chronic, degenerative diseases. Patients are taught how to live a healthful life and reduce their risks of major illness.

6. *Wellness*   This is inherent in everyone. If wellness is truly recognized and experienced, people will heal more quickly than they would through direct treatment of the "disease" alone.

7. *Doctor as teacher*   The original meaning of the word "doctor" is teacher. A main objective of naturopathic medicine is to educate the patient and emphasize responsibility for one's own health. Naturopathic physicians also recognize the therapeutic potential of the doctor–patient relationship.

Today, few people would disagree with some of these basic precepts of naturopathy. Moderation is the key in the pursuit of health and wellness. In naturopathy you are encouraged to get rid of unhealthy habits and avoid excesses, whether they are food, alcoholic drinks, drugs, the use of coffee or meat eating. Healthy living the naturopathic way also means getting enough sleep, having a normal sex life, enjoying your social life and not allowing yourself to be overburdened by life's worries. Once you are living a balanced life, naturopathic physicians are able to use therapies to enhance your body's inherent healing power; this is at the core of natural healing.

Dr. Joseph Pizzorno, president and founder of Bastyr University, the only accredited college of naturopathic medicine in the United States, urges people to care for themselves. The human body has such tremendous self-healing potential, he says, that in upwards of 70 percent of all cases, people recover from illness without ever seeing their doctors. He maintains that it is when people become too fixated on their symptoms that they sometimes lose their natural ability to detect the body's help signals. Dr. Pizzorno also believes that symptoms are more than just signals of disease; they reflect a patient's lifestyle and environmental challenges. The best naturopaths, he adds, are those who can understand the natural healing processes and recognize what is needed for their patients to have faith in their innate healing abilities.

Much of this is right in keeping with the philosophy behind HQ. I share many of the same goals as naturopaths, and I am not alone. Other medical practitioners are starting to endorse naturopathic techniques of lifestyle change supplemented by small doses of multivitamins and safe herbal tonics. It is likely that this trend will continue and there will be more scientific research in the field.

Other contemporary non-mainstream techniques

Chiropractic   Developed by Daniel David Palmer in the United States in the late nineteenth century, the origins of chiropractic medicine lie in ancient Greece. Chiropractic science is concerned with investigating the relationship between the structure (primarily related to the spine) and the function (primarily related to the nervous system) of the human body to restore and preserve health. Chiropractic medicine applies such knowledge to diagnosing and treating structural dysfunctions that can affect the nervous system. Chiropractors consider disease to be the result of a disturbance in the nervous system. It is thought that misalignments in the spine, "the centre of the nervous system," affect people's health. Chiropractors correct these displacements through direct manipulation, using manual procedures and interventions, creating the conditions for the body to heal itself. Chiropractic treatment is a popular approach to lower-back pain. All chiropractors must be licensed in order to practise.

Homeopathy   Homeopathic medicine is practised worldwide, especially in Europe, Latin America, Asia and North America. This therapy was started by Samuel Hahneman, a German physician, in the eighteenth century. He believed that disease signifies a disturbance in the body's ability to heal itself. Thus, symptoms are a manifestation of the body's natural response. The underlying principle of homeopathy is that a remedy can cure a disease only if it is able to produce symptoms similar to that of the disease in a healthy person. Homeopathic remedies are extremely diluted natural substances that are chosen with reference to each patient and the physical symptoms. The remedies, made from naturally occurring plant, animal or mineral substances, are thought to stimulate the body to heal itself. They come in tablets, pills, capsules and sachets of powder. The exact dose required depends on the intensity of the symptom. Homeopathy is used to treat acute and chronic health problems as well as in disease prevention and health promotion. Recent clinical trials suggest that homeopathic medicines have a positive effect on allergic rhinitis and influenza.

Herbal medicine Many plants have known medicinal effects that can be used to treat symptoms and restore health by stimulating the body's normal functions, enabling it to heal itself. Many herbal remedies have been used for thousands of years. Treatments are made from whole plants, parts of a plant (such as the leaves, stem, flowers or seeds) or extracts of plants. Herbal remedies can be taken in many forms: tablets, teas, mixtures, suppositories or creams. A single remedy might use one plant or many plants in combination.

The use of herbs has become one of complementary medicine's most popular practices. For example, just look at the number of people who swear by herbal tea instead of regular orange pekoe or coffee. Herbal advocates believe that nothing was put on this earth without a purpose. Chickweed, for instance, one of the most common plants in the world, is supposed to help cure many ailments. Some of these plant uses may be debatable and are not scientifically proven, but people are enthusiastically trying all kinds of herbs anyway. Witness the recent success of the plant St. John's wort, which many are calling a wonder drug that can counteract minor and moderate depression. The word gets around fast on the informal grapevine. Echinacea, good for treating colds and flu, has been selling like hotcakes in health food stores and is now stocked on the shelves of your local pharmacy and supermarket.

Gardeners and green-thumbers have taken to growing their own herbs. There are dozens of books devoted to herbs on the shelves and a whole explosion of Web pages on the Internet. A gentle reminder: use your HQ and be careful—some of those herbs can be harmful.

Massage therapy Developed in different parts of the world, this is one of the oldest known forms of physical treatment. This therapy uses the scientific manipulation of the soft body tissues to return those tissues to their normal state. Massage consists of a group of manual techniques that include applying fixed or movable pressure and holding the body and causing it to move. The hands are used primarily, but sometimes forearms, elbows and feet are employed also. Massage therapy encompasses the concept of helping the body to heal itself, and it aims to increase health and well-being through the medium of touch. There are many kinds of massage therapy techniques, including Swedish massage, deep-tissue massage, sports massage and neuro-muscular massage. Other physical healing methods include reflexology, zone therapy, tuina, acupressure, Rolfing, Trager, Feldenkrais method and Alexander technique.

Osteopathic medicine One of the earliest health-care systems in the United States to use manual healing methods was developed by Andrew Taylor Still in the late nineteenth century. Osteopathy is based on the belief that health is determined by the structure of the skeleton. An extensive body of work supports the use of osteopathic techniques for musculo-skeletal problems. Treatment is based on the idea that blood should flow freely throughout the body, and it uses a variety of techniques to correct posture and the alignment of the spine.

Environmental medicine An extension of modern biomedicine, it developed from allergy treatment. Dr. Theron Randolph in the 1940s identified a variety of common foods and chemicals that were able to trigger the onset of acute and chronic illness even when exposure was at relatively low levels. Environmental medicine recognizes that illness can be caused by a broad range of allergy-aggravating substances, including foods, chemicals found at home and in the workplace, and chemicals in air, water and food. Today, there are three thousand physicians worldwide practising environmental medi-cine. There are several environmental control units in the United States and Canada, where patients' sensitivities are unmasked through fasting and complete avoidance of potentially problematic chemicals.

The Future of Non-Mainstream Medicine

Make no mistake: complementary medicine is destined to become even more popular in the new millennium. In a recent U.S. survey (Eisenberg et al., 1998), the increased use was shown to be staggering. The estimated number of visits to "alternative" medicine practitioners rose dramatically, from 427 million in 1990 to 629 million in 1997, and only 38.5 percent of those who used "alternative" therapies discussed them with their physicians. Total out-of-pocket costs for people using alternative medicine in 1997 were estimated at $27 billion—a significant increase from an estimated $13.7 billion in 1990.

Clearly, people are looking for alternatives, and their enthusiasm is beginning to arouse the attention of the media, governments, and the insurance and pharmaceutical industries. This will lead to the integration of proven complementary therapies into mainstream standard health practice—something I strongly support.

The growing interest in complementary therapies is also acting as a catalyst for change in the relationship between physicians and patients. A more collaborative relationship, which empowers patients to become actively involved in their own health care, allows them to reap the rewards of feeling in firmer control of their lives. Meanwhile, a shift in emphasis from treating patients to teaching them would encourage physicians to act as guides and mentors rather than paternalistic "experts." Patient care can then become a more fulfilling partnership.

I sincerely hope to see complementary medicine gradually become an integral part of mainstream medical practice. An idle dream? I don't think so. Some mainstream institutions in North America are already beginning to undertake interesting research on complementary therapies. I've mentioned the Office of Alternative Medicine in the United States. This now has a healthy budget as well as a healthy outlook, and it has been able to fund studies of complementary therapies at ten major academic centres, including the Harvard, Stanford and Columbia university medical schools. Our own Tzu Chi Institute for Complementary and Alternative Medicine, within the Vancouver Hospital and Health Sciences Centre (in partnership with all the other hospitals in Vancouver), will promote research and education on mind/body and complementary medicine. As the founder of the institute, I'll make sure it does! Meanwhile, many insurance companies in the United States are offering special plans that include complementary therapies.

More enlightened people in the medical community have begun to discover the advantages of using complementary therapies to assist their conventional health care. They have discovered that these sometimes work better, especially for patients with chronic conditions. As you have seen, complementary therapies could improve the health of the population and curb the upward spiral in health-care costs. This is also right in line with my HQ philosophy and goals. Use of the world's healing traditions and complementary care arises from a wider vision of what medicine can and should be, for the better health of all.

Tom Harkin, a U.S. senator from Iowa, pushed hard to elevate the status of complementary medicine and helped raise the Office of Alternative Medicine to "Center" status at the National Institutes of Health in Washington. He also created a national commission on alternative health care, which will generate more money for research into complementary medicine. The Center will initially receive $50 million in support. The purpose of the Center is not only to conduct basic research into complementary and alternative treatments but also to study the "integration of alternative treatment, diagnostic and prevention systems, modalities, and disciplines with the practice of conventional medicine as a complement to medicine and into health care delivery systems in the United States." Sounds like a lofty ambition, but it's very simple: as we head into the new century, the United States is about to look seriously at complementary health care. That is what this book has been suggesting: integration of the best of both disciplines.

NON-MAINSTREAM MEDICINE

- Use of non-mainstream medicine is a health reformation already in progress as people around the globe flock to the burgeoning array of complementary therapies.

- Generally, the medical establishment and the scientific world have been caught off guard by this phenomenon, and many traditional physicians are skeptical about the credibility and scientific merit of the alternatives.

- In 1992, the United States National Institutes of Health launched a grant program to do global research into complementary therapies. It has classified seven categories of therapies to study. A similar group has been established by the European Commission.

- Already, some of the complementary or alternative health-care systems have gained some recognition for their philosophies and approaches. Among these are acupuncture, acupressure, Tai Chi, qigong and herbs, from traditional Chinese medicine; and dietary counselling, micronutrient supplements and healthy lifestyle practices, from naturopathic medicine.

- Traditional Chinese medicine has gained a great deal of attention and interest from the West. It is a unique health-care system not only in terms of its holistic approach, historical background, clinical methods and philosophy but also because of the methods employed. In this system, an ancient art of healing is based on the belief that individuals can achieve health and well-being by harmonizing the mind, body and spirit. TCM also places strong emphasis on self-care, including qigong, Tai Chi, acupressure, meditation, spirituality focus, diet, habits, supplements, emotional intelligence and self-healing.

- Unfortunately, most of the complementary approaches lack standardization, quality control, and regulation for their safety and efficacy. Mind/body medicine, on the other hand, seems to have outgrown its alternative status to become an important adjunct or part of mainstream medicine through research and development.

- In the future, an enthusiastic public will drive the media, drug companies, governments, insurance companies and the traditional medical establishment to pay attention to this rapidly developing area of medical knowledge.

- We still need thorough and painstaking research into the safety and effectiveness of non-mainstream medicines and to sort out the genuine therapies from the hogwash. Our own Tzu Chi Institute for Complementary and Alternative Medicine at the Vancouver Hospital and Health Sciences Centre has a clear role to play in the ongoing debate.

- Mainstream and non-mainstream enthusiasts need to co-operate towards their common goals of extending health expectancy, improving quality of life and reducing suffering.

- Complementary medicine is a strong component of the HQ approach to health and health care.

CHAPTER 9

MANAGING YOUR ILLNESS THE HQ WAY

This is it. I've saved the best till last. In more than one sense, this chapter brings it all together for you on your HQ journey. It is the culmination of all the new insight you have gained from the previous pages. HQ medicine—how to manage your health the HQ way—is all about integration, blending the best of East and West, old and new, in your quest for personal health. Most important, it puts you at the centre; you are in charge of your health. After all, is there anyone who knows you better than yourself?

HEALTH GOALS FOR EVERYONE

- Stay healthy and well. Do everything you can to be full of vitality and to avoid disease.

- Do your best to recover fully from any illness that does occur, and reduce your likelihood of becoming disabled by disease.

- Make a point of improving your quality of life, especially any health-related aspects you can change for the better.

- Live longer and better! Why not set your sights on living as long and full a life as you can in the best possible health?

How can you make effective use of all the tools around you to improve your current health, future health and quality of life? In this chapter I'll help you understand how to manage your own health care, the HQ way. It's an exciting new realm of opportunity, combining the accumulated wisdom of the ages with all the blessings of modern-day medicine and the most up-to-date computer technology, literally at your fingertips.

Your HQ in the Information Age

In the industrial age of health care, the whole domain of lay medicine was largely ignored. A huge health resource of informed and experienced lay people, well able to prevent or manage their own health problems, was overlooked or sometimes actively discouraged. Enter computers, and everything changed. The old rules of the game are gone. Suddenly, that grand database of professional medicine is available to everyone. People are becoming aware that the mighty medical establishment no longer has a monopoly on health care. This has been described as the medical equivalent of breaking down the Berlin Wall.

We are living in the era of "the healing computer," and believe me, this will have an enormous impact on our personal health and health-care systems around the world. I am enthusiastic about what this technological future has in store because it empowers people to take charge of their own health care—an underlying principle of my HQ philosophy. I also believe that people will need a high HQ to participate fully in the new health information age. We need to start now to equip people to use the tools within their grasp and to play their part in the emerging health environment. This involves far more than teaching them how to look for the best health sites on the Internet. I would like to see some of the basic skills of self-examination and self-help treatment taught in our schools. Life skills classes should also include lessons on how to create a health Web page and how to set up and operate a self-help network of support.

Let's look ahead to see how medicine might unfold in the health information age. I foresee a future where the health-conscious consumer, the supportive family caretaker, the online newsgroup co-ordinator, the corporate wellness professional and perhaps other key players yet to evolve will become the next generation of primary health practitioners. This health reformation comes at a crucial time, as many of our existing health services are in disarray and screaming for more money. There simply are not enough resources to go around. Using online health systems can lead to huge savings and at the same time actually improve the quality of care. Health networks that connect ordinary people to doctors or specialists, and self-helpers to each other, have a unique ability to transform patients into providers and problems into resources. At a time when the demands on professional health-care services outpace what nations can afford, we would be foolish to ignore the potential of computer-generated health. As we move into the next millennium, we should be giving it the same amount of attention, respect and support that in the past we have given to professional mainstream care.

Of course, every change brings with it new challenges. Not least of these is the overwhelming amount of health-care information available online. People will need to be skilled to sort out what is true and trustworthy among the medical overload. People with HQ knowledge will be able to use their common sense and will make a point of checking everything they are not sure about. Also, it's a sad reality that unscrupulous scammers roam the Net in search of vulnerable victims. They are adept at disguise and can sneak into regular chat lines or health networks. You will be wary, of course, of anyone promising cures or miracle treatments. Also, when surfing for health information, watch out for the so-called friend who tries to gain your confidence by pretending to share your symptoms. You may be tempted to divulge confidential information to someone that you have never met. In fact, this "friend" might be in search of potential customers for a particular health product or service. Genuine products would not need to advertise themselves in this way. Take a look at the resources section, chapter 10, where I have included a list of ten dangers of using the Internet, taken from an invaluable book, *Good Health Online* by J. Carroll and R. Broadhead.

As usual, we are playing catch-up when it comes to regulating online health information. As more people turn to computer-based health experts, we need to address the issues of liability and confidentiality right now, so that they don't impede the progress of this valuable tool.

As a doctor, I understand that many of my colleagues may find it difficult to adjust to the information age. Perhaps they feel threatened by the loss of power that will result from their patients having more choice and self-determination in health matters. Or they may simply be afraid of losing their livelihood as people turn to their computers for the information and advice that in the past would have taken them to their doctor's office. Only time will reassure these physicians that they do indeed still have a vital role in the new health reality, particularly in the area of diagnosis and treatment. In the meantime, the train of computer health is relentlessly speeding along and there are a thousand opportunities for those willing to get on board. I predict that before too long a highly qualified "Net doctor" will surface, who could have a great influence in the future of health-care delivery.

A new-millennium scenario

Let's look at an example of how a typical patient—a woman who suspects that her symptoms may be due to an undiagnosed ulcer—could use computer-based care. Right off the bat she should go to see her family physician for accurate diagnosis, recommendation and guidance, including drug and surgical treatments. She could also read online information and talk with experienced self-helpers on an ulcer support forum. She could view an online video illustrating her condition and find out about preventive self-help measures, such as changing her diet and managing stress. Online research would enable her to find out about local doctors with special training and hospitals that treat ulcer patients, and she could look into their preferred treatments, success rates and consumer satisfaction ratings. She might also want to access her online medical records someday to review earlier symptoms and drugs she had used in the past. She could record her findings and plans in a special "patient's notes" section. After reviewing her options, she could collaborate with her doctor of choice in selecting a treatment plan and keep track in her records of how the therapy is progressing. As long as she needed it, she would be able to participate in a self-help group for people with ulcers, getting support and advice, and sharing her own knowledge and expertise with others.

This is an exciting and challenging scenario, and it may not be too far off. Already there is a workstation for people with AIDS; an interactive system that helps men who have been diagnosed with an enlarged prostate decide whether to have surgery; a psychological spreadsheet for people experiencing stressful life events; and a voicemail-based system for creating self-help networks. There is even an information system in Cleveland serving drug-abusing pregnant women, who can phone in for the help that they need. All of this has spawned a new field of research called "consumer health informatics," which is devoted to the study, development and implementation of the use of computers and telecommunications for health consumers. These online health resources will surely help to reduce the long lineups in hospital emergency rooms and the demands on busy health professionals. Perhaps the word "patient" will gradually slip out of fashion, as people will no longer have to wait patiently to be seen. Instead, they will become responsible providers of their own health care. In many ways this will be a bonus to physicians, who will no longer face the frustration of trying to guide passive people who are unaware of their capacity to help themselves, and treating minor illnesses. It may also be a relief for health professionals to share the controversies that in the past they have felt obliged to keep to themselves.

Obviously, having a good HQ is vital if you are to become health literate in the modern world. In the resources section in chapter 10, I have included Carroll and Broadhead's list of ten good reasons why you should use the Internet for your own health care. There are many more. No magic wand is going to appear to save our beleaguered health-care services. As waiting lists for medical care grow longer, self-help will become a necessity. Carroll and Broadhead say, and I wholeheartedly agree with them, that people who learn how to take advantage of the vast medical resources online will cope far better with this new reality.

The Internet can prove a powerful ally if you are being sent home from the hospital to recover from illness or surgery, or if a loved one faces a serious medical situation. It also excels as a tool for researching the potential courses of action in health management. The global body of medical knowledge is expanding at such a rapid pace that the Internet is vital to keep you up to date with developments. For example, the rare affliction necrotizing fasciitis, widely known as the flesh-eating disease, is not likely to be found in your family medical book. Nevertheless, there is a wide range of information about it on the Internet. The Internet can also bring together or assist people who suffer from particularly rare conditions or diseases. Carroll and Broadhead point out that, as society ages, there will be increased pressure on long-term health care. Many people will opt for providing such care at home, and the Internet will help to support them and answer the many questions that will arise. For example, people struggling to cope at home with a family member who has Alzheimer's or a similar debilitating disease can find themselves physically and mentally drained. They might think that they are alone in their exhausting situation. The Internet provides them with a place to find the emotional support that they need. Carroll and Broadhead also urge people to use the Internet to get involved in the public debate over health issues. There is so much at stake as to how our health services will evolve that it is vital for everyone to become knowledgeable and make their voices heard.

All of this makes so much sense that I would like to endorse the computer as both a catalyst and an invaluable tool for HQ medicine. There can be no doubt that we are in for a sea change in attitudes, which will put you at the helm of your health care. The old mindset of running to the doctor's office for every minor ache or ailment is outdated. People are demanding more proactive care, and computers are rapidly filling the void. It's high time to learn what technology has to offer. You don't want to be left out of the loop when it comes to your health. Don't worry: HQ medicine will be there for sure, for it represents the best of all health worlds.

HQ, the Best of All Health Worlds

HQ medicine is a turning point in health care. It's a whole new system with a completely new set of values and a new, intelligent attitude to personal health. But in essence, it is not complicated or hard to understand. Basically, HQ medicine has four main characteristics: it is *holistic*, taking the whole person into account; it is *integrative*, embracing the best of all medical worlds; it is *self-caring*, recognizing that you are your own best health resource; and it is *evidence-based*, representing the most up-to-date scientific knowledge. Take a look at the diagram below to get a picture of how your health revolves around these HQ initiatives.

HQ INITIATIVES ON HEALTH AND HEALTH CARE
An Intelligent Approach to Getting Well and Staying Healthy

Wellness Model
(HQ health culture)

Achieving Maximum
Well-being and Optimal Health

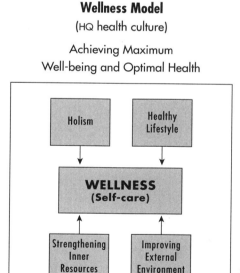

Integrative Health Care
(HQ medicine)

Using the Best from All
Health-care Systems for Healing

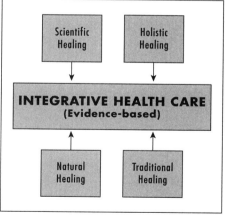

This diagram shows a wellness model in which your holistic and self-care approaches to health operate in tandem with your personal efforts to strengthen your inner resources and improve your environment. The resulting balance gives you the absolute best health and well-being. The HQ initiatives also include the integrative health-care model—HQ medicine. The integrative approach brings together the best evidence-based healing practices from all health-care systems based on the evidence and the most up-to-date knowledge of ways to prevent disease and manage illness.

The holistic view

Holism is the belief that the human body should be viewed as one organic entity, a complete system of mind, body and spirit, and that each whole person should be seen as unique. In terms of health care, this view places far greater emphasis on the patient than on the healer.

There is much to be gained if health-care professionals go beyond attending to just the physical symptoms and think about the overall experience facing their sick patients. It makes sense to treat the whole person. How does the disease affect the patient's mental state, emotional reactions and spirit? Is he or she under stress? Could mind/body techniques help to reduce the effects? I believe this is far more than just a fanciful idea, which would be "nice if we had the time." In my view it has become essential to treat people's emotions and their emotional distress as a high priority in their overall care. Holism is a necessity, not a luxury. It is a concept whose time has come.

Integrative care

Integrative healing brings the best of all health-care systems or healing practices to the management of your illness. If mind/body medicine, the ancient healing arts and complementary medicine are combined with mainstream health care, you really do have the best of all worlds. You will have a better chance to recover from illness, a potentially much healthier life and, more important, a better quality of life. Integration leads to a greater understanding of health and illness, with all professionals working together towards their common goal of making people well.

Imagine, if you will, a perfect HQ world, where you can pick from various systems, approaches and so on. Integrative medicine means you can look through the whole package of health-care systems and opt for the choices that work best for you. That's what it is all about: finding the right combination of care for your unique situation. It won't necessarily mean that the same treatment that works for your neighbours or your friends will work for you, even if you share a similar illness or set of symptoms; so it helps if you can be as fully aware of your personal health situation as possible.

Self-care

By now you are well aware of all those important ways to take good care of yourself, and you have a thorough review of your health with the HQ Profile! You also need to co-ordinate your self-care with your personal health team. Yes, you have a team. It includes your doctor, of course, but maybe you also call on a dietitian or nutritionist for assistance, use a fitness expert at the gym or a health support network on the Internet. All of these people are part of your personal health entourage. The more people you have on your team, the better. Don't be shy of taking advantage of what society has to offer when it comes to your health. There is a vast array of resources to help you look after yourself—everything from social networks and self-help groups to your trained reference librarian, who can point out the books, journals and Internet sites that may be helpful to your particular situation. While taking control of your health care, you will need to know how to work hand in hand with your doctor and the other members of your team. Good communication is a valuable skill in self-care. I have already talked about having a better doctor–patient relationship and noted that you may need to learn better techniques for talking to your doctor. Assert yourself when necessary, ask questions and be involved. For a complete picture, your doctor must be aware of all the health services you are receiving when he or she compiles your medical history, so remember that communication works both ways.

Today's doctors and medical students definitely need more training in communicating with patients. It's not easy for them, either. Imagine having to break bad news to people or elicit vital information from reluctant patients. They also need to be non-judgmental when asking about the health assistance you are getting from other places, such as complementary health-care services. At times, doctors and other health-care providers have to be circumspect in asking delicate questions. Your GP may need to assess your cultural, social and economic circumstances in order to help you weigh up the risks and benefits of treatment. Then you can reach a decision together about what needs to be done. This is the ideal health scenario, but most physicians are so busy that it doesn't usually happen. In fact, most of the complaints against physicians originate from poor communication. In my new HQ world this will change. People who are more knowledgeable and responsible about their health will no longer be crowding the surgery waiting rooms. The days of the traditional paternalistic doctor are numbered. Every day we are moving closer to a consumer-oriented situation, where you and your doctor are partners in your care. It's a powerful change.

Evidence-based medicine

Evidence-based medicine is one of the revolutions taking place in medicine today, with more and more physicians embracing the idea. It means, at its most basic level, keeping up to speed. David L. Sackett, a professor of medicine at

Oxford University and one of the discipline's founders, defines it as "the conscientious, explicit and judicious use of current best evidence in making decisions about the care of individual patients." The evidence-based movement also seeks to discover ways to ensure that physicians can be confident they really are doing something that will improve patient health.

The idea is that health-care decision making should reflect more clearly the results of scientific research. It de-emphasizes intuition and requires new qualities in the physician. Not only does he or she require top-notch medical skills, but the general practitioner, intern or surgeon needs to have skills in information technology, the ability to search scientific journals, and an ever-inquiring mind. It's not enough to say, "Well, I learned this in medical school." Now, every treatment has to be based on up-to-date scientific evidence, because the medical literature is forever changing. There's also, somewhat controversially, a belief that the longer a doctor is out of medical school, the less knowledgeable he or she becomes about current best practices.

The movement is still in its infancy, but I would highly recommend that you raise the subject with your physician. The patient with a good HQ will ask, "Do you believe in evidence-based medicine?" And when the doctor suggests a certain treatment, the patient will ask, "What's the most recent scientific evidence about this kind of treatment? Have there been clinical trials? Have you studied the most recent medical literature on the subject?"

I embrace evidence-based medicine as a tool of the future. Knowledge is power. And that, whether you're a doctor or a patient, is at the root of HQ.

Treating Chronic Disease the HQ Way

Half a century ago, most people died before the age of fifty; now, the majority live well beyond that age. Average life expectancy at birth reached sixty-five years in 1996. While increasing global longevity is a desirable goal in itself, how much better would be the blessing if it could be accompanied by freedom from additional years of pain or disability. Unfortunately, for many millions of people, there is as yet no such freedom. The quality of human life is just as important as its quantity. People are entitled to be as concerned about health expectancy as about life expectancy.

Regrettably, as we have seen, in this world of cultural and technological transition we can expect worldwide epidemics of chronic diseases in the decades to come. It is urgent to find ways of reducing the impending burden on health care. Many issues need to be addressed in society: poverty, genetic predisposition to

THE HQ MODEL OF HOLISTIC MEDICINE

MAINSTREAM MEDICINE

Mainstream medicine is considered the scientific medicine, applying science and technology and putting emphasis on molecular and structural abnormality in diagnosis and treatment.

MIND/BODY MEDICINE

Mind/body medicine includes a variety of approaches—meditation, relaxation and social-support groups—that are designed to enlist the mind in achieving both psychological and emotional well-being and physical health.

COMPLEMENTARY MEDICINE

Traditional Chinese medicine is a form of healing art applied to harmonize the mind, body and spirit. Naturopathic medicine places emphasis on natural healing. Many other contemporary complementary approaches focus on a specific concept and techniques.

INTEGRATIVE, HOLISTIC HEALTH CARE
Evidence-based Medicine

PATIENT-CENTRED CARE
Self-care Approach

OPTIMAL HEALTH CARE
HQ Medicine

disease, occupational hazards, poor living environment and stressful working conditions. Much of the suffering and many premature deaths from chronic disease are closely linked to significant lifestyle changes that are happening everywhere. I'm talking about the transition from physical, outdoor labour to sedentary work; from rural to urban life; from traditional healthful diets to consumption of fatty or sweet fast food; from negligible intake of alcohol and tobacco to daily or heavy consumption of one or both; and from leisurely to more stressful daily living. Each of these changes takes its toll. In later life hundreds of millions of adults suffer from mental illnesses ranging from chronic depression to dementia, and untold numbers may be disabled for years by rheumatoid arthritis and osteoporosis. It doesn't have to be this way. At every stage throughout the entire human lifespan, opportunities exist for prevention or treatment, for cure or for care of chronic diseases. It all comes back to the HQ model of holistic medicine, integrating the best from all the health worlds for your personal care. Think about my three-part plan for dealing with chronic diseases:

1. Consult your physician for diagnosis and recommendation of treatment.
2. Use the Internet, books or any other source to find out how each of the health-care systems can help you. Specifically, to recap, mainstream medicine addresses diagnosis and treatment of chronic diseases and their symptoms; mind/body medicine treats stress-related problems or psychological stress caused by diseases; and non-mainstream medicine enhances natural self-healing power by changes in behaviour and the use of foods, herbs and manipulations.
3. Take your HQ medicine by improving your HQ score, practising relaxation and meditation, making lifestyle changes and taking supplements if necessary. There's more. You also need to approach your illness with the idea of integrated care; work with your health-care team to find integrated holistic therapies and then stick to your treatment plan.

So far, all this sounds good in theory, but what about in practice? I have chosen coronary heart disease, one of the major chronic illnesses of our age, to give you a better idea of how someone with a high HQ might approach the management of a chronic disease.

Managing coronary heart disease

Coronary heart disease—an illness in which your lifestyle and position in life play a major role—accounted for more than 7 million deaths worldwide in 1996. It was responsible for about one-third of all deaths in industrialized countries. In spite of some improvement, it is still the leading cause of death and disability in the United States. As I have mentioned, heart disease is now increasing in developing countries as their populations age and people adopt the unhealthy habits of the affluent West.

Look to your children: they may appear healthy enough, but the insidious process of heart disease may already have begun. Atherosclerosis—the narrowing of the coronary arteries due to fatty deposits—can start early in life. Its initial stages often occur in children and young people, and it tends to progress silently and without symptoms, until illness strikes. Yet, while the disease may be creeping up on people unawares, health experts are now well acquainted with the how and why. Years of research have made it abundantly clear that it is our dangerous lifestyles and unhealthy diets and habits, beginning in early childhood, that lead us slowly and relentlessly to that moment of devastation. A heart attack is an earth-shattering, sometimes fatal shock to your system—the body's alarm signal, which cannot be ignored. A deadly band of villains conspire to bring about this menace. I think that after reading this book you will recognize them: high blood pressure, cigarette smoking, dietary habits (particularly excessive intake of saturated fat), elevated blood cholesterol and homocysteine levels, lack of physical activity, obesity and diabetes. And lurking in the background are the genetic factors that interact with your environment to bring about added risk.

Nevertheless, you can fight back! Even after heart disease strikes, there is plenty of hope through the use of HQ medicine and the HQ approach to restoring wellness. Of course, I understand that it is hard to think clearly in the midst of the anguish of diagnosis and the realization that you are facing this life-threatening disease. It probably doesn't even register when your physician first tells you what is happening in your body. There are various stages of the disease, and it is important to find out which one you are in. Medical treatment varies, depending on the severity of the disease, from a simple prescription of aspirin or other "clot-buster" drugs to surgery. Angioplasty, which opens up the blocked artery with a balloon distention, and bypass heart surgery are becoming common procedures.

That's only the beginning. There is a whole distinct dimension of health care for people recovering from heart attacks or heart surgery. It involves a combination of exercise, health education and counselling, and it can be set up in any community, however small. You don't have to live in a big city to recover well. The goal is to enable you to return to a useful and personally satisfying role in society.

In earlier chapters I discussed at some length how personal lifestyle and habits can affect your heart. This is good news for heart attack victims because it gives them plenty of opportunities to make changes that will help to prevent another attack. HQ abilities will help in this process. Here's one clue: in chapter 4, in the sections on lifestyle and diet, I described the Chinese puzzle—why is the incidence of cardiovascular disease in mainland China about one-fifth that in the developed world? It seems as though diet is the key, in particular flavonoids and folate, found in green tea, soy products and vegetables. Both folate and those mysterious flavonoids may also help protect the arteries from damage.

Now let me provide the heart attack victim with some more ideas. How much mainstream help do you need? How much mind/body and complementary medicine? Some of each? More of one? In dealing with this situation, the high-HQ person will learn the facts (old, new and on the horizon) about coronary heart disease; take personal action (self-care) to prevent the development or progression of the disease; and improve quality of life by finding ways to lessen suffering and enhance the chances of recovery.

Changing behaviour for the better

Heart disease, as you know, is caused or made worse by smoking, poor diet and physical inactivity, and by the risks inherent in social isolation, depression and hostility. High blood pressure is another significant risk that you can do something about, by tackling obesity, excessive intake of salt and alcohol, and your exposure to chronic stress. As you successfully lower your blood pressure levels, at the same time you are reducing the chance of having a repeat heart attack.

Improved survival rates have meant that there are now many people at risk for increasing disability because of their existing disease. Programs to change behaviour for the better are evolving and prove to be very promising. The preliminary evidence shows that an intensive program that combines stress management with dietary changes and exercise can even reverse the effects of heart disease.

Stick to your medical program and aim for a high quality of life

Two things are essential for improving your odds after a heart attack: aiming for a good quality of life and following your medical plan.

Quality of life is a subjective dimension that varies greatly from person to person. You have to take into account such things as your ability to take care of yourself, your mobility, whether your social needs are being met, your ability to work, and your overall feeling of satisfaction and fulfillment. The success of any treatment you take must be viewed in this wider context. The most important thing is whether you are satisfied that your quality of life is your personal best.

The ultimate success of your treatment depends a great deal on how closely you co-operate with your doctor in working out a program best suited to your needs. This partnership is especially important when treating chronic diseases. Statistics tell us that as many as 30 to 70 percent of patients may fail to follow their recommended treatments completely. When it comes to the tougher recommendations, such as to stop smoking, the failure rate is even higher, more like 80 percent. Others neglect to take their medications. Of course, these people are making a huge mistake and will likely suffer serious consequences. This is one of the reasons why it is important to have people around you who can support you.

Heart attack victims need lots of support

Don't try to go it alone if you are a heart attack survivor. You will need plenty of good support. In fact, recent data suggest that support will make all the difference to how long you will live after your first diagnosis of heart disease. This conclusion makes sense, because well-supported patients tend to comply better with their treatments and are more willing to make positive health changes. When people feel cherished and cared for, their emotional state is strengthened. In one clinical trial, socially isolated men who had experienced a heart attack and high life stress had a four times greater risk of death. In another study, patients who lived alone had a greater risk of mortality following a heart attack, as did patients who were unmarried or reported no close friends. Social isolation and lack of social support also had a measurable impact, causing a pattern of repeat attacks and a poor quality of life.

Change your life to heal your heart

The cardiologist Dean Ornish in his book *Reversing Heart Disease* shows how changing your life can heal your heart. An improved diet, stopping smoking, an exercise program and a positive outlook on life can all help. His reversal plan recommends a vegetarian diet, daily multivitamin supplements, moderate exercise of three hours accumulated per week, stress management through use of the relaxation response, meditation, and group support sessions to nurture patients and help them to develop more love and intimacy in their lives.

After a year, a group of twenty-eight people with heart disease who were on the Ornish reversal plan showed dramatic progress compared to people who followed conventional advice. The table on the next page shows the difference:

CONTROL GROUP		TREATMENT GROUP
−5.4 %	Total cholesterol	−243 %
−5.8 %	LDL-cholesterol	−37.2 %
+1.7 %	Body weight	−11.1 %
−6.4 %	Systolic blood pressure	−5.2 %
+165.5 %	Angina incidence	−91.2 %
+8 %	Size of arterial blockage	−5.5 %

Dr. Ornish's treatment fits in well with some aspects of the HQ concept. As a prominent cardiologist, Dr. Ornish has access to all the up-to-date knowledge about the mainstream approaches to heart disease, including sophisticated diagnostic techniques, drugs and surgery.

Two cardiovascular programs at the Beth Israel Deaconess Medical Center Mind/Body Medical Institute offer a method of helping patients at risk for developing heart disease (those with high blood pressure, a high cholesterol level and diabetes) and others already diagnosed with the illness. The philosophy of the programs is to provide comprehensive lifestyle management. This includes self-empowerment skills that stimulate self-care and make possible a shift in attitude, allowing people to view life in a more positive and open way. Each program is based on the relaxation response combined with nutrition, exercise and mind therapy.

Personal actions bring about the best results

You can tell already that there is plenty of scope for you to find out which therapies or combination of therapies will work best for you. I can't stress enough how much your personal actions will make a difference to the healing of your heart. This is one area where self-care can reap rich rewards.

Essentially, changing your habits can help you to control or overcome heart disease. Positive life changes will boost your nervous system, thus protecting your heart and decreasing your susceptibility to the disease. Switching to a healthy diet and maybe taking a multivitamin supplement, as well as getting regular exercise, can actually bring about a turnaround of the dangerous buildup of fatty deposits in the arteries. This will significantly reduce your chance of having a repeat attack. Your outlook can be even better if you deal positively with your stress through mind/body medicine. Whatever you do, if you find yourself getting depressed, get some help; people suffering from depression and anxiety are more likely to have recurring heart attacks and suffer more pain.

I have emphasized the need to take an integrated approach to handling your heart care. This should include the gamut of everything that conventional and complementary medicine can offer in terms of therapies to minimize your risks. Clearly, it will require personal actions and efforts to make the program successful. The table below outlines the highlights of each medical system:

MAINSTREAM MEDICINE	MIND/BODY MEDICINE	COMPLEMENTARY MEDICINE
Diagnosis: angiogram, cardiac imaging, enzyme measurement, blood cholesterol homocysteine level Drugs: Aspirin, nitroglycerine, streptokinase, beta blockers, blood-pressure-lowering drugs Surgery: angioplasty, bypass Rehabilitation program: lifestyle changes, weight control, stop smoking, diet, exercise, monitoring cardiac function	Holistic approach Stress reduction: relaxation response, meditation (yoga) Behavioural change Social group support Use of emotional intelligence Treatment of depression	Enhancing natural healing Food as medicine: natural, organic products, Asian food pyramid, lowering homocysteine level with dietary folic acid, moderate alcohol, nutritional counselling Supplements: folic acid, multivitamins, antioxidants, herbs as tonic Exercise: qigong, Tai Chi, walking, aerobics

The Future with HQ

Before I move on from this discussion of HQ medicine and chronic diseases, I would like to answer a couple of questions that may be buzzing in your brain. If the world is going to advance so dramatically, isn't its technology going to save us from the effects of chronic disease? And if we'll be born healthier and live longer, surely technology will enable us to live better too?

The answer to both is yes—but only as far as it goes. Optimistically, we'll experience a dazzling technological future where designer drugs are made to order to treat individual patients, where microchip implants can release needed medicines into the body, or in which virtual-reality therapy can provide patients with relief from their condition in a computer-generated

---

KEY SELF-CARE SUGGESTIONS FOR PEOPLE WITH CHRONIC DISEASE

- Improve your HQ score.

- Enhance self-healing.

- Improve your quality of life.

- Adhere to your treatment program.

- Make lifestyle changes: commit yourself to exercising, a healthy diet (HQ diet), drinking no excessive alcohol, stopping smoking and maintaining normal body weight.

- Practise the relaxation response and other mind/body techniques.

- Practise Tai Chi or qigong regularly.

- Be a partner with your doctors and health-care providers.

- Identify associated clinical conditions.

- Learn about self-monitoring.

- Keep informed, using online information (consumer health informatics).

- Join a self-help network.

---

fantasy world. High technology, however, cannot exist alone. A patient on a high-tech life support system isn't exactly living a life of high quality. We may find the future health outlook exciting, but in reality most people will eventually develop sickness, experience suffering and require health care.

Our current health-care safety net is full of holes. In spite of all our high-tech achievements, we still cannot deal with all illnesses satisfactorily, and pain often becomes chronic. We need a new plan. In the early part of this book I emphasized the value of enhancing the quality of our lives by embracing wellness, increasing our health chances, living a healthy lifestyle and practising self-care. Now, a twenty-first-century health-care plan is needed to repair the holes and ensure the safety net for our future society. I believe that HQ medicine is indeed such a health-care system. Integrative, holistic and embracing the new self-caring reality, HQ medicine is just what the doctor ordered!

My HQ concept was born out of the realization that the old ways are not working for us and that there is a better way. I hope that you have not found my HQ medicine too hard to take! It's the best medicine for an ailing world, and a prescription for health that I would like to make available to all. I'm happy that you have come this far on your HQ health journey and now have the knowledge and resources you need to look forward to a healthier new millennium.

HIGHLIGHTS OF HQ HEALTH CARE

- Become familiar with the four main goals of personal health care: staying healthy, recovering fully from illness to avoid lasting disability, improving quality of life, and living longer in better health.

- Grab hold of the computer health loop; it may be the lifeline you need. Don't let go until you have found out the myriad of ways it can help you to improve your health. Check out the resources section of this book (in chapter 10) for a list of ten excellent reasons for seeking health online—and ten reasons why you should be careful of what you find there.

- The four key characteristics that define HQ medicine are holistic, integrative, self-caring, and evidence-based.

- Consider your personal health team. Do you need more health helpers onside? These might include a nutrition adviser, a fitness expert or personal trainer, a self-help group, or even your friends and family members if they are prepared to support your fitness goals.

- Chronic diseases are the scourge of our modern, self-indulgent world. Tackle them the HQ way with my three-part plan: consult your doctor, research the best therapies from all the choices available to you, and take your HQ medicine. That means improving your HQ score, practising relaxation and meditation, making lifestyle changes and taking supplements if necessary.

- Each chronic disease has unique features that require different management strategies. Integrative HQ-style medicine enables you to have an endless variety of combinations of different therapies from the choices available in mainstream, mind/body and complementary medicines. Regardless of what combination of approaches is used, it is imperative to practise self-care and to take control of and responsibility for your personal state of health.

- Coronary heart disease is an all too common killer. You can't begin too early to find ways to combat its devastating potential. The choices you make regarding your diet, lifestyle and habits may well decide whether you become a victim or you vanquish this insidious disease.

- The health-care system is at a crossroads. In spite of remarkable advances in science, medicine and technology, our current system is outdated and a burden on society. Dissatisfied consumers are demanding reform and new approaches to care. The overall HQ model is a new direction in medicine that can fill this void.

SECTION IV

NOW THAT YOU'RE HQ AWARE—WHAT'S NEXT?

CHAPTER 10

HQ ACTION FOR STAYING HEALTHY AND GETTING WELL

Create Your Personal Action Plan

You now have many of the tools you need to develop true HQ, or to become an active health consumer. You have an accurate portrait of how healthy—or unhealthy—you really are. You know about the various health options that are open to you. You're well versed in the concept of self-care, or realistically caring for yourself, and becoming a healthier, happier person. And you know you want to improve your life and your health.

Now for the most difficult part: how do you make it all happen?

If you want this book to really work for you, I strongly urge you to develop a personal action plan; that's the only way you're going to reap the full benefits of the information you've gathered so far. The worst thing you could do right now is to put this book aside, to say to yourself, "That was interesting," and then forget everything you've learned within a week. It's vitally important for you as an individual, as someone who cares about quality of life, to work to improve your HQ score—and your life.

Simply by reading this book, you've taken a giant leap along the road to good health. But how do you ensure you're going to stay with the program? Three things are essential: willpower, discipline and time management.

Willpower and discipline are, I know, two of the most prickly words in the English language. Ask any smoker to give up cold turkey and you begin to appreciate the enormous importance of willpower. It's never easy to kick willpower into gear. But willpower starts with a specific goal. The smoker knows that he is short of breath, knows she is spending an enormous amount of money to fuel her habit, knows that there's an ongoing risk of emphysema, cancer, lung defect or even heart disease. Yet many smokers continue—because it's easier. Willpower only works when you look beyond the moment. It requires motivation. For the smoker, it's asking what life would be like without smoking. How about a walk with your children or grandchildren without puffing and wheezing on an uphill climb? How about having a longer life? How about escaping the guilt every time a match hits the end of a cigarette? How about more money in your pocket? (Some ex-smokers I know save all the money they would have spent on cigarettes for one year and then splurge on a trip—a perfect celebration.) Willpower comes down to this: trying. That's an easier word to handle. Simply deciding to try, to give it your best shot, is that first key step on the road to success. Willpower, always with an eye on the prize, is an extension of trying as hard as you can to achieve your goal.

Then there's discipline. The difference between the couch potato, who gets home at the end of the day and flops in front of the TV, and the active person, who goes out for a walk or a game of tennis, often comes down to discipline. Sure, you're tired after a long day of work or looking after the kids, and really, all you want to do is crash onto that sofa. But simply having the discipline to do something on a certain day—a walk, a swim, a jog—will help turn your health and your life around. Having the discipline to resist that doughnut and eat a carrot stick instead will in time—believe me—make you a happier human being. One way to make discipline easier is to create a habit and share it with a friend. It may be less disagreeable if you play squash one night a week with a buddy than if you try to do some other form of exercise by yourself. Or maybe get into the rhythm of walking to work or taking the stairs up to your office instead of the elevator. Every little bit extra you do will help your health.

And then there's time management. They teach long courses to managers and executives about how to handle their time effectively in the workplace, but time management is just as crucial at home. You must make time for yourself and your health. Working yourself to a standstill, living in a world of stress and fatigue, is a recipe for disaster. Of course, I understand that modern life often requires a major juggling act around the demands of children, work and home. "I don't have time" is an all too familiar refrain. But busy people can usually make time for the things that matter, and your health should not be at the bottom of that list; it should be a top priority. Don't put it off, because "later" may be too late. If you take the time now, you will have the time—and the best health—later.

So, how do I get there? By reading this book, you have learned the importance of adopting a new set of habits. Each of us learns and approaches change in his or her own way. Developing an awareness of yourself and your behaviour will enable you to take increased responsibility for your choices. You must decide which habits you wish to change. Then you must develop short-term and long-term action plans that allow you to continually evaluate, re-evaluate and readjust your plans to meet your goals.

Step one: set a long-term goal

On a piece of paper, set out what you wish to achieve in the long term; this could be three, six or twelve months. I recommend three for now. After three months you can check back and then set another three-month timetable; after that, six months. Look at your HQ score and identify the areas that need improvement. For instance, if you're overweight, simply write:

Goal: lose weight.

Beneath that, write the reason why you'd like to lose some pounds. Ask yourself what your true motivation is.

I'd really like to lose some weight so that I can be attractive to other people.

or

I'd really like to lose some weight so that I can wear fashionable clothes.

or

I feel embarrassed when I look in the mirror each morning and would like to lose weight.

Be honest with yourself. If you really, deep down, want to be attractive to the opposite sex, say so. If you hate the way you look, own up.

If you want to give up smoking cigarettes, write:

Goal: quit smoking.

Again, fill out your motivation.

I don't have as much breath as I once had.

or

I smell like an ashtray and I'm unattractive to people.

You can write down one, two, three or more long-term goals and the motivation for reaching those goals. But beware: setting the bar too high can be discouraging if you fall short. So set realistic goals.

Step two: set short-term actions

The actions or strategies you now write down will enable you to reach your long-term goal(s). So, on that same piece of paper, carefully list the actions that will be required to achieve the long-term goal, your HQ destination. If you want to lose weight, commit yourself to eliminating fatty foods, such as pizza and hamburgers, from your diet for the next three-month period.

Here's one way you may wish to structure a three-month plan:

LONG-TERM GOAL	REASONS	SHORT-TERM GOALS
Become fitter	I'm feeling lackadaisical and frumpy I want to look leaner and younger	Walk the dog three times a week Use the stairs at the office instead of the elevator Swim every Sunday afternoon Go for a two-mile walk every two weeks

I've made the above example as easy as possible; yours may be much more sophisticated. You may already be much farther along the HQ journey, depending on your HQ score.

Complete each of your action plans on a separate piece of paper. *Then— and read this carefully—sign it. This is your commitment to a better HQ.*

If you're willing to share your action plan with a family member or close friend, have that person sign it too. Reinforcement is a powerful thing. If your friend or relative also has an action plan, so much the better: you can sign each other's and support and encourage one another over the time frame you have chosen.

Now, hang your action plan on the wall, on the fridge or somewhere prominent. Each week, assess how well you have done. Did you really walk the dog? Did you go for that swim? If you didn't, simply go back to the beginning and read your entire action plan again. Look for more motivation and ask yourself what you need to change in your life to reach that elusive goal. Perhaps you can choose a less difficult aspect of your life to change, to make your first goal easier to attain. For instance, if you know you are not getting adequate sleep, instead of aiming to go to bed earlier every night, pick one or two nights a week that will work for you. Reward your efforts somehow, perhaps by allowing yourself to read a couple of chapters of a good book before you turn off your light. Be careful, though, that you don't get so engrossed in the story that you are still reading at two in the morning.

Let me give you an example of an action plan that worked. I know of a middle-aged man who kept saying he wanted to spend more time with his children. He was a successful businessman, a workaholic, and he kept complaining he had too little time for his kids. He loved them dearly but was pushed hard by his career and by the need to make money to pay for his house, cars and other accoutrements of a successful life. The point is, he kept promising to spend more time with his family—and never did. Then, one day, he had a heart attack. It wasn't a serious attack, but like many cardiac scares, it proved to be a wake-up call. It made him reassess what was really important in his life. Prestige and power paled in comparison with the idea of family.

After some discussions with friends and professionals, he filled out an action plan. He had three long-term goals: (1) to spend more time with his family; (2) to remove as much stress from his life as possible; and (3) to find time to stop and smell the roses. He wrote down his short-term goals, including leaving work early on Thursdays to play badminton with his family at a local recreation centre, and—I particularly liked this one—making Saturday sacrosanct, a day for walking, picnicking, skiing or family activities. Now, a decade later, he's fit, healthy and happier than he's ever been. And, most important of all, he still fills out an action plan every three months, after reassessing and re-evaluating his life and deciding what changes he'd like to make. *His heart is in great shape—in more ways than one!*

Making the action plan work

Without an action plan, the task ahead will often seem too large, too difficult. Here are some ideas on how to make your action plan workable—and the goal achievable.

1. **Be patient.** Rome wasn't built in a nanosecond. Swearing off doughnuts will not make you lose ten pounds in a week. Giving up smoking won't make you breathe much more easily for some time (the lungs take a long time to recover). You will get there eventually. Remember: it will take time.
2. **Monitor your progress.** Check regularly to see how you're doing. A weekly reality check will make all the difference.
3. **Don't procrastinate.** Don't put things off until it's too late.
4. **Rewards motivate.** Make sure you give yourself a treat to celebrate each achievement. If you've lowered the stress in your life, buy yourself a CD or a book you've always wanted. If you've given up smoking, or reduced the amount you smoke, use the money you've saved for a self-indulgent gift. If you've lost precious pounds off those hips, buy a new dress or pants; you may have to!

5.   **Project forward.** Think of the person you want to be a year from now. Visualize a better life, a healthier life, the kind of life you'd like to lead. Close your eyes and picture yourself in your perfect situation and ask yourself how you can get there.

Aiming to fully integrate HQ into your life should be an underlying theme of your action plan. How can you change your attitude to ensure that you take advantage of the lessons you've learned in this book? How can you enhance your health in the short and long term? How can you become more holistic, less dependent on traditional health care? Below, you'll find a number of resources that can be of particular use to you. I urge you to read the list carefully and decide whether any of them will help you to reach that not-so-elusive goal of perfect health. First, though, an idea to help you get motivated.

How to build up your HQ bank account

Good health, as I said at the beginning of this book, is more valuable than having millions of dollars in the bank. Now I would like you to consider the concept of an HQ "bank account" where you make deposits in your personal health. Every time you take a positive, health-building action, it is a deposit in your health account. You will be withdrawing from your personal health balance every time you make unhealthy choices. The odd withdrawal from time to time won't matter so much if you have made frequent deposits and maintain a healthy balance. In fact, if you have made regular deposits over a long period of time and have good reserves in your health savings account, well done! It means your health is probably in excellent shape and you have made yourself less susceptible to illness. Unfortunately, just as being constantly overdrawn at a regular bank will eventually lead to bankruptcy and financial disaster, too many withdrawals from your health account will make you increasingly vulnerable to health problems and serious disease. You wouldn't deliberately make yourself bankrupt, so why knowingly put your health in danger?

In the same way that it requires effort and self-control to stay on top of your financial affairs, you will need to take responsibility and show initiative to build up your health account. Think of it: you could become a "health millionaire." I guarantee you will feel like one!

KEY POINTS FOR CREATING YOUR PERSONAL ACTION PLAN

- The three qualities required to take the information in this book and make it work for you are willpower, discipline and time management skills.

- Decide which habits you want to change and develop short-term and long-term action plans, allowing for constant re-evaluation. Be realistic.

- Commit your plan to paper, carefully listing the actions and strategies you need to reach your goals. Sign it and display it in a prominent place in your home or workplace—or both!

- If possible, share your action plan with a close friend or family member; this will help to boost your morale and reinforce your intentions. All the better if your buddy has an action plan too!

- Monitor your progress, but be patient: major changes in your life may take many months. Reward each achievement, however small, and keep on track by constantly visualizing the healthy person you are aiming to become.

- Whatever you do, *start now!* It's all too easy to keep putting things off until tomorrow.

- Invest in yourself by making deposits in your personal "health account." Build up your long-term savings for a healthy balance. At the end of the day you will reap health riches that will be more valuable to you than the money in your bank account.

- Use the wealth of resources available to you on-line, while being watchful for false or inaccurate information. Read everything you can that pertains to your health, and find out which groups, organizations and institutions might be helpful to you.

- Repeat the HQ Profile questionnaire, make a commitment to progress, and take action to improve your scores as a means of building up your health account.

Resources

I. Online

The World Wide Web is a treasure trove of health and lifestyle information, and a convenient source for improving your HQ efficiently and quickly. Health-related sites abound on the Web, from easy-to-understand consumer health sites to complex medical home pages. The challenge is using the Internet effectively. Yes, there's good information, but there are also pages of potentially damaging drivel, produced by the modern equivalent of snake-oil salesmen and witch doctors. Even well-intentioned health advice on the Net may be full of inaccuracies, which can be dangerous if used to manage your own health care. You could easily be misled into making a wrong decision. In particular, I don't recommend the Net as a reliable tool for diagnosing your own ailments and illnesses. Use your own judgment and, when necessary, check your findings with a trusted physician. An editorial in the *Journal of the American Medical Association* warns: "When it comes to medical information the Internet too often resembles a cocktail conversation rather than a tool for effective health care communication and decision."

A safety standard is needed to rate health information on the Net and to guide consumers to specific medical sites approved for layperson use. I anticipate that this will be set up before too long. Appendix 1 lists useful Web sites.

II. Groups, organizations and institutions

In general, these are support groups for people with specific illnesses, organizations that can help you find skilled practitioners of a particular discipline, or organizations that provide information on a particular topic. A partial list of groups, organizations and institutions is provided in appendix 2. The organizations and clinics listed have not, however, been evaluated or endorsed by the author or publisher.

III. Reading resources

Appendix 3 lists some excellent publications on health and health care at a level appropriate to the general reader. They are presented in the five major categories that are the basic components of the HQ Profile.

THE INTERNET: A MIXED BLESSING

The book *Good Health Online*, by J. Carroll and R. Broadhead, is full of all kinds of good advice about surfing the Net for health-care information. It presents ten reasons for using the Internet for your health care and ten inherent risks of using it.

TEN REASONS WHY YOU SHOULD USE THE INTERNET FOR YOUR OWN HEALTH CARE

1. You should learn to cope in a world where there are increasing demands on the health-care system.
2. You should learn how to use the concept of preventive health care to your benefit.
3. You should educate yourself to overcome your feelings of lack of awareness with respect to certain medical situations and conditions.
4. You should seek information that will help you to better understand your alternatives.
5. You should learn to keep yourself up to date on important medical issues that affect you.
6. You should learn to take advantage of more specialized health-care information.
7. You should prepare for a world in which long-term home care will become more common.
8. You should learn how to improve communications with the medical professionals with whom you deal.
9. You can learn more in order to become involved in the debate about health-care services.
10. You should learn the benefits of on-line emotional support.

TEN RISKS IN USING THE INTERNET FOR YOUR OWN HEALTH CARE

1. You could misdiagnose yourself or use a Web site that makes a misdiagnosis.
2. You may encounter information that is fraudulent.
3. You may encounter information that is clearly biased in nature.
4. You may rely on information that is just plain wrong.
5. You may find and use information that is not relevant or applicable to Canada and the Canadian health-care system.
6. You could become a target of the modern-day form of snake-oil salesperson.
7. You could come to believe in the quick fix.
8. You could turn into a new form of hypochondriac: a Net hypochondriac.
9. You may not find what you are looking for or may not be able to comprehend what you do find.
10. You can waste a lot of time (and money).

Source: Reprinted, by permission of Jim Carroll and Rick Broadhead, from Jim Carroll and Rick Broadhead, *Good Health Online*.

THE HQ HEALTH CULTURE

We are entering a breathtaking, almost anarchic period in the evolution of human health. People care more passionately about their health than ever before. Society is insisting on taking ever greater responsibility for its well-being, and many are simply not satisfied with the conventional options. The last few years have seen a burgeoning of alternatives: wellness and fitness centres, natural-food and health stores, and a mind-boggling smorgasbord of complementary therapies.

We are beginning to see our doctors not as invincible miracle workers but as flesh-and-blood human beings. There is worry everywhere about rising health-care costs, and growing concern that some drugs, surgeries, technologies and procedures may be unnecessary. Clearly, people do not always use medical services in appropriate ways. All these perceptions make it obvious that people have to change the way they view their health. Immigration and the widening multicultural diversity of our society, in which we share knowledge, ideas and customs, are fuelling our skepticism. Add to that globalization, the explosion of media communications and the power of the Internet to break down the old barriers of the medical establishment, and we seem to be careening at giddy speed towards a revolution in health.

Into this volatile scenario comes HQ—your health quotient, health intelligence and more. It is a new health culture beaming a powerful beacon of light through the present turmoil to a healthy new future. This bright and strong source of light is made up of your health intelligence, your sense of wellness, self-care, a healthy lifestyle, your knowledge of resources, and your respectful understanding of the link between mind and body and between quality of life and health. I trust I have given you an understanding of the HQ concept and the resources you need to launch yourself into this revolutionary new health world.

The HQ health culture starts early in life. You need to know more about yourself, including your genetic makeup and your environment, in order to determine how to adjust your habits and lifestyle to achieve good health and wellness. The good news is that you can do most of this yourself; that's what this book has been all about. Self-care, an essential part of HQ health culture, involves determining your own health strategies and accepting responsibility for them through attention to proper food and nutrition, exercise, stress management and the development of good lifestyle habits. It means understanding the different health issues at various stages of the life cycle, and finding out about and becoming familiar with mainstream, non-mainstream and mind/body medicine.

Self-care is all about your ability to look after yourself in maintaining health and wellness, in preventing disease, and also in the treatment of minor illnesses. The person who practises good self-care doesn't rush off to the doctor or the emergency waiting room at the first sign of a sniffle or sore throat; he or she is confident about taking prudent and direct action in dealing with illness or disease when it occurs. Through self-knowledge and self-care education, you're able to seek out and use the best medical services intelligently. Self-care begins with the recognition that the most important steps on the road to achieving optimal health are those you take yourself.

In HQ medicine you play a key role as a primary health-care provider for yourself. In addition, you should be willing to consult with your physician for diagnosis and with other health-care professionals, and be able to identify the competent ones. You should have the confidence to create a health team for your needs, one that is under your control and co-ordination. You should have knowledge of how to use appropriate self-care products and technologies wisely. These might include self-care books and CD-ROM/Internet/software resources, attending credible health seminars, and making wise use of prescribed or over-the-counter medications and services.

Health knowledge is critical to your lifelong quest for your best health. You need a good grasp of the concepts of health, illness and a healthy lifestyle. You should not only understand mainstream medicine but also pursue information on a range of health systems and strategies, such as mind/body medicine, integrated and holistic medicine, disease prevention/injury prevention, and the importance of diet, nutrition, vitamins, minerals, herbs and drugs. You need to know how to cope with stress and how to use relaxation techniques. Routinely, you practise qigong or Tai Chi. All of these things you can begin to appreciate by taking the HQ Profile questionnaire in the first part of this book and then applying it to your life with the wisdom you gain from the later sections.

Hopefully, all this will mean more to you than simply a couple of new health techniques to add to your repertoire. The HQ culture is far more than that. It means adopting new attitudes and a whole new way of life and health that will affect everything you do and every decision you make. In my new health culture, you won't be taking your good health for granted any more. I want to see working at health become second nature, as much a part of every-day life as breathing. This health culture can come to pass as you tackle your risk for disease and illness, focus on caring for yourself, appreciate your innate self-healing abilities, and learn the skills you need to take an integra-tive, holistic approach to managing your own health care.

Remember, HQ culture challenges genetics. We used to think that health destiny was predetermined by our genes. Now we know that, by changing our lifestyle and practising good self-care, to some extent we can trick our bodily mechanisms into redrawing the genetic map.

Public fixation on global environmental issues—air pollution, industrial pollution, deforestation, ozone degradation and other similar concerns—has led us almost to ignore the importance of indoor physical environments, such as the home, public buildings and the workplace. Urban living conditions, smoking and contaminants in foods are finally beginning to be looked upon as truly significant to health. The HQ health culture promises to spotlight both kinds of environmental issues.

Family breakdown, the prevalence of sexually transmitted diseases, failed interpersonal relationships and workplace difficulties are all having a tremen-dous impact on our society. The HQ health culture realizes the importance of family units, better community support, a more caring society and a balanced, healthy lifestyle. We all need to reflect on what is really essential in life. We have to move on from the self-indulgence of the past decades.

Human civilization has passed from survival and mere existence to expec-tations of something better. That "something better" is not the driven, fast-paced, fast-food society that has produced poor eating habits, stress and time pressures, which deliver victims into the hands of disease. My HQ health culture urges changes that would return our priorities to a more wholesome way of life: thoughtful selection and preparation of food, healthy eating, phys-ical activity, making time for family and friends, and enjoyment of life's true blessings.

Having a gold-standard quality of life, brimming with vitality and well-being, comes down to living in healthful harmony with yourself and the world around you. It will lead to a life full of meaningfulness and happiness. Your health is a resource for everyday living and for a lifetime of satisfaction. It is a conscious and conscientious choice, not merely a random outcome attained by heredity, coincidence, luck or fate.

The actions of each one of us reverberate in the world at large. Good health is the very fabric of society's safety net. As the world rapidly evolves, we have an obligation to ensure that the net is well woven and strong. Furthermore, a healthy population is better equipped to deal with the challenges of the new century and millennium, whatever they turn out to be.

Put yourself in the future and imagine a world in which good health is honoured as your highest achievement, more important to your status than having a good job, a house or lots of money in the bank. I'm hopeful that that will be the health culture of tomorrow. It will be an all-embracing health culture, where no one is excluded. It will be a fusion of the best of every health system in the world. As I told you at the beginning, it will be a health culture that will quietly revolutionize the world. Congratulations on being in at the beginning. There are still many miles to go for you and for society at large. I wish you well on your journey, and good health—the best health.

APPENDIX 1

HEALTH ON-LINE

Finding reliable health information on the Internet can be difficult. The list I have provided is not comprehensive, but it will provide you with a starting point on your search for information. Official government sites and sites with the HONcode seal are your best bet to begin with. The HONcode was launched in 1996 by the Health On the Net Foundation to help standardize the accuracy of medical and health information available on the Web. The blue-and-red HONcode seal identifies sites with trustworthy information.

American Medical Association Health Insight

www.ama-assn.org/consumer.htm

Developed and maintained by the AMA, this site provides on-line health information for everyone, and covers general health topics, as well as various specific conditions.

America Online

www.aol.com/webcenters/health/home.adp

This site contains health advice, information about illnesses and diseases, diet tips, calorie and body mass calculators, and chats and message boards.

Canadian Health Network

www.canadian-health-network.ca

Funded by Health Canada, this Web site is a national bilingual Internet-based health information service and features twenty-six health centres that are focused on major health topics and population groups. The site provides easy access to reliable health information from over five hundred organizations across Canada.

Canadian Centre for Occupational Health and Safety
www.ccohs.ca
This Web site provides information and advice about occupational health and safety.

Centers for Disease Control and Prevention
www.cdc.gov
The Atlanta-based CDC is an agency of the U.S. Department of Health and Human Services. It publishes the journal *Emerging Infectious Diseases* through the Internet. This is one of the most important publications for the global medical community. The entire contents of each issue are available free on the Internet through CDC's Web site, which also provides links to many other information networks and resources.

CNN
www.cnn.com/HEALTH
At this site one can read the health news or find in-depth information on disease and nutrition. It also includes CNN health program details and links to other health related Web sites.

Discovery Health
www.discoveryhealth.com
The site provides up-to-the-minute information about health, medicine and fitness concerns.

U.S. Food and Drug Administration
www.fda.gov
This site contains helpful information on both conventional and complementary medicines. The "food" icon refers to information on topics such as dietary supplements.

WebDoctor™
www.gretmar.com/webdoctor
WebDoctor has been designed specifically by physicians for physicians to assist them in navigating the Internet as quickly and effectively as possible to research medical information.

HealthAnswers®

www.healthanswers.com

A site that contains extensive information on specific medical conditions and diseases, as well as such topics as fitness, mental health and medical tests. The health centers provide particularly useful information.

Health A to Z

www.healthAtoZ.com

This site provides medical and health resources for patients, their families, health care workers and physicians. It features information on women's health, expectant moms and men's health.

Healthfinder®

www.healthfinder.org

This is a consumer health information site developed by the U.S. Department of Health and Human Services, through which you can locate reliable health information from selected on-line publications, databases and Web sites.

HealthGate®

www.healthgate.com

This site provides free access to Medline, HealthSTAR, and cancer- and AIDS-related databases. Medline is the best-known biomedical database for health-care professionals. It also includes information on wellness topics, daily headlines, and articles from the Reuters Health eLine.

HealthWWWeb™

www.healthwwweb.com

This is a resource page devoted to health information and tools for wellness. It contains many links to other resource pages on the Web.

Health on the Net Foundation

www.hon.ch

This site provides patient education, a library, a medical image gallery, Internet medical support communities and newsgroups, answers to frequently asked questions and healthcare conference details.

Mayo Clinic

www.mayoclinic.com

This site provides a number of health centers, each of which provides headlines, quizzes and links to other sites broken down by clinical area. In addition, the site provides an extensive searchable drug database.

MedExplorer™

www.medexplorer.com

This site has information on diseases and links to Web sites on alternative medicine, community health, emergency services, health insurance, mental health, medical news and health publications.

Mediconsult

www.mediconsult.com

This site is probably one of the largest medical reference sources on the Internet. For any specific medical condition, you can find educational material, drug information, related Web sites, support groups, on-line conferences, related topics and other information.

Medscape®

www.medscape.com

Three versions of this medical reference are available for doctors, patients and other professionals. As it notes on-line, it "covers all but the most obscure disorders, in addition to describing symptoms, common clinical procedures and laboratory tests." The Merck Health Infopark is a comprehensive disease-oriented area of the Web site that allows for easy navigation through a graphical interface.

National Center for Complementary and Alternative Medicine

www.nccam.nih.gov/

The National Center for Complementary and Alternative Medicine (formerly the Office of Alternative Medicine) is a division of the U.S. National Institutes of Health. It provides access to Medline, which has indexed over 3,800 journals, including eighteen complementary medicine journals. It also provides a link to the National Center for Complementary and Alternative Medicine Clearinghouse.

U.S. National Institute of Environmental Health Sciences

www.niehs.nih.gov

This government agency is involved in research, prevention and public programs. This site provides facts about environment-related diseases and health risks.

U.S. National Institutes of Health

www.nih.gov/health

NIH is an agency of the U.S. Department of Health and Human Services and one of the world's foremost medical research centres. This site provides comprehensive health resources available at the U.S. National Institutes of Health, and information on publications, clinical trials, health hotlines, health literature references, special programs and other resources.

U.S. National Library of Medicine

www.nlm.nih.gov

This site provides free access to Medline and many other useful health-related databases.

U.S. Department of Health and Human Services

www.os.dhhs.gov

This is the official Web site of the U.S. government's principle agency for protecting the health of all Americans and providing essential human services. The site provides comprehensive links to major health sites.

Reuters Health

www.reutershealth.com

This site features medical news, a drug database and a news archive.

Scorecard

www.scorecard.org

This site provides information about toxic chemicals in the United States: where they come from, what their health effects are, and what actions you can take.

Stayhealthy.com

www.stayhealthy.com

This site offers a comprehensive drug information database; a physicians, hospitals, treatment centres, and services locator; extensive original health, nutrition and fitness content; reviews and rankings of more than four thousand health-related Web sites.

WebMD Health

www.webmd.lycos.com
This site provides comprehensive health resources for consumers, physicians, nurses and educators. It includes news, chat forums, health quizzes and consumer product updates.

World Health Organization

www.who.org
This is the official Web site of WHO. It provides links to major programs, an archive of WHO statements, and guidelines for international health and travel.

Yahoo!®

www.ca.yahoo.com/Health
Contains "Today's News: Health and Wellness," a daily update of medical news.

MAJOR GROUPS, ORGANIZATIONS AND INSTITUTIONS RELATED TO HUMAN HEALTH

Organizations targeted at patient-centred care

As people become more interested in playing an active role in their health care, some new organizations are developing programs to help them do so.

Self-help clearinghouses can assist in a number of ways. They may be able to provide current information on your particular medical concern or condition and in some cases advise you of any existing self-help groups focused on that medical topic. If no suitable group exists in your local area, they can help interested parties to start their own.

National Self-Help Clearinghouse
Graduate School and University Center of the City University of New York
365 Fifth Ave., Suite 3300
New York, NY 10016
Tel: (212) 817-1822
Email: info@selfhelpweb.org
www.selfhelpweb.org

Major organizations associated with specific subjects on health and illness

American College of Sports Medicine
401 W. Michigan St.
Indianapolis, IN 46202-3233
Tel: (317) 637-9200
Fax: (317) 634-7817
www.acsm.org

American Dietetic Association
216 W. Jackson Blvd.
Chicago, IL 60606-6995
Tel: (312) 899-0040
www.eatright.org

American Medical Association
515 N. State St.
Chicago, IL 60610
Tel: (312) 464-5000
www.ama-assn.org

American Pharmaceutical Association
2215 Constitution Ave. NW
Washington, DC 20037-2985
Tel: 800-237-APHA / (202) 628-4410
Fax: (202) 783-2351
www.aphanet.org

The Association of Occupational & Environmental Clinics
1010 Vermont Ave. NW, Suite 513
Washington, DC 20005
Tel: (202) 347-4976
Fax: (202) 347-4950
Email: AOEC@AOEC.ORG
www.aoec.org

Canadian Medical Association
1867 Alta Vista Dr.
Ottawa, ON K1G 3Y6
Tel: (613) 731-9331
Email: public_affairs@cma.ca
www.cma.ca

Center for Nutrition Policy and Promotion
U.S. Department of Agriculture
1120 Twentieth St. NW, Suite 200
North Lobby, Washington, DC 20036
Tel: (202) 418-2312
Fax: (202) 208-2321
www.usda.gov/cnpp/center.htm

Food and Nutrition Information Center
National Agricultural Library
U.S. Department of Agriculture
10301 Baltimore Ave.
Beltsville, MD 20705-2351
Tel: (301) 504-5719
Fax: (301) 504-6409
Email: fnic@nal.usda.gov
www.nal.usda.gov/fnic

Genetic Alliance
4301 Connecticut Ave. NW, Suite 404
Washington, DC 20008-2304
Tel: 800-336-GENE / (202) 966-5557
Fax: (202) 966-8553
Email: info@geneticalliance.org
www.geneticalliance.org/

La Leche League International
1400 N. Meacham Rd.
Schaumburg, IL 60173-4840
Tel: (847) 519-7730
Fax: (847) 519-0035
www.lalecheleague.org

U.S. Food and Drug Administration
Center for Biologics Evaluation and Research
1401 Rockville Pike
Rockville, MD 20852-1448
Tel: 800-835-4709 / (301) 827-1800
Fax: (301) 827-3843
www.fda.gov/cber

One important question is, how can you determine if a physician is a certified specialist or subspecialist in North America? The American Board of Medical Specialties has a toll-free number you can call to verify certification status: 800-776-2378. You can also use their Web site: www.certifieddoctor.org.

Major Organizations and Associations on Major Diseases and Conditions

Heart disease

Support groups can play an important role in helping heart disease patients cope better with their illness. Nearly every hospital of any size has a cardiac rehabilitation program that includes a support group in addition to the standard components of supervised exercise and guidance in reducing risk factors. If your local hospital does not have such a program, you can obtain information about sources of help by contacting The Mended Hearts.

The Mended Hearts, Inc.
7272 Greenville Ave.
Dallas, TX 75231
Tel: 800-AHA USA1 / (214) 706-1442
Fax: (214) 706-5231
Email: dbonham@heart.org
www.mendedhearts.org

Cancer

The National Cancer Institute, the American Cancer Society and the Canadian Cancer Society provide general information on the various aspects of cancer and cancer treatment. They may also be able to give you information on community resources for people with cancer in your area.

American Cancer Society
1599 Clifton Rd. NE
Atlanta, GA 30329-4251
Tel: 800-ACS-2345 / (404) 320-3333
Fax: (404) 325-9341
www.cancer.org

Canadian Cancer Society
10 Alcorn Ave., Suite 200
Toronto, ON M4V 3B1
Tel: 888-939-3333 / (416) 961-7223
Fax: (416) 961-4189
www.cancer.ca

National Cancer Institute
Building 31, Room 10A03
31 Center Dr., MSC 2580
Bethesda, MD 20892-2580
Tel: (301) 435-3848
Fax: (301) 402-0894
www.cancer.gov

Cancer Information Services
Tel: 800-4-CANCER
cis.nci.nih.gov/

The following organizations provide various kinds of support for people with cancer and their families:

The Candlelighters Childhood Cancer Foundation
3910 Warner St.
Kensington, MD 20895
Tel: 800-366-2223 / (301) 962-3520
Fax: (301) 962-3521
Email: info@candlelighters.org
www.candlelighters.org

The National Hospice and Palliative Care Organization
1700 Diagonal Rd., Suite 300
Alexandria, VA 22314
Tel: (703) 837-1500
Email: info@nhpco.org
www.nhpco.org

Commonweal Cancer Help Program
PO Box 316
Bolinas, CA 94924
Tel: (415) 868-0970
Fax: (415) 868-2230
www.commonweal.org

Chronic diseases and conditions

American Chronic Pain Association
PO Box 850
Rocklin, CA 95677
Tel: (916) 632-0922
Fax: (916) 632-3208
Email: ACPA@pacbell.net
www.theacpa.org

American Psychiatric Association
1400 K St. NW
Washington, DC 20005
Tel: 888-357-7924
Fax: (202) 682-6850
Email: apa@psych.org
www.psych.org

The American Diabetes Association
1701 North Beauregard St.
Alexandria, VA 22311
Tel: 800-342-2383
Fax: (703) 549-6995
www.diabetes.org

American Psychological Association
750 First St. NE
Washington, DC 20002-4242
Tel: 800-374-2721 / (202) 336-5500
www.apa.org

Arthritis Foundation
1330 W. Peachtree St.
Atlanta, GA 30309
Tel: 800-283-7800 / (404) 872-7100
Fax: (404) 872-0457
Email: help@arthritis.org
www.arthritis.org

Asthma and Allergy Foundation of America
1233 Twentieth St. NW, Suite 402
Washington, DC 20036
Tel: 800-7-ASTHMA
Fax: (202) 466-8940
Email: info@aafa.org
www.aafa.org

International Association for the Study of Pain
909 Forty-third St. NE, Suite 306
Seattle, WA 98105-6020
Tel: (206) 547-6409
Fax: (206) 547-1703
Email: IASP@locke.hs.washington.edu
www.halcyon.com/iasp

International Foundation for Functional Gastrointestinal Disorders
PO Box 170864
Milwaukee, WI 53217-8076
Tel: 888-964-2001 / (414) 964-1799
Email: iffgd@iffgd.org
www.iffgd.org

Multiple Sclerosis Foundation
6350 N. Andrews Ave.
Fort Lauderdale, FL 33309-2130
Tel: 800-441-7055 / (954) 776-6805
Fax: (954) 938-8708
Email: support@msfacts.org
www.msfacts.org

Organizations that focus on mind/body approaches

The Mind/Body Medical Institute programs are designed to help people with chronic illness or stress-related physical symptoms better manage their conditions. The approach combines conventional medical treatment and awareness of how behaviour and attitude can affect health. Mind/body medicine programs are available to:

- reduce medical symptoms—headaches, gastrointestinal disorders, anxiety, fatigue, insomnia;
- reduce effects of HIV and AIDS and cancer;
- reduce or eliminate general stress-related physical symptoms, such as infertility and insomnia;
- provide cardiac rehabilitation and risk reduction;
- deal with symptoms of menopause;
- deal with symptoms of infertility;
- counsel patients undergoing chemotherapy and radiation therapy.

Mind/Body Medical Institute
Beth Israel Deaconess Medical Center
110 Francis St., Suite 1A
Boston, MA 02215
Tel: (617) 632-9530
www.mindbody.harvard.edu

Affiliate mind/body programs of the Mind/Body Medical Institute

Affiliate programs of the Mind/Body Medical Institute have created partnerships with teaching hospitals throughout the United States and the world to promote and integrate mind/body medicine in these institutions. To date, these are the affiliates:

The Mind/Body Medical Institute
Allen Memorial Hospital
1825 Logan Ave.
Waterloo, IA 50703-1999
Tel: (319) 235-3967
Fax: (319) 235-3192
www.allenhospital.org/special/index.htm
(medical symptom reduction)

The Mind/Body Medical Institute
Maryland Center for Integrative Medicine
at Greater Baltimore Medical Center
6701 N. Charles St., Suite 5200
Baltimore, MD 21204
Tel: (410) 828-3585
Fax: (410) 828-8674
(infertility, healthy lifestyles)

The Mind/Body Medical Institute
Bon Secours Richmond Health System
2006 Bremo Rd., Suite 102A
Richmond, VA 23226
Tel: (804) 288-5415
Fax: (804) 282-8606
Email: tom_wojick@bshsi.com
*(medical symptom reduction,
cardiac wellness)*

The Mind/Body Medical Institute
Harvard University Health Services
75 Mt. Auburn St., 2 East
Cambridge, MA 02138
Tel: (617) 496-9005
Fax: (617) 495-1135
Email: mindbody@uhs.harvard.edu
www.uhs.harvard.edu
(medical symptom reduction)

**The Mind/Body Medical Institute of
Care**
New England Wellness Center
2191 Post Rd.
Warwick, RI 02886
Tel: (401) 732-3066
Fax: (401) 732-3094
(cardiac rehab)

The Mind/Body Medical Institute
Memorial Hermann Healthcare System
7500 Beechnut, Suite 321
Houston, TX 77074
Tel: (713) 776-5020
Fax: (713) 776-5512
www.mhhs.org
(cardiac wellness, healthy lifestyles)

Multicare Mind/Body Medical Institute
A227-1901 South Union Ave.
Tacoma, WA 98405
Tel: (253) 403-2349
Fax: (253) 403-5620
Email: paige.fury@multicare.org
www.multicare.com
(medical symptom reduction)

The Mind/Body Medical Institute
The Queen's Medical Center
1301 Punchbowl St.
Honolulu, HI 96813
Tel: (808) 547-4603
Fax: (808) 547-4259
(cardiac wellness, healthy lifestyles)

The Mind/Body Medical Institute
Sisters of Charity Healthcare
75 Vanderbilt Ave.
Staten Island, NY 10304
Tel: (718) 354-5190 / (718) 354-6000
Fax: (718) 354-6011
Email: dhopkins@schsi.org
www.nymindbody.org
(medical symptom reduction)

The Mind/Body Medical Institute
St. Joseph's Regional Medical Center
410 N. Notre Dame Ave.
South Bend, IN 46617
Tel: (219) 239-6107 / 888-237-7360
Fax: (219) 237-7725
www.sjmed.com/mindbody.html
(cardiac wellness, cancer, pain)

Outpatient clinical programs that focus on mind/body medicine

There are now pioneering multidisciplinary clinical outpatient programs for the treatment of symptoms and diseases caused or aggravated by stress, including model programs for general medical conditions caused or exacerbated by stress. The major areas focused on by these clinical programs are healthy lifestyles, pre-surgery, cancer, AIDS, cardiovascular risk reduction, cardiovascular rehabilitation and reversal, insomnia, chronic pain, infertility and menopause.

Integrative programs featuring mind/body medicine are offered in three major general hospitals in New York City. These hospitals are risking millions of dollars and their reputations to try to establish these clinical programs based on a belief that patients recover more quickly and less traumatically with the use of support groups, meditation, a variety of relaxation techniques and cognition therapy.

Columbia-Presbyterian Medical Center
622 W. 168th St.
New York, NY 10032
Tel: (212) 305-2500
cpmcnet.columbia.edu/

Mount Sinai Medical Center
One Gustave Levy Pl.
New York, NY 10029
Tel: (212) 241-6500
www.mountsinai.org

Memorial Sloan-Kettering International Center
1429 First Ave.
New York, NY 10021
Tel: (212) 639-4900
www.mskcc.org
Physician Referral Service

Stress reduction clinic

An eight-week mindfulness-training program aimed at improving a range of physical symptoms is offered at

University of Massachusetts Medical Center
55 Lake Ave. N.
Worcester, MA 01655
Tel: (508) 334-1000
Email: mindfulness@umassmed.edu
www.umassmed.edu/cfm

Complementary health-care organizations

The following organizations can provide information to verify the certification status of your complementary health-care providers.

Acupressure Institute
1533 Shattuck Ave.
Berkeley, CA 94709
Tel: 800-442-2232 / (510) 845-1059
Email: info@acupressure.com
www.acupressure.com

Acupuncture Foundation of Canada
2131 Lawrence Ave. E., Suite 204
Scarborough, ON M1R 5G4
Tel: (416) 752-3988
Fax: (416) 752-4398
Email: info@afcinstitute.com
www.afcinstitute.com

American Academy of Medical Acupuncture
4929 Wilshire Blvd., Suite 428
Los Angeles, CA 90010
Tel: 800-521-2262 / (323) 937-5514
Email: jdowden@prodigy.net
www.medicalacupuncture.org

American Association of Naturopathic Physicians
8201 Greensboro Dr., Suite 300
McLean, VA 22102
Tel: (703) 610-9037
Fax: (703) 610-9005
Email: info@aanp.com
www.naturopathic.org

American Association of Oriental Medicine
433 Front St.
Catasauqua, PA 18032
Tel: 888-500-7999 / (610) 266-1433
Fax: (610) 264-2768
Email: aaoml@aol.com
www.aaom.org

American Massage Therapy Association
820 Davis St., Suite 100
Evanston, IL 60201-4444
Tel: (847) 864-0123
Fax: (847) 864-1178
www.amtamassage.org

American Osteopathic Association
142 E. Ontario St.
Chicago, IL 60611
Tel: 800-621-1773 / (312) 202-8000
Fax: (312) 202-8200
Email: info@aoa-net.org
www.aoa-net.org
www.aoa-net.org

Ayurvedic Institute
11311 Menaul Blvd. NE
Albuquerque, NM 87112
Tel: (505) 291-9698
Fax: (505) 294-7572
www.ayurveda.com

Canadian Massage Therapist Alliance
365 Bloor St. E., Suite 1807
Toronto, ON M4W 3L4
Tel: (416) 968-2149
Fax: (416) 968-6818
www.collinscan.com/~collins/clientspgs/cmtai.
html

Canadian Osteopathic Association
575 Waterloo St.
London, ON N6B 2R2
Tel: (519) 439-5521
Fax: (519) 439-2616

Federation of Chiropractic Licensing Boards
901 Fifty-fourth Ave., Suite 101
Greeley, CO 80634-4400
Tel: (970) 356-3500
Fax: (970) 356-3599
Email: fclb@fclb.org
www.fclb.org

International Chiropractors Association
1110 N. Glebe Rd., Suite 1000
Arlington, VA 57222
Tel: 800-423-4690 / (703) 528-5000
Fax: (703) 528-5023
Email: chiro@chiropractic.org
www.chiropractic.org

National Acupuncture and Oriental Medicine Alliance
14637 Starr Rd. SE
Olalla, WA 98359
Tel: (253) 851-6896
Fax: (253) 851-6883
www.acupuncturealliance.org

National Center for Homeopathy
801 N. Fairfax St., Suite 306
Alexandria, VA 22314
Tel: 877-624-0613 / (703) 548-7790
Fax: (703) 548-7792
Email: info@homeopathic.org
www.homeopathic.org

Canadian Chiropractic Association
1396 Eglinton Ave. W.
Toronto, ON M6C 2E4
Tel: 800-668-2076 / (416) 781-5656
Fax: (416) 781-7344
Email: dbegin@ccachiro.org
www.ccachiro.org

Canadian Naturopathic Association
1255 Sheppard Ave. E.
North York, ON M2K 1E2
Tel: 877-628-7284 / (416) 496-8633
Email: info@naturopathicassoc.ca
www.naturopathicassoc.ca

PUBLISHED RESOURCES AND SUGGESTED READINGS

Self-care

Harden, B.L., and C.R. Harden. *Alternative Health Care—The Canadian Directory*. Toronto: Noble Ages Publishing Ltd., 1997.

Inlander, C.B., and the staff of the People's Medical Society. *The People's Medical Society Health Desk Reference*. New York: Hyperion, 1995.

Lorig, K., H. Holman, D. Bobel, D. Laurent, V. Gonzalez, and M. Minor. *Living a Healthy Life with Chronic Conditions*. Palo Alto, CA: Bull Publishing Co., 1994.

Marion, M., and P. Eve. *Triumph: Getting Back to Normal When You Have Cancer*. New York: Avon Books, 1990.

Reiner Foundation. *I Am Your Child*. Toronto: CICH, MHPL, 1998.

White, B.J., and E.J. Madara. *The Self-help Source Book: Your Guide to Community and Online Support Groups*. New Jersey: Northwest Covenant Medical Center, 1997.

Knowledge

Collinge, W. *Complete Guide to Alternative Medicine*. New York: Warner Books, 1996.

Gordon, J.S. *Manifesto for a New Medicine*. Menlo Park, CA: Addison-Wesley, 1996.

Hobbs, C. *Herbal Remedies for Dummies*. Toronto: IDG Books, 1998.

Laszlo, J. *Understanding Cancer*. New York: HarperCollins, 1998.

Lerner, M. *Choices in Healing: Integrating the Best of Conventional and Complementary Approaches to Cancer*. Cambridge, MA: MIT Press, 1996.

Micozzi, M.S. *Fundamentals of Complementary and Alternative Medicine*. New York: Churchill Livingstone Inc., 1996.

Morton, M., and M. Morton. *Five Steps to Selecting the Best Alternative Medicine: A Guide to Complementary and Integrative Health Care*. Novato, CA: New World Library, 1996.

Ott, R.W., and W.J. Roberts. "Everyday Exposure to Toxic Pollutants." *Scientific American* (February 1998).

Pizzorno, J. *Total Wellness: Improve Your Health by Understanding the Body's Healing Systems*. Rocklin, CA: Prima Publishing, 1996.

Scientific American (September 1996). Special issue on cancer.

Shorter, E. *The Health Century*. New York: Doubleday, 1987.

Tyler, V.E. *Herbs of Choice*. New York: Haworth Press, 1994.

Weil, A. *Spontaneous Healing*. New York: Fawcett Columbine, 1996.

Williams, T. *Chinese Medicine*. Dorset, England: Element Books, 1997.

World Health Organization. *The World Health Report*. Geneva: WHO, 1997, 1998.

Xie Zhufan. *Best of Traditional Chinese Medicine*. Beijing: New World Press, 1995.

Lifestyle

American College of Sports Medicine Staff. *ACSM Fitness Book*. Windsor, Ont.: Human Kinetics Canada, 1997.

Lu, C.H. *Chinese System of Food Cures—Prevention and Remedies*. New York: Sterling Publishing Co., 1986.

Mitchell, M.K. *Nutrition Across Life Span*. Philadelphia: WUB Founders Company, 1997.

Oakley, G.P., Jr. "Eat Right and Take a Multivitamin." *New England Journal of Medicine* 338, no. 15 (April 9, 1998): 1060–61.

Ornish, D. *Dr. Dean Ornish's Program for Reversing Heart Disease*. New York: Ivy Books, 1996.

Packer, L., and C. Colman. *The Antioxidant Miracle*. New York: John Wiley and Sons, 1999.

Rowe, J.W., and R.L. Kahn. *Successful Aging*. New York: Pantheon Books, 1998.

Wong, S. *HeartSmart Chinese Cooking*. Vancouver: Douglas & McIntyre, 1996.

Mind

Benson, H., and E.M. Stuart. *The Wellness Book*. New York: Simon and Schuster, 1993.

Davis, M., E.R. Eshelman, and M. McKay. *The Relaxation & Stress Reduction Workbook*. Oakland, CA: New Harbinger Publications, 1997.

Goleman, D., and J. Gurin. *Mind/Body Medicine: How to Use Your Mind for Better Health*. Yonkers, NY: Consumer Reports Books, 1993.

Goleman, D. *Emotional Intelligence*. New York: Bantam Books, 1995.

Goleman, D. *Healing Emotions*. Boston and London: Shambhala, 1997.

Gordon, J.S., D. Jaffe, and D. Bresler, eds. *Mind, Body and Health: Toward an Integral Medicine*. New York: Human Science Press Inc., 1984.

Gordon, J.S., *Stress Management*. New York: Chelsea House, 1990.

Moyers, B. *Healing and the Mind*. New York: Doubleday, 1993.

Pelletier, K.R. *Mind as Healer, Mind as Slayer*. New York: Delacorte, 1997.

Stoltz, P.G. *Adversity Quotient*. New York: John Wiley and Sons, 1997.

Life skills

Carroll, J., and R. Broadhead. *Good Health Online*. Scarborough, Ont.: Prentice Hall Canada, 1997.

Ferguson, T. *Health Online*. Menlo Park, CA: Addison-Wesley Publishing Company, 1996.

National Heart, Lung and Blood Institute. *Report of the Task Force on Behavioral Research in Cardiovascular Lung and Blood Health and Disease*. U.S. Department of Health and Human Services (February 1998).

Ware, J.E., K.K. Snow, and M. Konnan. *SF36 Health Survey General and Interpretation Guide*. Boston: New England Medical Center, 1993.

World Health Organization, *Lifeskill Programs for Child and Adolescent: An Overview*. Geneva: WHO, 1997.

World Health Organization, *WHOQOL-100, Measuring Quality of Life*. Geneva: WHO, 1997.

FOODS WITH THE MOST VITAMINS AND MINERALS

FOODS HIGH IN FOLIC ACID

Okra
Orange juice
Spinach
White beans
Red kidney beans
Soybeans
Wheat germ
Asparagus
Turnip greens
Brussels sprouts

FOODS HIGH IN BETA-CAROTENE

Brightly coloured fruits and vegetables

Apricots
Peaches
Sweet potatoes
Carrots
Collard greens
Kale
Spinach
Pumpkin
Cantaloupe

FOODS HIGH IN VITAMIN C

Abundant in fruits and vegetables

Guava
Sweet pepper
Cantaloupe
Papaya
Strawberries
Brussels sprouts
Grapefruit
Kiwi fruit
Oranges
Tomatoes
Broccoli
Cabbage

FOODS HIGH IN VITAMIN D

Eels
Pilchards
Sardines
Herring
Salmon
Mackerel
Tuna
Milk

Source: Modified and reprinted, by permission of HarperCollins Publishers, Inc., from Jean Carper, *Food—Your Miracle Medicine* (New York: HarperPaperbacks, 1993).

FOODS HIGH IN VITAMIN E

Vitamin E is fat-soluble and concentrated in vegetable oils, nuts and seeds. Legumes and brans also contain fairly high amounts. Vitamin E is almost non-existent in animal foods. It is nature's master antioxidant.

Nuts and seeds	Brans and legumes	Oils	Vegetables
Sunflower seeds	Wheat germ	Wheat germ	Asparagus
Walnuts	Soybeans	Soybean	Spinach
Almonds	Rice bran	Corn	Peas
Hazelnuts	Lima beans	Sunflower	Broccoli
Cashews	Wheat bran	Safflower	
Peanuts		Sesame	
Brazil nuts		Peanut	
Pecans			

FOODS HIGH IN CALCIUM

Parmesan cheese
Milk
Yogurt, no-fat
Dried figs
Tofu, firm
Turnip greens
Kale
Broccoli
Baked beans

FOODS HIGH IN SELENIUM

Selenium is an essential component of antioxidant enzymes.

Brazil nuts
Puffed wheat
Sunflower seeds
Oysters
Wheat flour, whole grain
Garlic
Onions
Red grapes
Broccoli

FOODS HIGH IN ZINC

Zinc has a strong immune enhancement property.

Oysters
Crabmeat
Pot roast
Turkey, dark meat
Pumpkin and squash seeds
Cereals

Source: Modified and reprinted, by permission of HarperCollins Publishers, Inc., from Jean Carper, *Food—Your Miracle Medicine* (New York: HarperPaperbacks, 1993).

GLYCEMIC INDEX OF SOME COMMON FOODS

GI = Glycemic index

Glucose has a GI of 100.

FOOD GROUP	HIGH-GI FOODS (+50)	LOW-GI FOODS (−50)
Grains, Breads, Cereals, Bakery Products	Buns	Whole rice
	White bread	Oat and bran bread
	French bread	Mixed grain bread
	Rye bread	Sponge cake
	Instant rice	Wheat grain
	Cornflakes	Barley grain
	Croissant	Whole grain pasta
	Puffed wheat	Rye grain
	Brown rice	All-Bran
	Macaroni and cheese	Parboiled rice
	Spaghetti, durum	Rice pasta, brown
	Cake—angel food, banana, pound	Fettuccine
	Crumpet	Linguine
	Doughnut, cake-type	Macaroni
	Pastry	Spaghetti, white
	Waffles	Vermicelli
	Muffins	

Source: Reprinted, by permission of *The American Journal of Clinical Nutrition,* from Kaye Foster-Powell and Jeanette Brand Miller, "International Tables of Glycemic Index," *The American Journal of Clinical Nutrition* 62 (1995): 871s–93s.

FOOD GROUP	HIGH-GI FOODS (+50)	LOW-GI FOODS (−50)
Vegetables and Legumes	Parsnips	Green peas
	Carrots	Black-eyed peas
	Potatoes—instant, baked, mashed	Dried beans, lentils
	French fries	Green beans
	Beets	Lima beans
	Sweet potatoes	Kidney beans
	Yams	Soybeans
	Sweet corn	Chickpeas
	Rutabaga	Butter beans
	Pumpkin	
Fruits and Fruit Products	Watermelon	Apples
	Pineapples	Oranges
	Raisins	Apricots
	Mangoes	Grapefruit
	Kiwi fruit	Cherries
	Grapes	Tomatoes
	Peaches, canned	Peaches, fresh
	Papayas	Pears
	Orange juice	Plums
	Fruit cocktail, canned	Grapefruit juice, unsweetened
	Bananas	Apple juice, unsweetened
Miscellaneous	Ice cream	Yogurt, with added fruit
	Maltose (as in beer)	Milk—whole, skimmed, chocolate
	Glucose	Yogurt, plain, no sugar
	Refined sugar	Nuts
	Pretzels	Peanuts
	Honey	Fructose
	Sucrose	Lactose
	Cookies	Fish fingers
	Crackers	Sausages
	Corn chips	
	Popcorn	
	Jelly beans	
	Life Savers	
	Soft drinks	

Source: Reprinted, by permission of *The American Journal of Clinical Nutrition,* from Kaye Foster-Powell and Jeanette Brand Miller, "International Tables of Glycemic Index," *The American Journal of Clinical Nutrition* 62 (1995): 871s–93s.

Substituting Low-GI Foods for High-GI Foods

HIGH-GI FOOD	LOW-GI ALTERNATIVE
Bread—whole meal or white	Bread containing a high proportion of whole grains
Processed breakfast cereal	Unrefined cereal such as oats (muesli or porridge) or Kellogg's All-Bran
Plain cookies and crackers	Cookies made with dried fruit and grains such as oats
Cakes and muffins	Look for those made with fruit, whole grains
Tropical fruits such as bananas	Temperate-climate fruits such as apples and stone fruit
Potatoes	Pasta or legumes
Rice	Use basmati or other high-amylose rices

Source: Reprinted, by permission of the American Diabetes Association, from Jennie Brand Miller, Stephen Colagiuri and Kaye Foster-Powell, "The Glycemic Index Is Easy and Works in Practice," *Diabetes Care* 20, no.10(1997):1628.

FACTS ABOUT FAT

Saturated fat

Saturated fats tend to raise LDL-cholesterol levels. The main food sources are meat, poultry, dairy products, butter, lard, and palm and coconut oil.

Monounsaturated fat

This type of fat seems to lower LDL-cholesterol levels and may also increase HDL-cholesterol. Monounsaturated fats are primarily found in olive and canola oils, soft margarines and nuts (hazelnuts, almonds, pistachios, pecans and cashews).

Polyunsaturated fat

Polyunsaturated fats help lower the LDL-cholesterol levels in your blood. This type of fat also contains essential fatty acids, which are mainly found in vegetable oils, such as safflower, sunflower, corn, soybean, sesame seed and most nut oils; soft margarines made with these oils; nuts (walnuts, chestnuts, Brazil nuts, and pine nuts); and seeds (sesame and sunflower). Using vegetable oils for your cooking will help to keep your bad cholesterol down.

Omega-3 fatty acids are a type of polyunsaturated fat found mainly in fatty fish, such as salmon, mackerel, trout and herring. These fish oils promote heart health by reducing the stickiness or clotting tendency of blood. There is strong evidence that fish oils play a role in preventing the formation of blood clots. Fish adds variety to your diet and may lower your risk for heart disease.

Trans fat

Some trans fatty acids occur naturally in foods while others are formed by a chemical process called hydrogenation, which makes liquid vegetable oils into solid vegetable shortening. Processed foods made with shortening, such as cookies, crackers, snack foods, deep-fried foods, some peanut butters and many (not all) margarines are the main sources of trans fatty acids. Even though trans fatty acids are unsaturated, they raise the bad cholesterol level, like saturated fat, and should therefore be avoided.

STRESSFUL LIFE EVENTS THAT AFFECT YOUR HEALTH

To estimate how much stress you have experienced, add up the numbers listed for life events you have undergone within the last year. If you score more than 200, you have a 50 percent chance of becoming ill from stress; a score of 300 or more raises your chances of illness to 80 percent.

LIFE EVENT	SCORE	LIFE EVENT	SCORE
Death of spouse	100	Son or daughter leaving home	29
Divorce	73	Trouble with in-laws	29
Marital separation	65	Outstanding personal achievement	28
Jail term	63	Spouse begins or stops work	26
Death of close family member	63	Begin or end school	26
Personal injury or illness	53	Change in living conditions	25
Marriage	50	Change in personal habits	24
Being fired	47	Trouble with boss	23
Marital reconciliation	45	Change in work hours or conditions	20
Retirement	45	Change in residence	20
Change in health of family member	44	Change in schools	20
Pregnancy	40	Change in church activities	19
Sex difficulties	39	Change in recreation	19
Having a baby	39	Change in social activities	18
Business readjustment	39	Small mortgage in relation to income	17
Change in financial state	38	Change in sleeping habits	16
Death of close friend	37	Change in number of family get-togethers	15
Change to different line of work	36	Change in eating habits	15
Change in number of arguments with spouse	35	Vacation	13
Mortgage, large in relation to income	31	Christmas	12
Foreclosure of mortgage or loan	30	Minor violations of the law	11
Change in responsibilities at work	29		

Source: Reprinted, by permission of Elsevier Science, from Thomas H. Holmes and Richard H. Rahe, "Social Readjustment Rating Scale," *Journal of Psychosomatic Research* 11 (1967).

INSTRUCTIONS FOR INTERNAL QIGONG PRACTICE

Preparation

1.   You should not be influenced or disturbed by the environment. Your mind should be clear of thought.
2.   In any position, sitting or lying, the clothes should be loose so that respiration and blood circulation are free from restraint. The posture should be natural, without squaring the shoulders or pulling in the abdomen.

Instructions

1.   **Relaxation**

     Physical relaxation: Drink some water, empty the bowels and bladder, take off any hat, wristwatch or glasses, loosen your belt and relax your whole body, including your head, trunk and limbs.

     Mental relaxation: Begin with an easy mind.

2.   **Posture**   Select a comfortable and natural posture. The form selected is not important.

     Lying down: Lie on the side (either the right or the left) with the head slightly bent forward and placed comfortably on a pillow. If lying on the right side, extend the left arm naturally along the left (upper) side of the trunk with the left palm facing downward, placed on the left hip. Bend the right arm at the elbow with the right palm facing upward and the fingers separated, placed on the pillow about six to seven centimetres from the head. Bend the waist a little bit, extend the right leg naturally with a slight bend at the knee; bend the left leg 120 degrees and rest it on the right leg.

     Sitting up: Sit upright on a bench with the legs apart at shoulder width and knees bent at a ninety-degree angle. Place the feet flat on the floor. The palms, facing upward, are placed on the middle third of the thighs, with the elbows naturally bent and relaxed.

3. **Breathing** Two different abdominal breathing techniques can be used:
    Inhale and exhale through the nose. Lift the tongue to touch the palate while inhaling and lower it while exhaling. Inhalation should be natural, without exertion.
    Inhale through the mouth, using the mouth to guide the air to the lower abdomen. Exhale naturally through the nose, followed by a pause for the sentence, during which time the tongue is touching the palate. After reciting the sentence, lower the tongue and inhale again.

4. **Concentration of the mind** The mind should be free from all distractions. Recite a short sentence in your mind. Start with a sentence of three words or a few syllables and gradually increase the number. Though there is no fixed pattern, those commonly used are: "I am still," "I am sitting (lying) still," "I am sitting (lying) very still," and so on. Recitation should be co-ordinated with respiration. There are two methods: inhale with the first word and exhale with the last, holding the breath in between; or recite the whole sentence in the pause between inhalation and exhalation. Either way, the more words in a sentence, the longer the pause in respiration. After repeated practice of silent recitation, a tranquil state will be reached.

Source: Reprinted, by permission of the publisher, from Xie Zhufan, *The Best of Traditional Chinese Medicine* (Beijing: New World Press, 1995).

REFERENCES

Chapter 2: Your Genetic Endowment and Your Environment

Albers, J.W. "Understanding Gene–Environment Interactions, Environmental Health Perspectives." *NIEHS News* 105, no. 6 (June 1997).

D'Arcy, C. "Unemployment and Health: Data and Implications." *Canadian Journal of Public Health*, 77, suppl. 1 (May/June 1986): 124.

Dockely, D.W., et al. "An Association between Air Pollution and Mortality in Six U.S. Cities." *New England Journal of Medicine* 329, no. 24 (1993): 1753–59.

Ott, W.R., and J.W. Roberts. "Everyday Exposure to Toxic Pollutants." *Scientific American* (February 1998).

Chapter 3: The Healthy Mind

Benson, H., and E. Stuart. *The Wellness Book.* New York: Simon and Schuster, 1993.

Frasure-Smith, N., F. Lesperance, and M. Talejic. "Depression Following Myocardial Infarction: Impact on 6-month Survival." *JAMA* 270, no. 15 (1993): 1819–25.

Friedman, H.S., and S. Booth-Kewley. "The 'Disease-prone Personality.'" *American Psychologist* 42 (1987): 539–55.

Goleman, D. *Emotional Intelligence.* New York: Bantam Books, 1995.

Gordon, J.S. *Stress Management.* New York: Chelsea House, 1990.

House, J.S., K.R. Landis, and D. Umberson. "Social Relationships and Health." *Science* 241 (1998): 540–45.

Kabat-Zinn, Jon. *Where You Go, Where You Are: Mindfulness Meditation in Everyday Life.* New York: Hyperion, 1994.

Langer, E.J., and J. Rodin. "The Effects of Choice and Enhanced Responsibility for the Aged: A Field Experiment in an Institutional Setting." *Journal of Personality and Social Psychology* 34 (1976): 191–98.

Mark, D. "High Hopes Help Heart Patients Recover, Study Finds." *Minneapolis Tribune*, April 16, 1994, 7A.

Myers, D.G. *Psychology.* 5th ed. New York: Worth Publishers, 1998.

Ornish, D. *Dr. Dean Ornish's Program for Reversing Heart Disease.* New York: Ivy Books, 1996.

Pert, C.B., H.E. Dreher, and M.R. Ruff. "The Psychosomatic Network: Foundations of Mind/Body Medicine." *Alternative Therapies in Health and Medicine* 4, no. 4 (1998): 30–41.

Peterson, C., M.E. Seligman, and G.E. Vaillant. "Pessimistic Explanatory Style Is a Risk Factor for Physical Illness: A Thirty-five-Year Longitudinal Study." *Journal of Personality and Social Psychology* 55, no. 1 (1998): 23–27.

Spiegel, D., et al. "Effect of Psychosocial Treatment on Survival of Patients with Metastatic Breast Cancer." *Lancet* 2 (1989): 888–91.

Stoltz, P.G. *Adversity Quotient.* New York: John Wiley and Sons, 1997.

Wells-Federman, C.L. *Provider's Manual Clinical Training in Mind/Body Medicine.* Boston: The Mind/Body Medical Institute, 1995.

Williams, R., and V. Williams. *Anger Kills: Several Strategies for Controlling the Hostility that Can Harm Your Health.* New York: Harper Books, 1993.

Williams, R.B., and M.A. Chesney. "Psychosocial Factors and Prognosis in Established Coronary Artery Diseases: The Need for Research on Interventions." *JAMA* 270, no. 15 (1993): 1860–61.

Chapter 4: Lifestyle and Health

Blair, S.N., et al. "Changes in Physical Fitness and All-Cause Mortality: A Prospective Study of Healthy and Unhealthy Men." *JAMA* 273, no. 14 (1995): 1093–98.

Blair, S.N., et al. "Influences of Cardiorespiratory Fitness and Other Precursors on Cardiovascular Disease and All-Cause Mortality in Men and Women." *JAMA* 276, no. 3 (1996): 205–10.

Campbell, T.C., B. Parpia, and J. Chen. "Diet, Lifestyle, and the Etiology of Coronary Artery Disease: The Cornell China Study." *American Journal of Cardiology* 82, no. 108 (1998): 18T–21T.

Canadian Society for Exercise Physiology. *Handbook for Canada's Physical Activity Guide to Healthy Active Living.* Ottawa: Health Canada, 1998.

Lee, I.M., and R.S. Paffenbarger Jr. "Physical Activity and Stroke Incidence: The Harvard Alumni Health Study." *Stroke* 29, no. 10 (October 1998); 2049–54.

Matheson G.O., et al. "Musculoskeletal Injuries Associated with Physical Activity in Older Adults." *Medicine and Science in Sports and Exercise* 21, no. 4 (1989): 379–85.

Mitchell, A. *The Nine American Lifestyles.* New York: Macmillan, 1983.

Oakley, G.P., Jr. "Eat Right and Take a Multivitamin." *New England Journal of Medicine* 338, no. 15 (1998): 1060–61.

Pate, R.R., et al. "Physical Activity and Public Health: A Recommendation from the Centers for Disease Control and Prevention and the American College of Sports Medicine." *JAMA* 273, no. 5 (1995): 402–7.

Pearson, T.A. "AHA Science Advisory: Alcohol and Heart Disease." *Circulation* 94, no. 11 (1996): 3023–25.

Thun, M.J., et al. "Alcohol Consumption and Mortality among Middle-aged and Elderly U.S. Adults." *New England Journal of Medicine* 337, no. 24 (1997): 1705–14.

Volkow, N.D., et al. "Decreased Striatal Dopaminergic Responsiveness in Detoxified Cocaine-Dependent Subjects." *Nature* 386 no. 6627 (1997): 830–33.

Wolf, S.L. et al. "Reducing Frailty and Falls in Older Persons." *Journal of the American Geriatrics Society* 44, no. 5 (1996): 489–97.

Wolfson, L., et al. "Balance and Strength Training in Older Adults: Intervention Gains and Tai Chi Maintenance." *Journal of the American Geriatrics Society* 44, no.5 (1996): 498–506.

Woo, K.S., et al. "Chinese Adults are Less Susceptible than Whites to Age-related Endothelial Dysfunction." *Journal of the American College of Cardiologists* 30, no. 1 (1997): 113–18.

Chapter 5: HQ and Life's Journey

Brody, E.J., and Reporters of *The New York Times*. *The New York Times Book of Health: How to Feel Fitter, Eat Better, and Live Longer*. New York: Random House, 1997.

Davidson, M.H., et al. "Weight Control and Risk Factor Reduction in Obese Subjects Treated for Two Years with Orlistat: A Randomized Controlled Trial." *JAMA* 281, no. 3 (January 20, 1999): 235–42.

Goleman, D. *Emotional Intelligence*. New York: Bantam Books, 1995.

Greenberg, S.A. American Diabetes Association's 58th Annual Scientific Sessions. Chicago, June 14, 1998.

Gunby, P. "'Life Begins' for Baltimore Longitudinal Study of Aging—Research Group Has 40th Birthday." *JAMA* 279, no. 13 (1998): 982–83.

National Heart, Lung and Blood Institute. *Clinical Guidelines on Overweight and Obesity*. U.S. National Institutes of Health, 1998.

Rowe, J.W., and R.L. Kahn. *Successful Aging*. New York: Pantheon Books, 1998.

Chapter 6: Mainstream Medicine

Collins, F.S., et al. "New Goals for the U.S. Human Genome Projects: 1998–2003." *Science* 282 (1998): 682–89.

Lazarou, J., B.H. Pomeranz, and P.N. Corey. "Incidence of Adverse Drug Reactions in Hospitalized Patients." *JAMA* 279, no. 15 (1998): 1200–1205.

National Institutes of Health. *NIH Consensus Development Conference Statement: Genetic Testing for Cystic Fibrosis*. Bethesda, MD: National Institutes of Health,

1997.

Stern, M.P. American Diabetes Association's 58th Annual Scientific Sessions. Chicago, June 14, 1998.

Watson J.D., J. Tooze, and D.T. Kurtz. *Recombinant DNA: A Short Course.* New York: Scientific American Books, 1983.

World Health Organization. *Life in the 21st Century: A Vision for All.* Geneva: WHO, 1998.

Chapter 7: Mind/Body Medicine

Goleman, D., and J. Gurin. *Mind/Body Medicine: How to Use Your Mind for Better Health.* Yonkers, N.Y.: Consumer Reports Books, 1993.

Penninx, B.W., et al. "Chronically Depressed Mood and Cancer Risk in Older Persons." *Journal of the National Cancer Institute* 90, no. 24 (December 1998): 1888–93.

Chapter 8: Non-mainstream Medicine

Bensoussan, A., et al. "Treatment of Irritable Bowel Syndrome with Chinese Herbal Medicine: A Randomized Controlled Trial." *JAMA* 280, no. 18 (1998): 1585–89.

Cardini, F., and H. Weixin. "Moxibustion for Correction of Breech Presentation: A Randomized Controlled Trial." *JAMA* 280, no. 18 (1998): 1580–84.

Eisenberg, D.M., et al. "Trends in Alternative Medicine Use in the United States, 1990–1997: Results of a Follow-up National Survey." *JAMA* 280, no. 18 (1998): 1569–75.

Micozzi, M.S. *Fundamentals of Complementary and Alternative Medicine.* New York: Churchill Livingstone, 1996.

Ornish, D. *Dr. Dean Ornish's Program for Reversing Heart Disease.* New York: Ivy Books, 1996.

Weil, A. *Spontaneous Healing.* New York: Fawcett Columbine, 1996.

Chapter 9: Managing Your Illness the HQ Way

Carroll, J., and R. Broadhead. *Good Health Online.* Scarborough, Ont.: Prentice Hall Canada, 1997.

Ornish, D. *Dr. Dean Ornish's Program for Reversing Heart Disease.* New York: Ivy Books, 1996.

ACKNOWLEDGEMENTS

I wish to thank the following individuals for their significant contributions to the first health book in the HQ series: Ms. Diane Barei, Dr. Herbert Benson, Dr. T. Berry Brazelton, Ms. Margaret Catley-Carlson, Dr. Theresa Chiang, Mrs. Janet Craig, Mr. David Devine, Mr. Richard K. Gallop, Mr. James O. Hall, Mrs. Elizabeth Haysom, Mr. Ian R. Haysom, Dr. Joseph Z. Losos, Dr. Joseph E. Pizzorno, Dr. Joseph Tai, Mr. Bruce Westwood and Ms. Susan Zhizhong Xu. In particular I am indebted to an exceptionally talented group of individuals—Ian, Elizabeth, Janet, Diane, Theresa and Joseph Tai—who have helped to make the writing style of this book suitable for the general reader. Both James and Bruce have worked endlessly to promote the book. Dr. Benson's pioneer work in mind/body medicine has provided inspiration in the development of the concept of HQ, the Health Quotient. Dr. Minzhang Chen, the late minister of health of China and a dear friend, provided advice and encouragement during the writing process but unfortunately passed away before seeing the published edition. And to the many others who have helped but have not been mentioned here I also owe a great deal of gratitude.

PERMISSIONS

Grossbart, Ted A., "The Skin: Matters of the Flesh" from *Mind/Body Medicine*, edited by Daniel Goleman and Joel Gurin. Reprinted by permission of Ted A. Grossbart.

Holland, Jimmie C., and Sheldon Lewis, "Emotions and Cancer: What Do We Really Know?" from *Mind/Body Medicine*, edited by Daniel Goleman and Joel Gurin. Reprinted by permission of Jimmie C. Holland and Sheldon Lewis.

Kabat-Zinn, Jon, "Mindfulness Meditation: Health Benefits of an Ancient Buddhist Practice" from *Mind/Body Medicine*, edited by Daniel Goleman and Joel Gurin. Reprinted by permission of Jon Kabat-Zinn.

Micozzi, Marc S., ed., *Fundamentals of Complementary and Alternative Medicine*. Copyright © 1996. Reprinted by permission of W.B. Saunders Company.

Mrazek, David A., "Asthma: Stress, Allergies, and the Genes" from *Mind/Body Medicine*, edited by Daniel Goleman and Joel Gurin. Reprinted by permission of David A. Mrazek.

Nash, Justin M. and Dennis C. Turk, "Chronic Pain: New Ways to Cope" from *Mind/Body Medicine*, edited by Daniel Goleman and Joel Gurin. Reprinted by permission of Justin M. Nash and Dennis C. Turk.

Ott, Wayne R. and John W. Roberts, "Everyday Exposure to Toxic Pollutants" from *Scientific American* (February 1998). Reprinted by permission of Scientific American, Inc.

Pelletier, Kenneth R., "Between Mind and Body: Stress, Emotions, and Health," from *Mind/Body Medicine*, edited by Daniel Goleman and Joel Gurin. Reprinted by permission of Kenneth R. Pelletier.

Pincus, Theodore, "Arthritis and Rheumatic Diseases: What Doctors Can Learn from Their Patients" from *Mind/Body Medicine*, edited by Daniel Goleman and Joel Gurin. Reprinted by permission of Theodore Pincus.

INDEX

Half-Angle Identities

$$\sin \frac{\alpha}{2} = \pm \sqrt{\frac{1 - \cos \alpha}{2}}$$

$$\cos \frac{\alpha}{2} = \pm \sqrt{\frac{1 + \cos \alpha}{2}}$$

$$\tan \frac{\alpha}{2} = \pm \sqrt{\frac{1 - \cos \alpha}{1 + \cos \alpha}}$$

$$= \frac{1 - \cos \alpha}{\sin \alpha}$$

$$= \frac{\sin \alpha}{1 + \cos \alpha}$$

The Law of Sines

In any triangle ABC, $\dfrac{\sin A}{a} = \dfrac{\sin B}{b} = \dfrac{\sin C}{c}$.

The Law of Cosines

For any triangle ABC, $a^2 = b^2 + c^2 - 2bc \cos A$,

$$b^2 = a^2 + c^2 - 2ac \cos B,$$
$$c^2 = a^2 + b^2 - 2ab \cos C.$$

Reference Angle/ASTC Procedure

To find the exact value of a trigonometric function
for a nonquadrantal angle whose reference angle is

$30° \left(\dfrac{\pi}{6}\right)$, $45° \left(\dfrac{\pi}{4}\right)$ or $60° \left(\dfrac{\pi}{3}\right)$:

1. Find the value of the reference angle.
2. Find the value of the appropriate trigonometric ratio for
   the reference angle (use the table of certain
   trigonometric values).
3. Determine the sign of this value using the ASTC rule.

Certain Trigonometric Values

	sine	cosine	tangent
$30°, \dfrac{\pi}{6}$	$\dfrac{1}{2}$	$\dfrac{\sqrt{3}}{2}$	$\dfrac{\sqrt{3}}{3}$
$45°, \dfrac{\pi}{4}$	$\dfrac{\sqrt{2}}{2}$	$\dfrac{\sqrt{2}}{2}$	1
$60°, \dfrac{\pi}{3}$	$\dfrac{\sqrt{3}}{2}$	$\dfrac{1}{2}$	$\sqrt{3}$

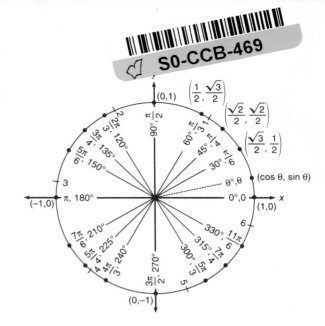

ASTC Rule

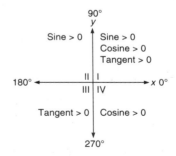

TRIGONOMETRY
WITH APPLICATIONS

SECOND EDITION

TRIGONOMETRY

WITH APPLICATIONS

SECOND EDITION

TERRY H. WESNER
HENRY FORD COMMUNITY COLLEGE

PHILIP H. MAHLER
MIDDLESEX COMMUNITY COLLEGE

WGB **Wm. C. Brown Publishers**
Dubuque, Iowa•Melbourne, Australia•Oxford, England

Book Team

Editor *Paula-Christy Heighton*
Developmental Editor *Theresa Grutz*
Production Editor *Eugenia M. Collins*
Designer *K. Wayne Harms*
Cover designer *Anna Manhart*
Photo Editor *Carrie Burger*

Wm. C. Brown Publishers
A Division of Wm. C. Brown Communications, Inc.

Vice President and General Manager *Beverly Kolz*
Vice President, Publisher *Earl McPeek*
Vice President, Director of Sales and Marketing *Virginia S. Moffat*
National Sales Manager *Douglas J. DiNardo*
Marketing Manager *Julie Joyce Keck*
Advertising Manager *Janelle Keeffer*
Director of Production *Colleen A. Yonda*
Publishing Services Manager *Karen J. Slaght*
Permissions/Records Manager *Connie Allendorf*

Wm. C. Brown Communications, Inc.

President and Chief Executive Officer *G. Franklin Lewis*
Corporate Senior Vice President, President of WCB Manufacturing *Roger Meyer*
Corporate Senior Vice President and Chief Financial Officer *Robert Chesterman*

Cover photo © Bill Brooks/Masterfile

Copyedited by Patricia Steele

Copyright © 1994 by Wm. C. Brown Communications, Inc. All rights reserved

A Times Mirror Company

Library of Congress Catalog Card Number: 93–71068

ISBN 0–697–12292–1

Printed in the United States of America by Wm. C. Brown Communications, Inc.,
2460 Kerper Boulevard, Dubuque, IA 52001

10 9 8 7 6 5 4 3 2 1

To Robert Shannon Wesner

Dad

To my students

Philip Mahler

Contents

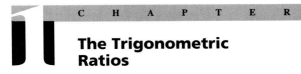
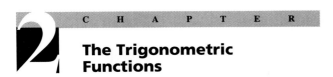

CHAPTER 5
Trigonometric Equations

CHAPTER 6
Oblique Triangles and Vectors

CHAPTER 7
Complex Numbers and Polar Coordinates

Preface

Intent

This text is designed to serve as a one-semester introduction to trigonometry and its applications for college students.

Assumptions

It is assumed that students have basic skills in solving linear and quadratic equations, working with radicals, and simple graphing as well as some acquaintance with, and access to, a scientific calculator.

There is no separate chapter of review material. Most students react negatively to such a chapter, and many teachers get bogged down in unnecessary details in such a chapter. In this book, material is reviewed as it is encountered during the exposition of the new material. Focusing on old skills when they become necessary provides a more interesting sequence for students. The best motivation for reviewing something is the fact that it is needed to learn something new. Examples go out of their way to review the algebraic skills being applied, as they first arise.

Calculators

It is assumed that students have constant access to a modern scientific/engineering calculator. In terms of approximate calculations, the text is completely calculator oriented. However, the usual exact radian/degree values, for $\frac{\pi}{6}(30°)$, $\frac{\pi}{4}(45°)$, and their multiples, are explicitly used as well.

Many students today have access to graphing calculators. The book is designed to be used *without* these calculators, but their use is encouraged. The text shows how to use these calculators for the many graphs that occur in trigonometry. The TEXAS INSTRUMENTS TI-81 is used to illustrate within the text. Appendix B, *Further uses for graphing calculators and computers,* shows further detail on using the TI-81 and also presents material on using the CASIO *fx*-7000 graphing calculator.

Content

Chapter 1 reviews the basic geometric foundations of right triangle trigonometry, followed by the trigonometry of the right triangle. The term trigonometric *ratio* is used to distinguish the definitions made in terms of the right triangle from those made in chapter 2 in terms of points in the plane. We begin with right triangle trigonometry for at least the following four reasons. First, a survey of mathematics teachers indicated a clear preference for this approach. Second, this allows students to start the course in territory that is probably familiar, degree measure and right triangles. Third, applications in this area can be drawn from everyday experience. Fourth, this approach is most helpful to those students who may be starting a physics or other technical course at the same time.

The secant, cosecant, and cotangent functions are defined as reciprocals of the cosine, sine and tangent functions. In this way students are exposed to identities immediately, and, after all, this is the way we view these functions in advanced applications.

The use of the calculator, including a basic use of the inverse trigonometric functions, is covered in this chapter.

The chapter ends with a section that introduces trigonometric equations, both conditional and identities. It is important for students to see equations involving trigonometric functions early and throughout the course. The topic of conditional equations is revisited in the context of radian measure in chapter 2. In this way, the inevitable chapter on trigonometric equations (chapter 5) becomes simply an expansion of previous material, instead of the cold shock it often is for students.

Chapter 2 begins with a review of *functions,* which are introduced in terms of sets of ordered pairs. This approach combines mathematical precision with pedagogical simplicity (as opposed to a long statement about rules associating something with something else). It also permits a much simpler, more natural development of the concepts of one-to-one and inverse functions and has no negative impact on acquiring ability with $f(x)$ terminology. In addition, this approach helps avoid the documented problem that most students cannot separate the concept of a function from a defining expression (i.e., an equation).

This chapter then covers the trigonometry of angles in standard position. In this exposition of analytic trigonometry, we refer to trigonometric *functions* not ratios. The topic is first completely covered with familiar angle measure. Radians are then introduced, and the topic is revisited in these terms, including the solution of simple conditional equations in terms of radians.

Chapter 3 gives a more in-depth treatment of the properties of the trigonometric functions as functions from the real numbers to the real numbers. Domains, ranges, and graphs are stressed. An uncommon method of graphing periodic functions is introduced here. Period and phase shift are not treated separately but are integrated into one step. It is our experience that this independently discovered the method of graphing quite complicated functions is easily and quickly taught and learned. It also provides a basis for understanding what makes periodic functions intrinsically different from nonperiodic functions.

This chapter also supports the use of graphing calculators to obtain graphs, for those who have access to these calculators.

Chapter 4 discusses the inverse of any function, then fully treats the inverse trigonometric functions. Students will have some feeling for these functions from earlier chapters, where they were explicitly mentioned in the context of finding unknown angles and solving conditional equations. The simplification of expressions involving these functions, using reference triangles, is stressed. This skill is very important in a calculus course.

The definitions of the inverse cosecant and secant functions are made in terms of the inverse sine and cosine functions. Although less common than other possible definitions, this is in keeping with other sources and provides a great simplicity in learning and using these functions. Some calculus texts define the ranges of these functions differently than as presented here (for good reason, in that context), but the additional complexity is not pedagogically warranted for

an introduction. The definitions here, by the way, agree with those used in at least one popular symbolic algebra computer package.

Chapter 5 is a full treatment of trigonometric identities and conditional equations. The modern depth of coverage and the introduction in earlier chapters of most of the concepts should provide the basis for success for both teachers and students. Section 5–0 is explicitly designed to widen the scope of how students understand an expression to include trigonometric functions.

Chapter 6 presents topics that are applications of the previous material. The laws of sines and cosines are presented, and analytic vectors are introduced. The way in which the law of sines is presented should eliminate confusion for most students. The important fact that no triangle has more than one obtuse angle is stressed and used to solve triangles in a directed way.

Chapter 7 covers complex numbers, including De Moivre's theorem, and polar coordinates. The graphing of polar coordinates includes an independently discovered approach to the graphing of certain polar equations using the rectangular coordinate graph as a guide. This is a nontraditional approach, which the authors have used with success. It is easy to use, promotes a "feeling" for polar graphs, and reviews the graphing of trigonometric equations in rectangular coordinates.

Appendixes

Appendix A discusses using addition of ordinates for graphing. This topic is of much less practical value in the age of the electronic graphing device, but it can be a valuable pedagogical tool to promote the understanding of functions.

Appendix B presents more material on using graphing calculators. It can be used to enhance a course where every student has access to these wonderful devices.

Appendix C is the lengthy algebraic development of an identity, which may or may not be used in the course. This development has been set aside in an appendix because its inclusion within the text does not promote students' reading of the text or even a better understanding of the material.

Appendix D provides graphical material which the student may want to reproduce and have handy as an aid in studying.

Appendix E provides the answers to odd-numbered exercise problems, all chapter review problems, and all chapter test problems. Solutions are also provided for those trial exercise problems whose number is boxed in the exercise sets.

Exposition of the Material

We have attempted to write the exposition of the material in clear, understandable prose, in a logical order of development. Each section of a chapter is designed to provide accessible reading for students and clear examples of the skills that students are expected to master in that section. We have also tried to provide a cross section of *applications,* mainly in the exercises. These are designed to put the subject in a wider context of knowledge and therefore to pique students' interest. In particular, we have tried to show that trigonometry has become more important than ever in the age of the digital computer.

Each section of every chapter ends with a list of *mastery points,* which clearly states what students should know from that section. The exercise sets are designed to enable students to apply the material learned in the examples within the text, which attempt to provide a clear outline of the skills that the student must master. The exercise sets reinforce these skills explicitly, with many problems similar to the examples. Some problems require that students synthesize what has been learned, and a few require above-average efforts to solve. These are marked with the symbol ⬤ . The complete solutions to those problems whose numbers are contained in boxes, called *trial problems,* are given in Appendix E.

A set of core problems are indicated in each exercise set by having their numbers in color. These problems exemplify each of the mastery points. Thus, if students can do these problems without error or difficulty then they have mastered the skills presented in that section. This is provided for those students who do not have the time to work a larger subset of the exercises. All students are still well advised to do the more difficult less skill oriented problems at the end of the exercise set when assigned.

Each chapter ends with a *chapter summary, chapter review,* and *chapter test.* The summary serves as a memory jogger, to be occasionally reviewed after the chapter is completed. The review consists of problems that enable students to practice the skills acquired throughout the chapter; these problems are keyed by section. The test is designed to allow students to practice a chapter test before seeing one in class. The material in the chapter test is removed from its exposition—this is the opportunity for students to see the material out of context, which is the situation when taking an in-class test.

Text Features

Some of the themes which we believe make this text special include the following.

- Algorithmic   The text is explicit about procedures for accomplishing the skills required. These procedures are highlighted in the text. The examples explicitly follow these procedures.
- Detailed   Skills and knowledge that are often assumed of students, but that in fact are not present, are explicitly covered. Rationalizing denominators is shown many times, as are many other algebraic manipulations, in the examples. Another example of this is the explicit coverage of the manipulation of the fractions involved in the radian measures, which are multiples of $\dfrac{\pi}{6}$ and $\dfrac{\pi}{4}$, and achieving a feeling for the location on the unit circle of these measures. Still another is the algebraic manipulations often used in solving identities.
- Gradual skill building   The level of algebraic competence required builds through the chapters. For example, solving equations in which a product equals zero is covered early, whereas factoring is postponed until the chapter on identities.

    Identities and conditional equations are difficult, so they are introduced early, and revisited lightly in the chapters preceding the chapter on trigonometric equations.

Solving right triangles is so basic to trigonometry at all levels of abstraction that it must be second nature. For this reason, right triangles are stressed not only in the applications and theoretical development but also as a means of finding the values of trigonometric functions when given the value of one of them. This is most important in a calculus course.

- Repetition of themes   There are many themes that are revisited over and over in the chapters. Examples include solving conditional equations and manipulating identities, solving right triangles, and the idea of reference angles. In addition, a great deal of material is explicitly repeated when radian measure is covered in the last third of chapter 2.

    Vectors in two dimensions, complex numbers in polar form, and polar coordinates have a great deal of similarity in skills required, particularly in conversions between rectangular and polar forms. We have stressed these similarities.

- Balance of concrete versus abstract   Most attention is paid to numeric manipulations, as in solving triangles and finding the values of trigonometric functions when given the value of one trigonometric function, but attention is paid to symbolic manipulation as well. Using these skills with symbolic manipulation is important in a calculus course, and they have not been short changed.

    Some of the exercises, always toward the end of each exercise set, also stress more abstract thinking, as well as the investigation of related ideas.

Changes from the Previous Edition

All references to tables of values have been deleted in this edition. This simplifies the material in the earlier chapters, allowing some material to migrate toward the front of the text. Functions are now explicitly reviewed earlier, at the beginning of chapter 2. This better provides the setting for the introduction of the trigonometric functions.

The topic of radian measure occurs earlier, in chapter 2 also. This provides the setting for reviewing the trigonometric functions in a new context.

A section on graphing by addition of ordinates is moved to the appendixes. Introductory material on the inverse trigonometric functions and trigonometric equations is more thoroughly integrated into the earlier chapters.

The chapter on identities is refashioned to include a more explicit review of equation solving and algebraic manipulation. Several sections were combined, which allows a more coherent presentation of the material.

In the previous edition, vectors and complex numbers each got two sections. The material on vectors was simplified by lessening the stress on geometric vectors and proceeding more quickly to analytic vectors. Thus, vectors are now treated in one section. It also seemed pedagogically appropriate and feasible to combine the two sections on complex numbers into one, with only minor adjustments in coverage, at no loss of depth. A section on graphing polar equations has been added.

The appendix on graphing calculators is new, as is the discussion of these calculators within the text. It is only a matter of time and economics before these devices are universally used in mathematics courses, and they can certainly be used with this text.

An appendix was added containing material students may want to reproduce xerographically. In particular, rectangular and polar coordinate templates are provided.

Supplements

For the instructor

The *Instructor's Manual* includes an introduction to the text, a guide to the supplements that accompany *Trigonometry,* and reproducible chapter tests. Also included are a complete listing of all mastery points and suggested course schedules based on the mastery points. The final section of the *Instructor's Manual* contains answers to the reproducible materials.

The *Instructor's Solutions Manual* contains completely worked-out solutions to all of the exercises in the textbook.

Selected *Overhead Transparencies* are available to enhance classroom presentations.

WCB Computerized Testing Program provides you with an easy-to-use computerized testing and grade management program. No programming experience is required to generate tests randomly, by objective, by section, or by selecting specific test items. In addition, test items can be edited and new test items can be added. Also included with the *WCB Computerized Testing Program* is an on-line testing option which allows students to take tests on the computer. Tests can then be graded and the scores forwarded to the grade-keeping portion of the program.

The *Test Item File* is a printed version of the computerized testing program that allows you to examine all of the prepared test items and choose test items based on chapter, section, or objective. The objectives are taken directly from *Trigonometry*.

For the student

The *Student's Solutions Manual* introduces the student to the textbook and includes solutions to every-other odd-numbered section exercise and odd-numbered end-of-chapter exercise problems. It is available for student purchase.

Videotapes covering the major topics in each chapter are available. Each concept is introduced with a real-world problem and is followed by careful explanation and worked-out examples using computer-generated graphics. These videos can be used in the math lab for remediation or even the classroom to motivate or enhance the lecture. The videotapes are available free to qualified adopters.

The concepts and skills developed in *Trigonometry* are reinforced through the interactive *Software*.

The Plotter is software for graphing and analyzing functions. This software simulates a graphing calculator on a PC. You may use it to do the technology exercises even if you don't have a graphics calculator. A manual is included that describes operations and includes student exercises. The software is menu driven and has an easy-to-use window-type interface. The high-quality graphics can also be used for classroom presentation and demonstration. Students who go on to calculus classes will want to keep the software for future use.

Acknowledgments

The authors wish to acknowledge the many reviewers of this text, both in its initial form and again after their many constructive suggestions and criticisms had been addressed. In particular, we wish to acknowledge Judy Barclay, Cuesta College; Glenn R. Boston, Catawba Valley Community College; Barbara Cohen, West Los Angeles College; Daniel B. McCallum, University of Arkansas at Little Rock; Peggy Miller, University of Nebraska at Kearney; and Mary Jane Still; Annette Trujillo, New Mexico State University. We need to acknowledge Ruth Mikkelson who did a great deal of fine work to try to make the text error free. Our thanks to Linda J. Murphy, Carol Hay, and Nancy K. Nickerson of Northern Essex Community College for carefully and conscientiously checking the accuracy of the entire typeset text. We also wish to acknowledge Patricia Steele who did an outstanding job as copy editor, and who often went beyond what was required and gave excellent editorial suggestions.

Throughout the development, writing, and production of this text, two WCB employees have been of such great value they deserve special recognition: Theresa Grutz and Eugenia M. Collins.

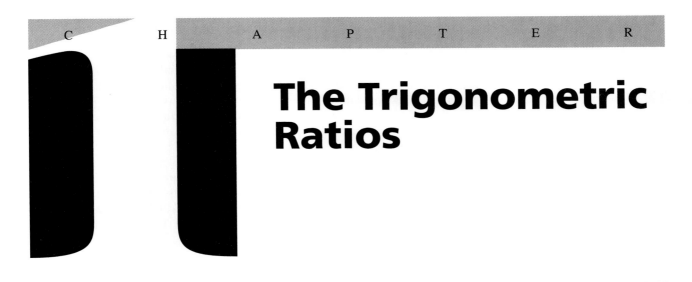

The Trigonometric Ratios

1–0 Introduction

Initially trigonometry was developed to express relationships between the sizes of the arcs in circles and the chords determining those arcs. (An arc is a portion of the circumference of a circle; a chord is a line segment going from one point on a circle to another.) These relationships were used in astronomy more than two thousand years ago to study what is called the celestial sphere. In fact, until the fifteenth century, trigonometry was mostly applied to spheres. This part of trigonometry is now called spherical trigonometry, and it is still used in navigation and astronomy.

After the fifteenth century, trigonometry was also used to relate the measure of angles in a triangle to the lengths of the sides of the triangle. The word "trigonometry," which means "triangle measurement," is credited to Bartholomaus Pitiscus (1561–1613). Besides being used in surveying, trigonometry became important for the physics being developed by Sir Isaac Newton and others. Practically all the ideas of trigonometry had been developed by the eighteenth century.

Over the next two hundred years, trigonometry became more and more important as it was used to describe many physical phenomena, such as electricity, magnetism, and sound.

Today, in the age of the computer, trigonometry is being used even more. The computer can control manufacturing machines to great precison, but only if trigonometry is used to describe where this precision is to be applied. This whole area of engineering, called numerical control, relies heavily on the ideas we will study in this book. Computer graphics use aspects of projective geometry, which again uses the concepts of trigonometry. Voice recognition by computers uses a concept in mathematics called Fourier transforms, which again is built on these same ideas.

From medicine to manufacturing, from solar design to computer art, the ideas we study here are found over and over again.

In this chapter we learn how trigonometry provides a method for telling us a great deal about a right triangle from limited information. These simple ideas, widely applied in science, engineering, and mathematics, lay the groundwork for some of the more advanced ideas we will eventually need.

Students are expected to have access to engineering or scientific calculators to facilitate many of the calculations throughout this text. Many calculations are followed by the notation $\boxed{\text{CS } n}$, where n is an integer. This indicates that the appropriate calculator steps are shown at the end of that section. Steps are shown for a generic algebraic calculator (one with an $\boxed{=}$ key, indicated by Ⓐ) and for a generic postfix notation calculator (indicated by Ⓟ). The latter calculator has no $\boxed{=}$ key but has an $\boxed{\text{ENTER}}$ or $\boxed{\uparrow}$ key instead. Steps are also shown for the Texas Instruments TI-81 calculator. These are indicated by $\boxed{\text{TI-81}}$.

Some preliminary words are in order about calculating with a calculator. It is difficult to give a general rule for the number of digits that should appear in the final result of a calculation, and a discussion of this is outside the scope and intent of this book. The number of digits to which an approximate number should be rounded is specified throughout the text. The number of digits is chosen to represent a reasonable, if sometimes arbitrary, value.

Also, we will apply the most straightforward rounding rule to values. That is, if the first discarded digit is 5 or above we round up, otherwise we do not. Thus, 2.349 rounds to 2.35 to two decimal places, and to 2.3 to one decimal place.

1–1 Angle measurement, the right triangle, and the Pythagorean theorem

Angle measurement

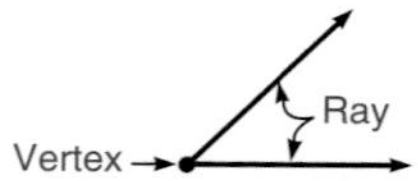

An **angle** is composed of two rays, both beginning at what is called the **vertex** of the angle. Figure 1–1 shows a representation of an angle.

In modern geometry a method of angle measurement is assumed. We will assume that angles can be measured in **degrees.** The notation for degrees is °. A common and useful interpretation of angle measure is ''the amount of rotation'' of one ray away from the other. In this context, 90° corresponds to a quarter-rotation, 180° to a half-rotation, 270° to a three-quarter rotation, and 360° to a full rotation. Naturally, the measurement of an angle does not necessarily imply any actual rotation. See figure 1–2.

Vertex →   Ray

Figure 1–1

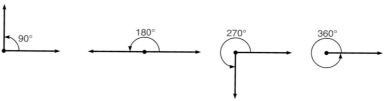

Figure 1–2

An angle with measure between 0° and 90° is said to be **acute;** an angle with measure 90° is **right;** an angle with measure between 90° and 180° is **obtuse;** and an angle with measure 180° is a **straight angle.**

One degree is divided into smaller units in two ways: using the degree, minute, second system and using the decimal degree system.

In the **degree, minute, second (DMS) system** a degree is divided into 60 equal parts called *minutes,* and each minute is divided into 60 equal parts called *seconds.* This is analogous to the way in which hours are divided into minutes and seconds on the clock. The notation for minutes is ′ and the notation for seconds is ″. For example, 51°18′22″ means 51 degrees, 18 minutes, and 22 seconds.

In the **decimal degree system** the degree measure is written in decimal notation. For example, 2.53° is in decimal degrees and means 2 and 53 hundredths of a degree.

Calculators will generally not perform operations on values in the DMS system, so we must be able to convert from this system to decimal form. Many calculators are programmed to do this. They typically use keys marked $\boxed{\circ\ ′\ ″}$ or $\boxed{\rightarrow\text{H}}$. This is illustrated in example 1–1 A for two typical calculators. Also note that we use the fact that there are 60 minutes in one degree, and $60^2 = 3{,}600$ seconds in one degree.

■ *Example 1–1 A*

Convert 46°42′27″ to decimal degrees to the nearest 0.001°.

Manually:

$$46° + \left(\frac{42}{60}\right)° + \left(\frac{27}{3600}\right)°$$

Rewrite minutes and seconds as fractional parts of a degree

46.7075° $\boxed{\text{CS 1}}$

46.708°   Round to the nearest 0.001°

Calculator A:

46 $\boxed{\circ\ ′\ ″}$ 42 $\boxed{\circ\ ′\ ″}$ 27 $\boxed{\circ\ ′\ ″}$

Calculator B:

46.4227 $\boxed{\rightarrow\text{H}}$ "H" stands for hours   ■

The right triangle

A closed figure composed of three straight sides will always include three angles, and these figures are therefore called **triangles**[1] (*tri* is from the Latin for three). (Actually the angles are formed by extending the sides, which are line segments, to form rays.)

A useful property of triangles is that *the measures of the three angles of a triangle always add up to 180°.* This fact was known thousands of years ago and its first known demonstration appears in Euclid's *Elements,* an ancient Greek book on geometry. This allows us to find the measure of the third angle in a triangle if we know the measures of the other two: if we add the measures

---

[1]Note that, unless otherwise specified, all references to lines, triangles, etc., are to these concepts as they occur in plane, or Euclidean, geometry. Fortunately, this is the geometry with which the reader is most likely to be familiar, but it is worth mentioning that mathematics recognizes other "types" of geometry, called non-Euclidean geometries. In fact, several of these geometries find applications in modern physics.

of the two known angles and subtract this from the known total, 180°, the result must be the measure of the third angle.

Note   We often denote angles using Greek letters. The letters most often used are α (alpha), β (beta), γ (gamma), and θ (theta).

■ *Example 1–1 B*

Find the measure of angle α in the triangle in the figure.

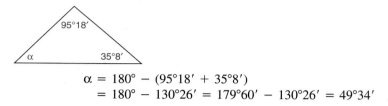

$$\alpha = 180° - (95°18' + 35°8')$$
$$= 180° - 130°26' = 179°60' - 130°26' = 49°34'$$ ■

When we say that a side of a triangle is **opposite** to an angle, we are referring to the side that is not used to form the angle. When we say that a side of a triangle is **adjacent** to an angle, we mean that the side actually forms one side of the angle. For example, in triangle *ABC* in figure 1–3, we would say that side *BC* is opposite to angle *A,* while sides *AB* and *AC* are each adjacent to angle *A.*

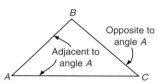

Figure 1–3

A **right triangle** is a triangle in which one of the angles is a right angle (90°). In such a triangle, two of the angles must be acute (less than 90°), since their measures must add up to 90°. The side of a right triangle that is opposite the right angle is called the **hypotenuse,** and the sides that are adjacent to the right angle are sometimes called **legs.** See figure 1–4.

One particular way to label right triangles is widely used. Unless we are told otherwise, in a right triangle we always label the right angle *C* and the two acute angles *A* and *B.* The lengths of the legs are always labeled *a* and *b,* with *a* opposite angle *A* and *b* opposite angle *B.* The hypotenuse is always labeled *c.* This is illustrated in figure 1–5.

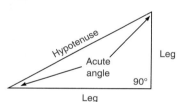

Figure 1–4

Note   The symbol ⌐ denotes a right angle.

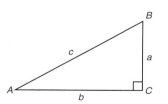

Figure 1–5

The Pythagorean theorem

We often use the following theorem.[2] It is one of the most important facts in mathematics.

> **The Pythagorean theorem**
> In a right triangle with legs having lengths *a* and *b* and hypotenuse having length *c,*
> $$a^2 + b^2 = c^2$$

We use the Pythagorean theorem to find the length of the hypotenuse of a right triangle if we know the lengths of the two legs.

[2]The word *theorem* means a statement that has been proved to be true, and the proof of this theorem is credited to the Greek mathematician Pythagoras (sixth century B.C.), who is said to have sacrificed an ox as an offering of thanks. In the last two thousand years literally hundreds of proofs of this theorem have been given.

■ *Example 1–1 C*

If the two legs of a right triangle have lengths 6 and 8, what is the length of the hypotenuse?

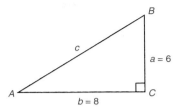

To use the Pythagorean theorem, we label one leg a and the other b. See the figure. Let $a = 6$ and $b = 8$ and use the theorem as follows:

$$a^2 + b^2 = c^2 \text{ so } 6^2 + 8^2 = c^2$$
$$100 = c^2$$

To find c we take the principal square root of 100:

$$\sqrt{100} = c$$
$$10 = c$$ ■

The Pythagorean theorem also provides a way to find the length of one leg of a right triangle if the hypotenuse and the other leg are known.

■ *Example 1–1 D*

If one leg of a right triangle has length 7, and the hypotenuse has length 14, find the length of the other leg. Find the answer both exactly and to the nearest tenth.

Let $a = 7$ and b be the unknown side, as in the figure. Then,

$$a^2 + b^2 = c^2$$

so

$$7^2 + b^2 = 14^2$$
$$49 + b^2 = 196$$
$$b^2 = 147$$
$$b = \sqrt{147}$$
$$b = \sqrt{(49)(3)}$$
$$b = \sqrt{49}\sqrt{3}$$
$$b = 7\sqrt{3} \qquad \text{Exact solution}$$
$$b \approx 12.1 \qquad \text{Approximate solution}[3] \boxed{\text{CS 2}}$$ ■

It can also be shown that *if $a^2 + b^2 = c^2$, then that triangle is a right triangle, and the right angle is opposite side c.*

[3]When we write something like $7\sqrt{3} \approx 12.1$, we mean that $7\sqrt{3}$ is *approximately* 12.1. This use of the symbol $\approx$ is adhered to in this text to signify approximate values.

■ *Example 1–1 E*

1. Is the triangle in the figure a right triangle?

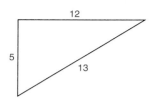

If the triangle is a right triangle, then the hypotenuse would be the side having length 13 (*the hypotenuse of a right triangle is always the longest side*). Therefore the legs would have lengths 5 and 12. We now add the squares of the lengths of the legs and see if this sum equals the square of the hypotenuse, 13.

$$5^2 + 12^2 = 25 + 144 = 169, \text{ and}$$
$$13^2 = 169$$

Thus, $a^2 + b^2 = c^2$ and, therefore, the triangle is a right triangle.

Note   In part 1 of example 1–1 E, we stated that the hypotenuse of a right triangle is always the longest side. This is because *in any triangle,* whether or not it is a right triangle, *the longest side is always opposite the largest angle.* Similarly, the shortest side is always opposite the smallest angle.

2. The sides of a triangle have lengths 32, 53, and 62. Is the triangle a right triangle?

Using the Pythagorean theorem,

$$32^2 + 53^2 = 1{,}024 + 2{,}809 = 3{,}833 \text{ and } 62^2 = 3{,}844$$

Since $a^2 + b^2 \neq c^2$, we see that the triangle is not a right triangle.   ■

As we said earlier, the Pythagorean theorem is one of the most important facts in mathematics because it has so many applications to practical situations and technical problems. Many situations in science and technology can be described, or modeled, using right triangles. If we know that a physical situation can be described in terms of right triangles, then all of the mathematics that applies to right triangles can be used to learn more about the situation or to solve a given problem.

In practice we must often make simplifying assumptions about the situation. For example, we may assume that a telephone pole makes a right angle with the ground, when in fact it is unlikely that the angle is exactly 90°, or we may assume that the earth is flat, that ''level'' roads are perfectly level, etc.

■ *Example 1–1 F*

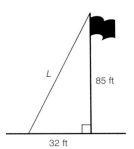

1. A guy wire is to be attached to the top of a flagpole and anchored in the ground at a point 32 feet from the base of the flagpole. If the pole is 85 feet high, how long will the guy wire have to be, to the nearest foot?

   We first draw a figure to describe the problem, as shown. We assume that a flagpole is constructed to form as close to a 90° angle with the ground as possible. Also, we ignore the fact that the wire will actually sag somewhat and therefore is not a true straight line.

   We can see from the figure that the unknown length of the guy wire L is the hypotenuse of a right triangle in which the legs have lengths 85 and 32. Thus, the Pythagorean theorem provides the answer.

$$85^2 + 32^2 = L^2$$
$$8{,}249 = L^2$$
$$\sqrt{8{,}249} = L$$
$$90.8 \approx L \qquad \boxed{\text{CS 3}}$$

   To the nearest foot, the guy wire must be 91 feet long.

2. In the theory of alternating current[4] in electronics, the total **circuit impedance** Z in an inductive circuit can be found if we know the **inductive reactance** X_L and the **resistance** R by using the impedance diagram shown in the figure.

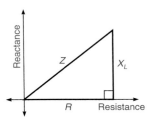

   Suppose $R = 320$ ohms and $X_L = 160$ ohms. Find Z to the nearest ten ohms.

   Using the Pythagorean theorem,

$$Z^2 = R^2 + X_L^2$$
$$Z^2 = 320^2 + 160^2$$
$$Z^2 = 128{,}000$$
$$Z = \sqrt{128{,}000}$$
$$Z \approx 357.8$$
$$Z \approx 360 \text{ ohms, to the nearest ten ohms}$$

---

[4]As in many other examples and problems in this text, the reader may not be familiar with the terminology and/or the facts involved in the application being illustrated. Please note, however, that where the necessary background is not provided, the problem is phrased so that it is clear to the reader which mathematical operation is required to achieve the desired result.

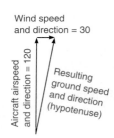

Wind speed
and direction = 30

Aircraft airspeed
and direction = 120

Resulting
ground speed
and direction
(hypotenuse)

3. An aircraft is flying with an airspeed of 120 knots[5] and a heading of due north. A 30-knot wind is blowing from the west. What is the aircraft's ground speed, to the nearest knot?

It is a fact of physics that we can represent the speeds and directions given above in a right triangle as illustrated in the figure. The ground speed of the aircraft is the length of the hypotenuse. Solving the triangle shows that the ground speed is 124 knots:

$$(\text{ground speed})^2 = 120^2 + 30^2 = 15{,}300$$
$$\text{ground speed} = \sqrt{15{,}300}$$
$$\approx 124$$

■

Calculator steps

1. Ⓐ 46 $\boxed{+}$ 42 $\boxed{÷}$ 60 $\boxed{+}$ 27 $\boxed{÷}$ 3600 $\boxed{=}$ Display $\boxed{46.7075}$

Ⓟ 46 $\boxed{\text{ENTER}}$ 42 $\boxed{\text{ENTER}}$ 60 $\boxed{÷}$ $\boxed{+}$ 27 $\boxed{\text{ENTER}}$ 3600 $\boxed{÷}$ $\boxed{+}$

$\boxed{\text{TI-81}}$ 46 $\boxed{+}$ 42 $\boxed{÷}$ 60 $\boxed{+}$ 27 $\boxed{÷}$ 3600 $\boxed{\text{ENTER}}$

2. Ⓐ 7 $\boxed{×}$ 3 $\boxed{\sqrt{x}}$ $\boxed{=}$ Display $\boxed{12.12435566}$

Ⓟ 7 $\boxed{\text{ENTER}}$ 3 $\boxed{\sqrt{x}}$ $\boxed{×}$

$\boxed{\text{TI-81}}$ 7 $\boxed{×}$ $\boxed{\sqrt{\ }}$ 3 $\boxed{\text{ENTER}}$

3. Ⓐ 85 $\boxed{x^2}$ $\boxed{+}$ 32 $\boxed{x^2}$ $\boxed{=}$ $\boxed{\sqrt{x}}$ Display $\boxed{90.82400564}$

Ⓟ 85 $\boxed{x^2}$ 32 $\boxed{x^2}$ $\boxed{+}$ $\boxed{\sqrt{x}}$

$\boxed{\text{TI-81}}$ $\boxed{\sqrt{\ }}$ $\boxed{(}$ 85 $\boxed{x^2}$ $\boxed{+}$ 32 $\boxed{x^2}$ $\boxed{)}$ $\boxed{\text{ENTER}}$

Mastery points

Can you

- State whether a given angle is acute, right, straight, or obtuse?
- Convert from the degree, minute, second system to the decimal degree system?
- Find the third angle of any triangle when you know the other two angles?
- Give the definition of right triangle and draw and label one using the conventional notation?
- State the Pythagorean theorem?
- Use the Pythagorean theorem to find one side of a right triangle when you know the other two sides?

[5]One knot means one nautical mile per hour. A nautical mile is $\frac{1}{60}$ of a degree on the earth's circumference. It is approximately 6,080.27 feet. Nautical miles are often used in the navigation of ships and aircraft.

Exercise 1–1

Convert each angle to its measure in decimal degrees. Round the answer to the nearest 0.001° where necessary. Also, state whether each angle is acute, obtuse, straight, or right.

1. 13°25′
2. 111°56′
3. 0°12′
4. 42°37′
5. 25°33′19″
6. 87°2′13″
7. 165°47′
8. 19°15′
9. 33°5′55″
10. 0°19′12″
11. 159°59′
12. 20°1′

13. Draw a representation of a right triangle and label it using the conventional labeling (using *A*, *B*, *C*, *a*, *b*, *c*).

14. State the Pythagorean theorem from memory.

In the following problems find the measure of the angle θ.

15.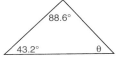

16.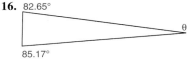

17.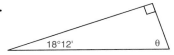

18.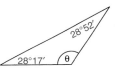

19.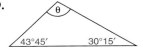

20.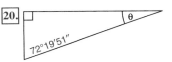

In the following problems state whether each triangle is a right triangle or not; if the triangle is a right triangle, state the length of the hypotenuse.

21.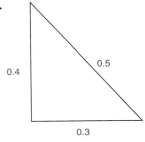

22.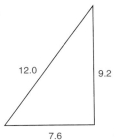

23.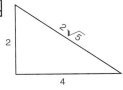

24.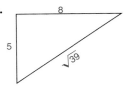

25.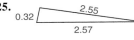

26.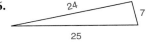

In the following problems two of the three sides of a right triangle are given. Use the Pythagorean theorem to calculate the length of the missing side; leave your answer in exact form and also approximate your answer to the same number of decimal places as the data (if necessary).

	a	*b*	*c*		*a*	*b*	*c*		*a*	*b*	*c*
27.	9	12	?	28.	10	?	26	29.	?	8	10
30.	5	10	?	31.	12	?	18	32.	?	6.8	9.2
33.	$\sqrt{5}$	3	?	34.	13.2	19.6	?	35.	100	150	?
36.	0.66	1.42	?	37.	$\sqrt{7}$	3	?	38.	4	?	$\sqrt{23}$
39.	6.3	?	15.0	40.	2	?	3	41.	$3\sqrt{2}$	$4\sqrt{5}$	?
42.	$3\sqrt{2}$	?	$4\sqrt{5}$	43.	?	19	28	44.	1,002	3,512	?
45.	1	1	?	46.	30	?	50				

Solve the following problems.

47. A flagpole is 55 feet tall and is supported by a wire attached at the top of the pole and to the ground 26 feet from the base of the pole. How long is the wire, to the nearest foot?

48. A flagpole is 93 feet tall and is supported by a guy wire that is 157 feet long, attached at the top of the pole and to the ground some distance from the base of the pole. Find the distance of the wire's ground attachment point from the base of the pole, to the nearest foot.

49. A surveyor has made the measurements shown in the diagram in order to compute the width of a pond. How wide is the pond, to the nearest 0.1 foot?

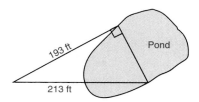

This diagram is called an impedance diagram. It is used to compute total impedance in a certain electronic circuit. X_L means inductive reactance, R is resistance, and Z is impedance. All units are ohms.

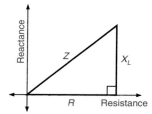

50. If X_L is 40.0 ohms and R is 56.6 ohms, calculate the total impedance Z to the nearest 0.1 ohm.

51. Suppose that X_L is 5.68 ohms and R is 19.25 ohms. Find Z to the nearest 0.01 ohm.

52. If $Z = 213$ ohms and $R = 183$ ohms, find X_L to the nearest ohm.

53. If $X_L = 2,150$ ohms and $Z = 4,340$ ohms, find R to the nearest 10 ohms.

54. A triangular piece of land has been surveyed and the results are shown in the diagram. What can you say about the accuracy of the survey? Give a reason for your answer.

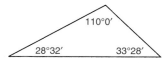

55. A rectangular piece of land has been surveyed and the results are shown in the diagram. What can you say about the accuracy of the survey? Give a reason for your answer.

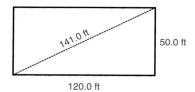

56. A machinist has to cut a rectangular piece of steel along its diagonal. The saw that will be used can cut this type and thickness of steel at the rate of 0.75 inch per minute. If the piece is 13.8 inches long and 9.6 inches wide, calculate how many minutes (to the nearest minute) it will take to cut the piece.

57. Do problem 56 but assume that the piece is 15.0 centimeters (cm) long and 10.5 cm wide and that the saw will cut at 0.8 cm per minute.

58. The ladder on a fire truck can extend 125 feet. If the truck is 25 feet from a building, how high up the building can the ladder reach, to the nearest tenth of a foot?

59. If the fire truck of problem 58 moves 5 more feet from the building (to 30 feet), does the height up the building that the ladder can reach decrease by 5 feet? If not, how much does it decrease, to the nearest tenth of a foot?

60. Find the ground speed, to the nearest knot, of an aircraft flying with a heading due east and an airspeed of 132 knots if there is a wind blowing from the north at 23 knots.

61. Find the ground speed, to the nearest knot, of an aircraft flying with a heading due west and an airspeed of 105 knots if there is a wind blowing from the north at 18 knots.

62. Find the ground speed, to the nearest knot, of an aircraft flying with a heading due south and an airspeed of 178 knots if there is a wind blowing from the east at 25 knots.

63. Find the speed relative to the ground, to the nearest knot, of a boat heading directly across a river at 16 knots if the current is moving at 4.3 knots.

64. To the nearest $\frac{1}{4}$ inch, find the length of the diagonal of an $8\frac{1}{2}$-inch by 11-inch piece of paper.

65. In the ''Mathematics of Warfare'' by F. W. Lanchester (from *The World of Mathematics* by James R. Newman), Mr. Lanchester presents the idea that, all other things being equal, the strengths of fighting forces add in a manner proportional to the squares of their numbers. Referring to the diagram, this means that a force of size *B* is equal to two forces of sizes *a* and *b;* that *C* is equal to the combined strengths of *a, b,* and *c;* etc. Assuming

that forces *a, b, c, d,* and *e* are of size 20, 5, 12, 8, and 10, respectively, find the size of force *E* that is equivalent to the combined strengths of these forces. Find this force to the nearest unit.

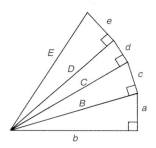

1–2 *The trigonometric ratios*

Trigonometry has existed in one form or another for more than two thousand years. The creator of trigonometry is said to have been the Greek Hipparchus of the second century B.C. The Hindus and, primarily, the Arabs continued developing the subject. In the fifteenth and sixteenth centuries, the Germans developed trigonometry into the form presented here.

The primary trigonometric ratios

We first define the **sine, cosine,** and **tangent** ratios, abbreviated sin, cos, and tan, respectively. We refer to these as the primary trigonometric ratios.

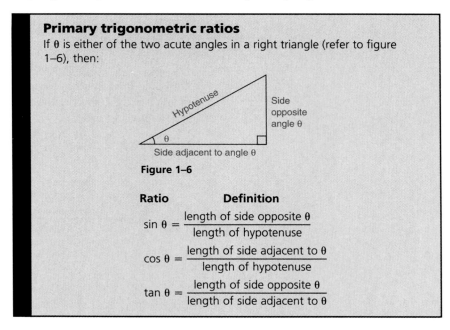

Primary trigonometric ratios

If θ is either of the two acute angles in a right triangle (refer to figure 1–6), then:

Figure 1–6

Ratio	Definition
$\sin \theta =$	$\dfrac{\text{length of side opposite } \theta}{\text{length of hypotenuse}}$
$\cos \theta =$	$\dfrac{\text{length of side adjacent to } \theta}{\text{length of hypotenuse}}$
$\tan \theta =$	$\dfrac{\text{length of side opposite } \theta}{\text{length of side adjacent to } \theta}$

Note   "sin θ" means "the sine of angle θ" and is read "sine theta."
"cos θ" means "the cosine of angle θ" and is read "cosine theta."
"tan θ" means "the tangent of angle θ" and is read "tangent theta."

An abbreviated version of these definitions is

$$\sin \theta = \frac{\text{opp}}{\text{hyp}}$$

$$\cos \theta = \frac{\text{adj}}{\text{hyp}}$$

$$\tan \theta = \frac{\text{opp}}{\text{adj}}$$

These ratios are used in astronomy, surveying, engineering, science, and mathematics. In fact, there is virtually no area of science and technology that does not use them.

■ *Example 1–2 A*

1. Find the sine, cosine, and tangent ratios for angles A and B in right triangle ABC, where $a = 3$ and $b = 6$.

Recall that the right angle is always labeled C, side a is opposite angle A, and side b is opposite angle B. We show this and the given data in the figure.

First, we find c by the Pythagorean theorem.

$$a^2 + b^2 = c^2$$
$$3^2 + 6^2 = c^2$$
$$45 = c^2$$
$$\sqrt{45} = c$$
$$\sqrt{(9)(5)} = c$$
$$\sqrt{9}\sqrt{5} = c$$
$$3\sqrt{5} = c$$

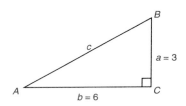

Now find the sine ratio for each angle A and B. Since the sine ratio for an angle is the length of the side opposite the angle over the length of the hypotenuse, we have

$$\sin A = \frac{\text{side opposite angle } A}{\text{hypotenuse}} = \frac{a}{c} = \frac{3}{3\sqrt{5}} = \frac{1}{\sqrt{5}}$$

$$= \frac{1}{\sqrt{5}} \cdot \frac{\sqrt{5}}{\sqrt{5}} = \frac{\sqrt{5}}{5}$$

$$\sin B = \frac{\text{side opposite angle } B}{\text{hypotenuse}} = \frac{b}{c} = \frac{6}{3\sqrt{5}} = \frac{2}{\sqrt{5}}$$

$$= \frac{2}{\sqrt{5}} \cdot \frac{\sqrt{5}}{\sqrt{5}} = \frac{2\sqrt{5}}{5}$$

To find the cosine ratio we form the ratios of the sides adjacent to each angle over the length of the hypotenuse.

$$\cos A = \frac{\text{side adjacent to angle } A}{\text{hypotenuse}} = \frac{b}{c} = \frac{6}{3\sqrt{5}} = \frac{2}{\sqrt{5}} = \frac{2\sqrt{5}}{5}$$

$$\cos B = \frac{\text{side adjacent to angle } B}{\text{hypotenuse}} = \frac{a}{c} = \frac{3}{3\sqrt{5}} = \frac{1}{\sqrt{5}} = \frac{\sqrt{5}}{5}$$

The tangent of an angle is the length of the side opposite the angle over the length of the side adjacent to the angle. Thus,

$$\tan A = \frac{\text{side opposite angle } A}{\text{side adjacent to angle } A} = \frac{a}{b} = \frac{3}{6} = \frac{1}{2}$$

$$\tan B = \frac{\text{side opposite angle } B}{\text{side adjacent to angle } B} = \frac{b}{a} = \frac{6}{3} = 2$$

2. Find the sine, cosine, and tangent ratios, in terms of the values x and y only, for the angle labeled X in the right triangle in the figure.

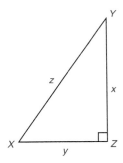

Using the Pythagorean theorem, we find the hypotenuse:

$$z^2 = x^2 + y^2$$
$$z = \sqrt{x^2 + y^2}$$

Since the sine of an acute angle in a right triangle is the length of the side opposite the angle divided by the length of the hypotenuse, then

$$\sin X = \frac{x}{\sqrt{x^2 + y^2}} \text{; similarly, } \cos X = \frac{y}{\sqrt{x^2 + y^2}} \text{ and } \tan X = \frac{x}{y}. \qquad \blacksquare$$

The reciprocal trigonometric ratios

The final three trigonometric ratios are called the **cosecant** (csc), **secant** (sec), and **cotangent** (cot) of an acute angle of a right triangle. These ratios are the reciprocals of the three ratios above.

> **Reciprocal trigonometric ratios**
> If θ represents either acute angle of a right triangle, then
> $$\csc \theta = \frac{1}{\sin \theta}, \quad \sec \theta = \frac{1}{\cos \theta}, \quad \cot \theta = \frac{1}{\tan \theta}$$

Note   The definitions of csc θ, sec θ, and cot θ given here are equivalent to the following definitions:

$$\csc \theta = \frac{\text{hyp}}{\text{opp}}, \quad \sec \theta = \frac{\text{hyp}}{\text{adj}}, \quad \cot \theta = \frac{\text{adj}}{\text{opp}}$$

We could use these as the definitions for these three ratios.

It is worth stressing that the following pairs of ratios are reciprocals:

cosine and secant

sine and cosecant

tangent and cotangent

This means that if we know one ratio, we can invert it to find the other ratio in the pair.

■ *Example 1–2 B*

1. $\sin A = \frac{2}{3}$. Find csc A.
    Invert $\frac{2}{3}$, giving $\csc A = \frac{3}{2}$

2. $\cot B = 5$. Find tan B.
    Invert $\frac{5}{1}$ to get $\tan B = \frac{1}{5}$

3. $\sec A = 1.6$. Find cos A.
    Invert 1.6 to get $\frac{1}{1.6}$, or 0.625, so $\cos A = 0.625$.   ■

■ *Example 1–2 C*

1. Given the triangle in the figure, find the six trigonometric ratios of θ.

    Since we are not told the length of the hypotenuse, we calculate it, using the Pythagorean theorem:

    $$3^2 + 4^2 = 9 + 16 = 25, \text{ and } \sqrt{25} = 5$$

    $$\sin \theta = \frac{\text{opp}}{\text{hyp}} = \frac{3}{5}, \cos \theta = \frac{\text{adj}}{\text{hyp}} = \frac{4}{5}, \tan \theta = \frac{\text{opp}}{\text{adj}} = \frac{3}{4},$$

    $$\csc \theta = \frac{1}{\sin \theta} = \frac{1}{\frac{3}{5}} = \frac{5}{3}, \sec \theta = \frac{1}{\cos \theta} = \frac{1}{\frac{4}{5}} = \frac{5}{4},$$

    $$\cot \theta = \frac{1}{\tan \theta} = \frac{1}{\frac{3}{4}} = \frac{4}{3}$$

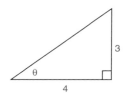

2. Find sin B and cos B for the triangle in the figure.

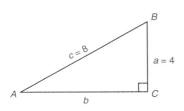

First we find the length of side b, using the Pythagorean theorem:
$a^2 + b^2 = c^2$ so $16 + b^2 = 64$, or $b^2 = 48$, so $b = \sqrt{48} = \sqrt{(16)(3)} = 4\sqrt{3}$.

$$\sin B = \frac{b}{c} = \frac{4\sqrt{3}}{8} = \frac{\sqrt{3}}{2}$$

$$\cos B = \frac{a}{c} = \frac{4}{8} = \frac{1}{2}$$

■

The fundamental identity of trigonometry

Recall that an identity is an equation that is true for any valid replacement of the variable. The following trigonometric identity is so important that it is often called the **fundamental identity of trigonometry.**

> ### The fundamental identity of trigonometry
> If θ is either acute angle in a right triangle, then
> $$\sin^2\theta + \cos^2\theta = 1$$
>
> ***Concept***
> If we square both the sine and the cosine ratios for a given angle and add these quantities, we always get 1.

Note   1. In chapter 2 we see that θ does not have to be acute.
   2. The notation $\sin^2\theta$ means $(\sin \theta)^2$, and $\cos^2\theta$ means $(\cos \theta)^2$.

■ *Example 1–2 D*

1. Show that the fundamental identity of trigonometry applies to the results of part 2 of example 1–2 C.

Recall that in part 2 of example 1–2 C the angle is called B, not θ. Also, $\sin B = \dfrac{\sqrt{3}}{2}$ and $\cos B = \frac{1}{2}$.

$$\sin^2 B + \cos^2 B = (\sin B)^2 + (\cos B)^2$$
$$= \left(\frac{\sqrt{3}}{2}\right)^2 + \left(\frac{1}{2}\right)^2$$
$$= \tfrac{3}{4} + \tfrac{1}{4}$$
$$= 1$$

2. Prove that the fundamental identity of trigonometry applies to angle A in any right triangle ABC.

$$\sin^2 A + \cos^2 A = (\sin A)^2 + (\cos A)^2$$
$$= \left(\frac{a}{c}\right)^2 + \left(\frac{b}{c}\right)^2$$
$$= \frac{a^2}{c^2} + \frac{b^2}{c^2}$$
$$= \frac{a^2 + b^2}{c^2}$$

and, since $a^2 + b^2 = c^2$,

$$= \frac{c^2}{c^2}$$
$$= 1 \qquad \blacksquare$$

Finding other trigonometric ratios from a known ratio

If we know one of the trigonometric ratios of an angle, we can construct a right triangle with an angle for which that ratio is true. We can use this triangle to compute the other five trigonometric ratios.

■ **Example 1–2 E**

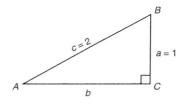

In right triangle ABC, $\sin A = \frac{1}{2}$. Draw a triangle in which $\sin A$ is $\frac{1}{2}$, and use this to compute the other five trigonometric ratios for angle A.

Since $\sin A$ is $\dfrac{a}{c}$, we see that $\dfrac{a}{c} = \dfrac{1}{2}$. Thus, a right triangle in which $a = 1$ and $c = 2$ would work. This is shown in the figure. We then compute b by the Pythagorean theorem,

$$a^2 + b^2 = c^2$$
$$1^2 + b^2 = 2^2$$
$$b^2 = 3$$
$$b = \sqrt{3}$$

and then compute the other five ratios for angle A:

$$\cos A = \frac{\sqrt{3}}{2}, \ \tan A = \frac{1}{\sqrt{3}} \text{ or } \frac{\sqrt{3}}{3}, \ \sec A = \frac{2}{\sqrt{3}} \text{ or } \frac{2\sqrt{3}}{3},$$
$$\csc A = 2, \ \cot A = \sqrt{3} \qquad \blacksquare$$

A logical question is whether any other triangles would work in example 1–2 E; the answer is yes. In fact, since $\frac{2}{4}$ reduces to $\frac{1}{2}$, we could use the triangle in figure 1–7. However, our values for the six ratios would not change.

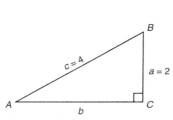

Figure 1–7

For example, we find that $b = \sqrt{12}$, or $2\sqrt{3}$; thus, $\cos A = \dfrac{2\sqrt{3}}{4}$, which reduces to the same value, $\dfrac{\sqrt{3}}{2}$. The other ratios will also reduce to the same values we already obtained.

Similarly, we could start with any fraction that is equivalent to $\frac{1}{2}$. This means that we could use an unlimited number of triangles in such problems. This is true because of the properties of similar triangles, discussed in section 1–3.

■ *Example 1–2 F*

1. $\cot B = 3$. Draw a right triangle for which this is true and compute the other five trigonometric ratios for B.

   We know that if $\cot B = 3$, then $\tan B = \frac{1}{3}$ (see example 1–2 B) and $\tan B = \dfrac{\text{opp}}{\text{adj}} = \dfrac{b}{a}$. Thus, a triangle in which $b = 1$ and $a = 3$ would work. This is shown in the figure.

   Using the Pythagorean theorem, we find c:

   $$c^2 = a^2 + b^2 = 3^2 + 1^2 = 10$$
   $$c = \sqrt{10}$$

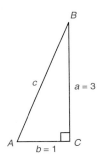

   With this we can now compute the four remaining ratios:

   $$\sin B = \frac{1}{\sqrt{10}} = \frac{\sqrt{10}}{10}, \quad \cos B = \frac{3}{\sqrt{10}} = \frac{3\sqrt{10}}{10},$$
   $$\sec B = \frac{\sqrt{10}}{3}, \quad \csc B = \sqrt{10}$$

2. In right triangle ABC, $\cos A = x$. Draw a right triangle for which this is true and find $\tan B$ in terms of x.

   If we think of x as $\dfrac{x}{1}$ we see that $\cos A$ in the triangle shown in the figure is x.

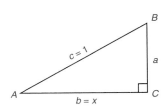

   From the Pythagorean theorem we find a:

   $$c^2 = a^2 + b^2$$
   $$1^2 = a^2 + x^2$$
   $$1 - x^2 = a^2$$
   $$\sqrt{1 - x^2} = a$$

   Now we can find $\tan B$:

   $$\tan B = \frac{b}{a} = \frac{x}{\sqrt{1 - x^2}}$$ ■

Mastery points

Can you
- State the definitions of the six trigonometric ratios?
- Find the six trigonometric ratios of an angle in a right triangle when you know the lengths of the sides?
- State and use the fundamental identity of trigonometry?
- Find the remaining five ratios for an angle if given one of the six ratios for an angle in a right triangle?

Exercise 1–2

1. Draw a right triangle, label it in the standard way (using A, B, C, a, b, c), and use it to define the six trigonometric ratios for both acute angles.

In the following problems you are given parts of right triangle ABC; use this information to compute the six trigonometric ratios for the angle specified.

	a	b	c	Find ratios for this angle		a	b	c	Find ratios for this angle
2.	3	4		A	**3.**	3	4		B
4.	5		13	A	**5.**	1	3		B
6.	4	$\sqrt{10}$		A	**7.**	5	$\sqrt{7}$		B
8.		2	$\sqrt{13}$	A	**9.**	2		$\sqrt{5}$	B
10.	4		7	A	**11.**	12	13		B
12.	5	12		A	**13.**	6		10	A
14.	10		15	A	**15.**	$\sqrt{3}$	4		A
16.	x	y		A	**17.**	x		z	B
18.	1	1		A	**19.**	1		2	B
20.		5	8	A	**21.**	9	5		B

22. You will learn in section 1–3 that if the sine ratio for an acute angle is more than 0.5, then the angle is larger than 30°. In a right triangle, $a = 3$ and $c = 5$; is angle B more or less than 30°?

In the following problems you are given one of the trigonometric ratios for an angle. Use this to sketch a triangle for which the ratio is true, and then use this triangle to find the other five trigonometric ratios for that angle.

23. $\sin A = \frac{4}{5}$ 24. $\cos B = \frac{1}{4}$ 25. $\cos A = 0.5$ 26. $\tan B = 4$

27. $\sec A = 3$ 28. $\cot B = 0.2$ 29. $\sin A = \frac{5}{13}$ 30. $\csc B = 1.6$

31. $\cos A = 0.9$

Solve the following problems.

32. Show that the fundamental identity of trigonometry applies to the results of problems 27 and 29.

33. Show that the fundamental identity of trigonometry applies to angle B in any right triangle ABC.

34. In right triangle ABC, $\sin A = x$. Sketch a triangle for which this is true and use it to find $\sin B$ in terms of the variable x. $\left(\text{Hint: } x = \dfrac{x}{1}. \right)$

35. In right triangle ABC, $\tan A = x$. Sketch a triangle for which this is true and use it to find $\sin B$ in terms of the variable x. (See the hint for problem 34.)

36. In right triangle ABC, $\sec A = x$. Sketch a triangle for which this is true and use it to find $\sec B$ in terms of the variable x.

37. In right triangle ABC, $\tan B = x$. Sketch a triangle for which this is true and use it to find $\tan A$ in terms of the variable x.

1–3 *Angle measure and the values of the trigonometric ratios*

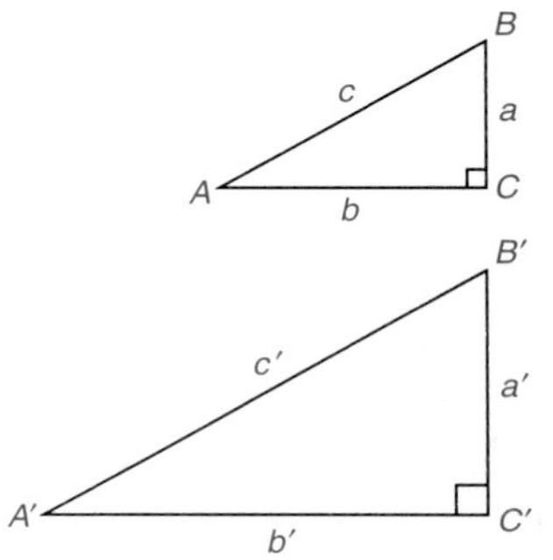

Trigonometric ratios for equal angles are equal

It is possible to have angles of the same measure in different right triangles. Angles A and A' in figure 1–8 are examples. The trigonometric ratios will have the same value for these angles. This is because these triangles are *similar*—that is, they have the same shape, but perhaps different sizes. It is a theorem of geometry that corresponding ratios in similar figures are equal. Thus, in figure 1–8, $\dfrac{a}{c} = \dfrac{a'}{c'}$, so sin A = sin A'. For the same reasons, the other five trigonometric ratios are also equal.

Note Read A' as "A-prime," B' as "B-prime," etc.

These facts mean that the values of the trigonometric ratios for an acute angle do not depend upon the particular right triangle in which it appears. *For an acute angle with a given measure, the values of the trigonometric ratios will always be the same.*

Values for angles of measure 30°, 45°, and 60°

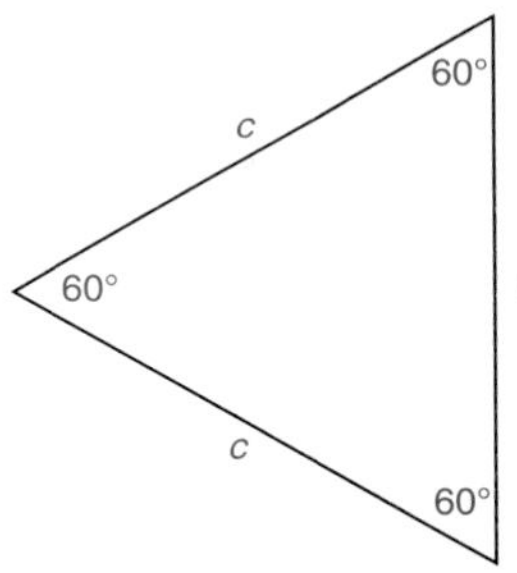

We now find the trigonometric ratios for some special angles—30°, 45°, and 60°. Figure 1–9 shows an equilateral triangle, which is a triangle in which all sides have equal length. We label this length c.

We construct the line AC, as shown in figure 1–10, which forms a right triangle with acute angles $A = 30°$ and $B = 60°$. The length a is half of c, so $a = \dfrac{c}{2}$. We find b next.

$$b^2 = c^2 - a^2 = c^2 - \left(\frac{c}{2}\right)^2 = \frac{4c^2}{4} - \frac{c^2}{4}$$

$$b^2 = \frac{3c^2}{4}$$

$$b = \frac{\sqrt{3}}{2}c$$

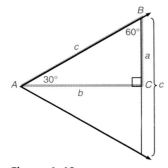

Figure 1–8

Figure 1–9

Figure 1–10

Angle A is a 30° angle, so we will write sin 30° to mean the value of the sine ratio associated with an angle of measure 30°. Thus,

$$\sin 30° = \frac{a}{c} = \frac{\frac{c}{2}}{c} = \frac{1}{2}$$

$$\cos 30° = \frac{b}{c} = \frac{\frac{\sqrt{3}}{2}c}{c} = \frac{\sqrt{3}}{2}$$

$$\tan 30° = \frac{a}{b} = \frac{\frac{c}{2}}{\frac{\sqrt{3}}{2}c} = \frac{1}{\sqrt{3}} = \frac{\sqrt{3}}{3}$$

The values for a 60° angle can be obtained from angle B in figure 1–10.

$$\sin 60° = \frac{b}{c} = \frac{\frac{\sqrt{3}}{2}c}{c} = \frac{\sqrt{3}}{2}$$

$$\cos 60° = \frac{a}{c} = \frac{\frac{c}{2}}{c} = \frac{1}{2}$$

$$\tan 60° = \frac{b}{a} = \frac{\frac{\sqrt{3}}{2}c}{\frac{c}{2}} = \sqrt{3}$$

In the exercises we will compute the sine, cosine and tangent ratios for a 45° angle; these are shown in table 1–1, along with the values obtained above.

	Sine	Cosine	Tangent
30°	$\frac{1}{2}$	$\frac{\sqrt{3}}{2}$	$\frac{\sqrt{3}}{3}$
45°	$\frac{\sqrt{2}}{2}$	$\frac{\sqrt{2}}{2}$	1
60°	$\frac{\sqrt{3}}{2}$	$\frac{1}{2}$	$\sqrt{3}$

Table 1–1

General values

It is actually impossible to find the exact values of the trigonometric ratios for most angles. Tables of approximate values were calculated long ago. The earliest known table of trigonometric values, for the equivalent of the sine ratio, was created by Hipparchus of Nicaea about 150 B.C. In the second century A.D. Ptolemy constructed a table of values of the sine ratio for acute angles in increments of one-quarter degree. Today we use calculators to approximate these values. When using a calculator it is important that the calculator be in **degree mode.** This means that the calculator is expecting the measure of the angle in decimal degrees. *Check your calculator's manual to make sure it is in degree mode.* This is usually done with a key marked $\boxed{\text{DRG}}$ or simply $\boxed{\text{DEG}}$. "DRG" means degrees, radians, grads. We discuss radian measure in a later section. Grads, or grades, is the metric measure for an angle. There are 100 grads in a right angle. We will not use this measure in this text.

To select degree mode on the Texas Instruments TI-81 it is necessary to select "Deg" under the $\boxed{\text{MODE}}$ feature. To do this, select $\boxed{\text{MODE}}$, darken in the "Deg" mode indicator (use the four cursor-moving "arrow" keys) and select $\boxed{\text{ENTER}}$.

■ *Example 1–3 A*

Find each value rounded to four decimal places.

1. sin 34.51°   34.51 $\boxed{\text{sin}}$ Display $\boxed{0.5665500655}$

   sin 34.51° ≈ 0.5666 $\boxed{\text{TI-81}}$ $\boxed{\text{SIN}}$ 34.51 $\boxed{\text{ENTER}}$

2. tan 84.6°   84.6 $\boxed{\text{tan}}$ Display $\boxed{10.57889499}$

   tan 84.6° ≈ 10.5789 $\boxed{\text{TI-81}}$ $\boxed{\text{TAN}}$ 84.6 $\boxed{\text{ENTER}}$

3. sec 33.5°

   Since there is no secant key on a calculator we use the fact that sec 33.5° $= \dfrac{1}{\cos 33.5°}$. Compute cos 33.5° and divide it into one; the $\boxed{1/x}$ key is designed for this type of situation.

   33.5 $\boxed{\text{cos}}$ $\boxed{1/x}$ Display $\boxed{1.199204943}$

   $\boxed{\text{TI-81}}$ $\boxed{(\,}$ $\boxed{\text{COS}}$ 33.5 $\boxed{)}$ $\boxed{x^{-1}}$

   $\boxed{\text{ENTER}}$

   Note that on the TI-81 the $\boxed{1/x}$ key is the $\boxed{x^{-1}}$ key.
   sec 33.5° ≈ 1.1992

4. cot 87.23°   cot 87.23° $= \dfrac{1}{\tan 87.23°}$, so use

   87.23 $\boxed{\text{tan}}$ $\boxed{1/x}$

   Display $\boxed{0.04838332158}$

   $\boxed{\text{TI-81}}$ $\boxed{(\,}$ $\boxed{\text{TAN}}$ 87.23 $\boxed{)}$ $\boxed{x^{-1}}$

   $\boxed{\text{ENTER}}$

   cot 87.23° ≈ 0.0484

5. cos 13°43′

Recall that angles in the DMS system must be converted to decimal degrees. We show the calculation with and without special calculator keys. (See also example 1–1 A.)

No special keys: 13 $\boxed{+}$ 43 $\boxed{÷}$ 60 $\boxed{=}$ $\boxed{\cos}$

Display $\boxed{0.9714801855}$

Calculator A: 13 $\boxed{°\,'\,''}$ 43 $\boxed{°\,'\,''}$ $\boxed{\cos}$

Calculator B: 13.43 $\boxed{→H}$ $\boxed{\cos}$

$\boxed{\text{TI-81}}$ $\boxed{\cos}$ $\boxed{(}$ 13 $\boxed{+}$ 43 $\boxed{÷}$ 60 $\boxed{)}$

$\boxed{\text{ENTER}}$

cos 13°43′ ≈ 0.9715   ∎

Finding an angle from a known trigonometric ratio

It is important to be able to reverse the operations discussed above. For example, if θ is an acute angle and sin θ = $\frac{1}{2}$, what is θ? We can see from table 1–1 that θ must be 30°. The calculator is programmed to solve this problem. This is done with the **inverse trigonometric ratios** called the inverse sine ($\sin^{-1}$), inverse cosine ($\cos^{-1}$) and inverse tangent ($\tan^{-1}$) ratios. The superscript −1 does *not* indicate a reciprocal value in the way that, say, $2^{-1} = \frac{1}{2}$. We will study these ratios in more detail later. For now we illustrate how to find the acute angle whose sine, cosine, or tangent value is known.

For this, most calculators use the appropriate key (sin, cos, tan), prefixed by another key such as $\boxed{\text{SHIFT}}$, $\boxed{\text{2nd}}$, $\boxed{\text{INV}}$ or $\boxed{\text{ARC}}$. The appropriate function is generally shown above the key itself. The *result is always an angle in decimal degrees* (when the calculator is in degree mode). We will show the necessary two keystrokes as one.

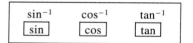

■ *Example 1–3 B*

Find θ in the following problems using the calculator. Assume θ is an acute angle. Round the answer to the nearest 0.01°.

1. cos θ = 0.4602

We need to calculate $\cos^{-1}0.4602$.

0.4602 $\boxed{\cos^{-1}}$ Display $\boxed{62.59998611}$

$\boxed{\text{TI-81}}$ $\boxed{\cos^{-1}}$ .4602 $\boxed{\text{ENTER}}$

θ ≈ 62.60°

2. tan θ = 1.2231

Calculate $\tan^{-1}1.2231$.

1.2231 $\boxed{\tan^{-1}}$ Display $\boxed{50.73075144}$

$\boxed{\text{TI-81}}$ $\boxed{\tan^{-1}}$ 1.2231 $\boxed{\text{ENTER}}$

θ ≈ 50.73°

3. csc $\theta = 1.0551$

We use the fact that if csc $\theta = 1.0551$, then $\sin \theta = \dfrac{1}{1.0551}$. Thus we

compute $\sin^{-1}\left(\dfrac{1}{1.0551}\right)$. Use the $\boxed{1/x}$ key. (On the TI-81 the $\boxed{1/x}$

key is the $\boxed{x^{-1}}$ key.)

1.0551 $\boxed{1/x}$ $\boxed{\sin^{-1}}$ Display $\boxed{71.40162609}$

$\boxed{\text{TI-81}}$ $\boxed{\text{SIN}^{-1}}$ 1.0551 $\boxed{x^{-1}}$ $\boxed{\text{ENTER}}$

$\theta \approx 71.40°$ ■

Solving right triangles

One application of trigonometry that occurs in many situations is *solving right triangles*—this means *discovering the lengths of all sides and the measures of all angles* of the triangle. We will round the values we compute to the same number of decimal places as the given data.

These types of situations fall into two categories, ones in which we know one side and one acute angle and others in which we know two sides and no angles. Each category is illustrated in example 1–3 C.

■ *Example 1–3 C*

Solve the following right triangles.

1. $A = 35.6°$, $a = 13.6$ (one side, one angle)

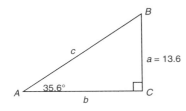

To solve this triangle we need to find the lengths of sides b and c and the measure of angle B. Since angle C is always 90°, angles A and B total 90°. Thus, angle B is $90° - 35.6° = 54.4°$. We now note that

$$\sin A = \frac{a}{c}, \text{ so that}$$

$$\sin 35.6° = \frac{13.6}{c}$$

$$c \sin 35.6° = 13.6 \qquad \text{Multiply each member by } c$$

$$c = \frac{13.6}{\sin 35.6°} \qquad \text{Divide each member by } \sin 35.6°$$

$$c \approx 23.4 \qquad \boxed{\text{CS 1}}$$

Now we find b by noting that $\tan A = \dfrac{a}{b}$.

$$\tan 35.6° = \frac{13.6}{b}$$

$$b \tan 35.6° = 13.6 \qquad \text{Multiply each member by } b$$

$$b = \frac{13.6}{\tan 35.6°} \qquad \text{Divide each member by } \tan 35.6°$$

$$b \approx 19.0 \qquad \boxed{\text{CS 2}}$$

Since we know the lengths of all sides and all angles we have solved the triangle. To summarize, $a = 13.6$, $b \approx 19.0$, $c \approx 23.4$, $A = 35.6°$, $B = 54.4°$, $C = 90°$.

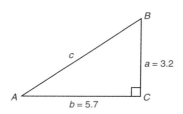

2. $a = 3.2$, $b = 5.7$ (two sides)

We can find the length of side c by the Pythagorean theorem.

$$c^2 = a^2 + b^2$$
$$c^2 = 3.2^2 + 5.7^2$$
$$c^2 = 42.73$$
$$c = \sqrt{42.73}$$
$$c \approx 6.5$$

We can find angle A by noting that $\tan A = \dfrac{a}{b}$.

$$\tan A = \frac{3.2}{5.7}$$

$$A = \tan^{-1}\left(\frac{3.2}{5.7}\right) \qquad \boxed{\text{CS 3}}$$

$$A \approx 29.3°$$

We know that the sum of the measures of A and B is 90°, so $B = 90°$ $- 29.3° = 60.7°$. This completes the process of finding the lengths of all sides and measures of all angles. Thus, $a = 3.2$, $b = 5.7$, $c \approx 6.5$, $A \approx 29.3°$, $B \approx 60.7°$, $C = 90°$.

3. A tag on a 25-foot ladder states that, for safety reasons, the angle that the ladder makes with the ground should not exceed 65°. How high can the ladder reach without exceeding this angle, to the nearest 0.1 feet?

We need to find h in the figure. If we observe that h is opposite the known angle and that the length of the hypotenuse of the triangle is known, we see that we can use the sine ratio.

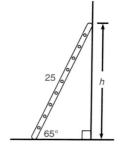

$$\sin 65° = \frac{h}{25}$$

$$25 \sin 65° = h \qquad \text{Multiply each member by 25}$$

$$22.7 \approx h \qquad \boxed{\text{CS 4}}$$

The ladder can reach a height of approximately 22.7 feet without exceeding a 65° angle with the ground.   ∎

Calculator steps

1. Ⓐ 13.6 $\boxed{÷}$ 35.6 $\boxed{\sin}$ $\boxed{=}$ Display $\boxed{23.36276130}$

Ⓟ 13.6 $\boxed{\text{ENTER}}$ 35.6 $\boxed{\sin}$ $\boxed{÷}$

$\boxed{\text{TI-81}}$ 13.6 $\boxed{÷}$ $\boxed{\text{SIN}}$ 35.6 $\boxed{\text{ENTER}}$

2. Ⓐ 13.6 $\boxed{÷}$ 35.6 $\boxed{\tan}$ $\boxed{=}$ Display $\boxed{18.99627899}$

Ⓟ 13.6 $\boxed{\text{ENTER}}$ 35.6 $\boxed{\tan}$ $\boxed{÷}$

$\boxed{\text{TI-81}}$ 13.6 $\boxed{÷}$ $\boxed{\text{TAN}}$ 35.6 $\boxed{\text{ENTER}}$

3. Ⓐ   3.2 $\boxed{\div}$ 5.7 $\boxed{=}$ $\boxed{\tan^{-1}}$ Display $\boxed{29.31000707}$

    Ⓟ   3.2 $\boxed{\text{ENTER}}$ 5.7 $\boxed{\div}$ $\boxed{\tan^{-1}}$

    $\boxed{\text{TI-81}}$ $\boxed{\text{TAN}^{-1}}$ $\boxed{(}$ 3.2 $\boxed{\div}$ 5.7 $\boxed{)}$ $\boxed{\text{ENTER}}$

4. Ⓐ   25 $\boxed{\times}$ 65 $\boxed{\sin}$ $\boxed{=}$ Display $\boxed{22.65769468}$

    Ⓟ   25 $\boxed{\text{ENTER}}$ 65 $\boxed{\sin}$ $\boxed{\times}$

    $\boxed{\text{TI-81}}$ 25 $\boxed{\times}$ $\boxed{\text{SIN}}$ 65 $\boxed{\text{ENTER}}$

Mastery points

Can you

- Compute the value of the trigonometric ratios for a given acute angle, using a calculator?
- Compute the value of an acute angle, given the value of a trigonometric ratio, using a calculator?
- Solve a right triangle when given one side and one acute angle?
- Solve a right triangle when given two sides?

Exercise 1–3

Use a calculator to find four-decimal-place approximations for the following.

1. sin 31.28°	**2.** cos 85.23°	**3.** tan 11.95°	**4.** sec 40.08°
5. cot 28.87°	**6.** csc 5.15°	**7.** sin 40.28°	**8.** tan 76.23°
9. sec 66.47°	**10.** sin 35.56°	**11.** sin 78.33°	**12.** cos 17.45°
13. sin 78°33′	**14.** cos 17°45′	**15.** cos 85°28′	**16.** tan 40°41′
17. tan 35°8′	**18.** cos 23°24′	**19.** cos 56°24′	**20.** cot 13°3′
21. sin 48°8′	**22.** tan 33°38′	**23.** sec 86°22′	

24. A surveyor needs to compute R in the following formula as part of finding the area of the segment of a circle: $R = \dfrac{LC}{2 \sin I}$. Find R to three decimal places if $LC = 425.0$ feet and $I = 13.2°$.

25. Compute R using the formula of the previous problem if $LC = 611.1$ meters and $I = 18°20′$. Round the answer to two decimal places.

26. In the mathematical modeling of an aerodynamics problem the following equation arises:

$$y = x \cos A \cos B - x^2 \cos A \sin B - x^3 \sin A$$

Compute y to two decimal places if $x = 2.5$, $A = 31°$, and $B = 17°$.

27. Compute y to two decimal places using the formula of problem 26 if $x = 1.2$, $A = 10°$, and $B = 15°$.

28. The average power in an AC circuit is given by the formula $P = VI \cos \theta$. Compute P (in watts) if $V = 120$ volts, $I = 2.3$ amperes, and $\theta = 45°$, to the nearest 0.1 watt.

29. Compute P using the formula of problem 28 if $V = 42$ volts, $I = 25$ amperes, and $\theta = 45°$, to the nearest 0.1 watt.

30. A formula that relates the distance across the flats of a piece of hexagonal stock in relation to the distance across the corners is $f = 2r \cos \theta$. A machinist needs to compute f for a piece of stock in which $r = 28$ millimeters (mm) and $\theta = 30°$. Compute f to the nearest 0.1 mm.

31. Using the formula of problem 30 find r if $f = 21.4$ inches and $\theta = 25°$.

32. Using the formula of problem 30 find θ to the nearest 0.1 if $f = 36.8$ millimeters and $r = 24.0$.

33. Find the exact values for the sine, cosine, and tangent ratios for an angle of measure 45° by proceeding in the following manner. Draw an *isosceles* right triangle—a right triangle in which the two legs have the same length. Label this length one. Observe that the two acute angles must be 45°. Now find the length of the hypotenuse and use the definitions of the trigonometric ratios to find the desired values.

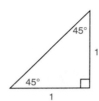

Find the unknown acute angle θ to the nearest 0.01°.

34. $\sin \theta = 0.3746$

35. $\sin \theta = 0.8007$

36. $\cos \theta = 0.1028$

37. $\tan \theta = 1.8807$

38. $\sin \theta = 0.9484$

39. $\cos \theta = 0.8515$

40. $\tan \theta = 1.0014$

41. $\sin \theta = \dfrac{35.9}{68.3}$

42. $\cos \theta = \dfrac{8.25}{12.5}$

43. $\tan \theta = 2$

44. $\csc \theta = 1.1243$

45. $\sec \theta = 4.8097$

46. $\cot \theta = 2.5$

47. $\sec \theta = \dfrac{6.45}{2.35}$

48. $\csc \theta = \sqrt{10.8}$

In the following problems you are given one side and one angle of a right triangle. Solve the triangle. Round all answers to the same number of decimal places as the data.

49. $a = 15.2, B = 38.3°$

50. $a = 12.6, B = 17.9°$

51. $a = 11.1, A = 13.7°$

52. $a = 5.25, A = 70.3°$

53. $b = 0.672, A = 29.4°$

54. $b = 15.2, A = 81.3°$

55. $b = 21.8, B = 78.0°$

56. $b = 2.14, B = 50.4°$

57. $c = 10.0, A = 15.0°$

58. $c = 3.45, A = 46.2°$

59. $c = 122, B = 65.5°$

60. $c = 31.5, B = 62.0°$

In the following problems you are given two sides of a right triangle. Solve the triangle. Round all lengths to the same number of decimal places as the data and all angles to the nearest 0.1°.

61. $a = 13.1, b = 15.6$

62. $a = 5.67, b = 8.91$

63. $a = 0.22, b = 1.34$

64. $a = 2.82, b = 1.09$

65. $a = 17.8, c = 25.2$

66. $a = 311, c = 561$

67. $b = 51.3, c = 111.0$

68. $b = 4.55, c = 5.66$

69. $a = 12.0, c = 13.0$

70. $a = 33.1, c = 41.0$

71. $b = 84.0, c = 90.1$

72. The figure illustrates an impedance diagram used in electronics theory. If Z (impedance) $= 10.35$ ohms and X_L (inductive reactance) $= 4.24$ ohms, find θ (phase angle) to the nearest degree and R (resistance) to the nearest 0.01 ohm.

73. Use the impedance diagram of problem 72 to find Z if $\theta = 24.2°$ and $X_L = 22.6$ ohms.

74. The diagram illustrates the measurements a surveyor made to find the width w of a pond; compute the width to the nearest foot.

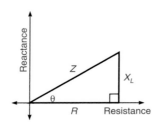

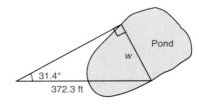

75. The diagram illustrates the tip of a threading tool; find angle θ to the nearest degree.

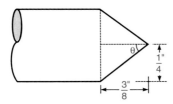

76. The diagram illustrates a piece of wood that is being mass produced to form the bottom of a planter. Find dimension a in the figure to the nearest 0.01 inch if $b = 8\frac{1}{4}$ inches. Note: angle θ is $\dfrac{360°}{7}$.

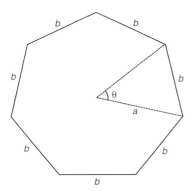

77. A formula found in electronics is $E = \dfrac{P}{I \cos \theta}$, where E is voltage, P is power, I is current, and θ is phase angle. Find E (in volts) if $P = 45.0$ watts, $I = 2.5$ amperes, and θ = 15°. Round the answer to the nearest 0.1 volt.

78. The diagram illustrates the wind triangle problem in air navigation. A plane has an airspeed of 155 mph and heading of due north. It is flying in a wind from the west with a speed of 30 mph. Find the ground speed S and the ground direction θ, each to the nearest unit.

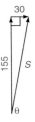

79. An **angle of elevation** is an angle formed by one horizontal ray and another ray that is above the horizontal. Angle θ in the diagram is the angle of elevation to an aircraft that radar shows has a slant distance of 12.4 miles from the radar site. If θ is 30.1°, find the elevation h of the aircraft, to the nearest 100 feet. Remember that 1 mile = 5,280 feet.

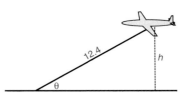

80. If it is known that an aircraft is flying at 28,500 feet and the angle of elevation of a radar beam tracking the aircraft is 8.2°, what is the slant distance d from the radar to the aircraft, to the nearest 100 feet?

81. The diagram illustrates the path of a laser beam on an optics table. Compute the total distance traveled by the beam to the nearest millimeter.

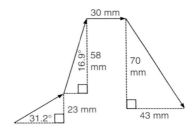

82. An **angle of depression** is an angle formed by one horizontal ray and another ray that is below the horizontal. Angle θ in the figure is the angle of depression formed by the line of sight of an observer in an airport control tower looking at a helicopter on the ground. If θ is 17.2° and the tower is 257 feet high, how far is the aircraft from the base of the tower, to the nearest foot.

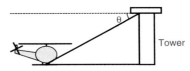

83. If an aircraft is 1.23 miles from the foot of the tower in problem 82, what is θ, to the nearest 0.1°? (Remember, 1 mile = 5,280 ft.)

84. The diagram is a top view of a portion of a spiral stair-case that an architect has designed. If $\theta_1 = \theta_2 = \theta_3$, find the length x to one decimal place. (Caution: Carry out your calculations to as many digits as practical to avoid an accumulation of errors.)

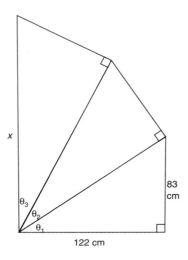

85. If the architect of problem 84 revises the plans so that $\theta_2 = \theta_1 + 5°$ and $\theta_3 = \theta_2 + 5°$, find x to one decimal place.

86. In right triangle ABC, $A = 45°$ and $b = 4$. Solve this triangle using exact values only. (Use the exact values for sin 45° etc., and do not approximate radicals as decimals.)

87. In right triangle ABC, $B = 60°$ and $b = 8$. Solve this triangle using exact values only. (Use the exact values for sin 60° etc., and do not approximate radicals as decimals.)

1–4 *Introduction to trigonometric equations*

This section introduces equations involving the trigonometric ratios. In chapter 2 we learn about the trigonometric *functions*. The material covered here applies to these functions as well.

Equations can be categorized as identities and conditional equations. An **identity** is an equation that is true for every allowed value of its variable (or variables). For example,

$$2(x + 3) = 2x + 6$$

is an identity, since the left member and right member of the equation represent the same value, regardless of the value of x. Similarly

$$\frac{3x^2}{3x} = x$$

is an identity; the left member equals the right member for every value of x for which both members are defined. Observe that the left member is not defined for the value 0, so the identity is true for all real values *except* zero.

A **conditional equation** is an equation that is true only for some, but not all, values that may replace the variable. For example,

$$6x = 12$$

is true if and only if x is replaced by 2, and

$$x^2 = 9$$

is true if and only if x is replaced by 3 or -3.

Identities

We have seen the reciprocal ratio identities

$$\csc\theta = \frac{1}{\sin\theta}, \sec\theta = \frac{1}{\cos\theta}, \cot\theta = \frac{1}{\tan\theta}$$

Similarly,

$$\sin\theta = \frac{1}{\csc\theta}, \cos\theta = \frac{1}{\sec\theta}, \tan\theta = \frac{1}{\cot\theta}$$

are identities.

Knowing these identities permits us to simplify certain trigonometric expressions.

■ Example 1–4 A

Simplify each trigonometric expression.

1. $\csc\theta \sin\theta$

$$\csc\theta \sin\theta$$

$$\frac{1}{\sin\theta} \cdot \sin\theta \qquad \csc\theta = \frac{1}{\sin\theta}$$

$$1$$

Thus, $\csc\theta \sin\theta = 1$.

2. $\dfrac{1 - \csc\theta}{\csc\theta}$

$$\frac{1 - \csc\theta}{\csc\theta}$$

$$\frac{1}{\csc\theta} - \frac{\csc\theta}{\csc\theta} \qquad \frac{a - b}{c} = \frac{a}{c} - \frac{b}{c}$$

$$\sin\theta - 1 \qquad \sin\theta = \frac{1}{\csc\theta}$$

Thus, $\dfrac{1 - \csc\theta}{\csc\theta} = \sin\theta - 1$. The right member is considered simpler because it is not a rational expression.   ■

Two more useful identities are

$$\tan\theta = \frac{\sin\theta}{\cos\theta}, \cot\theta = \frac{\cos\theta}{\sin\theta}$$

To see why the first is true consider angle A in figure 1–11. Note that

$$\tan A = \frac{a}{b}, \text{ and } \frac{\sin A}{\cos A} = \frac{\frac{a}{c}}{\frac{b}{c}} = \frac{a}{c} \cdot \frac{c}{b} = \frac{a}{b} \text{ also. It is left as an exercise to}$$

show that the same is true for angle B and that the second identity is true.

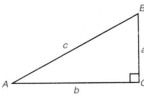

Figure 1–11

■ *Example 1–4 B*

Simplify each expression.

1. $\cot \alpha(\sin \alpha - \tan \alpha)$

$$\cot \alpha(\sin \alpha - \tan \alpha)$$

$$\cot \alpha \sin \alpha - \cot \alpha \tan \alpha \qquad a(b - c) = ab - ac$$

$$\frac{\cos \alpha}{\sin \alpha} \sin \alpha - \frac{1}{\tan \alpha} \tan \alpha \qquad \cot \alpha = \frac{\cos \alpha}{\sin \alpha}; \cot \alpha = \frac{1}{\tan \alpha}$$

$$\cos \alpha - 1$$

Note We replaced $\cot \alpha$ by $\frac{\cos \alpha}{\sin \alpha}$ in one term and by $\frac{1}{\tan \alpha}$ in another term. We use whichever identity better suits the rest of the term.

Thus, $\cot \alpha (\sin \alpha - \tan \alpha) = \cos \alpha - 1$.

2. $\sec \theta (\cos \theta - \cot \theta)$

$$\sec \theta(\cos \theta - \cot \theta)$$

$$\sec \theta \cos \theta - \sec \theta \cot \theta$$

$$\frac{1}{\cos \theta} \cos \theta - \frac{1}{\cos \theta} \cdot \frac{\cos \theta}{\sin \theta}$$

$$1 - \frac{1}{\sin \theta}$$

$$1 - \csc \theta$$

Thus $\sec \theta(\cos \theta - \cot \theta) = 1 - \csc \theta$. ■

We also use the fundamental identity of trigonometry (section 1–2):

$$\sin^2\theta + \cos^2\theta = 1$$

■ *Example 1–4 C*

1. Simplify the expression $\dfrac{1}{\sec^2\theta} + \dfrac{1}{\csc^2\theta}$.

$$\frac{1}{\sec^2\theta} + \frac{1}{\csc^2\theta}$$

$$\frac{1}{(\sec \theta)^2} + \frac{1}{(\csc \theta)^2} \qquad \sec^2\theta \text{ means } (\sec \theta)^2, \csc^2\theta \text{ means } (\csc \theta)^2$$

$$\left(\frac{1}{\sec \theta}\right)^2 + \left(\frac{1}{\csc \theta}\right)^2 \qquad \frac{1}{x^2} = \left(\frac{1}{x}\right)^2$$

$$(\cos \theta)^2 + (\sin \theta)^2 \qquad \frac{1}{\sec \theta} = \cos \theta, \frac{1}{\csc \theta} = \sin \theta$$

$$1 \qquad \text{The fundamental identity of trigonometry}$$

Thus, $\dfrac{1}{\sec^2\theta} + \dfrac{1}{\csc^2\theta} = 1$.

2. Simplify the expression $1 - \sin^2\beta$.

$$1 - \sin^2\beta$$

$$(\sin^2\beta + \cos^2\beta) - \sin^2\beta \qquad 1 = \sin^2\beta + \cos^2\beta$$

$$\cos^2\beta$$

Thus, $1 - \sin^2\beta = \cos^2\beta$.

3. Verify the fundamental identity of trigonometry for $\theta = 60°$.

$$\sin^2 60° + \cos^2 60° = \left(\frac{\sqrt{3}}{2}\right)^2 + \left(\frac{1}{2}\right)^2 \quad \sin 60° = \frac{\sqrt{3}}{2}, \cos 60° = \frac{1}{2}$$
$$= \tfrac{3}{4} + \tfrac{1}{4}$$
$$= 1 \quad\blacksquare$$

Conditional trigonometric equations

Section 1–3 showed that if we have an equation like $\tan \theta = 4$, then one value of θ is $\tan^{-1} 4 \approx 76°$. This is an example of a simple conditional trigonometric equation. Solutions to such equations rely on the inverse sine, cosine, and tangent functions as illustrated in section 1–3.

■ *Example 1–4 D*

Solve the following conditional equations to the nearest $0.1°$.

1. $2 \sin x = 1$
   $\quad \sin x = \tfrac{1}{2}$ Divide both members by 2
   $\quad x = 30°$ Table 1–1, section 1–3

2. $5 \sin x = 3$
   $\quad \sin x = \tfrac{3}{5}$ Divide both members by 5
   $\quad x = \sin^{-1}\tfrac{3}{5}$
   $\quad x \approx 36.9°$ $\boxed{\text{CS 1}}$

3. $\sin 5x = 0.8$
   $\quad 5x = \sin^{-1} 0.8$
   $\quad x = \dfrac{\sin^{-1} 0.8}{5}$ or $\tfrac{1}{5} \sin^{-1} 0.8$
   $\quad x \approx 10.6°$ $\boxed{\text{CS 2}}$

4. $4 \cos 3\alpha = 3$
   $\quad \cos 3\alpha = \tfrac{3}{4}$ Divide both members by 4
   $\quad 3\alpha = \cos^{-1}\tfrac{3}{4}$
   $\quad \alpha = \dfrac{\cos^{-1}\tfrac{3}{4}}{3}$ or $\tfrac{1}{3} \cos^{-1}\tfrac{3}{4}$ Divide both members by 3
   $\quad \alpha \approx 13.8°$ $\boxed{\text{CS 3}}$ ■

Observe in example 1–4 D when it is proper to divide, and when it is not. An expression like

$$10 \sin x$$

indicates the product of 10 and $\sin x$. Thus, for example, the expression

$$\frac{10 \sin x}{5} = \frac{10}{5} \sin x = 2 \sin x$$

However,

$$\frac{\sin 10x}{5}$$

would not reduce. This is because the 5 is not dividing a product. The expression ''$\sin 10x$'' does not represent multiplication.

An expression like $\sin \dfrac{10x}{5}$ can be simplified to $\sin 2x$, since the 5 is dividing the product $10x$.

Calculator steps

1. (A)   3 $\boxed{\div}$ 5 $\boxed{=}$ $\boxed{\sin^{-1}}$

 (P)   3 $\boxed{\text{ENTER}}$ 5 $\boxed{\div}$ $\boxed{\sin^{-1}}$

 $\boxed{\text{TI-81}}$ $\boxed{\text{SIN}^{-1}}$ $\boxed{(}$ 3 $\boxed{\div}$ 5 $\boxed{)}$ $\boxed{\text{ENTER}}$

2. (A)   .8 $\boxed{\sin^{-1}}$ $\boxed{\div}$ 5 $\boxed{=}$

 (P)   .8 $\boxed{\sin^{-1}}$ 5 $\boxed{\div}$

 $\boxed{\text{TI-81}}$ $\boxed{\text{SIN}^{-1}}$ .8 $\boxed{\div}$ 5 $\boxed{\text{ENTER}}$

3. (A)   3 $\boxed{\div}$ 4 $\boxed{=}$ $\boxed{\cos^{-1}}$ $\boxed{\div}$ 3 $\boxed{=}$

 (P)   3 $\boxed{\text{ENTER}}$ 4 $\boxed{\div}$ $\boxed{\cos^{-1}}$ 3 $\boxed{\div}$

 $\boxed{\text{TI-81}}$ $\boxed{\text{COS}^{-1}}$ $\boxed{(}$ 3 $\boxed{\div}$ 4 $\boxed{)}$ $\boxed{\div}$ 3 $\boxed{\text{ENTER}}$

Mastery points

Can you
- Simplify simple trigonometric expressions?
- Solve simple equations involving the trigonometric ratios?

Exercise 1–4

Simplify the following trigonometric expressions.

1. $\tan \theta \cot \theta$

2. $\sec \theta \cos \theta$

3. $\cos \theta(1 - \sec \theta)$

4. $\cot \alpha(\tan \alpha + \sin \alpha)$

5. $\sec \theta(\cot \theta + \cos \theta - 1)$

6. $\dfrac{\cos \theta - 1}{\sin \theta}$

7. $\dfrac{\cos \alpha - \sin \alpha}{\cos \alpha}$

8. $\dfrac{\sin \theta + \cos \theta - 2}{\cos \theta}$

9. $1 - \cos^2\theta$

10. $\cos \theta \cos \theta + \sin^2\theta$

11. $\cos \beta(\sec \beta - \cos \beta)$

12. $-\sin \theta(\sin \theta - \csc \theta)$

13. $(\cos \theta + \sin \theta)(\cos \theta - \sin \theta) + 2 \sin^2\theta$

14. Verify by computation that the fundamental identity is true when $\theta = 30°$.

15. Using approximate values check the fundamental identity when
    a. $\theta = 16°50'$ b. $\theta = 50°$

16. Use the two identities $\cot \theta = \dfrac{1}{\tan \theta}$ and $\tan \theta = \dfrac{\sin \theta}{\cos \theta}$ to show that $\cot \theta = \dfrac{\cos \theta}{\sin \theta}$.

17. Use approximate values to show that $\tan \theta = \dfrac{\sin \theta}{\cos \theta}$ when $\theta = 32°40'$.

18. Show that $\tan \theta = \dfrac{\sin \theta}{\cos \theta}$ when $\theta = 60°$ (use values from table 1–1).

Use identities to show that the left side of each equation can be simplified to become the right side.

19. $\tan x(\cot x + \csc x) = 1 + \sec x$

20. $\csc \alpha(\cos \alpha - \sin \alpha) = \cot \alpha - 1$

21. $\sin \beta(\cot \beta - \csc \beta + \sin \beta) = \cos \beta - \cos^2\beta$

22. $\dfrac{\sin x - \cos x}{\sin x} = 1 - \cot x$

23. $\cos \alpha(\csc \alpha + \sec \alpha) = \cot \alpha + 1$

24. $\tan \beta(\cot \beta - \cos \beta) = 1 - \sin \beta$

Solve the following conditional equations to the nearest 0.1°.

25. $2 \cos x = 1$

26. $\sqrt{3} \tan x = 1$

27. $2 \sin x = \sqrt{3}$

28. $\sqrt{2} \cos x = 1$

29. $5 \sin x = 1$

30. $3 \sin x = 2$

31. $2 \tan x = 9$

32. $4 \cot x = 3$

33. $\dfrac{\sin x}{3} = \dfrac{2}{11}$

34. $\dfrac{\csc x}{3} = 2$

35. $\sin 3x = \frac{1}{2}$

36. $\cos 2x = \frac{1}{2}$

37. $\tan 2x = \sqrt{3}$

38. $\sin 2x = 0.8$

39. $\csc 3x = 3$

40. $4 \sin 2x = 3$

41. $2 \cos 4x = 1$

42. $3 \sin 2x = 0.75$

43. $2 \tan 3x = 8$

44. $\frac{1}{2} \sin 3x = \frac{1}{4}$

45. Show that in any right triangle ABC $\tan \theta = \dfrac{\sin \theta}{\cos \theta}$ is true when angle θ is angle B.

Chapter 1 summary

- A degree can be divided into smaller parts in one of two ways—into minutes and seconds or into decimal parts.

- The sum of the measures of the three angles of any triangle is 180°.

- A right triangle is a triangle in which one of the angles is a right (90°) angle. The side of a right triangle that is opposite the right angle is called the hypotenuse, and the sides that form the right angle are called the legs.

- The standard method of labeling right triangles is to label the right angle C and the two acute angles A and B. The sides are always labeled a and b, with a opposite angle A and b opposite angle B. The hypotenuse is always labeled c.

- **The Pythagorean theorem** Given a right triangle with legs a and b and hypotenuse c, then $a^2 + b^2 = c^2$.

- If $a^2 + b^2 = c^2$ in a triangle, then that triangle is a right triangle, and the right angle is opposite side c.

- If θ is one of the two acute angles in a right triangle, then

$$\sin \theta = \frac{\text{length of leg opposite } \theta}{\text{length of hypotenuse}}$$

$$\cos \theta = \frac{\text{length of leg adjacent to } \theta}{\text{length of hypotenuse}}$$

$$\tan \theta = \frac{\text{length of leg opposite } \theta}{\text{length of leg adjacent to } \theta}$$

$$\sec \theta = \frac{1}{\cos \theta}, \; \csc \theta = \frac{1}{\sin \theta}, \; \cot \theta = \frac{1}{\tan \theta}$$

- **Fundamental identity of trigonometry** If θ is either acute angle in a right triangle, then

$$\sin^2\theta + \cos^2\theta = 1$$

- The following pairs of ratios are reciprocals:

  cosine and secant

  sine and cosecant

  tangent and cotangent

- If we know one of the trigonometric ratios of an angle, we can find a triangle for which that ratio is true. We can use this triangle to compute the other five trigonometric ratios for that angle.

- The value of a trigonometric ratio depends only on the measure of the angle and not on the right triangle in which it appears.

- A right triangle is said to be solved once the lengths of its three sides and the measures of its two acute angles are known. To solve a right triangle, we must already know at least one side and either another side or one acute angle.

- **Several important trigonometric identities** are

$$\sin \theta = \frac{1}{\csc \theta}, \; \cos \theta = \frac{1}{\sec \theta}, \; \tan \theta = \frac{1}{\cot \theta},$$

$$\tan \theta = \frac{\sin \theta}{\cos \theta}, \; \cot \theta = \frac{\cos \theta}{\sin \theta}$$

Chapter 1 review

[1–1] Convert each angle to its measure in decimal degrees. Round your answer to the nearest 0.01°. Also, state whether each angle is acute, obtuse, or right.

1. 17°34'17''   **2.** 84°9'   **3.** 125°37'   **4.** 39°45'43''

Find the measure of the missing angle, θ.

5.
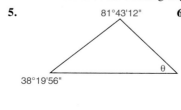
81°43'12"

38°19'56"

6.
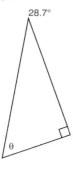
28.7°

In the following problems two of the three sides of a right triangle are given. Use the Pythagorean theorem to calculate the length of the missing side; give your answer in exact form and in approximate form, rounded to one decimal place if necessary.

	a	b	c
7.	8	12	?
8.	9	?	26
9.	?	8	13

10. A flagpole is 46 feet tall and is supported by a wire attached at the top of the pole and to the ground 25 feet from the base of the pole. How long is the wire (to the nearest foot)?

11. The diagram is called an impedance diagram and is used in computing total impedance in a certain electronics circuit. It shows that inductive reactance X_L is 40.0 ohms and that impedance Z is 56.6 ohms. Calculate the resistance R to the nearest tenth of an ohm.

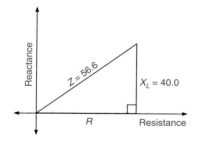

[1–2] In the following problems you are given parts of right triangle ABC. Use this information to compute the six trigonometric ratios for the angle specified.

	a	b	c	Find ratios for this angle
12.	3	7		A
13.	5		15	B
14.	2	$\sqrt{10}$		A

15. In right triangle ABC, sin $A = \frac{4}{5}$. Draw a triangle for which this is true and use it to find sin B.

16. In right triangle ABC, tan $A = 5$. Draw a triangle for which this is true and use it to find cos B.

17. In right triangle ABC, sec $A = 3$. Draw a triangle for which this is true and use it to find tan B.

18. In right triangle ABC, tan $B = 0.8$. Draw a triangle for which this is true and use it to find sec A.

[1–3] Use an electronic calculator to find four-decimal-place approximations for the following.

19. sin 15.5°   **20.** sec 68.2°   **21.** tan 17.9°
22. sin 40.8°   **23.** tan 16.3°   **24.** sec 25.7°
25. cot 31°20'   **26.** sec 85°40'   **27.** tan 31°30'
28. csc 43°10'   **29.** tan 63°30'   **30.** sec 86°40'

31. Find four-digit approximations for all six trigonometric ratios for
   a. 53.20°   **b.** 53°20'

32. A surveyor needs to compute R in the following formula as part of finding the area of the segment of a circle.
$$R = \frac{LC}{2 \sin I}.$$ Find R to three decimal places if $LC = 315.2$ meters and $I = 22.6°$.

Find the unknown acute angle θ to the nearest 0.1°.

33. sin θ = 0.6314   **34.** cos θ = 0.1382

35. tan θ = $\dfrac{35.9}{50.0}$ **36.** sec θ = 2.351

37. csc θ = 1.425   **38.** cot θ = 6.310

In the following problems two of the five values that must be known to solve right triangle ABC are given. Find the other three values. Round all answers to the same accuracy as the data.

	a	b	c	A	B
39.	23.3			56.1°	
40.		11.4	23.0		
41.	4.00	8.55			
42.			66.0		63.1°

43. Ground radar shows that an aircraft is 22.6 kilometers from the radar site, at an angle of elevation of 11.2°. Find the aircraft's altitude to the nearest 0.01 kilometer.

44. The diagram is a top view of a portion of a machine part. Find the length x to the nearest tenth of a millimeter.

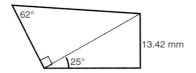

[1–4]

45. Show that the fundamental identity of trigonometry is true for an angle of measure 45°. (Use exact values.)

Simplify the following trigonometric expressions:

46. $\cot \theta \sec \theta$

47. $\csc \theta (\sin \theta - \tan \theta)$

48. $\dfrac{\sin \theta - 1}{\sin \theta}$

49. $\dfrac{\cos \alpha + 2 - \cot \alpha}{\cos \alpha}$

50. $(1 + \sin \theta)(1 - \sin \theta)$

51. Solve $3 \sin 2x = 2$ for x to the nearest 0.1°.

Chapter 1 test

1. Convert 26°27′43″ to its measure in decimal degrees. Round your answer to the nearest 0.001°.

2. Find the measure of the missing angle θ.

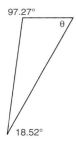

3. In right triangle ABC, $a = 6$ and $c = 12$. Find b. Leave your answer in exact form.

4. A flagpole is 46 feet tall and is supported by an 87-foot guy wire attached at the top of the pole and to the ground. How far from the base of the pole is the ground attachment point of the wire (to the nearest 0.1 foot)?

5. In right triangle ABC, $\sec A = \frac{5}{3}$. Draw a triangle for which this is true and use it to find $\tan B$.

Find approximations for the following, to four decimal places.

6. $\sin 25.5°$ **7.** $\sec 78.3°$ **8.** $\cot 31°50′$

9. The average power, in watts, in an AC circuit is given by the formula $P = VI \cos \theta$. Compute P (in watts) if $V = 220$ volts, $I = 4.1$ amperes, and $\theta = 48°$ (to the nearest 0.1 watt).

Find the unknown acute angle θ to the nearest 0.1°.

10. $\sin \theta = 0.1314$ **11.** $\sec \theta = 4.121$

12. In right triangle ABC, $a = 3.8$ and $A = 21.4°$. Solve the triangle, rounding answers to the nearest tenth.

13. In right triangle ABC, $a = 5.2$ and $b = 7.9$. Solve the triangle, rounding answers to the nearest tenth.

14. If the angle of depression from an aircraft to a ground point 13.6 miles away is 12.5°, how high is the aircraft flying, to the nearest ten feet?

15. Simplify the expression $\cos \theta (\sec \theta - \cos \theta)$.

16. Solve $\sec 5x = 5$ for x to the nearest 0.1°.

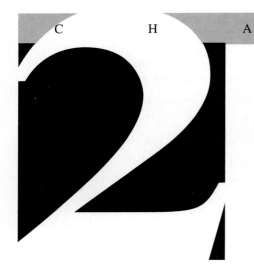

The Trigonometric Functions

In this chapter we widen the application of trigonometric concepts to include angles of any degree measure. We then learn about another method of angle measurement, called radian measure. This is the system of measurement most often used in higher mathematics, engineering, and the sciences. We begin by reviewing the idea of function.

2–1 Functions

The concept of a function is basic to higher mathematics. It provides a way to describe, or model, many real-world situations. For example, the temperature of a metal bar, heated at one end, varies with the distance from the heated end. We say that the temperature along the bar is a function of the distance along the bar. The number of pounds of tomatoes sold in a given geographic area may vary with the retail price per pound. We say that the number of pounds sold is a function of retail price. In short, any time a change in one measurable quantity can be linked to a change in another measurable quantity, the idea of function can be used to give precise meaning to the idea.

A useful definition of function is the following:

> **Function**
> A function is a set of ordered pairs having the property that no first element of the ordered pairs repeats.

For example, $f = \{(1,3), (4,9), (-2,6)\}$ is a function since, first, it is a set of ordered pairs and second, no first element of these ordered pairs repeats—that is, they are all different. However, $g = \{(1,3), (4,9), (4,6)\}$ is not a function since, although it is a set of ordered pairs, one of the first elements (4) is repeated.

If the weight of some type of steel bar is 1.5 pounds per foot and the bar comes in 1-, 2-, 5-, 8-, and 10-foot lengths, then a function that describes the weight of a bar would be {(1,1.5), (2,3), (5,7.5), (8,12), (10,15)}, where, of course, the first element of each pair is the length of the bar and the second element is the weight.

The set of all first elements of the ordered pairs in a function is called the **domain** of the function, and the set of all second elements is called the **range** of the function. The domain of f (above) is $\{-2,1,4\}$, and the range of f is $\{3,6,9\}$.

One to one

A function is said to be one to one if no second element of the ordered pairs repeats.

For example, the function f mentioned above is one to one, whereas the function $h = \{(1,5), (2,9), (3,9)\}$ is not one to one since there is a second element, 9, of the ordered pairs that repeats.

■ *Example 2–1 A*

For each set of ordered pairs listed,

    a. State whether the set is a function or not.
    b. If a function, state the domain and range.
    c. If a function, state whether it is one to one or not.

1. $\{(-2,8), (5,9), (100,19)\}$
    a. The set is a function since no first element repeats.
    b. The domain is $\{-2, 5, 100\}$, and the range is $\{8, 9, 19\}$.
    c. It is one to one since no second element repeats.

2. $\{(-20,-10), (-3,0), (-3,1), (22,15)\}$
    a. The set is not a function since the first element -3 repeats.

3. $\{(-5,3), (-1,9), (12,9), (256,256)\}$
    a. The set is a function since no first element repeats.
    b. The domain is $\{-5, -1, 12, 256\}$, and the range is $\{3, 9, 256\}$.
    c. The function is not one to one because the second element 9 is repeated. ■

If we reverse the first and second elements in each ordered pair of a one-to-one function f we get a new function. For example, consider the function f.

$$f = \{(2,3), (5,9), (7,16)\}$$

If we reverse the ordered pairs, we get

$$\{(3,2), (9,5), (16,7)\}$$

which is also a function. If we reverse the ordered pairs of the function

$$h = \{(1,5), (2,9), (3,9)\}$$

we get

$$\{(5,1), (9,2), (9,3)\}$$

which is not a function (because one of the first elements, 9, is repeated). This first element repeated because a second element repeated in function *h*. Note that *h* was not a one-to-one function.

Now consider the situation in a general way. If we reverse the elements of each ordered pair in a one-to-one function, then no first element in the resulting set will repeat since no second element in the original function was repeated. Thus, reversing the ordered pairs of a one-to-one function produces a function.

If we reverse the elements of each ordered pair in a function that is not one to one, the resulting set cannot be a function, since if the function was not one to one there was a second element that repeated, which becomes a repeated first element in the resulting set. Taken together these statements prove the following theorem:

Theorem
Reversing the elements of the ordered pairs of a function produces a function if and only if the function is one to one.

We call the function produced by reversing the ordered pairs of a one-to-one function *f* the **inverse function** f^{-1}.

Note   A symbol for function with a superscript "-1" does not mean the same thing as an expression with an exponent "-1." Although 3^{-1} means $\frac{1}{3^1}$ or $\frac{1}{3}$, and x^{-1} means $\frac{1}{x}$, the symbol f^{-1} does *not* mean $\frac{1}{f}$ if *f* represents a function.

■ *Example 2–1 B*

In each of the given sets of ordered pairs,

    a. Determine if the set is a function.
    b. If a function, state the domain and range.
    c. If a one-to-one function, state its inverse function.

1. $f = \{(1,3), (1,5), (2,5), (4,9)\}$
    a. *f* is not a function since a first element, 1, repeats.

2. $g = \{(-2,-8), (0,2), (2,3), (8,8)\}$
    a. *g* is a function since no first element repeats.
    b. The domain of *g* is $\{-2, 0, 2, 8\}$, and the range is $\{-8, 2, 3, 8\}$.
    c. *g* is one to one since no second element repeats. Therefore, it has an inverse.

$$g^{-1} = \{(-8,-2), (2,0), (3,2), (8,8)\}$$

3. $h = \{(-1,0), (0,0), (1,2)\}$
    a. *h* is a function since no first element repeats.
    b. The domain of *h* is $\{-1, 0, 1\}$, and the range is $\{0, 2\}$.
    c. *h* is not one to one because there is a second element, 0, which repeats. Therefore, *h* does not have an inverse function.   ■

Function notation

We often describe an ordered pair of a function by using "*f* of *x*," or "*f(x)*" notation. For example, in the function *f* is defined as *f* = {(−2,6), (1,3), (4,9)} we would say

$$f(-2) = 6 \qquad \text{"}f \text{ of } -2 \text{ is } 6\text{"}$$
$$f(1) = 3 \qquad \text{"}f \text{ of } 1 \text{ is } 3\text{"}$$
$$f(4) = 9 \qquad \text{"}f \text{ of } 4 \text{ is } 9\text{"}$$

Thus, *f(x)* notation is a way of describing what range element is associated with a given domain element.

Note *f*(−2) is read "*f* of −2" or "*f* at −2." Also, letters other than "*f*" can be used. We could write "*g(x)*" or "*h(x)*," for example.

■ *Example 2–1 C*

In the function *f* = {(−100,10), (−50,20), (0,30)} state

a. *f*(−50)   **b.** *f*(10)

a. *f*(−50) is 20, since the range element associated with −50 is 20.

b. *f*(10) does not exist. This is because 10 is not in the domain, so we have no way to relate it to some element in the range.   ■

Since most functions contain an infinite number of ordered pairs, we cannot describe them with a list. In these cases we use a rule. The rule is usually combined with *f(x)* notation. For example, we might describe a function *f* with the rule

$$f(x) = 5x - 3$$

This rule tells us that to form an ordered pair that belongs to the function, where the domain element is *x*, compute 5*x* − 3. This is the range element. If *x* = 2, then 5*x* − 3 becomes 5(2) − 3 = 7, so the ordered pair (2,7) is in the function *f*. Usually we write

$$f(x) = 5x - 3$$
$$f(2) = 5(2) - 3$$
$$f(2) = 7$$

The statement *f*(2) = 7, verbalized "*f* of 2 is 7," means that for the domain element 2 the range element is 7.

■ *Example 2–1 D*

1. If a function *f* is described by the rule

$$f(x) = -3x + 1$$

form the ordered pairs in *f* for the domain elements (a) −2, (b) 3, and (c) 5.

a. *f*(−2) = −3(−2) + 1
    f(−2) = 7, so (−2,7) is an ordered pair in *f*.
b. *f*(3) = −3(3) + 1
    f(3) = −8, so (3,−8) is an ordered pair in *f*.
c. *f*(5) = −14, so (5,−14) is an ordered pair in *f*.

2. If a function g is described by the rule

$$g(x) = x^2 - 2x + 3$$

form the ordered pairs in g for the domain elements (a) -5, (b) $\sqrt{2}$, and (c) 10.

a. $g(-5) = (-5)^2 - 2(-5) + 3$
$g(-5) = 38$, so $(-5,38)$ is an ordered pair in g.

b. $g(\sqrt{2}) = (\sqrt{2})^2 - 2(\sqrt{2}) + 3$
$g(\sqrt{2}) = 2 - 2\sqrt{2} + 3 = 5 - 2\sqrt{2}$,
so $(\sqrt{2}, 5 - 2\sqrt{2})$ is an ordered pair in g.

c. $g(10) = 10^2 - 2(10) + 3$
$g(10) = 83$, so $(10,83)$ is an ordered pair in g. ■

In these examples we never stated exactly what the domain of each function was. If we are not told what the domain is, we always use all real numbers for which the rule makes sense. This is called the **implied domain.**

For example, if the rule for a function f were $f(x) = \dfrac{3}{x - 2}$, then the domain would be every real number except 2, since $f(2)$ would be $\dfrac{3}{2 - 2} = \dfrac{3}{0}$, which is undefined. If $f(x) = \dfrac{x}{x^2 - 1}$ were the rule that described a function, the domain would be all the real numbers except ± 1, since either value would make the denominator of the expression 0.

The trigonometric ratios are functions in the sense of our definition. They can be viewed as sets of ordered pairs in which no first element repeats. For example the sine ratio can be described as the ordered pairs (degree measure of angle, sine of angle). It would include, for example, the ordered pairs $\left(30°, \dfrac{1}{2}\right)$, $\left(45°, \dfrac{\sqrt{2}}{2}\right)$, $\left(60°, \dfrac{\sqrt{3}}{2}\right)$, etc.

Mastery points

Can you
- State the definition of a function?
- Determine if a set is a function?
- State whether a function is one to one?
- State the inverse of a one-to-one function?
- Use $f(x)$ notation to form ordered pairs in a function?

Exercise 2–1

In each of the following sets of ordered pairs:
a. Determine if the set is a function.
b. If a function, state the domain and range.
c. If a one-to-one function, state the inverse.

1. $f = \{(3,5), (4,5), (6,9), (7,10)\}$
3. $h = \{(-2,-2), (3,4), (4,3)\}$

2. $g = \{(-4,-3), (-1,1), (1,3), (2,5)\}$
4. $f = \{(0.5,2), (1.5,3), (2,4), (2.5,5)\}$

5. $g = \{(1,4), (1,5), (5,9), (6,10)\}$
7. $f = \{(1,1), (2,2), (3,3), (4,4)\}$

6. $h = \{(-10,-5), (10,5), (12,20), (20,30)\}$
8. $g = \{(-3,5), (5,8), (8,13), (13,21)\}$

Assume $f = \{(-3,6), (-2,9), (-1,0), (0,19), (4\frac{1}{2},7), (2\pi,11), (200,220), (300,7)\}$ in problems 9 and 10.

9. Find
   a. $f(-2)$ **b.** $f(0)$ **c.** $f(2\pi)$ **d.** $f(7)$ **e.** $f(250)$

10. Find
   a. $f(-1)$ **b.** $f(4\frac{1}{2})$ **c.** $f(\pi)$ **d.** $f(300)$

In each of the following problems a rule that describes a function is given. Form the ordered pairs that this function contains for the following domain elements:

a. -2 **b.** 0 **c.** $\sqrt{3}$ **d.** $\frac{1}{2}$ **e.** 5

11. $f(x) = 5x - 3$
15. $g(x) = x^2 + x - 1$

12. $g(x) = 2 - 3x$
16. $h(x) = x^2$

13. $h(x) = (x - 3)(x + 2)$
17. $f(x) = 3x^4 - x^2 + 2$

14. $f(x) = x^2 - 2x + 3$
18. $g(x) = 1 - x^2$

19. $h(x) = \dfrac{x}{x + 3}$

20. $f(x) = \dfrac{4}{x^2 - 1}$

21. The statement $t(x) = 500 - 2x$ states the functional relationship between the temperature t of an iron rod at a point x centimeters from the heated end. Find the temperature (in degrees centigrade) for points that are (a) 3 cm, (b) 12 cm, and (c) 104 cm from the heated end.

2–2 *The trigonometric functions—definitions*

There are many situations where we have to think of angles as being nonacute. This is often a situation in which we wish to describe an amount of rotation. For example, a ship may turn through an angle of 215°, a computed tomography (CT) scanner used in medical diagnosis may move through an angle of 360°, or a surveyor may find the measure of the angle at one corner of a piece of land to be 165°20′. For these situations, we often place the angle in a rectangular (*x-y*) coordinate system.

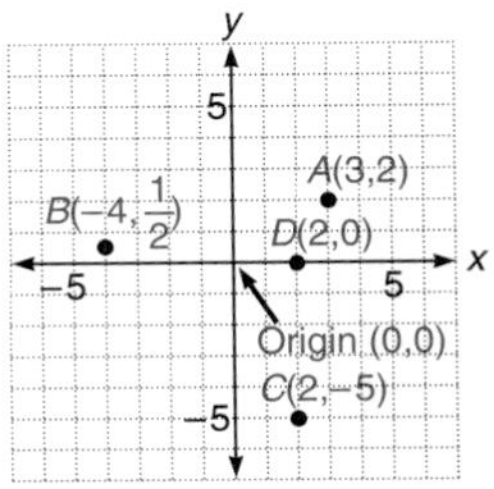

The *x-y* (rectangular) coordinate system

We graph using the *x-y* rectangular coordinate system. Recall that an **ordered pair** is a pair of numbers listed in parentheses, separated by a comma. In the ordered pair (x,y) x is called the **first component** and y is called the **second component**; $(5,-3)$, $(9,3)$, and $(4,\frac{2}{3})$ are examples of ordered pairs. The graphing system we use is formed by sets of vertical and horizontal lines; one vertical line is called the *y*-axis, and one horizontal line is called the *x*-axis. The geometric plane (flat surface) that contains this system of lines is called the **coordinate plane.** See figure 2–1.

The **graph** of an ordered pair is the geometric point in the coordinate plane located by moving left or right, as appropriate, according to the first component of the ordered pair, and vertically a number of units corresponding to the second component of the ordered pair. The graphs of the points $A(3,2)$, $B(-4,\frac{1}{2})$, $C(2,-5)$, and $D(2,0)$ are shown in the figure. The first and second elements of the ordered pair associated with a geometric point in the coordinate plane are called its **coordinates.**

Figure 2–1

Angles in standard position

> **Angle in standard position**
> An angle in standard position is formed by two rays, one of which always lies on the nonnegative portion of the x-axis. This ray is called the **initial side.** The second ray is called the **terminal side.** It may be in any quadrant or along any axis.

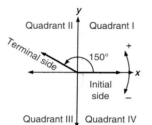

Figure 2–2

Figure 2–2 shows an angle in standard position, with measure 150°. Observe the labeling of the quadrants formed by the x-axis and the y-axis. They are called quadrants I through IV as shown. We generally use the word ''angle'' instead of the phrase ''angle in standard position.''

If the measure of the angle is *positive,* we picture the terminal side as having moved away from the initial side in a *counterclockwise* direction; if the measure of the angle is *negative* we picture the terminal side as having moved away from the initial side in a *clockwise* direction. If an angle's measure is greater than 360° or less than −360° we consider the angle to have ''gone around'' more than once. Several examples of angles in standard position are shown in figure 2–3. In part c we show the angle as a 360° revolution, followed by an additional 200° turn.

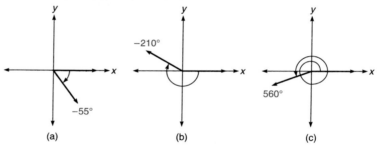

Figure 2–3

Angles which have the same terminal side are said to be **coterminal.** (All angles in standard position have the same initial side.) The 150° angle in figure 2–2 and the −210° angle in figure 2–3 (b) are coterminal. We can see this when we realize that in each case the angle formed by the negative side of the x-axis and the terminal side of each angle is 30°. Since ±360° represents one complete revolution, coterminal angles are angles whose degree measures differ by an integer multiple of 360°. This forms the basis for our definition.

> **Coterminal angles**
> Two angles[1] α and β are said to be coterminal if
> $$\alpha = \beta + k(360°), k \text{ an integer.}$$
> *Concept*
> Two angles are coterminal if the difference of their degree measures is evenly divisible by 360°.

[1]Remember, α is the Greek letter alpha, and β is the Greek letter beta.

■ *Example 2–2 A*

In each case find a coterminal angle with measure x such that $0° \leq x < 360°$.

1. 875°

$$875° - 360° = 515° \qquad \text{Subtract } 360° \text{ until } x \text{ is found}$$
$$515° - 360° = 155° \qquad \text{The required angle is } 155°$$

We could have done this more elegantly by computing $875° - 2(360°)$.

2. −1,000°

$$-1,000° + 360° = -640° \qquad \text{Add } 360° \text{ until } x \text{ is found}$$
$$-640° + 360° = -280°$$
$$-280° + 360° = 80°$$

Or solve by computing $-1,000° + 3(360°) = -1,000° + 1,080° = 80°$.■

The trigonometric functions

We now define the six trigonometric functions. They have the same names as the six trigonometric ratios, and the same abbreviations. The trigonometric ratios are functions with domain the set of *acute* angles. The trigonometric functions have the set of *all* angles as their domain. We used the word ratio to distinguish the two sets of functions. For acute angles the trigonometric functions are essentially the same as the trigonometric ratios. The following definition refers to figure 2–4.

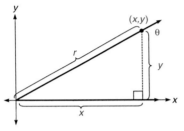

Figure 2–4

The trigonometric functions

Let θ be an angle in standard position, and let (x,y) be any point on the terminal side of the angle, except $(0,0)$. Let $r = \sqrt{x^2 + y^2}$ be the distance from the origin to the point. Then,

$$\sin \theta = \frac{y}{r}, \qquad \cos \theta = \frac{x}{r}, \qquad \tan \theta = \frac{y}{x}$$

$$\csc \theta = \frac{r}{y}, \qquad \sec \theta = \frac{r}{x}, \qquad \cot \theta = \frac{x}{y}$$

Note
1. We define r so that $r > 0$.
2. If x or y in the point (x,y) is zero, then those ratios with x or y in the denominator are not defined.
3. Unlike the trigonometric ratios, the trigonometric functions can take on negative values.
4. We sometimes call the cosecant, secant, and cotangent functions the *reciprocal trigonometric functions.*

It can be proven that for a given angle, *it does not matter what point on the terminal side is chosen; the values of the trigonometric functions will be the same.* This is illustrated in example 2–2 D.

It can also be seen that *coterminal angles have the same values for the trigonometric functions.* This is because two coterminal angles have the same terminal side, and the definitions depend solely on a point on the terminal side.

The definitions of the trigonometric functions imply the following identities for all values of θ for which any denominator is nonzero. These identities look identical to those for the trigonometric ratios; however, those were shown to be true only for acute angles in right triangles.

Reciprocal function identities

$$\csc \theta = \frac{1}{\sin \theta}, \qquad \sin \theta = \frac{1}{\csc \theta}$$

$$\sec \theta = \frac{1}{\cos \theta}, \qquad \cos \theta = \frac{1}{\sec \theta}$$

$$\cot \theta = \frac{1}{\tan \theta}, \qquad \tan \theta = \frac{1}{\cot \theta}$$

To see that the first reciprocal function identity is true observe that $\csc \theta = \dfrac{r}{y} = \dfrac{1}{\dfrac{y}{r}} = \dfrac{1}{\sin \theta}$. It is left as an exercise to show that the rest of these are true.

Using the reciprocal function identities we can usually find the values of the cosecant, secant, and cotangent functions by finding the reciprocal of the sine, cosine, and tangent functions.

Two other identities that can be useful are the following; again, they are true only for those values of θ for which no denominator is 0.

Tangent/cotangent identities

$$\tan \theta = \frac{\sin \theta}{\cos \theta}, \qquad \cot \theta = \frac{\cos \theta}{\sin \theta}$$

■ *Example 2–2 B*

Show that $\tan \theta = \dfrac{\sin \theta}{\cos \theta}$ is an identity for the trigonometric functions.

We show that each member of the equation is equivalent to the same thing.

$\tan \theta$	$\dfrac{\sin \theta}{\cos \theta}$	
$\dfrac{y}{x}$	$\dfrac{\dfrac{y}{r}}{\dfrac{x}{r}}$	Apply the definitions
	$\dfrac{y}{r} \cdot \dfrac{r}{x}$	Algebra of division
	$\dfrac{y}{x}$	Reduce $\dfrac{ry}{rx}$

Thus, $\tan \theta = \dfrac{y}{x}$ and $\dfrac{\sin \theta}{\cos \theta} = \dfrac{y}{x}$, so $\tan \theta = \dfrac{\sin \theta}{\cos \theta}$. ■

Example 2–2 C illustrates finding values of the trigonometric functions for an angle in standard position, given a point on the terminal side of the angle.

■ *Example 2–2 C*

In each problem a point on the terminal side of an angle θ is given. Use it to find the trigonometric functions for that angle. Also, make a sketch of the angle.

1. $(3,-4)$

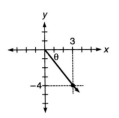

$$r = \sqrt{x^2 + y^2} \qquad \text{Definition}$$
$$= \sqrt{3^2 + (-4)^2} \qquad \text{Replace } x, y$$
$$= 5$$

$$\sin \theta = \frac{y}{r} = -\frac{4}{5}, \ \csc \theta = \frac{1}{\sin \theta} = -\frac{5}{4}$$

$$\cos \theta = \frac{x}{r} = \frac{3}{5}, \ \sec \theta = \frac{1}{\cos \theta} = \frac{5}{3}$$

$$\tan \theta = \frac{y}{x} = -\frac{4}{3}, \ \cot \theta = \frac{1}{\tan \theta} = -\frac{3}{4}$$

2. $(-8,-2)$

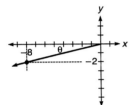

$$r = \sqrt{x^2 + y^2} \qquad \text{Definition}$$
$$= \sqrt{(-8)^2 + (-2)^2} \qquad \text{Replace } x, y$$
$$= \sqrt{68} = 2\sqrt{17}$$

$$\sin \theta = -\frac{2}{2\sqrt{17}} = -\frac{1}{\sqrt{17}} = -\frac{\sqrt{17}}{17}, \ \csc \theta = -\sqrt{17}$$

$$\cos \theta = -\frac{8}{2\sqrt{17}} = -\frac{4}{\sqrt{17}} = -\frac{4\sqrt{17}}{17}, \ \sec \theta = -\frac{\sqrt{17}}{4}$$

$$\tan \theta = \frac{-2}{-8} = \frac{1}{4}, \ \cot \theta = 4$$

3. $(0,-3)$

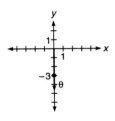

$$r = \sqrt{0^2 + (-3)^2} = 3$$

$$\sin \theta = \frac{y}{r} = \frac{-3}{3} = -1, \ \csc \theta = \frac{1}{\sin \theta} = -1$$

$$\cos \theta = \frac{x}{r} = \frac{0}{3} = 0, \ \sec \theta = \frac{1}{\cos \theta} = \frac{1}{0}, \ \text{undefined}$$

$$\tan \theta = \frac{y}{x} = \frac{-3}{0}, \ \text{undefined}; \ \cot \theta = \frac{\cos \theta}{\sin \theta} = \frac{0}{-1} = 0$$

As illustrated here, when the tangent function is undefined the cotangent function is defined. In this one case it is useful to use the appropriate tangent/cotangent identity or equivalently $\cot \theta = \dfrac{x}{y}$.

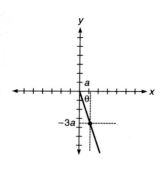

4. $(a, -3a)$, $a > 0$

Since the x-coordinate is positive the angle is in quadrants I or IV; since the y-coordinate is negative, we choose quadrant IV for our sketch.

$$r = \sqrt{a^2 + (-3a)^2} = \sqrt{10a^2} = a\sqrt{10}$$

$$\sin \theta = -\frac{3a}{a\sqrt{10}} = -\frac{3}{\sqrt{10}} = -\frac{3\sqrt{10}}{10}, \csc \theta = -\frac{\sqrt{10}}{3}$$

$$\cos \theta = \frac{a}{a\sqrt{10}} = \frac{1}{\sqrt{10}} = \frac{\sqrt{10}}{10}, \sec \theta = \sqrt{10}$$

$$\tan \theta = -\frac{3a}{a} = -3, \cot \theta = -\frac{1}{3}$$ ■

Example 2–2 D illustrates that the value of the trigonometric functions for a given angle depend only on the measure of the angle and not on the point that is chosen on its terminal side.

■ *Example 2–2 D*

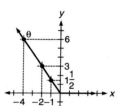

The point $(-2,3)$ is on the terminal side of an angle θ in standard position. Find two other points that would also be on the terminal side of this angle and then compute the value of the sine, cosine, and tangent functions with all three points.

We can find other points on the terminal side of this angle by multiplying both values, -2 and 3, by the same amount. Thus, if we double them we obtain the point $(-4,6)$. If we take half of each we obtain $(-1,1\frac{1}{2})$. All three points are shown in the figure.

The computations for the three points are shown in the table. The same results are obtained regardless of which point is used to perform the calculation.

Point	x	y	r	$\sin \theta$	$\cos \theta$	$\tan \theta$
$\left(-1,1\frac{1}{2}\right)$	-1	$\frac{3}{2}$	$\frac{\sqrt{13}}{2}$	$\frac{\frac{3}{2}}{\frac{\sqrt{13}}{2}} = \frac{3\sqrt{13}}{13}$	$\frac{-1}{\frac{\sqrt{13}}{2}} = -\frac{2\sqrt{13}}{13}$	$\frac{\frac{3}{2}}{-1} = -\frac{3}{2}$
$(-2,3)$	-2	3	$\sqrt{13}$	$\frac{3}{\sqrt{13}} = \frac{3\sqrt{13}}{13}$	$\frac{-2}{\sqrt{13}} = -\frac{2\sqrt{13}}{13}$	$\frac{3}{-2} = -\frac{3}{2}$
$(-4,6)$	-4	6	$2\sqrt{13}$	$\frac{6}{2\sqrt{13}} = \frac{3\sqrt{13}}{13}$	$\frac{-4}{2\sqrt{13}} = -\frac{2\sqrt{13}}{13}$	$\frac{6}{-4} = -\frac{3}{2}$

■

Mastery points

Can you
- When given an angle θ, find a positive coterminal angle with measure x such that $0° \leq x < 360°$?
- Sketch an angle and find the values of the six trigonometric functions when given a point on the terminal side of the angle?

Exercise 2–2

In problems 1–17,
   a. Draw the initial and terminal side of the given angle.
   b. State the measure of the smallest nonnegative angle that is coterminal with the given angle.

1. 420°	**2.** −40°	**3.** 230°	**4.** 1,000°	**5.** 1,800.6°
6. 1,260°	**7.** 547.9°	**8.** 2,000°	**9.** −870°	**10.** 625°
11. 525°	**12.** −610°	**13.** −1,530.3°	**14.** 390°	**15.** −720°
16. −11.9°	**17.** −313°			

18. An automobile engine is timed to fire the spark plug for cylinder 1 at 8° BTDC (before top dead center), which, for our purposes, is −8°. Assuming this engine rotates in a counterclockwise direction, what is the equivalent amount ATDC (after TDC) (i.e., the least nonnegative angle coterminal with it)?

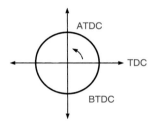

19. If an automobile engine is timed to fire at 13° BTDC, what is the equivalent amount ATDC?

20. If an automobile engine is timed to fire at 8.6° BTDC, what is the equivalent amount ATDC?

21. If an automobile engine is timed to fire at 6.1° BTDC, what is the equivalent amount ATDC?

22. In an electronic circuit with an inductive component to the impedance, the current follows the voltage. For example, the current may follow the voltage by 15°, in which case we could say the phase angle of the current is −15°, relative to the voltage. We could just as easily say that the phase angle of the voltage is 345°, relative to the current. Find the phase angle of the voltage relative to the current if the phase angle of the current relative to the voltage is (a) −88°, (b) −24.33°, (c) −35°56′, (d) −16.56° (e) −0°14′, (f) −0.14°. (Find the least nonnegative coterminal angle in each case.)

In the following problems you are given a point that lies on the terminal side of an angle in standard position. In each case, compute the value of all six trigonometric functions for the angle.

23. (3,6)	**24.** (−2,5)	**25.** (−5,8)	**26.** (−7,−8)	**27.** (2,−2)
28. (3,0)	**29.** (−1,4)	**30.** (0,−4)	**31.** (−10,−15)	**32.** $(3,\sqrt{5})$
33. $(-\sqrt{2},6)$	**34.** $(3,-\sqrt{6})$	**35.** $(-\sqrt{3},-\sqrt{2})$	**36.** $(1,-\sqrt{3})$	**37.** $(\sqrt{6},-\sqrt{10})$

In the following problems you are given a point that lies on the terminal side of an angle in standard position. In each case, compute the value of all six trigonometric functions for the angle. Assume $a > 0$, $b > 0$.

38. $(b,-2b)$	**39.** $(2a,-a)$	**40.** $(-a,-a)$	**41.** $(\sqrt{2}b,b)$	**42.** $(3a,\sqrt{3}a)$
43. $\left(\dfrac{b}{2},b\right)$	**44.** $\left(-\dfrac{a}{3},\dfrac{a}{2}\right)$			

45. Show that the identity $\sec\theta = \dfrac{1}{\cos\theta}$ is true, except where $\cos\theta = 0$.

46. Show that the identity $\cot\theta = \dfrac{1}{\tan\theta}$ is true, except where $\tan\theta = 0$.

47. Show that the identity $\cot\theta = \dfrac{\cos\theta}{\sin\theta}$ is true, except where $\sin\theta = 0$.

48. Show that the identity $\cos\theta = \dfrac{1}{\sec\theta}$ is true.

49. Show that the identity $\sin\theta = \dfrac{1}{\csc\theta}$ is true.

To solve the following two problems, we must recall that the equation of a nonvertical straight line can be put in the form $y = mx + b$, where m is the slope and b is the y-intercept. If a straight line passes through the origin then $b = 0$ and the equation becomes $y = mx$.

50. Show that if two different points lie on the terminal side of an angle in standard position, then using either point gives the same value for the sine function. For the sake of simplicity assume the terminal side is not vertical or horizontal. Represent the points as (x_1, y_1) and (x_2, y_2). Note that these points lie on the same line. The equation of any line that passes through the origin is of the form $y = mx$, so we know that for the same value of m, $y_1 = mx_1$ and $y_2 = mx_2$. This means that the points (x_1, y_1) and (x_2, y_2) can be rewritten as (x_1, mx_1) and (x_2, mx_2). Use these versions of the points to compute the length r for each point. Then show that the value of the sine function is the same when computed using either point.

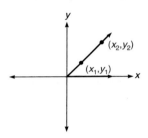

51. Show that if the trigonometric function values are the same for two points, then these points lie on the terminal side of the same angle. Assume for simplicity that these points are not located on either the x-axis or the y-axis. To show that the points lie on the terminal side of the same angle we must show that both points lie on the same line and are in the same quadrant. Let (x_1, y_1) and (x_2, y_2) represent the two points, and consider the value of the tangent function as given by each point. This can be used to show that $y_1 = mx_1$ and $y_2 = mx_2$ (for the same value of m). This means that the two points lie on the same line. Now explain why they must be in the same quadrant.

52. Fill in the table below. One way to do this is to choose points on the terminal side of each angle and apply the definitions of each function. For example, a point on the terminal side of an angle of measure 0° is (1,0).

θ	$\sin \theta$	$\cos \theta$	$\tan \theta$	$\csc \theta$	$\sec \theta$	$\cot \theta$
0°						
90°						
180°						
270°						

2–3 *Values for any angle—the reference angle/ASTC procedure*

The values of the trigonometric functions for an angle of any measure are related to the values for the acute angles of the first quadrant. These values (for the first quadrant) are the same as those for the trigonometric ratios for acute angles. The values of the trigonometric functions for any angle have a sign and a "size" (absolute value). We first discuss the sign of the basic trigonometric functions, then the size.

The ASTC rule—the signs of the trigonometric functions by quadrant

The **sign** of the value of a trigonometric function for an angle *depends on the quadrant in which the angle terminates.* Figure 2–5 shows the quadrants in which the sine, cosine, and tangent functions are positive. (They are negative in the other quadrants.)

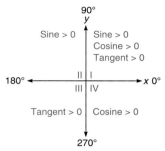

Figure 2–5

The figure shows that the sine function is positive in quadrants I and II, and therefore negative in quadrants III and IV. This is because the sine function is defined by the ratio $\dfrac{y}{r}$; since r is always positive this ratio is positive where y is positive, in quadrants I and II. Since the cosine function is $\dfrac{x}{r}$ and $r > 0$, the cosine is positive where x is positive: quadrants I and IV. The tangent function is defined by $\dfrac{y}{x}$, so it is positive where x and y are both positive (quadrant I) or both negative (quadrant III).

Figure 2–5 should be memorized; it represents the ASTC rule.

The ASTC rule	
In quadrant I,	**A**ll the trigonometric functions are positive.
In quadrant II, the	**S**ine function is positive.
In quadrant III, the	**T**angent function is positive.
In quadrant IV, the	**C**osine function is positive.

One memory aid is the sentence ''**A**ll **S**tudents **T**ake **C**alculus.''

Since the sign of the reciprocal of a value is the same as the value, the sign of the cosecant function is the same as the sign of the sine function, that of the secant function is the same as that of the cosine function, and the sign of the cotangent function is the same as that of the tangent function.

The ASTC rule can be used to determine in which quadrant a given angle terminates.

■ *Example 2–3 A*

Determine in which quadrant the given angle θ terminates.

1. sin θ < 0, tan θ > 0

   If sin θ < 0 then θ terminates in quadrants III or IV.
   If tan θ > 0 then θ terminates in quadrants I or III.

Thus, for both conditions to be true, θ must terminate in quadrant III.

2. cos θ < 0, sin θ > 0

   cos θ < 0 means θ terminates in quadrant II or III.
   sin θ > 0 means θ terminates in quadrant I or II.

Thus, θ terminates in quadrant II.   ■

Reference angles

Angles whose degree measures are integer multiples of 90°, such as 0°, ±90°, ±180°, ±270°, etc. are called **quadrantal angles** because their terminal sides fall between two quadrants. All other angles are nonquadrantal angles. A **reference angle** for a nonquadrantal angle is the acute angle formed by the terminal side of the angle and the *x*-axis. A reference angle is not defined for

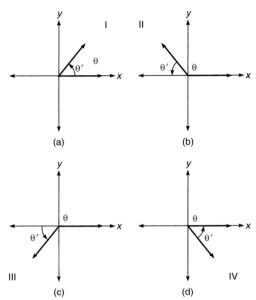

Figure 2–6

quadrantal angles. Figure 2–6 shows a reference angle, θ′ (theta-prime) for an angle θ terminating in each quadrant.

A reference angle is always acute (between 0° and 90°) *and is always formed by the terminal side of the angle and the x-axis* (never the *y*-axis). As will be illustrated in example 2–3 B, a good way to find a reference angle is to sketch the angle itself. This should make clear what computation to perform.

■ *Example 2–3 B*

Compute and sketch the reference angle for each angle.

1. 47°

This angle terminates in quadrant I. The reference angle is the same as the angle itself, 47°.

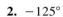

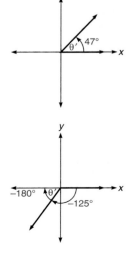

2. −125°

This angle terminates in quadrant III. The positive difference between −125° and −180° is 180° − 125° = 55°, which is the value of the reference angle.

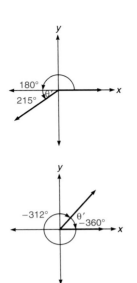

3. 215°

This angle terminates in quadrant III also. Here the reference angle is $215° - 180° = 35°$.

4. −312°

This angle terminates in quadrant I. The value of the reference angle is the positive difference between $-312°$ and $-360° = 360° - 312° = 48°$.   ■

It can be seen that if $0° < \theta < 360°$ then the reference angle θ' can be found according to the following formulas.

$$\begin{aligned} \theta \text{ in quadrant I:} &\quad \theta' = \theta \\ \theta \text{ in quadrant II:} &\quad \theta' = 180° - \theta \\ \theta \text{ in quadrant III:} &\quad \theta' = \theta - 180° \\ \theta \text{ in quadrant IV:} &\quad \theta' = 360° - \theta \end{aligned}$$

The absolute value of the trigonometric functions for any angle

The **absolute value** of a trigonometric function for any angle is the same as the trigonometric ratio for the corresponding reference angle. Figure 2–7 illustrates this idea for the angle 150°. If an angle of measure 150° is in standard position, then we find the values of the trigonometric functions by taking a point on its terminal side (the point $B(x,y)$ in the figure), and using the definitions of these functions in terms of x, y, and r.

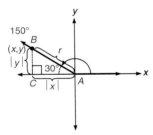

Figure 2–7

As seen in the figure, the absolute value of sin 150° is $\dfrac{|y|}{r}$. This is also the value of the trigonometric ratio for the reference angle, with measure 30°: $\sin 30° = \dfrac{\text{length of side opposite } 30°}{\text{length of hypotenuse}}$. We know from section 1–3 that $\sin 30° = \frac{1}{2}$. Thus, in absolute value, $|\sin 150°| = \sin 30° = \frac{1}{2}$. Since we know that the sine function is positive in quadrant II, $\sin 150° = \frac{1}{2}$.

The reference angle/ASTC procedure

The facts discussed in the previous paragraphs provide a method for finding the *exact* values of the basic trigonometric functions for any nonquadrantal angle whose reference angle is 30°, 45°, or 60°. We call this the reference angle/ASTC procedure.

> **Reference angle/ASTC procedure**
> To find the exact value of a trigonometric function for a nonquadrantal angle whose reference angle is 30°, 45°, or 60°:
> 1. Find the value of the reference angle.
> 2. Find the value of the appropriate trigonometric ratio for the reference angle from table 1–1, section 1–3.
> 3. Determine the sign of this value using the ASTC rule (figure 2–5).

For convenience, the needed table and figure are repeated here (see table 2–1 and figure 2–8).

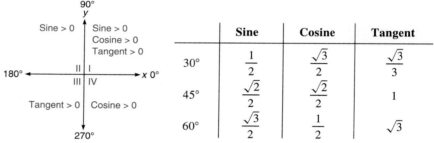

	Sine	**Cosine**	**Tangent**
30°	$\dfrac{1}{2}$	$\dfrac{\sqrt{3}}{2}$	$\dfrac{\sqrt{3}}{3}$
45°	$\dfrac{\sqrt{2}}{2}$	$\dfrac{\sqrt{2}}{2}$	1
60°	$\dfrac{\sqrt{3}}{2}$	$\dfrac{1}{2}$	$\sqrt{3}$

Figure 2–8   **Table 2–1**

■ *Example 2–3 C*

Find the exact value of the given trigonometric function for the given angle.

1. $\cos 210°$

$$\theta' = 210° - 180° = 30°$$ Find the value of the reference angle

$$\cos 30° = \frac{\sqrt{3}}{2}$$ Table 2–1 (memorized value)

$$\cos 210° = -\frac{\sqrt{3}}{2}$$ A 210° angle terminates in quadrant III, where the cosine function is negative

2. $\tan(-45°)$

$$\theta' = 45°$$ Find the value of the reference angle
$$\tan 45° = 1$$ Table 2–1 (memorized value)
$$\tan(-45°) = -1$$ A −45° angle terminates in quadrant IV, where the tangent function is negative

3. $\tan 840°$

$$840° - 2(360°) = 120°$$ 120° and 840° are coterminal
$$\theta' = 180° - 120° = 60°$$ Reference angle for 840°
$$\tan 60° = \sqrt{3}$$ Memorized value
$$\tan 840° = -\sqrt{3}$$ 840° terminates in quadrant II, where the tangent function is negative   ■

The values of the trigonometric functions for quadrantal angles can be found by selecting any point on the terminal side of the angle and using the definitions.

■ Example 2–3 D

Find the values of the six trigonometric functions for the angle with measure 900°.

$900° - 2(360°) = 180°$, so 900° and 180° are coterminal angles.

The point $(-1,0)$ is on the terminal side of a 180° angle, and is therefore on the terminal side of a 900° angle. Use this point to find the values for 900°.

$$r = \sqrt{(-1)^2 + 0^2} = 1, x = -1, y = 0.$$

$$\sin 900° = \frac{y}{r} = \frac{0}{1} = 0, \csc 900° = \frac{1}{\sin 900°} = \frac{1}{0} ; \text{undefined}$$

$$\cos 900° = \frac{x}{r} = \frac{-1}{1} = -1, \sec 900° = \frac{1}{\cos 900°} = \frac{1}{-1} = -1$$

$$\tan 900° = \frac{y}{x} = \frac{0}{-1} = 0, \cot 900° = \frac{1}{\tan 900°} = \frac{1}{0} ; \text{undefined} \quad ■$$

Approximate values of the trigonometric functions—calculators

Approximate values of the trigonometric functions are calculated using the same calculator keys as for the trigonometric ratios; for acute angles the ratios and functions have the same values. Recall from section 1–3 that the calculator must be in degree mode when entering angle measure in degrees.

■ Example 2–3 E

Find four decimal place approximations to the following function values.

Make sure the calculator is in degree mode.

1. sin 133°   133 [sin]   Display [0.731353701]

  sin 133° ≈ 0.7314   [TI-81] [SIN] 133 [ENTER]

2. tan (−18°)   18 [±] [tan]   Display [−0.324919696]

  tan (−18°) ≈ −0.3249   [TI-81] [TAN] [(−)] 18 [ENTER]

3. sec (−335.6°) $\sec(-335.6°) = \dfrac{1}{\cos(-335.6°)}$

  335.6 [±] [cos] [1/x]

  [TI-81] [(] [COS] [(−)] 335.6 [)]

  [x^{-1}] [ENTER]

  sec (−335.6°) ≈ 1.0981   Display [1.098076141]   ■

Solutions to trigonometric equations

Recall from chapter 1 that we use the inverse trigonometric functions to solve trigonometric equations of the form $\sin \theta = k$, $\cos \theta = k$, $\tan \theta = k$, where k is a known constant. In particular, to find one value of θ in each equation, we use the following facts:

$$\text{if } \sin \theta = k, \text{ then one solution for } \theta \text{ is } \theta = \sin^{-1} k$$
$$\text{if } \cos \theta = k, \text{ then one solution for } \theta \text{ is } \theta = \cos^{-1} k$$
$$\text{if } \tan \theta = k, \text{ then one solution for } \theta \text{ is } \theta = \tan^{-1} k$$

In chapters 4 and 5 we will examine this situation in more depth, but for now we will simply rely on these facts, and on the fact that these inverse trigonometric functions are programmed into calculators as seen in section 1–3.

■ *Example 2–3 F*

Find one solution to each trigonometric equation, to the nearest 0.1°.

1. $\sin \theta = -0.8500$
$$\theta = \sin^{-1}(-0.8500) \approx -58.2°$$

2. $\cos \theta = -0.8500$
$$\theta = \cos^{-1}(-0.8500) \approx 148.2°$$ ■

Mastery points

Can you
- Determine in which quadrant an angle terminates when given the signs of two of the trigonometric function values for that angle?
- Compute and sketch the reference angle for a given nonquadrantal angle θ with given degree measure?
- Find the exact value of any trigonometric function for an angle whose reference angle is 30°, 45°, or 60°, using the reference angle/ASTC procedure?
- Find the exact value of any trigonometric function for a quadrantal angle?
- Find the approximate value of any trigonometric function using a calculator?
- Find the approximate value of one solution to an equation of the form $\sin \theta = k$, $\cos \theta = k$, $\tan \theta = k$?

Exercise 2–3

In the following problems you are given the sign of two of the trigonometric functions of an angle in standard position. State in which quadrant the angle terminates.

1. $\sin \theta > 0$, $\cos \theta < 0$
2. $\sec \theta < 0$, $\tan \theta > 0$
3. $\cos \theta > 0$, $\tan \theta > 0$
4. $\cot \theta < 0$, $\csc \theta > 0$
5. $\tan \theta < 0$, $\csc \theta < 0$
6. $\sec \theta > 0$, $\csc \theta < 0$
7. $\csc \theta > 0$, $\cos \theta < 0$
8. $\tan \theta > 0$, $\sin \theta < 0$
9. $\sec \theta > 0$, $\sin \theta < 0$
10. $\cot \theta > 0$, $\sin \theta > 0$
11. $\sin \theta < 0$, $\sec \theta < 0$

For each of the following angles, find the measure of the reference angle θ'.

12. 39.3°   **13.** 164.2°   **14.** 213.2°   **15.** 427.1°   **16.** −16.8°
17. −255.3°   **18.** −100.4°   **19.** 130.7°   **20.** −671.3°   **21.** −181.0°
22. 512.8°   **23.** −279.5°   **24.** 292.3°   **25.** −252°   **26.** 312°

Find the exact trigonometric function value for each angle.

27. sin 135°   **28.** cos 120°   **29.** sin 210°   **30.** cos 330°   **31.** tan 300°
32. sin 240°   **33.** sin(−120°)   **34.** cos(−315°)   **35.** cos 660°   **36.** csc(−315°)
37. cot 300°   **38.** sin 450°   **39.** cos(−450°)   **40.** tan(−540°)   **41.** csc 90°
42. sin 840°   **43.** sin(−690°)   **44.** cot 215°   **45.** sec 150°   **46.** tan 330°

Find the trigonometric function value for each angle to four decimal places.

47. sin 113.4°   **48.** cos 88.2°   **49.** tan 214.6°   **50.** csc 345°10′   **51.** cot 412°
52. tan 527.2°   **53.** sec(−13°)   **54.** sin(−88°)   **55.** cos(−355°20′)   **56.** tan(−248.6°)
57. csc 285.3°   **58.** sec 211°   **59.** cos(−133.2°)   **60.** sin(−293°50′)

Find one approximate solution to each equation, to the nearest 0.1°.

61. $\sin \theta = 0.25$ **62.** $\sin \theta = \frac{1}{3}$ **63.** $\cos \theta = -0.5$ **64.** $\cos \theta = 0.813$ **65.** $\tan \theta = -\frac{8}{5}$
66. $\tan \theta = 3$ **67.** $\sin \theta = -0.59$ **68.** $\cos \theta = -0.18$

69. In a certain electrical circuit the instantaneous voltage E (in volts) is found by the formula $E = 156 \sin (\theta + 45°)$. Compute E to the nearest 0.01 volt for the following values of θ:
   a. 0°   **b.** 45°   **c.** 100°   **d.** −200°   **e.** 13.3°   **f.** −45°

70. In a certain electrical circuit the instantaneous current I (in amperes) is found by the formula $I = 1.6 \cos(800t)°$. Find I to the nearest 0.01 ampere for the following values of t:
   a. 0   **b.** 0.25   **c.** 0.85   **d.** 1   **e.** −1   **f.** −2.5   **g.** −0.02

71. If a force of 200 pounds is applied to a rope to drag an object, the actual force tending to move the object horizontally is $f(\theta) = 200 \cos \theta$, where θ is the angle the rope makes with the horizontal. Compute the force tending to move the object horizontally if the angle of the rope is
   a. 0°   **b.** 25°   **c.** 50°

72. If a rocket is moving through the air at a speed of 1,200 mph, at an angle of $\theta°$ with the horizontal, then the rate at which it is rising is $v(\theta) = 1200 \sin \theta$. Find the rate at which a rocket moving at 1200 mph is rising if the angle it makes with the horizontal is
   a. 50°   **b.** 60°   **c.** 70°   **d.** 80°

73. Use the values 30° and 60° to see if the statement $\sin(2\theta) = 2 \sin \theta$ is true. (Let θ be 30°.)

74. Use the values 30° and 60° to see if the statement $\sin \frac{\theta}{2} = \frac{\sin \theta}{2}$ is true. (Let θ be 60°.)

75. Use the values 30°, 60°, 90° to see if the statement $\sin(\alpha + \beta) = \sin \alpha + \sin \beta$ is true.

2–4 *Finding values from other values—reference triangles*

Finding a general angle from a value and quadrant

In sections 1–3 and 1–4 we learned how to find the degree measure of an acute angle if we know the value of one of the trigonometric ratios for that angle. We used the inverse sine, cosine, or tangent function as appropriate. We are now dealing with angles of any measure, but the same procedure can be used to find the value of a reference angle. From this we can find the least nonnegative measure for an angle.

As is illustrated in example 2–4 A, we *always find a reference angle* θ' *by finding the inverse sine, cosine, or tangent function value for a positive value.* We use a positive value to obtain an acute angle (all reference angles are acute). We could summarize the procedure as follows.

Finding the least nonnegative measure of an angle from a trigonometric function value and information about a quadrant.

1. If necessary use the ASTC rule[2] to determine the quadrant for the terminal side of the angle.
2. Use $\sin^{-1}$, $\cos^{-1}$, or $\tan^{-1}$ to find θ'. Use the absolute value of the given trigonometric function value.
3. Apply θ' to the correct quadrant to determine the value of θ.

Note We find the "least nonnegative value." There are actually an unlimited number of values, since the trigonometric values are the same for all coterminal angles.

In section 2–3 we saw formulas that find θ' if $0° < \theta < 360°$. These formulas can be solved for θ if necessary and thus provide a formula for finding θ given θ'.

Relationship between θ and θ' if $0° < \theta < 360°$

θ in Quadrant I:	$\theta' = \theta$	$\theta = \theta'$
θ in Quadrant II:	$\theta' = 180° - \theta$	$\theta = 180° - \theta'$
θ in Quadrant III:	$\theta' = \theta - 180°$	$\theta = \theta' + 180°$
θ in Quadrant IV:	$\theta' = 360° - \theta$	$\theta = 360° - \theta'$

It is interesting to observe that the formulas are the "same" when solved for θ and θ' for every quadrant except quadrant III.

■ *Example 2–4 A*

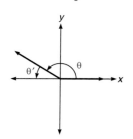

Find the least nonnegative measure of θ to the nearest 0.1°.

1. $\sin \theta = 0.5150$ and $\cos \theta < 0$

   Since $\sin \theta > 0$ and $\cos \theta < 0$, θ terminates in quadrant II (see the figure). We find the acute reference angle θ' just as we did in section 1–2.

$$\theta' = \sin^{-1} 0.5150 \approx 31.0°$$

   Thus, $\theta \approx 180° - 31.0° = 149.0°$.

   Note The calculator can be used to verify our result by checking that $\sin 149° \approx 0.5150$ and that $\cos 149° < 0$.

[2]Section 2–3.

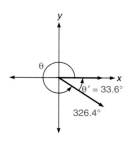

$\theta' = 33.6°$

326.4°

2. $\tan \theta = -0.6644$ and $\sin \theta < 0$

Since $\tan \theta < 0$ and $\sin \theta < 0$, θ terminates in quadrant IV.

$$\theta' = \tan^{-1} 0.6644 \approx 33.6° \qquad \text{Note we use the positive value 0.6644}$$
$$\theta = 360° - \theta' \approx 326.4°$$

■

Example 2–4 B applies several of the things we have been studying.

■ **Example 2–4 B**

The point $(3, -8)$ is on the terminal side of θ.
  a. Draw a representation of θ.
  b. Find the exact value of the trigonometric functions for θ.
  c. Find the least nonnegative measure of θ, to the nearest $0.1°$.

a. The representation is shown in the figure.

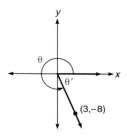

$(3, -8)$

b. Applying the definitions of section 2–2:

$$r = \sqrt{x^2 + y^2} = \sqrt{3^2 + (-8)^2} = \sqrt{73}$$

$$\sin \theta = \frac{y}{r} = \frac{-8}{\sqrt{73}} = -\frac{8\sqrt{73}}{73}, \qquad \csc \theta = \frac{1}{\sin \theta} = -\frac{\sqrt{73}}{8}$$

$$\cos \theta = \frac{x}{r} = \frac{3}{\sqrt{73}} = \frac{3\sqrt{73}}{73}, \qquad \sec \theta = \frac{1}{\cos \theta} = \frac{\sqrt{73}}{3}$$

$$\tan \theta = \frac{y}{x} = -\frac{8}{3}, \qquad \cot \theta = \frac{1}{\tan \theta} = -\frac{3}{8}$$

c. We can find θ' by using the fact that $\tan \theta' = |\tan \theta| = \frac{8}{3}$, so that

$$\theta' = \tan^{-1} \tfrac{8}{3} \approx 69.4°, \text{ so}$$
$$\theta \approx 360° - 69.4° = 290.6°$$

■

There are many places in science and technology where we find applications for trigonometric functions. With the advent of numerically controlled, or computer-controlled, machines these applications are becoming more common.

■ *Example 2–4 C*

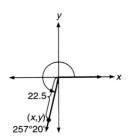

A technician is setting up a numerically controlled grinding wheel. The starting position for the wheel must be at an angle of 257°20′ and must be 22.5 inches from the origin (assuming the machine uses our usual x-y coordinate system). Find the x- and y-coordinates of the point at which the grinding wheel must start, to the nearest tenth of an inch.

The figure illustrates the situation. We have $r = 22.5$ inches and $\theta = 257°20′$. By definition, $\sin \theta = \dfrac{y}{r}$ and $\cos \theta = \dfrac{x}{r}$, so we find x and y as follows:

$$\sin 257°20′ = \frac{y}{22.5}$$
$$y = 22.5 \sin 257°20′$$
$$y \approx -22.0 \text{ inches} \qquad \boxed{\text{CS 1}}$$
$$\cos 257°20′ = \frac{x}{22.5}$$
$$x = 22.5 \cos 257°20′$$
$$x \approx -4.9 \text{ inches}$$

Thus, the starting coordinates, in inches, for the grinder are $(-4.9, -22.0)$. ■

Exact values of the trigonometric functions from a known value—reference triangles

There are many situations in which we know the exact value of one of the trigonometric functions for a given angle and need to find the exact value of one or more of the remaining five trigonometric functions for the same angle. We can do this by using a reference triangle, which is a convenient way of combining the idea of reference angle and right triangle. A **reference triangle** is a right triangle with one leg on the x-axis and one leg parallel to the y-axis. The acute angle on the x-axis is the reference angle for the angle in question. *The lengths of the legs of a reference triangle are treated as directed distances (i.e., positive or negative); the hypotenuse is always positive.* This is illustrated in example 2–4 D. Figure 2–9 shows a reference triangle for each quadrant.

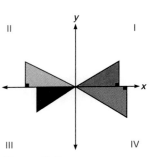

Figure 2–9

■ *Example 2–4 D*

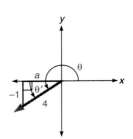

In each case draw a representation of angle θ and use a reference triangle to help find the values of the other five trigonometric functions. Also, find the least positive value of θ to the nearest 0.1°.

1. $\sin \theta = -\frac{1}{4}$ and $\tan \theta > 0$

We know θ terminates in quadrant III since $\sin \theta < 0$ and $\tan \theta > 0$. We construct a right triangle in quadrant III in which one acute angle is a reference angle. This is shown in the figure. We label the hypotenuse 4 and the directed side opposite $\theta′$ as -1. Thus,

$$\sin \theta′ = \frac{\text{length of side opposite } \theta′}{\text{length of hypotenuse}} = -\frac{1}{4}.$$

$a^2 + (-1)^2 = 4^2$ Find the value of $|a|$ using the Pythagorean theorem; since we
$a^2 = 15$ are squaring values this theorem works for directed distances
$a = \pm\sqrt{15}$

We choose $a = -\sqrt{15}$ since it is negative as a directed distance.

We can now use the definitions of the trigonometric ratios for θ' along with the directed distances to find the remaining trigonometric function values for θ.

$$\cos\theta = \frac{\text{adjacent}}{\text{hypotenuse}} = -\frac{\sqrt{15}}{4}, \quad \tan\theta = \frac{\text{opposite}}{\text{adjacent}} = \frac{-1}{-\sqrt{15}} = \frac{\sqrt{15}}{15}$$

$$\csc\theta = \frac{1}{\sin\theta} = -4, \qquad \sec\theta = \frac{1}{\cos\theta} = -\frac{4}{\sqrt{15}} = -\frac{4\sqrt{15}}{15}$$

$$\cot\theta = \frac{1}{\tan\theta} = \sqrt{15}$$

We now find an approximation to θ.

$$\sin\theta' = \tfrac{1}{4}, \text{ so } \theta' = \sin^{-1}\tfrac{1}{4} \approx 14.5°, \text{ so } \theta \approx 180° + 14.5° = 194.5°.$$

Note   The reference triangle works because it is equivalent to finding a point on the terminal side of θ and applying the definitions of the trigonometric functions (section 2–2). The reference triangle above was equivalent to finding the point $(-\sqrt{15}, -1)$ to be on the terminal side of angle θ. (Figure 2–10)

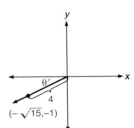

Figure 2–10

2. $\cot\theta = -\dfrac{1}{4}$ and $270° < \theta < 360°$

If $\cot\theta = -\tfrac{1}{4}$ then $\tan\theta = -4$. The figure shows a reference triangle for an angle in quadrant IV with tangent -4.

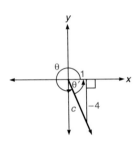

$$c^2 = 1^2 + (-4)^2$$
$$c = \sqrt{17}$$

$$\sin\theta = \frac{\text{opposite}}{\text{hypotenuse}} = \frac{-4}{\sqrt{17}} = -\frac{4\sqrt{17}}{17}, \quad \cos\theta = \frac{1}{\sqrt{17}} = \frac{\sqrt{17}}{17},$$

$$\csc\theta = \frac{1}{\sin\theta} = -\frac{\sqrt{17}}{4}, \quad \sec\theta = \frac{1}{\cos\theta} = \sqrt{17},$$

$$\tan\theta' = 4, \text{ so } \theta' = \tan^{-1}4 \approx 76.0°, \text{ and } \theta = 360° - \theta' \approx 284°.$$

3. $\sin\theta = u$ and θ terminates in quadrant II

The figure shows a reference triangle in quadrant II, where $\sin\theta' = u$.

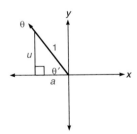

$$u^2 + a^2 = 1^2 \qquad \text{Find the value of side } a$$
$$a = \pm\sqrt{1 - u^2}$$
$$a = -\sqrt{1 - u^2} \qquad \text{Choose } a < 0 \text{ as a directed distance}$$

$$\cos\theta = \frac{a}{1} = a = -\sqrt{1 - u^2},$$

$$\tan\theta = \frac{u}{a} = \frac{u}{-\sqrt{1 - u^2}} = -\frac{u}{\sqrt{1 - u^2}},$$

$$\sec\theta = \frac{1}{\cos\theta} = -\frac{1}{\sqrt{1 - u^2}}, \quad \csc\theta = \frac{1}{\sin\theta} = \frac{1}{u},$$

$$\cot\theta = \frac{1}{\tan\theta} = -\frac{\sqrt{1 - u^2}}{u}$$

Since we do not know the actual value of u we cannot make a determination of an approximate value for angle θ.   ■

Calculator steps

1. (A)   22.5 $\boxed{\times}$ $\boxed{(}$ 257 $\boxed{+}$ 20 $\boxed{\div}$ 60 $\boxed{)}$ $\boxed{\sin}$ $\boxed{=}$

Display $\boxed{-21.9524013}$

(P)   22.5 $\boxed{\text{ENTER}}$ 257 $\boxed{\text{ENTER}}$ 20 $\boxed{\text{ENTER}}$ 60

$\boxed{\div}$ $\boxed{+}$ $\boxed{\sin}$ $\boxed{\times}$

$\boxed{\text{TI-81}}$ 22.5 $\boxed{\times}$ $\boxed{\text{SIN}}$ $\boxed{(}$ 257 $\boxed{+}$ 20 $\boxed{\div}$ 60 $\boxed{)}$

$\boxed{\text{ENTER}}$

Mastery points

Can you
- Find an approximation to the least nonnegative measure of an angle, given the value of one of the trigonometric functions and the sign of a second for that angle?
- Apply the definitions of the trigonometric functions in appropriate situations?
- Use reference triangles to find the exact values of the remaining trigonometric functions for a given angle, when given the value of one of the trigonometric functions of that angle?

Exercise 2–4

Find the measure of the least nonnegative angle that meets the conditions given in the following problems, to the nearest 0.1°.

1. $\sin \theta = 0.8251$, $\cos \theta > 0$
2. $\cos \theta = -0.1771$, $\sin \theta < 0$
3. $\tan \theta = 0.6569$, $\sec \theta > 0$
4. $\sin \theta = -0.6508$, $\tan \theta > 0$
5. $\sec \theta = -1.0642$, $\sin \theta < 0$
6. $\csc \theta = -1.3673$, $\tan \theta > 0$
7. $\tan \theta = -0.0349$, $\csc \theta < 0$
8. $\cos \theta = -0.2222$, $\sin \theta > 0$
9. $\sin \theta = \frac{3}{8}$, $\cos \theta > 0$
10. $\sin \theta = \frac{3}{8}$, $\cos \theta < 0$
11. $\cot \theta = -5$, $\sin \theta > 0$
12. $\tan \theta = -5$, $\sin \theta < 0$
13. $\cos \theta = -\frac{5}{7}$, $\tan \theta > 0$
14. $\cos \theta = -\frac{5}{7}$, $\tan \theta < 0$

In each case (a) draw a representation of angle θ and (b) use a reference triangle to help find the values of the other trigonometric functions. Also, (c) find the reference angle θ' and the least positive value of θ to the nearest 0.1°.

15. $\sin \theta = \dfrac{3}{4}$, $\cos \theta > 0$
16. $\sin \theta = \dfrac{4}{5}$, $\cos \theta < 0$
17. $\cos \theta = -\dfrac{1}{2}$, $\tan \theta > 0$

18. $\cos \theta = -\dfrac{5}{13}$, $\tan \theta < 0$
19. $\sin \theta = 1$
20. $\cos \theta = 1$

21. $\tan \theta = 2$, $\cos \theta < 0$
22. $\tan \theta = 3$, $\cos \theta > 0$
23. $\csc \theta = -5$, $\sec \theta < 0$
24. $\csc \theta = -2$, $\sec \theta > 0$
25. $\csc \theta = -1$
26. $\sec \theta = -1$
27. $\sin \theta = -\frac{3}{4}$, $\tan \theta > 0$
28. $\sin \theta = -\frac{2}{5}$, $\tan \theta < 0$
29. $\sec \theta = 4$, $\csc \theta > 0$

30. $\sec \theta = \sqrt{6}$, $\csc \theta < 0$
31. $\cot \theta = \dfrac{\sqrt{2}}{3}$, $\sin \theta < 0$
32. $\cot \theta = \frac{1}{3}$, $\sin \theta > 0$

33. $\cos \theta = -\frac{5}{13}$, $\sin \theta > 0$
34. $\cos \theta = -\dfrac{3}{\sqrt{10}}$, $\sin \theta < 0$
35. $\tan \theta = \frac{7}{2}$, $\sec \theta < 0$

36. $\tan \theta = \frac{7}{3}$, $\sec \theta > 0$

37. $\sec \theta = 5$, $\tan \theta > 0$

38. $\sec \theta = 4$, $\tan \theta < 0$

39. $\sin \theta = \dfrac{1}{\sqrt{5}}$, $\tan \theta < 0$

40. $\sin \theta = \dfrac{1}{\sqrt{3}}$, $\tan \theta > 0$

Solve the following problems.

41. The point $(2, -5)$ is on the terminal side of θ.
   a. Find the exact value of each of the trigonometric functions for θ.
   b. Find the least nonnegative measure of θ, to the nearest $0.1°$.

42. The point $(-3, -9)$ is on the terminal side of θ.
   a. Find the exact value of each of the trigonometric functions for θ.
   b. Find the least nonnegative measure of θ, to the nearest $0.1°$.

43. A numerically controlled drill is being set up to drill a hole in a piece of steel 6.8 millimeters from the origin at an angle of $135°30'$. To the nearest 0.01 millimeter, what are the coordinates of this point?

44. Suppose the hole in problem 43 must be 10.25 inches from the origin at an angle of $13°20'$. Find the coordinates of this point to the nearest 0.01 inch.

45. Suppose the hole in problem 43 must be 8.25 centimeters from the origin at an angle of $-134.4°$. Find the coordinates of this point to the nearest 0.01 centimeter.

46. A numerically controlled drill must drill four holes on a circle whose center is at the origin with radius 17.8 centimeters, as shown in the diagram. The holes must be drilled wherever on this circle the x-coordinate is ±10.0 centimeters. Find the y-coordinate and angle (to the nearest $0.1°$) for each of these four holes.

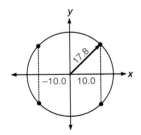

47. Suppose in problem 46 four additional holes must be drilled wherever the y-coordinate is ±15.5 cm. Find the x-coordinate and angle for each of these holes.

48. A technician is aligning a laser device that is used to cut patterns out of cloth. The device is positioned at an angle of $135.20°$ and at a distance 5.50 feet from the origin. What should the x- and y-coordinates be at this point, to the nearest 0.01 foot?

49. A scanning device used in medical diagnosis has a moving part that moves with great precision in a circle around the patient. Assume the y-axis is perpendicular to the top of the table on which the patient lies and the x-axis is at right angles to the length of the table. The diameter of the machine is 4 feet 3.5 inches. Find the coordinates of the moving part when the angle is $211.5°$, to the nearest 0.1 inch.

In problems 50–55 find values of the other five trigonometric functions in terms of u.

50. $\cos \theta = u$ and θ terminates in quadrant I.

51. $\tan \theta = u$ and θ terminates in quadrant I.

52. $\cos \theta = u$ and θ terminates in quadrant III.

53. $\tan \theta = u$ and θ terminates in quadrant III.

54. $\sin \theta = u + 1$ and θ terminates in quadrant I.

55. $\cos \theta = 1 - u$ and θ terminates in quadrant I.

56. In the June 1980 issue of *Popular Science* magazine Mr. R. J. Ransil presented several formulas for calculating saw angles for compound miters. The formulas are:

$$\text{angle } A = 90° - \frac{180°}{\text{number of sides}}$$
$$\tan(\text{arm angle}) = \cot(A) \cdot \sin(\text{slope})$$
$$\sin(\text{tilt angle}) = \cos(A) \cdot \cos(\text{slope})$$

Arm angles and tilt angles are acute.
   Calculate the arm angle and tilt angle to the nearest $0.1°$ for the following numbers of sides and slopes:

Number of sides	Slope (in degrees)
3	5
5	5
7	25
7	30
6	35
8	35

57. A surveying manual describes how to find distance *BP* in the figure. The distance *AP* can be found, but trees prevent measuring angle *a*. Angle *b* can be measured, but not distance *BP*. The manual instructs the surveyor to find *BP* by solving the following sequence of formulas:

$$\sin p = \frac{AB \sin b}{AP}$$

$$a = 180° - (b + p)$$

$$BP = \frac{AP \sin a}{\sin b}$$

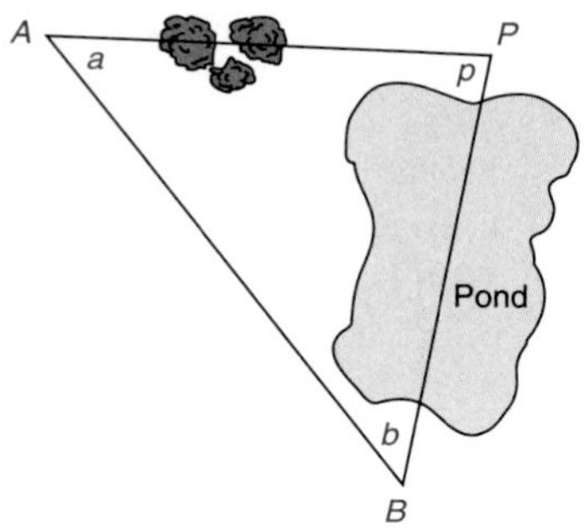

Note that the first formula does not give angle *p* but only sin *p*. Also, assume *p* is acute. Solve the sequence of formulas to compute the distance *BP* to the nearest 0.1 foot if *AB* = 512.4 feet, *AP* = 322.6 feet, and *b* = 28.3°.

58. Find *BP* in problem 57 to the nearest 0.1 meter if *AB* = 319.2 meters, *AP* = 225.7 meters, and *b* = 31.6°.

2–5 Radian measure—definitions

The unit circle

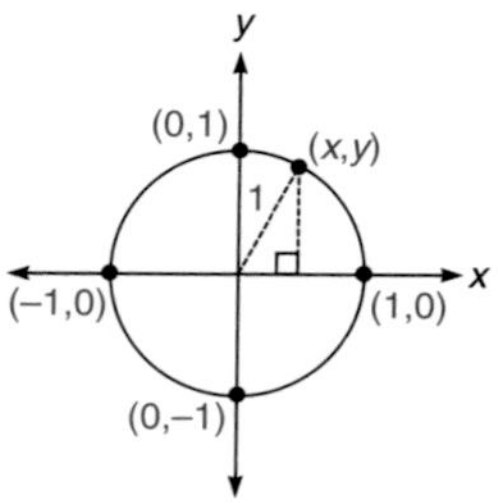

The circle with radius one and center at the origin is described by the equation

$$x^2 + y^2 = 1$$

It is called the unit circle. See figure 2–11. Observe that the absolute values of the *x*- and *y*-coordinates of any point not on an axis describe the lengths of two sides of a right triangle with hypotenuse of length one. The Pythagorean theorem shows that for these points $x^2 + y^2 = 1$. Those points of the circle that are on an axis also satisfy this equation.

The circumference *C* of a circle with radius *r* is the distance around the circle. This distance is found using the relation $C = 2\pi r$. Since the radius *r* for the unit circle is one, its circumference is $C = 2\pi$ (about 6.28 units).

Figure 2–11

Note The constant π is approximately 3.14159. It is a much-used number, about which entire books have been written. It is an irrational number, and has been approximated to over a billion digits![3]

Radian measure

A second system of angle measurement is called **radians.** This system is used extensively in engineering and scientific applications, as well as in the calculus. We will use it throughout the rest of this book. To define this system of angle measurement we use the unit circle.

Let θ be an angle in standard position, and let *s* represent the distance from the point (1,0) along the circumference of the unit circle to the terminal

---

[3]An interesting book on π is *A History of* π by Petr Beckmann, Golem Press, Boulder, Colo., 1977. Gregory V. and David V. Chudnovsky of Columbia University calculated 1,011,196,691 digits of π in 1989.

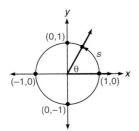

Figure 2–12

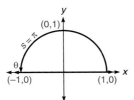

Figure 2–13

side of θ. The distance *s* is called the **arc length** (see figure 2–12). If the distance is measured in a clockwise direction we say *s* is positive, and if in a counterclockwise direction *s* is negative.

We define the radian measure of an angle to be this arc length *s*.

Radian measure of an angle in standard position

Let θ be an angle in standard position. Let *s* be the corresponding arc length on the unit circle. Let *s* be positive if measured in the counterclockwise direction, and negative if measured in the clockwise direction.

Then *s* is the radian measure of the angle θ.

For example, an angle of degree measure 180° has an arc length that corresponds to half the circumference of the unit circle. Thus, the corresponding radian measure is half of the circumference, or one-half of 2π, which is π. Thus, the radian measure of an angle that corresponds to a rotation of one-half a circle, in the counterclockwise direction, is π (see figure 2–13).

Conversions between radian and degree measure

Since 360° corresponds to a full revolution, and the circumference of the unit circle (2π) also corresponds to a complete revolution about the unit circle, the following relation is true.

$$\frac{\text{arc length } (s)}{\text{circumference } (2\pi)} = \frac{\text{measure of angle in degrees}}{360°}$$

If we multiply each member by 2 we obtain the same true statement, but with smaller denominators of π and 180°.

We use this proportion[4] to convert between degree and radian measure.

Radian/degree proportion

Let θ be an angle in standard position with degree measure θ° and radian measure *s*. Then,

$$\frac{s}{\pi} = \frac{\theta°}{180°}$$

The radian measure of an angle is a real number, defined with no units in mind. We often add the word radians after such a measure, but this is not necessary where it is clear that the real number refers to the measure of an angle. Observe that in the radian/degree proportion the ratio of degrees to degrees is unitless also. For example, $\frac{90°}{180°}$ is the same as the unitless ratio $\frac{1}{2}$.

We can describe the measure of an angle in standard position by using degree measure or by stating the arc length to which the angle corresponds on the unit circle (its radian measure). The proportion above shows the relationship between these two systems.

---

[4]A proportion is a statement of equality between two ratios (fractions).

■ *Example 2–5 A*

Compute the radian or degree measure, given the measure for each angle in degrees or radians.

1. 90°

$$\frac{s}{\pi} = \frac{\theta°}{180°}$$ Radian/degree proportion

$$\frac{s}{\pi} = \frac{90°}{180°}$$ Replace $\theta°$ by 90°

$$s = \frac{90(\pi)}{180}$$ Multiply each member by π; drop the reference to degrees

$$s = \frac{\pi}{2}$$ Simplify the fraction

Thus, 90° corresponds to $\frac{\pi}{2}$ (radians).

2. −210°

$$\frac{s}{\pi} = \frac{\theta°}{180°}$$ Radian/degree proportion

$$\frac{s}{\pi} = \frac{-210°}{180°}$$ Replace $\theta°$ with −210°

$$s = \frac{-210(\pi)}{180°} = -\frac{7\pi}{6}$$

Therefore, −210° corresponds to $-\frac{7\pi}{6}$.

3. $\frac{7\pi}{5}$

$$\frac{s}{\pi} = \frac{\theta°}{180°}$$ Radian/degree proportion

$$\frac{\frac{7\pi}{5}}{\pi} = \frac{\theta°}{180°}$$ Replace s by $\frac{7\pi}{5}$

$$\frac{7\pi}{5} \cdot \frac{1}{\pi} = \frac{\theta°}{180°}$$ Division by π is the same as multiplication by $\frac{1}{\pi}$

$$\frac{7}{5} \cdot 180° = \theta°$$ Multiply each member by 180°

$$252° = \theta°$$

$\frac{7\pi}{5}$ (radians) corresponds to 252°.

4. 1

Note that this means $s = 1$ radian.

$$\frac{s}{\pi} = \frac{\theta°}{180°} \qquad \text{Radian/degree proportion}$$

$$\frac{1}{\pi} = \frac{\theta°}{180°}$$

$$\frac{180°}{\pi} = \theta° \qquad \text{Multiply each member by } 180°$$

$$\frac{180°}{\pi} = \theta°$$

$$57.30° \approx \theta° \qquad \text{Decimal approximation to } \frac{180}{\pi}$$

Thus, 1 radian corresponds to $\dfrac{180°}{\pi}$ or about 57.3°.   ■

Note It is useful to remember that 1 radian is a little less than 60°, and that 2π radians exactly equals 360°.

Common radian measures

The unit circle can be very helpful in getting a feeling for radian measure. Those values of radian measure that correspond to quadrantal angles (0°, 90°, 180°, etc.) and to angles with reference angles of 30°, 45°, and 60° are common. In particular, the following correspondences are useful: $\dfrac{\pi}{6}$ and 30°, $\dfrac{\pi}{4}$ and 45°, and $\dfrac{\pi}{3}$ and 60°. The unit circle can be conveniently marked in terms of multiples of $\dfrac{\pi}{6}$ radians (30°) and of multiples of $\dfrac{\pi}{4}$ radians (45°). This is shown in figure 2–14.

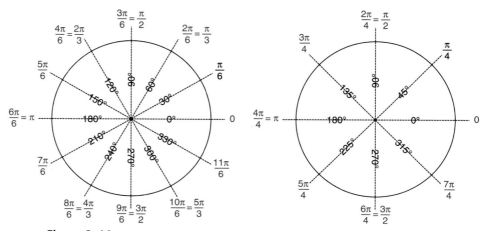

Figure 2–14

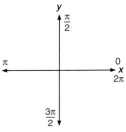

Figure 2–15

Coterminal and reference angles in radian measure

Figure 2–15 shows the smallest positive radian measure of the quadrantal angles, as well as the fact that a full revolution (circle) can be described by 2π radians. Observe that the quadrantal angles $0°$, $90°$, $180°$, $270°$, and $360°$ are, in radians, 0, $\dfrac{\pi}{2}$, π, $\dfrac{3\pi}{2}$, and 2π.

In degree measure, all angles that differ in measure by integer multiples of $360°$ are coterminal. For radian measure the difference is multiples of 2π. If k is an integer (positive, zero, or negative), then integer multiples of 2π are $k \cdot 2\pi$, or $2k\pi$.

> **Coterminal angles, radian measure**
> Two angles α and β are coterminal if $\alpha = \beta + 2k\pi$, k an integer.

Reference angles are found in the same manner as with degree measure (section 2–2) except that $180°$ becomes π and $360°$ becomes 2π. If the measure of θ in radians is positive and less than 2π, the following rules give the value of θ', the reference angle.

Quadrant in which θ terminates	Value of θ', the reference angle
I	$\theta' = \theta$
II	$\theta' = \pi - \theta$
III	$\theta' = \theta - \pi$
IV	$\theta' = 2\pi - \theta$

■ *Example 2–5 B*

For each angle θ find the least positive coterminal angle α (that is, $0 \leq \alpha < 2\pi$) and then find the reference angle θ'.

1. $\theta = \dfrac{7\pi}{6}$

It is difficult, at first, to deal with quantities like $\dfrac{7\pi}{6}$. This is because we are not used to radian measure, and because it can be difficult to compare the values of fractions.

If we convert 2π to $\dfrac{2\pi}{1} \cdot \dfrac{6}{6} = \dfrac{12\pi}{6}$, we can see that $\dfrac{7\pi}{6} < \dfrac{12\pi}{6}$, or $\dfrac{7\pi}{6} < 2\pi$, so that θ is already less than 2π, so $\alpha = \theta = \dfrac{7\pi}{6}$.

To determine the reference angle for θ we must determine in which quadrant $\dfrac{7\pi}{6}$ terminates. If you cannot see that it terminates in quadrant III then use the following method.

Rewrite the quadrantal angles in terms of denominators of 6, the denominator of $\dfrac{7\pi}{6}$:

Quadrant		I	II	III	IV
Quadrantal Angle	0	$\dfrac{\pi}{2}$	π	$\dfrac{3\pi}{2}$	2π
Denominator of 6	$\dfrac{0}{6}$	$\dfrac{3\pi}{6}$	$\dfrac{6\pi}{6}$	$\dfrac{9\pi}{6}$	$\dfrac{12\pi}{6}$

Now observe that $\dfrac{6\pi}{6} < \dfrac{7\pi}{6} < \dfrac{9\pi}{6}$ or $\pi < \dfrac{7\pi}{6} < \dfrac{3\pi}{2}$, so $\dfrac{7\pi}{6}$ is in quadrant III.

$$\theta' = \frac{7\pi}{6} - \pi = \frac{7\pi}{6} - \frac{6\pi}{6} = \frac{\pi}{6} \qquad \text{In quadrant III, } \theta' = \theta - \pi$$

Thus, the reference angle for $\dfrac{7\pi}{6}$ is $\dfrac{\pi}{6}$.

2. $\theta = \dfrac{11\pi}{3}$

Since $2\pi = \dfrac{6\pi}{3}$, we see that $\theta > 2\pi$. We must subtract multiples of 2π until we arrive at an angle α, $0 \le \alpha < 2\pi$.

$$\frac{11\pi}{3} - 2\pi = \frac{11\pi}{3} - \frac{6\pi}{3} = \frac{5\pi}{3}$$

Since $\dfrac{5\pi}{3} < 2\pi$, the angle α is $\dfrac{5\pi}{3}$. Thus, $\dfrac{11\pi}{3}$ is coterminal with $\dfrac{5\pi}{3}$. To locate in which quadrant the angle $\dfrac{5\pi}{3}$ terminates, rewrite $\dfrac{5\pi}{3}$ as $\dfrac{10\pi}{6}$ and the quadrantal angles in terms of denominators of 6. (It is not convenient to rewrite the quadrantal angles in terms of denominators of 3.)

Examining the values used in part 1 of this example we see that $\dfrac{9\pi}{6} < \dfrac{10\pi}{6} < \dfrac{12\pi}{6}$ so $\dfrac{3\pi}{2} < \dfrac{5\pi}{3} < 2\pi$ and $\dfrac{5\pi}{3}$ is in quadrant IV. Thus,

$$\theta' = 2\pi - \frac{5\pi}{3} = \frac{6\pi}{3} - \frac{5\pi}{3} = \frac{\pi}{3} \ .$$

3. $\theta = -\dfrac{13\pi}{4}$

We first add multiples of $2\pi = \dfrac{8\pi}{4}$ to obtain a positive valued coterminal

angle α. It is clear that one multiple of $\dfrac{8\pi}{4}$ will not give a positive result,

so we will add two multiples.

$$-\frac{13\pi}{4} + 2\left(\frac{8\pi}{4}\right) = -\frac{13\pi}{4} + \frac{16\pi}{4} = \frac{3\pi}{4} = \alpha$$

To find a reference angle we will use $\dfrac{3\pi}{4}$ instead of $-\dfrac{13\pi}{4}$. We rewrite

the quadrantal angles in terms of denominators of 4.

Quadrant		I	II	III	IV
Quadrantal Angle	0	$\dfrac{\pi}{2}$	π	$\dfrac{3\pi}{2}$	2π
Denominator of 6	$\dfrac{0}{4}$	$\dfrac{2\pi}{4}$	$\dfrac{4\pi}{4}$	$\dfrac{6\pi}{4}$	$\dfrac{8\pi}{4}$

Since $\dfrac{2\pi}{4} < \dfrac{3\pi}{4} < \dfrac{4\pi}{4}$, we see that $\dfrac{\pi}{2} < \dfrac{3\pi}{4}\pi$, so $\theta = \dfrac{3\pi}{4}$ is in

quadrant II, and $\theta' = \pi - \dfrac{3\pi}{4} = \dfrac{4\pi}{4} - \dfrac{3\pi}{4} = \dfrac{\pi}{4}$. ∎

Radian measure and arc length in any circle

A simple relation exists between the radian measure s of an angle θ and arc length L determined by that angle on the circumference of any circle (figure 2–16). Geometry tells us that corresponding parts of similar figures form equal ratios. This means, in this case, that $\dfrac{s}{1} = \dfrac{L}{r}$, or $L = rs$. Thus, *if s is the radian measure of an angle with vertex at the center of a circle of radius r, and L is the corresponding arc length,* then

$$L = rs$$

Thus, the arc length L on any circle equals the product of the radius of the circle and the radian measure of the related angle.

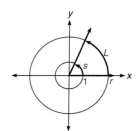

Figure 2–16

■ *Example 2–5 C*

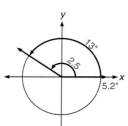

Use the relation $L = rs$ to solve each problem.

1. Find the length of the arc determined by a central angle of measure 2.5 radians on a circle of radius 5.2 inches.

$$L = rs$$
$$L = 5.2(2.5) \qquad \text{Replace } r \text{ with 5.2, } s \text{ with 2.5}$$
$$= 13 \text{ inches}$$

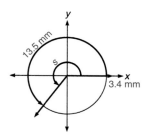

2. Find the measure in radians of the central angle corresponding to an arc length of 13.5 mm on a circle of diameter 6.8 mm.

$$r = 3.4 \text{ mm} \qquad \text{One-half the diameter}$$
$$L = rs$$
$$13.5 \text{ mm} = (3.4 \text{ mm})s \qquad \text{Substitute known values}$$
$$\frac{13.5}{3.4} = s$$
$$3.97 \approx s \qquad \text{Rounding to nearest 0.1}$$

Thus, the central angle measures 3.97 radians.

3. A railroad car has wheels with diameter 1.4 m (meters). If the wheels move through an angle of 200°, how far does the train move?

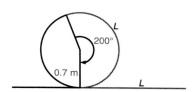

As illustrated, the distance the train will move is the same as the arc length L on the wheel. This length is determined by the central angle of 200°. We will find the measure of the central angle, θ, in radians, then use the relation $L = rs$.

$$\frac{200°}{180°} = \frac{s}{\pi} \qquad\qquad \frac{\theta°}{180°} = \frac{s}{\pi}$$

$$\frac{10}{9} = \frac{s}{\pi} \qquad\qquad \text{Reduce}$$

$$\frac{10\pi}{9} = s \qquad\qquad \text{Multiply each member by } \pi$$

$$L = rs$$

$$L = 0.7\left(\frac{10\pi}{9}\right) \qquad \text{The radius } r \text{ is half the diameter of 1.4 m; } s = \theta \text{ (in radians)}$$

$$L \approx 2.4 \text{ m}$$

Thus, the train moves 2.4 meters when the wheels move through an angle of 200°. ∎

Area of a sector of a circle

A sector of a circle is that part enclosed between two radii. See the shaded part of figure 2-17 for an example. The area A of a circle with radius r is determined by the equation $A = \pi r^2$. The area of a sector of a circle is proportional to the measure of the central angle θ determining the sector. Thus, the area of a sector with central angle θ with measure s radians is part of a circle determined by

$$\text{angle} \times \text{area of whole circle}$$

$$\frac{s}{2\pi} \times \pi r^2 = \frac{s}{2}r^2$$

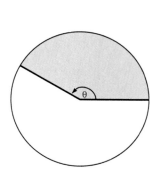

Figure 2-17

Thus, the area of a sector of a circle of radius r is

$$A_s = \frac{s}{2}r^2$$

■ *Example 2–5 D*

Use the formula for the area of a sector of a circle to solve the problem.

Find the area of a sector determined by a central angle of 2 radians in a circle of diameter 8.5''.

The radius r is half the diameter, or 4.25''.

$$A_s = \frac{s}{2}r^2 = \frac{2}{2}(4.25^2) \approx 18.06 \text{ square inches, rounded to the nearest } 0.01 \text{ in.}^2 \quad ■$$

Mastery points

Can you
- State the equation of the unit circle?
- Convert between degree and radian measure for angles?
- Mark off a unit circle in units of $\frac{\pi}{6}$ radians and in units of $\frac{\pi}{4}$ radians?
- Find the reference angle for an angle given in radian measure?
- Use the relation $L = rs$ to solve problems concerning arc length on any circle?
- Use the relation $A_s = \frac{s}{2}r^2$ to find the area of a sector of a circle?

Exercise 2–5

1. State the algebraic relation (equation) that describes the unit circle.

Convert the following degree measures to radian measures. Leave your answers both in exact form and approximated to two decimal places.

2. 30°	**3.** 45°	**4.** 60°	**5.** 100°	**6.** −200°	**7.** −300°
8. −135°	**9.** 270°	**10.** 750°	**11.** 127°	**12.** −422°	**13.** −305°

Convert the following radian measures into degree measures. Leave answers both in exact form and approximated to two decimal places.

14. $\frac{5\pi}{2}$	**15.** $\frac{11\pi}{6}$	**16.** $\frac{2\pi}{7}$	**17.** $\frac{3\pi}{5}$	**18.** $\frac{10\pi}{9}$	**19.** $\frac{2\pi}{9}$
20. $-\frac{5\pi}{3}$	**21.** $-\frac{17\pi}{6}$	**22.** $-\frac{5\pi}{7}$	**23.** $\frac{3}{2}$	**24.** $\frac{11}{6}$	**25.** $-\frac{12}{17}$
26. 1.5	**27.** 2	**28.** 3.25	**29.** −5	**30.** −6	

Find the reference angle for the following angles.

31. $\frac{2\pi}{3}$	**32.** $\frac{5\pi}{4}$	**33.** $\frac{11\pi}{6}$	**34.** $\frac{7\pi}{6}$	**35.** $\frac{4\pi}{3}$	**36.** $\frac{5\pi}{6}$
37. $\frac{3\pi}{4}$	**38.** $\frac{7\pi}{4}$	**39.** $\frac{5\pi}{3}$	**40.** $-\frac{\pi}{4}$	**41.** $-\frac{2\pi}{3}$	**42.** $-\frac{5\pi}{3}$
43. $-\frac{7\pi}{6}$	**44.** $-\frac{\pi}{6}$				

Solve the following problems.

45. The circle is marked off in units of $\frac{\pi}{6}$ (or 30°). Mark each angle shown with its appropriate measure. Reduce fractions.

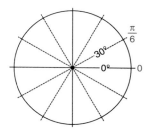

46. The circle is marked off in units of $\frac{\pi}{4}$ (or 45°). Mark each angle shown with its appropriate measure. Reduce fractions.

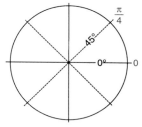

47. The circle is marked off in degrees. Also shown is the approximate location of 1 radian, which is approximately 57°. Mark off the approximate locations of 2, 3, 4, 5, and 6 radians.

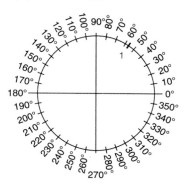

48. Find the length of the arc determined by a central angle of 2.1 (radians) on a circle of diameter 10 inches.

49. Find the measure, in radians, of a central angle on a circle of radius 4.5 mm (millimeter) determined by an arc length of 12 mm, to the nearest 0.1 radian.

50. Find the length of the arc determined by a central angle of 300° on a circle of diameter 12 mm.

51. Find the length of the arc determined by a central angle of 45° on a circle of radius 8.3 inches, to the nearest 0.1 inch.

52. Find the measure, in both radians and degrees, of the central angle determined by an arc length of 14.5 mm on a circle with diameter 10.3 mm. Round both answers to the nearest tenth.

53. The diameter of a wheel on an automobile is 32.4 inches. If the wheel moves through an angle of 85°, how far will the car move?

54. The diameter of a wheel that moves the cable of a ski lift is 5.75 meters, as shown in the diagram. Through what angle, in degrees, does the wheel have to move to advance one of the chairs a distance of 10 meters?

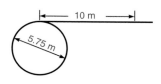

Find the area of the sector of a circle determined by the given angle and radius. Where necessary round the answer to two decimal places.

55. 4, 7 inches

56. $\frac{\pi}{3}$, 10 millimeters

57. $\frac{3\pi}{5}$, 6 centimeters

58. 2.4, 5 inches

59. $\frac{5}{12}$, 6 inches

60. $\frac{6\pi}{5}$, 22 centimeters

61. 15°, 9 millimeters

62. 135°, 24 inches

63. Find the radian measure of the central angle necessary to form a sector of area 14.6 cm² on a circle of radius 4.85 centimeters. Round the answer to two decimal places.

64. Find the *degree* measure of the central angle necessary to form a sector of area 200 in.² on a circle of diameter 50 inches. Round to the nearest 0.1°.

65. The figure shows a sector of a circle that was painted on the concrete in front of an airport terminal. The radius is now to be extended by 25 feet, to a total of 180 feet. The paint that will cover the unpainted area in the new, larger sector covers about 150 square feet per gallon. How many gallons will it take, to the nearest half gallon, to cover the new, unpainted area?

155 ft
73°

66. The alternator on an automobile engine is attached by a belt to a wheel on the engine. The wheel on the engine has a diameter of 14.88 cm (see the figure), and the wheel on the alternator has a diameter of 9.86 cm. If the wheel driven by the engine moves through an angle of 2.85 radians, through what angle does the alternator move, to the nearest 0.01 radian?

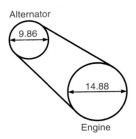

Alternator
9.86
14.88
Engine

67. A decal is being made to indicate timing marks on a wheel attached to the front of an engine (see the diagram). The radius of the wheel is 86.6 mm. What should the distance be between the −10° and 10° marks, to the nearest millimeter?

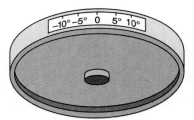

−10° −5° 0 5° 10°

2–6 *Radian measure—values of the trigonometric functions*

In this section we relate radian measure to the trigonometric functions. The concepts here are the same as seen in sections 2–2 through 2–4, concerning degree measure.

Relationship between points on the unit circle and the trigonometric function values

Recall that if (x,y) is a point on the terminal side of an angle θ (in standard position), and $r = \sqrt{x^2 + y^2}$, then $\sin \theta = \dfrac{y}{r}$ and $\cos \theta = \dfrac{x}{r}$. On the unit circle, $r = 1$, so $\sin \theta = y$, and $\cos \theta = x$. Thus, *if (x,y) is the point on the unit circle that intersects the terminal side of an angle θ, then $\sin \theta = y$ and $\cos \theta = x$.* Figure 2–18 shows this fact.

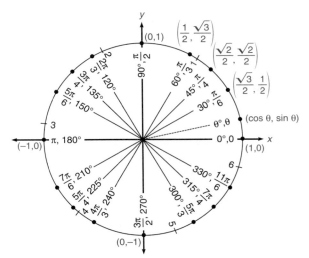

Figure 2–18

This figure is very useful because it shows the degree and radian measure for many common angles with measure between 0° and 360° (0 and 2π in radian measure). The angles shown are either quadrantal or have reference angles of measure 30° $\left(\dfrac{\pi}{6}\right)$, 45° $\left(\dfrac{\pi}{4}\right)$, or 60° $\left(\dfrac{\pi}{3}\right)$. The figure also shows the point on the terminal side of an angle where it meets the unit circle. As stated above, the (x,y) pair at each point on the unit circle is $(\cos\theta,\sin\theta)$ for the corresponding angle. Note that the radian measure is shown for the values $1, 2, 3, \ldots, 6$ as well as for the multiples of π mentioned above. For example, 2 (radians) is near $\dfrac{2\pi}{3} \approx 2.1$ (radians), or 120°.

Observe that you can find the sine or cosine value for any of the angles shown by observing the symmetries in figure 2–18. For example, the coordinates at $\dfrac{4\pi}{3}$ must be $\left(-\dfrac{1}{2},-\dfrac{\sqrt{3}}{2}\right)$. As seen in figure 2–19, traveling through the origin from one point on the unit circle to another simply changes the signs of the x- and y-coordinates. Thus, $\cos\dfrac{4\pi}{3}$ is $-\dfrac{1}{2}$ and $\sin\dfrac{4\pi}{3}$ is $-\dfrac{\sqrt{3}}{2}$.

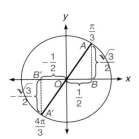

Figure 2–19

Similarly, the coordinates at $\dfrac{5\pi}{6}$ (figure 2–18) must have the same y-coordinate as at $\dfrac{\pi}{6}$, but the opposite of the x-coordinate. Thus, the coordinates there must be $\left(-\dfrac{\sqrt{3}}{2},\dfrac{1}{2}\right)$, and from this point we know that $\sin\dfrac{5\pi}{6}$ $= \sin 150° = y = \dfrac{1}{2}$, $\cos\dfrac{5\pi}{6} = \cos 150° = -\dfrac{\sqrt{3}}{2}$.

	Sine	Cosine	Tangent
$\dfrac{\pi}{6}$, 30°	$\dfrac{1}{2}$	$\dfrac{\sqrt{3}}{2}$	$\dfrac{\sqrt{3}}{3}$
$\dfrac{\pi}{4}$, 45°	$\dfrac{\sqrt{2}}{2}$	$\dfrac{\sqrt{2}}{2}$	1
$\dfrac{\pi}{3}$, 60°	$\dfrac{\sqrt{3}}{2}$	$\dfrac{1}{2}$	$\sqrt{3}$

Table 2–2

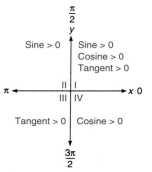

Figure 2–20

Using the reference angle/ASTC procedure with radian measure

The reference angle/ASTC procedure (section 2–3) can also be used instead of figure 2–18. It is restated here. Table 2–2 is the same as table 2–1 except that the radian measure of each angle is included. Figure 2–20 is the same as figure 2–5 except that the quadrantal angles less than 2π (360°) are shown in radian measure.

Reference angle/ASTC procedure for radian measure

To find the value of a trigonometric function for a nonquadrantal angle whose reference angle is $\dfrac{\pi}{6}$, $\dfrac{\pi}{4}$, or $\dfrac{\pi}{3}$:

1. Find the value of the reference angle.
2. Find the value of the appropriate trigonometric function for the reference angle from table 2–2.
3. Determine the sign of this value using the ASTC rule (figure 2–20).

■ *Example 2–6 A*

Use table 2–2 and the ASTC rule to find the exact value of each expression.

1. $\cos \dfrac{7\pi}{6}$

Step 1: $\theta' = \dfrac{\pi}{6}$ This was shown in part 1 of example 2–5 B

Step 2: $\cos \theta' = \cos \dfrac{\pi}{6} = \dfrac{\sqrt{3}}{2}$ Table 2–2

Step 3: $\cos \dfrac{7\pi}{6} < 0$ ASTC rule; $\cos \theta < 0$ in quadrant III

Thus, $\cos \dfrac{7\pi}{6} = -\dfrac{\sqrt{3}}{2}$.

2. $\sin \dfrac{11\pi}{3}$

Step 1: $\theta' = \dfrac{\pi}{3}$ Shown in part 2 of example 2–5 B

Step 2: $\sin \dfrac{\pi}{3} = \dfrac{\sqrt{3}}{2}$ Table 2–2

Step 3: $\sin \dfrac{5\pi}{3} < 0$ ASTC rule; $\sin \theta < 0$ in quadrant IV

Thus, $\sin \dfrac{5\pi}{3} = -\dfrac{\sqrt{3}}{2}$ and therefore $\sin \dfrac{11\pi}{3} = -\dfrac{\sqrt{3}}{2}$.

3. $\cot\left(-\dfrac{13\pi}{4}\right)$

$$\cot\left(-\frac{13\pi}{4}\right) = \frac{1}{\tan\left(-\dfrac{13\pi}{4}\right)}$$

In part 3 of example 2–5 B, we saw that $-\dfrac{13\pi}{4}$ and $\dfrac{3\pi}{4}$ are coterminal,

and the reference angle for either is $\dfrac{\pi}{4}$, so

$$\tan\left(-\frac{13\pi}{4}\right) = \tan\frac{3\pi}{4}$$

We proceed to find $\tan\dfrac{3\pi}{4}$:

Step 1:   The reference angle for $\dfrac{3\pi}{4}$ is $\dfrac{\pi}{4}$.

Step 2: $\tan\dfrac{\pi}{4} = 1$

Step 3: $\dfrac{3\pi}{4}$ terminates in quadrant II, where the tangent function is

negative, so $\tan\dfrac{3\pi}{4} < 0.$

Thus, $\tan\dfrac{3\pi}{4} = -1.$

Now we can finish the problem.

$$\cot\left(-\frac{13\pi}{4}\right) = \frac{1}{\tan\left(-\dfrac{13\pi}{4}\right)} = \frac{1}{-1} = -1 \qquad \blacksquare$$

Calculators are programmed to accept angle input in radian measure. All scientific calculators have a key, often marked ⬚DRG⬚ or ⬚MODE⬚ to tell the calculator to accept angles in radian measure. On the TI-81 use the ⬚MODE⬚ key to select the mode display. Then use the four cursor keys to darken Rad, and use ⬚ENTER⬚ to change to radian mode. Use ⬚QUIT⬚ (⬚2nd⬚ ⬚CLEAR⬚) to exit the mode display.

  Thus, for angles that are not coterminal with those in figure 2–18 we use the calculator, in radian mode. This is illustrated in example 2–6 B.

■ *Example 2–6 B*

Find the required value with a calculator; round the answer to four decimal places.

Make sure the calculator is in radian mode.

1. sin 1.2

$$1.2 \quad \boxed{\text{sin}} \qquad \text{Display} \quad \boxed{0.932039086}$$

$$\boxed{\text{TI-81}} \qquad \boxed{\text{SIN}} \quad 1.2 \quad \boxed{\text{ENTER}}$$

sin 1.2 ≈ 0.9320

2. cot(−0.7)

$$\cot(-0.7) = \frac{1}{\tan(-0.7)}$$

$$.7 \; \boxed{+/-} \; \boxed{\text{tan}} \; \boxed{1/x} \qquad \text{Display} \; \boxed{-1.187241832}$$

$$\boxed{\text{TI-81}} \qquad \boxed{(} \; \boxed{\text{TAN}} \; \boxed{(-)} \; .7 \; \boxed{)} \; \boxed{x^{-1}} \; \boxed{\text{ENTER}}$$

cot(−0.7) ≈ −1.1872 ■

As with degrees, we need to be able to find an angle in radians when given the value of one of the trigonometric functions for that angle, and information about the quadrant. As in section 2–3 we will restrict ourselves to the least (smallest value) nonnegative solution to trigonometric equations.

Since a reference angle is acute (between 0 and $\dfrac{\pi}{2}$ radians), and since the values of all the trigonometric functions are positive for acute angles (quadrant I, ASTC rule) we *always use a nonnegative value to find a reference angle.* This is illustrated in the following example.

In section 2–5 we saw formulas that give θ′ if 0 < θ < 2π. If these are solved for θ, we obtain formulas for finding θ given θ′ and the quadrant in which θ terminates.

Relationship between θ and θ′ if 0 < θ < 2π		
θ in Quadrant I:	θ′ = θ	θ = θ′
θ in Quadrant II:	θ′ = π − θ	θ = π − θ′
θ in Quadrant III:	θ′ = θ − π	θ = π + θ′
θ in Quadrant IV:	θ′ = 2π − θ	θ = 2π − θ′

■ *Example 2–6 C*

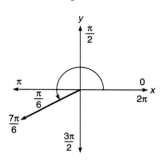

Find the least nonnegative value of θ, in radians. Round to two decimal places if necessary.

1. $\sin \theta = -\frac{1}{2}$, $\cos \theta < 0$

$\qquad \theta' = \sin^{-1}\frac{1}{2}$ Always use a nonnegative value to find a reference angle

$\qquad \theta' = \dfrac{\pi}{6}$ Table 2–2

θ is in quadrant III, since $\sin \theta < 0$ and $\cos \theta < 0$.

$\qquad \theta = \pi + \dfrac{\pi}{6}$ In quadrant III $\theta = \pi + \theta'$

$\qquad \theta = \dfrac{7\pi}{6}$ $\pi + \dfrac{\pi}{6} = \dfrac{6\pi}{6} + \dfrac{\pi}{6}$

2. $\cos \theta = -0.8$, $\tan \theta < 0$

$\qquad \theta' = \cos^{-1} 0.8$ Use the nonnegative value

$\qquad \theta' \approx 0.64$ radians 0.8 $\boxed{\cos^{-1}}$ (In radian mode.)

$\qquad\qquad\qquad\qquad$ $\boxed{0.6435011088}$

$\qquad\qquad\qquad\qquad$ $\boxed{\text{TI-81}}$ $\boxed{\text{COS}^{-1}}$ $.8$ $\boxed{\text{ENTER}}$

θ is in quadrant II since $\cos \theta < 0$, $\tan \theta < 0$.

$$\theta = \pi - \theta' \approx 2.50 \text{ radians} \qquad ■$$

Solutions to trigonometric equations

In sections 1–4 and 2–3 we examined solutions to equations involving the trigonometric ratios and functions in terms of degrees. Chapter 5 treats this subject in more depth, but this is a very important topic, so we revisit it here.

In the problems in example 2–6 D there are an unlimited number of answers. We will look for one basic answer in each case. By limiting the problems to practically all nonnegative values we can almost always find answers in the first quadrant in a very straightforward way.

The objective here is not to completely solve these equations, but to get used to the algebra involved in solving trigonometric equations. These equations use the following facts, which are presented in depth in chapters 4 and 5:

$$\text{if } \sin \theta = k, \text{ then one solution is } \theta = \sin^{-1}k$$
$$\text{if } \cos \theta = k, \text{ then one solution is } \theta = \cos^{-1}k$$
$$\text{if } \tan \theta = k, \text{ then one solution is } \theta = \tan^{-1}k$$

We will see some equations that use the **zero product property:** If a product is zero, then at least one factor is zero. For example, if

$$\sin x(\sin x - 1) = 0$$

then either

$$\sin x = 0$$

or

$$\sin x - 1 = 0$$

■ *Example 2–6 D*

Find a solution to each equation, in radians. Round to two decimal places when necessary.

1. $4 \cos x = 1$

$$4 \cos x = 1$$
$$\cos x = \tfrac{1}{4}$$
$$x = \cos^{-1}\tfrac{1}{4} \approx 1.32 \text{ (radians)}$$

2. $3 \sin 2x = 2$

$$3 \sin 2x = 2$$
$$\sin 2x = \tfrac{2}{3} \qquad \text{Divide both members by 3}$$
$$2x = \sin^{-1}\tfrac{2}{3}$$
$$x = \tfrac{1}{2} \sin^{-1}\tfrac{2}{3}$$
$$x \approx 0.36 \text{ (radians)}$$

1 ÷ 2 × (| 2 ÷ 3 |) sin⁻¹ =

TI-81 (| 1 ÷ 2 |) SIN⁻¹ (| 2 ÷

3 |) ENTER

3. $\tan\dfrac{x}{2} = 1.5$

$$\tan\frac{x}{2} = 1.5$$

$$\frac{x}{2} = \tan^{-1} 1.5$$
$$x = 2 \tan^{-1} 1.5$$
$$x \approx 1.97 \text{ (radians)}$$

4. $(2 \sin \theta - 1)(\sin \theta + 1) = 0$

This is a product that equals zero, so we apply the zero product property.

$$2 \sin \theta - 1 = 0 \quad \text{or} \quad \sin \theta + 1 = 0$$
$$2 \sin \theta = 1 \quad \text{or} \quad \sin \theta = -1$$
$$\sin \theta = \tfrac{1}{2} \qquad\qquad \theta = \frac{3\pi}{2}$$
$$\theta = \sin^{-1}\tfrac{1}{2}$$
$$\theta = \frac{\pi}{6}$$

Thus, there are two solutions, $\dfrac{\pi}{6}$ and $\dfrac{3\pi}{2}$. ■

Mastery points °

Can you
- Find the exact value of a trigonometric function for an angle whose reference angle is $\dfrac{\pi}{6}$, $\dfrac{\pi}{4}$, or $\dfrac{\pi}{3}$, as well as quadrantal angles?
- Find approximate values of the trigonometric functions with a calculator when the angle is given in radians?
- Find a solution, in radians, to certain trigonometric equations?

Exercise 2–6

Find the exact function values for the following angles.

1. $\sin \dfrac{2\pi}{3}$

2. $\tan \dfrac{5\pi}{4}$

3. $\cos \dfrac{11\pi}{6}$

4. $\tan \dfrac{7\pi}{6}$

5. $\cos \dfrac{4\pi}{3}$

6. $\sin \dfrac{5\pi}{6}$

7. $\sin \dfrac{3\pi}{4}$

8. $\cos \dfrac{7\pi}{4}$

9. $\tan \dfrac{5\pi}{3}$

10. $\sin\left(-\dfrac{\pi}{4}\right)$

11. $\tan\left(-\dfrac{2\pi}{3}\right)$

12. $\sec(-\pi)$

13. $\sin\left(-\dfrac{7\pi}{6}\right)$

14. $\cos\left(-\dfrac{\pi}{6}\right)$

Find the following function values where the angle is given in radian measure. Round your answers to four decimal places.

15. $\sin 0.9$ **16.** $\cos 1.1$ **17.** $\tan 0.5$ **18.** $\sec 1.4$ **19.** $\csc 0.7$ **20.** $\cot 1.5$

21. $\sin 2.3$ **22.** $\cos 3.5$ **23.** $\tan 4.1$ **24.** $\sec 5.2$ **25.** $\csc 2.5$ **26.** $\cot 1.9$

Find the least nonnegative value of θ, in radians. Round to two decimal places if necessary.

27. $\cos \theta = -\frac{1}{2}$, $\tan \theta > 0$

28. $\tan \theta = \sqrt{3}$, $\sin \theta < 0$

29. $\sin \theta = -\dfrac{\sqrt{3}}{2}$, $\tan \theta < 0$

30. $\sec \theta = \dfrac{2}{\sqrt{3}}$, $\sin \theta > 0$

31. $\cot \theta = -1$, $\sec \theta > 0$

32. $\tan \theta = -\sqrt{3}$, $\cos \theta > 0$

33. $\csc \theta = -2$, $\cos \theta > 0$

34. $\sin \theta = -0.5624$, $\tan \theta > 0$

35. $\tan \theta = -2.5$, $\csc \theta > 0$

36. $\cot \theta = -0.3$, $\sin \theta > 0$

37. $\cos \theta = -0.885$, $\tan \theta > 0$

38. $\sin \theta = -0.2258$, $\cos \theta > 0$

39. $\csc \theta = -3$, $\sec \theta < 0$

Find one solution to the following equations, in radians. Round to two decimal places if necessary.

40. $4 \cos 3\theta = 2$

41. $3 \sin 2\theta = 1$

42. $\frac{1}{3} \tan 2\theta = 1$

43. $2 \tan \theta = 5$

44. $2 \sin 3\theta = \sqrt{3}$

45. $\sin \dfrac{\theta}{2} = 1$

46. $2 \sec 3\theta = 6$

47. $\sin 3\theta = \frac{1}{2}$

48. $(2 \sin \theta - 1)(\sin \theta - 1) = 0$

49. $\cos \theta (2 \cos \theta - 1) = 0$

50. $\tan \theta(\tan \theta - 1) = 0$

51. $(2 \sin \theta - \sqrt{3})(\sin \theta - 1) = 0$

52. In a certain series circuit the applied voltage V in volts is determined by the function

$$V = 200 \sin(35t + 1)$$

where t represents time in milliseconds and the expression $35t + 1$ is in radians. Compute V to the nearest 0.1 volt for the following values of t:

a. 0   **b.** 0.1   **c.** 0.8   **d.** 1

53. The position d at the end of a spring, under certain initial conditions, as a function of time t in seconds, is

$$d = \tfrac{1}{3} \cos 8t - \tfrac{1}{4} \sin 8t$$

Compute d for the following values of t:

a. $\frac{1}{8}$ **b.** $\frac{1}{4}$

54. An equation that arises in finding the trajectory of a rocket is

$$r = \dfrac{p}{1 + e \cos(s - C)}$$

Find r if $p = 200$, $e = 1.5$, $C = 0.5$, and

a. $s = 1$ **b.** $s = 1.25$

55. In interpreting an electrocardiogram a cardiologist obtains values a and b from the heights of certain peaks, and the value of angle θ, which depends on where the electrodes are attached to the patient. Then the value V is calculated from the expression

$$V = \dfrac{\sqrt{a^2 + b^2 - 2ab \cos \theta}}{\sin \theta}.$$

The value of V helps the cardiologist diagnose specific heart abnormalities. Compute V if $a = 6.2$ cm, $b = 3.5$ cm, and $\theta = 2.6$ (radians). Round the answer to two decimal places. The units will be centimeters.

56. If a 100-pound force pushes on an object at an angle θ that is measured between the direction of the force and the direction of motion of the object, then the amount of force actually moving the object is given by the function

$$f(\theta) = 100 \cos \theta$$

Find the force f for the following values of θ (all in radians), to one decimal place:

a. 0.2   **b.** 0.4   **c.** 0.6   **d.** 1

57. An equation that can be used to compute $\sin x$, if x is in radians, is called the *Maclaurin series* for the sine function. It is

$$\sin x = x - \frac{x^3}{3!} + \frac{x^5}{5!} - \frac{x^7}{7!} + \frac{x^9}{9!} - \cdots,$$

where

$$3! = 1 \cdot 2 \cdot 3 = 6,$$
$$5! = 1 \cdot 2 \cdot 3 \cdot 4 \cdot 5 = 120,$$
$$7! = 1 \cdot 2 \cdot 3 \cdot 4 \cdot 5 \cdot 6 \cdot 7 = 5,040, \text{ etc.}$$

($n!$ is read "n factorial" and is defined as $1 \cdot 2 \cdot 3 \cdot 4 \cdot \cdots \cdot n$.)

Although the Maclaurin series goes on forever, good accuracy is obtained by using the first few terms. Use the first four of the five terms shown here to compute approximations to

a. $\sin 0.1$ **b.** $\sin 0.5$ **c.** $\sin 1$ **d.** $\sin \dfrac{\pi}{6}$

Check the results with the sine key of a calculator. (Some computers use a method similar to this for computing the trigonometric functions.)

58. (See problem 57.) The Maclaurin series for the cosine function, if x is in radians, is

$$\cos x = 1 - \frac{x^2}{2!} + \frac{x^4}{4!} - \frac{x^6}{6!} + \frac{x^8}{8!} - \cdots.$$

Use the first four of the five terms shown above to calculate approximations to

a. $\cos 0.8$ **b.** $\cos 1$ **c.** $\cos 1.3$
d. Approximate $\cos 10°$ by first converting $10°$ to radians.

Chapter 2 summary

- A function is a set of ordered pairs having the property that no first element of the ordered pairs repeats.

- A function is one to one if no second element of the ordered pairs repeats.

- A one-to-one function f has an inverse function f^{-1}.

- **An angle in standard position** is formed by two rays, one of which always lies on the nonnegative portion of the x-axis. This ray is called the initial side. The second ray is called the terminal side. It may be in any quadrant or along any axis.

- Two angles α and β are said to be coterminal if $\alpha = \beta + k(360°)$, k an integer.

- **The trigonometric functions** Let θ be an angle in standard position, and let (x,y) be any point on the terminal side of the angle, except $(0,0)$. Let $r = \sqrt{x^2 + y^2}$ be the distance from the origin to the point. Then

$$\sin \theta = \frac{y}{r}, \qquad \cos \theta = \frac{x}{r}, \qquad \tan \theta = \frac{y}{x}$$

$$\csc \theta = \frac{r}{y}, \qquad \sec \theta = \frac{r}{x}, \qquad \cot \theta = \frac{x}{y}$$

- **Tangent/cotangent identities**

$$\tan \theta = \frac{\sin \theta}{\cos \theta}, \quad \cot \theta = \frac{\cos \theta}{\sin \theta}.$$

- **The ASTC rule**

In quadrant I,	All the trigonometric functions are positive.
In quadrant II, the	Sine function is positive.
In quadrant III, the	Tangent function is positive.
In quadrant IV, the	Cosine function is positive.

- Angles whose degree measures are integer multiples of $90°$, such as $0°$, $\pm 90°$, $\pm 180°$, $\pm 270°$, etc., are called quadrantal angles.

- A reference angle for a nonquadrantal angle is the acute angle formed by the terminal side of the angle and the x-axis.

- If $0° < \theta < 360°$, then the following relate the reference angle θ' and the angle θ.

θ in Quadrant I:	$\theta' = \theta$	$\theta = \theta'$
θ in Quadrant II:	$\theta' = 180° - \theta$	$\theta = 180° - \theta'$
θ in Quadrant III:	$\theta' = \theta - 180°$	$\theta = 180° + \theta'$
θ in Quadrant IV:	$\theta' = 360° - \theta$	$\theta = 360° - \theta'$

- The absolute value of a trigonometric function for any angle is the same as the trigonometric ratio for the corresponding reference angle.

- **Reference angle/ASTC procedure** To find the exact value of a trigonometric function for a nonquadrantal angle whose reference angle is $30°$ $\left(\text{or } \dfrac{\pi}{6}\right)$, $45°$ $\left(\text{or } \dfrac{\pi}{4}\right)$, or $60°$ $\left(\text{or } \dfrac{\pi}{3}\right)$:
  1. Find the value of the reference angle.
  2. Find the value of the appropriate trigonometric ratio for the reference angle from the following table.
  3. Determine the sign of this value using the ASTC rule.

	Sine	Cosine	Tangent
$30°, \dfrac{\pi}{6}$	$\dfrac{1}{2}$	$\dfrac{\sqrt{3}}{2}$	$\dfrac{\sqrt{3}}{3}$
$45°, \dfrac{\pi}{2}$	$\dfrac{\sqrt{2}}{2}$	$\dfrac{\sqrt{2}}{2}$	1
$60°, \dfrac{\pi}{3}$	$\dfrac{\sqrt{3}}{2}$	$\dfrac{1}{2}$	$\sqrt{3}$

- Solutions to simple trigonometric equations:
  if $\sin\theta = k$, then one solution for θ is $\theta = \sin^{-1}k$
  if $\cos\theta = k$, then one solution for θ is $\theta = \cos^{-1}k$
  if $\tan\theta = k$, then one solution for θ is $\theta = \tan^{-1}k$

- Finding the least nonnegative measure of an angle from a trigonometric function value and information about a quadrant.
  1. If necessary use the ASTC rule to determine the quadrant for the terminal side of the angle.
  2. Use $\sin^{-1}$, $\cos^{-1}$, or $\tan^{-1}$ to find θ'. Use the absolute value of the given trigonometric function value.
  3. Apply θ' to the correct quadrant to determine the value of θ.

- **A reference triangle** is a right triangle with one leg on the x-axis and one leg parallel to the y-axis.

- The circle with radius one and center at the origin is described by the equation $x^2 + y^2 = 1$. It is called the unit circle.

- Let θ be an angle in standard position. Let s be the corresponding arc length on the unit circle. Let s be positive if measured in the counterclockwise direction, and negative if measured in the clockwise direction. Then s is the radian measure of the angle θ.

- **Radian/degree proportion** Let θ be an angle in standard position with degree measure $\theta°$ and radian measure s. Then $\dfrac{s}{\pi} = \dfrac{\theta°}{180°}$.

- Relationship between an angle θ, $0 < \theta < 2\pi$, and θ', its reference angle in radian measure.

Quadrant in which θ terminates		
I	$\theta' = \theta$	$\theta = \theta'$
II	$\theta' = \pi - \theta$	$\theta = \pi - \theta'$
III	$\theta' = \theta - \pi$	$\theta = \pi + \theta'$
IV	$\theta' = 2\pi - \theta$	$\theta = 2\pi - \theta'$

- If s is the radian measure of an angle with vertex at the center of a circle of radius r, and L is the corresponding arc length, then $L = rs$.

- The area of a sector of a circle of radius r is $A_s = \dfrac{s}{2}r^2$.

- If (x,y) is the point on the unit circle that intersects the terminal side of an angle θ, then $\sin\theta = y$ and $\cos\theta = x$.

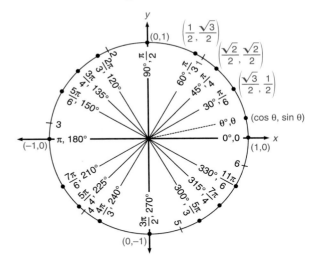

Chapter 2 review

[2–1] In each of the following sets of ordered pairs:
a. Determine if the set is a function.
b. If a function, state the domain and range.
c. If a one-to-one function, state the inverse function.

1. $\{(1,7),\ (4,5),\ (6,7),\ (7,10)\}$
2. $\{(-2,-3),\ (-1,1),\ (1,2),\ (2,5)\}$
3. $\{(1,3),\ (2,5),\ (2,9),\ (6,10)\}$

In each of the following problems a rule that describes a function is given. Form the ordered pairs that this function contains for the following domain elements:
a. -1 **b.** 0 **c.** $\sqrt{5}$ **d.** $\frac{1}{3}$

4. $f(x) = 4 - 2x$

5. $f(x) = 3x^2 - 2x + 3$

6. $f(x) = x^4 - 5$

7. $f(x) = \dfrac{3x}{x - 1}$

[2–2] In the following exercises draw the initial side and terminal side of the given angle. Also, state the measure of the smallest nonnegative angle that is coterminal with the angle.

8. $465°$ **9.** $-40.25°$ **10.** $-270°$
11. $1,800.6°$ **12.** $132°18'$ **13.** $547°26'$
14. $429.3°$ **15.** $-0°15'$

In the following problems you are given a point that lies on the terminal side of an angle in standard position. In each case draw a representation of the least positive angle that has the point on its terminal side and compute all six trigonometric functions for the angle.

16. $(5, -12)$ **17.** $(-5, 8)$ **18.** $(0, -3)$
19. $(2, \sqrt{5})$ **20.** $(-\sqrt{2}, 3)$ **21.** $(1, -\sqrt{6})$
22. $(a, -2a)$, $a > 0$

[2–3] In the following problems you are given the sign of two of the trigonometric functions of an angle in standard position. State in which quadrant the angle terminates.

23. $\sin \theta < 0$, $\cos \theta < 0$ **24.** $\sec \theta < 0$, $\tan \theta > 0$
25. $\cos \theta > 0$, $\tan \theta < 0$ **26.** $\cot \theta < 0$, $\csc \theta < 0$
27. $\csc \theta > 0$, $\cot \theta < 0$ **28.** $\tan \theta < 0$, $\cos \theta < 0$
29. $\tan \theta > 0$, $\csc \theta < 0$ **30.** $\sec \theta > 0$, $\csc \theta < 0$

In the following problems you are given the degree measure of an angle in standard position. For each indicate the measure of the reference angle θ'.

31. $46.3°$ **32.** $323°16'$ **33.** $421°48'$
34. $-22.7°$ **35.** $-248.7°$ **36.** $-105.15°$
37. $242.57°$

In the following problems you are asked to find a trigonometric function value for an angle. If the reference angle is $30°$, $45°$, or $60°$, give the exact answer. Otherwise find the required value to four decimal places.

38. $\sin 213.4°$ **39.** $\cos 240°$
40. $\tan(-114.6°)$ **41.** $\csc 870°$
42. $\cot 212.3°$ **43.** $\tan 213.9°$
44. $\sec 300°$ **45.** $\cos(-133°20')$
46. $\sin(-293°40')$

[2–4] In the following problems you are given a trigonometric function value of an angle in standard position, along with the sign of one of the other function values. Find the measure of the smallest nonnegative angle that meets these conditions, to the nearest $0.1°$.

47. $\sin \theta = 0.3251$, $\cos \theta < 0$
48. $\cos \theta = -0.7771$, $\sin \theta > 0$
49. $\tan \theta = 0.6306$, $\sec \theta < 0$
50. $\sin \theta = -0.9088$, $\tan \theta < 0$
51. $\sec \theta = -2.0642$, $\sin \theta > 0$
52. $\cot \theta = 4.1046$, $\sin \theta < 0$
53. $\sin \theta = \dfrac{\sqrt{3}}{2}$, $\cos \theta < 0$
54. $\tan \theta = -2$, $\sin \theta < 0$
55. $\cos \theta = -\dfrac{5}{13}$, $\tan \theta < 0$

In the following problems you are given the value of one trigonometric function and the sign of another function of an angle in standard position. Draw a representation of the least positive angle that meets these conditions and use it. Compute the exact value of the remaining five trigonometric functions.

56. $\sin \theta = \frac{4}{5}$, $\cos \theta > 0$ **57.** $\cos \theta = -\frac{1}{2}$, $\tan \theta > 0$
58. $\cos \theta = -\frac{5}{16}$, $\tan \theta > 0$ **59.** $\cos \theta = \frac{1}{4}$, $\cot \theta < 0$
60. $\tan \theta = -2$, $\cos \theta < 0$ **61.** $\csc \theta = -4$, $\sec \theta > 0$
62. $\sec \theta = 6$, $\csc \theta < 0$ **63.** $\cot \theta = 2$, $\sin \theta < 0$
64. $\cot \theta = \frac{2}{7}$, $\sin \theta < 0$ **65.** $\tan \theta = \frac{7}{2}$, $\sec \theta < 0$
66. $\tan \theta = 0$, $\cos \theta > 0$ **67.** $\sin \theta = 0.25$, $\cos \theta < 0$

68. $\sin \theta = z$ and θ terminates in quadrant II. Find $\tan \theta$ in terms of z.

69. $\tan \theta = z$ and θ terminates in quadrant IV. Find $\cos \theta$ in terms of z.

70. In a certain electrical circuit the instantaneous voltage E (in volts) is found by the formula

$$E = 120 \sin(\theta + 15°)$$

Compute E to the nearest 0.01 volt for the following values of θ:
a. $0°$ **b.** $45°$ **c.** $84.2°$ **d.** $-200°$
e. $-15°$ **f.** $-45°$

71. For a surveyor to locate a point by measuring an angle at one station and a distance from another one, the distance BP must be found by solving the following sequence of formulas:

$$\sin p = \frac{AB \sin b}{AP} \qquad (0° < p < 90°)$$

$$a = 180° - (b + p)$$

$$BP = \frac{AP \sin a}{\sin b}$$

Compute the distance BP to the nearest 0.1 meter if $AB = 211.5$ meters, $AP = 185.7$ meters, and $b = 29.6°$.

72. A machinist is setting up a numerically controlled drill. The drill must drill a hole in a piece of steel 9.0 millimeters from the origin at an angle of 125°30′. To the nearest 0.1 millimeter, what are the coordinates of this point?

73. Suppose the hole of problem 72 must be 8.075 inches from the origin at an angle of 10.2°. Find the coordinates of this point to the nearest 0.1 inch.

74. A technician is aligning a laser device used to cut patterns from cloth, and positions the device at an angle of −42.3° and a distance of 6.90 feet from the origin. What should the x- and y-coordinates be at this point to the nearest 0.1 foot?

[2–5] Convert the following degree measures into radian measures. Leave your answers both in exact form and approximated to two decimal places.

75. 120°   **76.** −215°   **77.** 430°

Convert the following radian measures into degree measures. Leave your answers both in exact form and approximated to two decimal places.

78. $\dfrac{7\pi}{2}$ **79.** $\dfrac{11\pi}{3}$ **80.** $-\dfrac{5\pi}{7}$

81. 2.5   **82.** −4.2

83. Find the length of the arc determined by a central angle of 3.9 (radians) on a circle of diameter 6.3 inches, to the nearest 0.1 inch.

84. Find the measure, in radians, of a central angle on a circle of radius 8.8 mm determined by an arc length of 20 mm, to the nearest 0.1 radian.

85. Find the length of the arc determined by a central angle of 150° on a circle of diameter 15 mm.

86. The diameter of a wheel on an automobile is 30 inches. If the wheel moves through an angle of 385°, how far will the car move?

Find the area of the sector determined by each of the following angles and radii. Give both the exact answer and a two-decimal-place approximation.

87. 30°, 9 inches   **88.** 240°, 8 mm

89. $\dfrac{11}{12}$, 6 mm   **90.** $\dfrac{2\pi}{5}$, 7 inches

[2–6] Find the following function values where the angle is given in radian measure. Round your answer to four decimal places.

91. sin 1.9   **92.** sec 2.4   **93.** tan 4.5

Find the exact function values for the following angles.

94. $\sin \dfrac{5\pi}{3}$ **95.** $\tan \dfrac{3\pi}{4}$ **96.** $\cos \dfrac{7\pi}{6}$

97. $\cos\left(-\dfrac{\pi}{6}\right)$ **98.** $\tan\left(-\dfrac{4\pi}{3}\right)$ **99.** $\sin\left(-\dfrac{5\pi}{6}\right)$

100. $\sec\left(-\dfrac{\pi}{4}\right)$

Find the least nonnegative value of θ in radians. Round to two decimal places if necessary.

101. $\sin \theta = -\frac{1}{2}$, $\cos \theta > 0$

102. $\tan \theta = -1.82$, $\sin \theta > 0$

Find one solution to the following equations, in radians. Round to two decimal places if necessary.

103. 2 sin θ = 0.84   **104.** 3 tan 2θ = 5

105. (2 cos θ − 1)(cos θ − 1) = 0

106. The position d at the end of a spring, under certain initial conditions, as a function of time t in seconds, is
$$d = \tfrac{1}{3}\cos 8t - \tfrac{1}{4}\sin 8t$$
Compute d if $t = \frac{1}{12}$.

Chapter 2 test

1. Draw the initial side and terminal side of the given angle. Also, state the measure of the least nonnegative angle that is coterminal with the given angle.
   a. 665°   **b.** −417°

In the following problems you are given a point that lies on the terminal side of an angle in standard position. In each case draw a representation of the least positive angle that has the point on its terminal side and compute all six trigonometric function values for the angle (leave answers exact).

2. (6, −12)   **3.** (−2, −6)   **4.** ($\sqrt{2}a, a$), a > 0

In the following problems you are given the value of one trigonometric function and the sign of another function of an angle in standard position. (a) Draw a representation of the least positive angle that meets these conditions. (b) Use a reference triangle to compute the exact value of the remaining five trigonometric functions. (c) Use one of the function values to find the least positive measure of the angle to the nearest 0.1°.

5. $\sin \theta = -\frac{1}{6}$, $\cos \theta > 0$ **6.** $\tan \theta = 8$, $\cos \theta < 0$

In the following problems you are given the degree measure of an angle in standard position. For each indicate the measure of the reference angle θ'.

7. 246.2°   **8.** $-55.6°$

In the following problems you are asked to find a trigonometric function value for an angle. Find the required value to four decimal places.

9. $\sin 116.4°$ **10.** $\tan(-14.8°)$ **11.** $\csc 115°20'$

In the following problems you are given a trigonometric function value of an angle in standard position, along with the sign of one of the other function values. Find the measure of the smallest nonnegative angle that meets these conditions to the nearest 0.1°.

12. $\sin \theta = -0.2961$, $\cos \theta < 0$
13. $\sec \theta = -2.0642$, $\sin \theta > 0$

14. In a certain electrical circuit the instantaneous current I is found by the formula $I = 5.4 \cos(\theta - 25°)$. Compute I to the nearest 0.1 ampere for $\theta = 45°$.

15. The arm of an industrial robot is positioned at 22.6 centimeters from the origin at an angle of 261.42°. To the nearest 0.1 centimeter, what are the coordinates of this point?

16. To align a precision laser that is part of an optical bench, a technician points the device at a test point with coordinates $(-211.5, 620.0)$ (inches). Assuming the bench is coordinatized in the usual way, with the laser at the origin, (a) what angle should the laser's indicator show to the nearest 0.1°, and (b) how far from the origin is the test point?

17. Convert 415° into radian measure. Leave your answer both in exact form and approximated to two decimal places.

18. Convert $\frac{7\pi}{12}$ into degree measure.

19. Find the length of the arc subtended by a central angle of 5.0 (radians) on a circle of diameter 8.2 inches, to the nearest 0.1 inch.

20. The diameter of a wheel on a pulley is 14 cm (see the diagram). If the wheel moves through an angle of 120°, how far will the belt that the wheel drives move?

21. Find a four-decimal-place approximation to $\csc 2.5$.

22. Find the exact value of $\cos \frac{5\pi}{6}$.

23. Find the area of the sector determined by a central angle of $\frac{\pi}{3}$ (radians) in a circle of diameter 32 mm, to the nearest 0.01 mm².

24. Let $f = \{(2,-3), (3,5), (5,6), (10,12)\}$.
   a. Is f a function?
   b. If so, is it one to one?
   c. Does f have an inverse? If so, state it.

25. If the function f is described by the rule $f(x) = x^2 - 3x + 5$, state the ordered pair that is an element of f when the domain element is (a) -4 and (b) $\sqrt{2}$.

Find the least nonnegative value of θ in radians. Round to two decimal places if necessary.

26. $\sin \theta = -\frac{1}{3}$, $\cos \theta > 0$
27. $\tan \theta = \sqrt{3}$, $\sin \theta < 0$

Find one solution to the following equations, in radians. Round to two decimal places if necessary.

28. $\frac{1}{2} \cos \theta = 0.20$ **29.** $2 \tan 3\theta = 4.2$
30. $\sin \theta(2 \sin \theta - 1) = 0$

31. The position d at the end of a spring, under certain initial conditions, as a function of time t in seconds, is $d = \frac{1}{3} \cos 4t - \frac{1}{4} \sin 4t$. Compute d if $t = \frac{\pi}{16}$.

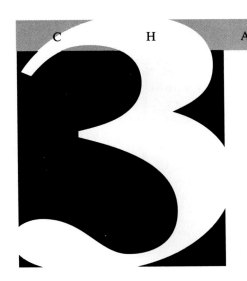

Properties of the Trigonometric Functions

To understand many applications of the trigonometric functions it is necessary to have a good understanding of the properties of these functions. As with any functions, we can gain a great deal of knowledge from their graphs. There are many graphing calculators and computer programs available today that are capable of graphing functions defined from equations. We will illustrate the graphing of trigonometric functions by two methods:

1. obtaining important information about the graph, then using this information to sketch the graph by hand, and

2. using a graphing calculator.

We use the TI-81 graphing calculator to illustrate using a graphing calculator. The process is practically the same with another brand or model.

Before going further, we show some basics of using the TI-81 graphing calculator. The reader can jump to section 3–1 if not using a graphing calculator.

3–0 TI-81 graphing basics

Setting the range for the screen

Graphing calculators have a way to describe which part of the coordinate plane will be displayed. It is called setting the RANGE. Using the $\boxed{\text{RANGE}}$ key shows a display similar to that in table 3–1. The Xmin and Xmax values refer to the range of x values which will be displayed. The Ymin and Ymax values refer to the range of y values which will be displayed. The Xscl and Yscl values refer to the tick marks which will appear on the screen. The Xres refers to the number of x values which will be calculated. It should be left at 1.

Throughout the text we will show the Xmin, Xmax, Xscl, Ymin, Ymax and Yscl values, in this order, in a box labeled RANGE. For the values shown in figure 3–1 we would write $\boxed{\text{RANGE } -10,10,1,-10,10,1}$. This omits the value for Xres, which we will assume is 1.

```
RANGE
Xmin=-10
Xmax=10
Xscl=1
Ymin=-10
Ymax=10
Yscl=1
Xres=1
```

Table 3–1

By entering numeric values and using the $\boxed{\text{ENTER}}$ key to move down the list, the values in the RANGE can be changed. Note that to obtain a negative number the $\boxed{(-)}$ (change sign) key is used, not the $\boxed{-}$ (subtract) key.

Figure 3–1 shows the screen appearance for various settings of Xmax, Xmin, Ymax, and Ymin. Xscl and Yscl are 1 except where labeled Yscl=3 and Xscl=2. After setting these values with the $\boxed{\text{RANGE}}$ key, use the $\boxed{\text{GRAPH}}$ key to show the screen. Using the $\boxed{\text{CLEAR}}$ button readies the calculator for numeric calculations again. The settings in part (a) of figure 3–1 are the "standard" settings, obtained by selecting $\boxed{\text{ZOOM}}$ 6.

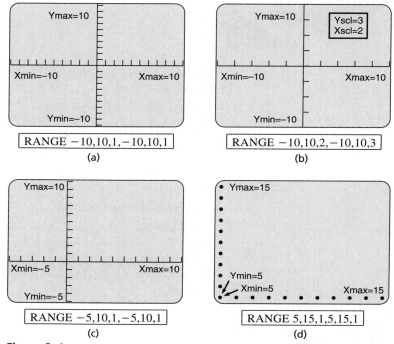

Figure 3–1

Observe that the distance between units are not the same on the screen. The calculator automatically makes horizontal units 1.5 times as long as vertical units. To have horizontal and vertical distances the same, use the $\boxed{\text{ZOOM}}$ function, where option 5 says SQUARE. This makes the screen use the same scale for distance vertically and horizontally by changing the values of Xmin and Xmax. In most cases, having equal horizontal and vertical scales will not be important.

When graphing trigonometric functions $\boxed{\text{ZOOM}}$ 7 (Trig) can be useful. It sets Range settings to

$$\boxed{\text{RANGE } -6.28\ (-2\pi),6.28\ (2\pi),1.57\left(\frac{\pi}{2}\right),-3,3,.25} \quad .$$

Graphing an equation in which *y* is described in terms of *x*

If an equation describes values for a variable y in terms of a variable x, the graphing calculator can be used to view the graph of the equation.

■ *Example 3–0 A*

x	$y\ (2x - 3)$
-3	-9
-2	-7
-1	-5
0	-3
1	-1
2	1
3	3

Graph each equation.

1. Graph $y = 2x - 3$

   This could be done without a graphing calculator with practically no knowledge of graphing by a table of values, by letting x take on many values, such as -3, -2, -1, 0, 1, 2, 3, etc., and computing y for each one. In fact, this table is shown here. The y-values are computed by computing $2x - 3$ for the given x-value. Each pair of values for x and y represents an ordered pair (x,y) (we always write the x-value first). If we plot enough of these values in a coordinate system we start to see a picture emerge. In this case it is a straight line.

   Of course the point of this section is to have the calculator automatically calculate the x- and y-values and plot them. Assuming the standard RANGE settings (obtained by $\boxed{\text{ZOOM}}$ 6) proceed as follows to obtain the graph:

   $\boxed{\text{Y=}}$ Allows us to enter up to four equations.

   $\boxed{2}$

   $\boxed{\text{X}\,|\,\text{T}}$ The variable x.

   $\boxed{-}$

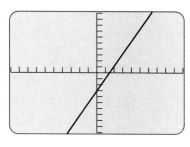

   $\boxed{3}$ The display looks like

:Y$_1$=2X−3
:Y$_2$=
:Y$_3$=
:Y$_4$=

   $\boxed{\text{GRAPH}}$

   Note If there are any equations already entered for Y$_1$ use the $\boxed{\text{CLEAR}}$ key before entering the equation. If there are any extra equations entered for Y$_2$, Y$_3$, or Y$_4$, move down with the down arrow key $\boxed{\triangledown}$ to that equation and use the $\boxed{\text{CLEAR}}$ key to clear that entry. Use $\boxed{\text{ZOOM}}$ 6 to obtain the standard Range settings. The figure shows what the display will look like.

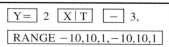

$\boxed{\text{Y=}}$ 2 $\boxed{\text{X}\,|\,\text{T}}$ $\boxed{-}$ 3,

$\boxed{\text{RANGE } -10,10,1,-10,10,1}$

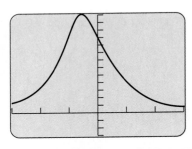

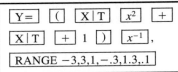

$$\boxed{Y=} \quad \boxed{(} \quad \boxed{X \mid T} \quad \boxed{x^2} \quad \boxed{+}$$
$$\boxed{X \mid T} \quad \boxed{+} \quad 1 \quad \boxed{)} \quad \boxed{x^{-1}},$$
$$\boxed{\text{RANGE} \; -3,3,1,-.3,1.3,.1}$$

2. Graph $y = \dfrac{1}{x^2 + x + 1}$

The following steps would produce a graph similar to that shown in the figure.

Steps	Explanation
$\boxed{\text{RANGE}}$	Enter the x- and y-axis limits.
$\boxed{(-)}$ 3 $\boxed{\text{ENTER}}$	Xmin becomes -3.
3 $\boxed{\text{ENTER}}$	Xmax becomes 3.
1 $\boxed{\text{ENTER}}$	Xscl becomes 1.
$\boxed{(-)}$ .3 $\boxed{\text{ENTER}}$	Ymin becomes -0.3.
1.3 $\boxed{\text{ENTER}}$	Ymax becomes 1.3.
.1 $\boxed{\text{ENTER}}$	Yscl becomes 0.1.

The $\boxed{x^{-1}}$ key is used to define a reciprocal (something divided into one).

$$\boxed{Y=} \; \boxed{(} \; \boxed{X \mid T} \; \boxed{x^2} \; \boxed{+} \; \boxed{X \mid T} \; \boxed{+} \; 1 \; \boxed{)} \; \boxed{x^{-1}} \; \boxed{\text{GRAPH}}$$

3. $y = \sin x + \cos x$

Make sure the calculator is in radian mode (with the $\boxed{\text{MODE}}$ key).

Steps	Explanation
$\boxed{Y=}$ $\boxed{\text{CLEAR}}$ $\boxed{\text{SIN}}$ $\boxed{X \mid T}$ $\boxed{+}$ $\boxed{\text{COS}}$ $\boxed{X \mid T}$	Enter graphing mode. Remove the previous function.
$\boxed{\text{ZOOM}}$ 7	Select standard settings for trigonometric functions. The graphing begins automatically after ZOOM 7 is selected.

$$\boxed{Y=} \quad \boxed{\text{SIN}} \quad \boxed{X \mid T} \quad \boxed{+}$$
$$\boxed{\text{COS}} \quad \boxed{X \mid T}$$
$$\boxed{\text{RANGE} \; -6.28,6.28,1.57,-3,3,.25}$$

In the remainder of this text we show how to enter the function and the Range settings for each graph, assuming the reader is using the TI-81 graphing calculator. The steps are practically the same for other brands and models.

3–1 *Graphs and properties of the sine, cosine, and tangent functions*

Graph of the sine function

The graph of $y = \sin x$ for x between 0 and 2π is shown in figure 3–2. This graph can be obtained by plotting points for various values of x. For example, the points for the following table of values are shown in the figure.

x (radians)	$\sin x$
0	0
$\dfrac{\pi}{6}$	$\dfrac{1}{2}$
$\dfrac{\pi}{4}$	$\dfrac{\sqrt{2}}{2}$ (0.7)
$\dfrac{\pi}{3}$	$\dfrac{\sqrt{3}}{2}$ (0.9)
$\dfrac{\pi}{2}$	1

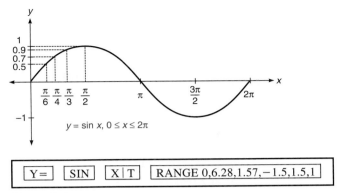

Figure 3–2

The graph in figure 3–2 repeats itself, as shown in figure 3–3, for other values of x because for values of x greater than 2π or less than 0 we have angles that are coterminal with values we have already plotted. Thus, every 2π units we find that the part of the graph that was shown in figure 3–3 is repeated. If we memorize the graph in figure 3–2, we can use it to reproduce the graph in figure 3–3.

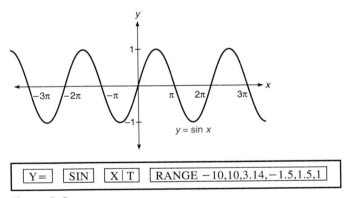

Figure 3–3

The repetitious nature of the sine function can be described with the identity

$$\sin x = \sin (x + k \cdot 2\pi), \ k \text{ any integer}$$

We say that *the sine function is 2π-periodic,* or is periodic with period 2π.

Note Any function that repeats the same pattern over and over is said to be **periodic**. The period is the length of the shortest pattern that produces the function when repeated. Algebraically, a function f is *p-periodic* if there is a number p, $p > 0$, such that

$$f(x + p) = f(x)$$

for all x in the domain, and p is the smallest such number.

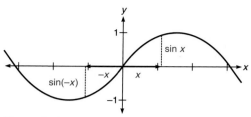

Figure 3–4

Several observations can be made by looking at the graph of $y = \sin x$ in figure 3–4. The domain of the sine function is all real numbers; that is, x can be any real number. The range of the sine function is restricted to the values between and including -1 to 1. In other words, if R represents the collection of all real numbers, then:

$$\text{Domain}_{\text{sine}}: R$$

and

$$\text{Range}_{\text{sine}}: -1 \leq y \leq 1$$

Note The domain is verbalized as "all real numbers"; the range is verbalized as "all real numbers y having the property that $y \geq -1$ and $y \leq 1$."

Another important point is that $\sin(-x) = -(\sin x)$ for any value x. This is illustrated in figure 3–4, where we see that if we go equal distances in the positive and negative directions along the x-axis, the value of the sine function at each place is of the same magnitude (absolute value) but of the opposite sign. Any function for which $f(-x) = -f(x)$ is true for all x in its domain is called an odd function; therefore, *sine is an odd function.*

Graph of the cosine function

Plotting various values of ordered pairs (x, y), where $y = \cos x$, and then connecting them with a smooth curve produces the graph shown in figure 3–5 for x between and including 0 and 2π. For example, we know that $\cos 0 = 1$, $\cos \dfrac{\pi}{6} = \dfrac{\sqrt{3}}{2}$, $\cos \dfrac{\pi}{3} = \dfrac{1}{2}$, $\cos \pi = -1$, etc. These values are shown in figure 3–5.

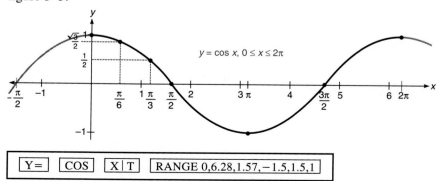

Figure 3–5

Just as with the sine function, the cosine function repeats after 2π units. The identity that states this algebraically is $\cos x = \cos(x + k \cdot 2\pi)$, k any integer. As with the sine function, we also say that *the cosine function is 2π-periodic.*

The graph of $y = \cos x$ is shown in figure 3–5. If we memorize the graph in figure 3–5, we can use it to reproduce the graph in figure 3–6.

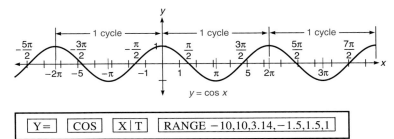

$$\boxed{\;Y=\;\;\;\boxed{COS}\;\;\boxed{X\,|\,T}\;\;\boxed{RANGE\;-10,10,3.14,-1.5,1.5,1}\;}$$

Figure 3–6

Several observations can be made by looking at the graph of $y = \cos x$ in figure 3–6. The domain of the cosine function is all real numbers; that is, x can be any real number. The range of the cosine function is restricted to the values between and including -1 to 1. These are, of course, the same as the domain and range of the sine function.

$$\text{Domain}_{\text{cosine}}:\; R$$
and
$$\text{Range}_{\text{cosine}}:\; -1 \le y \le 1$$

We also see that $\cos(-x) = \cos x$. This is illustrated in figure 3–7, where we see that if we go equal distances in the positive and negative directions along the x-axis, the value of the cosine function at each place is the same value. Any function for which $f(-x) = f(x)$ is true for all x in its domain is called an even function; therefore, *cosine is an even function.*

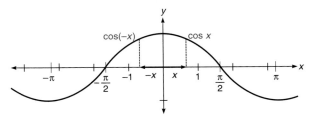

Figure 3–7

Finally, *the graphs of the sine and cosine functions have exactly the same shape;* either one becomes the other if it is shifted right or left a suitable amount. The smallest such amount is $\dfrac{\pi}{2}$, which is described in the statement that $\sin\left(x + \dfrac{\pi}{2}\right) = \cos x$. This statement is proved in chapter 5.

x	$\tan x$
0	0
$\dfrac{\pi}{6} \approx 0.52$	$\dfrac{\sqrt{3}}{3} \approx 0.6$
$\dfrac{\pi}{4} \approx 0.79$	1
$\dfrac{\pi}{3} \approx 1.05$	$\sqrt{3} \approx 1.7$
1.25	≈ 3.0
1.50	≈ 14.1
1.55	≈ 48.1
$\dfrac{\pi}{2} \approx 1.57$	undefined

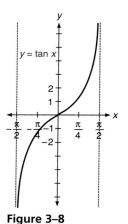

Figure 3–8

Graph of the tangent function

To obtain the graph of the tangent function, we also compute values and plot points. Some values for x between 0 and $\dfrac{\pi}{2}$ are shown in the table. Observe that as x gets closer to $\dfrac{\pi}{2}$, $\tan x$ gets larger. If we recall that $\tan x = \dfrac{\sin x}{\cos x}$, we can see why this is true. As x approaches $\dfrac{\pi}{2}$ (from below), $\sin x$ approaches 1, since $\sin \dfrac{\pi}{2} = 1$, and $\cos x$ approaches 0, since $\cos \dfrac{\pi}{2} = 0$. Now as the denominator, $\cos x$, gets smaller and smaller we divide it into values of $\sin x$, which are close to 1. Effectively we are calculating $\dfrac{1}{\cos x}$, or the reciprocal of $\cos x$. The smaller the absolute value of a number, the larger is its reciprocal. For example, the reciprocal of $\dfrac{1}{100}$ is 100, and of $\dfrac{1}{10,000}$ is 10,000. Thus, as $\cos x$ gets smaller, $\dfrac{1}{\cos x}$ gets larger and larger, and so $\tan x = \dfrac{\sin x}{\cos x}$ gets larger and larger. Since $\cos \dfrac{\pi}{2} = 0$, $\tan \dfrac{\pi}{2}$ is not defined. For the same reason, $\tan\left(-\dfrac{\pi}{2}\right)$ is not defined either. The graph of $y = \tan x$ is shown for $-\dfrac{\pi}{2} < x < \dfrac{\pi}{2}$ in figure 3–8. It can be proved that *the tangent function is π-periodic;* that is, for any x, $\tan x = \tan(x + k\pi)$, k any integer. The actual proof will be an exercise in chapter 5. This π-periodic property means that the graph of the tangent function repeats every π units. More of the graph of $y = \tan x$ is shown in figure 3–9. The vertical dashed lines indicate values

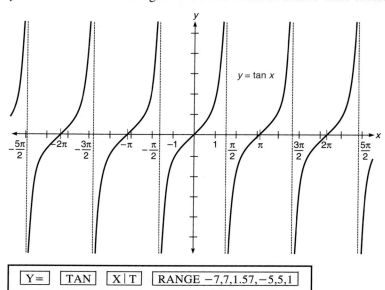

Figure 3–9

of x for which the tangent function is not defined. Since $\tan x = \dfrac{\sin x}{\cos x}$, we know that the tangent function is not defined wherever $\cos x = 0$. The vertical dashed lines are called **asymptotes** of the tangent function and occur wherever $\cos x = 0$.

The domain of the tangent function is all values of x except where $\cos x = 0$, and the range is all values of y.

$$\text{Domain}_{\text{tangent}}: x \neq \frac{\pi}{2} + k\pi, \ k \text{ any integer}$$

$$\text{Range}_{\text{tangent}}: R$$

It will also be an exercise to show that *the tangent function is an odd function;* that is, $\tan(-x) = -(\tan x)$ for any x in its domain.

Table 3–2 summarizes the properties of the three functions we have examined.

Function	Domain	Range	Period
$y = \sin x$	R	$-1 \leq y \leq 1$	2π
$y = \cos x$	R	$-1 \leq y \leq 1$	2π
$y = \tan x$	$x \neq \dfrac{\pi}{2} + k\pi$	R	π

$$\sin(-x) = -(\sin x) \text{ (odd)}$$
$$\cos(-x) = \cos x \text{ (even)}$$
$$\tan(-x) = -(\tan x) \text{ (odd)}$$

Table 3–2

We can use the odd-even properties of these functions to simplify some computations.

■ *Example 3–1 A*

1. Find $\tan\left(-\dfrac{5\pi}{6}\right)$.

Since tangent is an odd function, we know that

$$\tan\left(-\frac{5\pi}{6}\right) = -\left(\tan\frac{5\pi}{6}\right)$$

$\dfrac{5\pi}{6}$ terminates in quadrant II, so its reference angle is $\pi - \dfrac{5\pi}{6} = \dfrac{\pi}{6}$, and

$\tan\dfrac{\pi}{6} = \dfrac{\sqrt{3}}{3}$. Also, the tangent function is negative in quadrant II, so

$\tan\dfrac{5\pi}{6} = -\dfrac{\sqrt{3}}{3}$.

Therefore, $-\left(\tan\dfrac{5\pi}{6}\right) = -\left(-\dfrac{\sqrt{3}}{3}\right) = \dfrac{\sqrt{3}}{3}$ and $\tan\left(-\dfrac{5\pi}{6}\right) = \dfrac{\sqrt{3}}{3}$.

2. Find $\cos(-210°)$.

Since the cosine function is an even function, $\cos(-210°) = \cos 210°$.

The reference angle for $210°$ is $30°$, and $\cos 30° = \dfrac{\sqrt{3}}{2}$. Since $210°$

terminates in quadrant III where the cosine function is negative, $\cos 210°$

$= -\dfrac{\sqrt{3}}{2}$. Therefore, $\cos(-210°) = -\dfrac{\sqrt{3}}{2}$. ■

Mastery points

Can you
- Sketch the graphs of the sine, cosine, and tangent functions?
- State the domain, range, and period of the sine, cosine, and tangent functions?
- Use the odd-even properties to compute the values of sin x, cos x, and tan x for negative values of x?

Exercise 3–1

1. Sketch the graphs of
   a. $y = \sin x$ **b.** $y = \cos x$ **c.** $y = \tan x$

2. From memory, or using their graphs as an aid, state the domain, range, and period of each of the functions sine, cosine, and tangent.

3. Using the graph of $y = \sin x$ as a guide, describe all values of x for which sin x is
   a. 1   **b.** -1 **c.** 0

4. Using the graph of $y = \cos x$ as a guide, describe all values of x for which cos x is
   a. 1   **b.** -1 **c.** 0

5. Using the graph of $y = \tan x$ as a guide, describe all values of x for which tan x is 0.

Use the appropriate property, odd or even, to simplify the computation of the exact value of the (a) sine, (b) cosine, and (c) tangent functions for the following values.

6. $-\dfrac{\pi}{3}$

7. $-\dfrac{\pi}{6}$

8. $-45°$

9. $-\dfrac{5\pi}{3}$

In the text we stated that a function f is odd if $f(-x) = -f(x)$ for all x in its domain and is even if $f(-x) = f(x)$ for all x in its domain. An algebraic example of an odd function is $f(x) = x^3$, since

$$f(-x) = (-x)^3$$
$$= -x^3$$
$$= -f(x)$$

Thus, to illustrate this point, again using $f(x) = x^3$, we can see that $f(-2) = -8$, $f(2) = 8$, and so $f(-2) = -f(2)$.

An example of an even function is $f(x) = x^2$, since we can show that $f(-x) = f(x)$.

$$f(-x) = (-x)^2$$
$$= x^2$$
$$= f(x)$$

Some functions are neither odd nor even, such as $f(x) = x - 3$, since $f(-x) = -x - 3$, but $-f(x) = -(x - 3) = -x + 3$, so $f(-x)$ is neither $f(x)$ nor $-f(x)$, as we see when we compare

$$f(x) = x - 3$$
$$f(-x) = -x - 3$$
$$-f(x) = -x + 3$$

Compute $f(-x)$ and $-f(x)$ for each of the following functions, and state whether the function is odd, even, or neither.

10. $f(x) = x$ **11.** $f(x) = 3x$ **12.** $f(x) = 3x^2$ **13.** $f(x) = -x^2$

14. $f(x) = 2x^4 - 4x^2$ **15.** $f(x) = 3x^2 - 2x^4$ **16.** $f(x) = 2x^3 - 4x$ **17.** $f(x) = 3x - 2x^3$

18. $f(x) = 3 \sin x$ **19.** $f(x) = 2 \cos x$ **20.** $f(x) = \dfrac{x^2 - 1}{4}$ **21.** $f(x) = \dfrac{x^5 - x^3}{x}$

22. $f(x) = \sin^2 x$ **23.** $f(x) = \tan x$ **24.** $f(x) = \sin x + \cos x$ **25.** $f(x) = \dfrac{\sin x}{x}$

$\left(\textit{Hint:} \text{ Rewrite as } \dfrac{\sin x}{\cos x}. \right)$

3–2 *Graphs and properties of the reciprocal functions*

To graph the reciprocal functions cosecant, secant, and cotangent, we can use the graphs of the sine, cosine, and tangent functions as our guide.

The graph of the cosecant function

Remember that $\csc x = \dfrac{1}{\sin x}$. Thus, to graph $y = \csc x$ we first graph $y = \sin x$, and then examine the reciprocal values. Figure 3–10 shows the graph of $y = \sin x$ for $0 \leq x \leq 2\pi$, as well as dashed lines that represent the cosecant function values for these values of x.

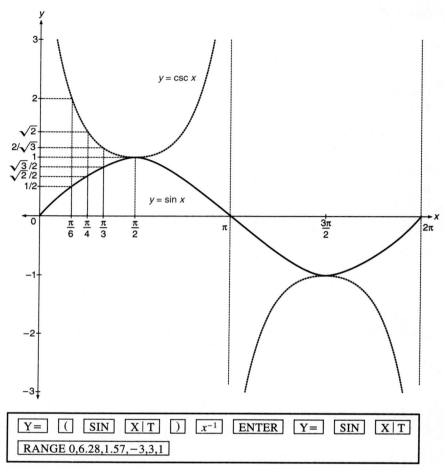

Figure 3–10

x	$\sin x$	$\csc x$
$\dfrac{\pi}{6}$	$\dfrac{1}{2}$	2
$\dfrac{\pi}{4}$	$\dfrac{\sqrt{2}}{2}$	$\sqrt{2}$ (1.4)
$\dfrac{\pi}{3}$	$\dfrac{\sqrt{3}}{2}$	$\dfrac{2\sqrt{3}}{3}$ (1.2)
$\dfrac{\pi}{2}$	1	1

To see that the dashed lines represent the values for the cosecant, consider the table, which shows both the sine and cosecant values for selected values of x. These selected values are also illustrated in figure 3–10.

Referring to figure 3–10 and the table, we see that as x increases from $\dfrac{\pi}{6}$ to $\dfrac{\pi}{2}$, $\sin x$ increases from $\frac{1}{2}$ to 1, and the reciprocal values, $\csc x$, decrease from 2 to 1. Also, as $\sin x$ decreases in absolute value (i.e., gets closer to the x-axis), the reciprocal gets larger in absolute value. Wherever $\sin x$ is 1 or -1, so is its reciprocal value, $\csc x$. Wherever $\sin x$ approaches 0, the absolute value of $\csc x$ approaches infinity (gets larger and larger). Note that if $\sin x$ approaches 0 through positive values, its reciprocal gets larger and larger, and wherever sin x approaches 0 through negative values, csc x becomes larger and larger in *absolute value,* although it is negative.

To graph $y = \csc x$, we can rely on the graph of $y = \sin x$ for our guide. The steps are:

1. Graph $y = \sin x$.

2. Wherever sin x is $+1$ or -1, so is csc x.

3. Wherever sin x is 0, draw vertical dashed lines (asymptotes).

4. As sin x approaches 0, draw csc x getting greater and greater in absolute value, positive or negative depending on the sign of the sine function.

The graph of $y = \csc x$ is shown in figure 3–11; the graph of $y = \sin x$ is shown as a dashed line.

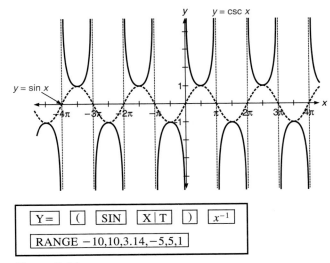

Figure 3–11

Note that the domain of the cosecant function is all x except where sin $x = 0$, and the range is all y greater than or equal to 1 in absolute value. This range reflects the fact that since sin x is less than or equal to 1 in absolute value, $\dfrac{1}{\sin x}$ must be greater than or equal to 1 in absolute value. Also, the cosecant function is 2π-periodic, just as the sine function is.

The graph of the secant function

The graph of $y = \sec x$ is analyzed in the same manner as the graph of $y = \csc x$, except that we are considering $y = \dfrac{1}{\cos x}$ instead of $y = \dfrac{1}{\sin x}$.

Thus, to graph $y = \sec x$, we can rely on the graph of $y = \cos x$ for our guide. The steps are the same as when graphing the cosecant function, except that the cosine function is our guide. This produces the graph of $y = \sec x$, which is shown along with the graph of $y = \cos x$ in figure 3–12.

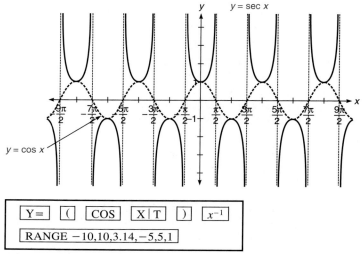

Figure 3–12

The domain is, of course, where $\cos x \neq 0$, and the range is the same as that of the cosecant function. The secant function is also 2π-periodic.

The graph of the cotangent function

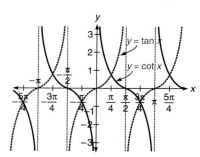

Figure 3–13

Since $\cot x = \dfrac{1}{\tan x}$ except where $\tan x = 0$, we can obtain the graph of $y = \cot x$ by analyzing the graph of $y = \tan x$ as we did previously for the other reciprocal functions. The graphs of both $y = \tan x$ and $y = \cot x$ are shown in figure 3–13. Note that wherever $\tan x$ is 0, we have a vertical asymptote, and wherever $\tan x$ approaches infinity or negative infinity, $\cot x$ approaches 0. This should make sense, since as a quantity gets greater and greater in absolute value, its reciprocal will get smaller and smaller in absolute value. Note that $y = \cot x$ is π-periodic as is the tangent function, its domain is all x except where $\sin x = 0$ $\left(\text{since } \cot x = \dfrac{\cos x}{\sin x}\right)$, and its range is all real numbers, as is the range of the tangent function.

Note   One way to remember where the vertical asymptotes are for the cotangent function is to sketch the graph of the sine function. Wherever $\sin x$ is 0, $\cot x$ does not exist, and instead "goes to infinity or negative infinity." This is where we draw the vertical asymptotes.

The graph of $y = \cot x$ is shown in figure 3–14.

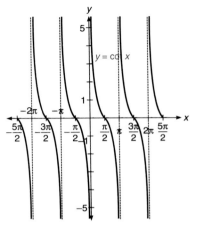

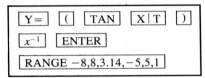

Figure 3–14

The properties of the three reciprocal trigonometric functions are summarized in table 3–3, where k is any integer.

Function	Domain	Range	Period
$y = \csc x$	$x \neq k\pi$	$|y| \geq 1$	2π
$y = \sec x$	$x \neq \dfrac{\pi}{2} + k\pi$	$|y| \geq 1$	2π
$y = \cot x$	$x \neq k\pi$	R	π

Table 3–3

Mastery points

Can you
- Sketch the graphs of the reciprocal functions?
- State the domain, range, and period of the reciprocal functions?

Exercise 3–2

1. Sketch the graphs of the three reciprocal trigonometric functions.

2. State the domain, range, and period for each of the three reciprocal trigonometric functions.

3. Use the identity $\csc x = \dfrac{1}{\sin x}$ to show that cosecant is an odd function.

4. Use the identity $\sec x = \dfrac{1}{\cos x}$ to show that secant is an even function.

5. Use the identity $\cot x = \dfrac{1}{\tan x}$ to show that cotangent is an odd function.

3–3 *Linear transformations of the sine and cosine functions*

In section 3–1 we developed the graphs of the sine and cosine functions. Most scientific and technological applications of these functions require that they be transformed in some way to fit measured or theoretical data. In this section we examine some of the ways in which this can be done. In particular, we will examine operations called **linear transformations.**

Graphically, linear transformations are operations that move a graph in some fixed direction, or "squeeze" or "expand" the graph uniformly. The linear transformations we examine are scaling factors and translations.

Vertical scaling factors and translations

Consider the graph of $y = 3 \sin x$, and what this equation tells us to do to compute y for a given value of x. First, we are to compute the value of $\sin x$, and then multiply this value by 3. Thus, for the same value of x, the expression $3 \sin x$ will be 3 times greater (in absolute value) than the expression $\sin x$. If we then compare the graph of $y = 3 \sin x$ with the graph of $y = \sin x$, the y-values of the first must be 3 times greater than the y-values of the second. See figure 3–15.

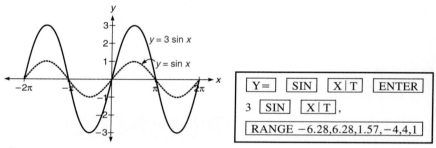

Figure 3–15

For the same reasons, the graph of $y = 2 \cos x$ is the same as that of $y = \cos x$, except that it reaches a magnitude of 2 instead of 1. See figure 3–16. Except for this vertical change in scale, the graph is the same as that of $y = \cos x$.

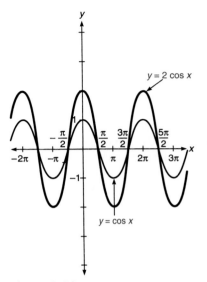

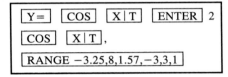

Figure 3–16

If the coefficient of the sine or cosine value is negative, a reflection about the horizontal axis occurs. Consider, for example, the graph of $y = -4 \cos x$ compared to the graph of $y = \cos x$. To compute a y-value in $y = -4 \cos x$, we first compute $\cos x$ and then multiply this value by -4. Multiplying by a negative value changes the sign of the value being multiplied. Thus, whenever y is negative in the graph $y = \cos x$, the y in $y = -4 \cos x$ is positive and scaled (multiplied) by a factor of 4. Also, whenever y is positive in the graph $y = \cos x$, the y in $y = -4 \cos x$ is negative and scaled by a factor of 4. See figure 3–17.

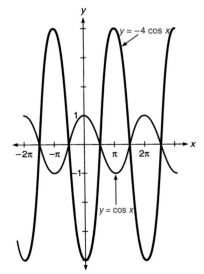

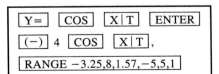

Figure 3–17

In general, the graphs of $y = A \sin x$ and $y = A \cos x$ are scaled vertically by a vertical scaling factor $|A|$. That is, the magnitude of the graph is changed from one to $|A|$. *Also, the graph is reflected about the horizontal (x) axis if $A < 0$.* $|A|$ is usually called the **amplitude** of the function. If the sine or cosine function describes sound waves in the air, then the amplitude corresponds to the loudness of the sound; indeed, we often use the word amplitude to describe this property of a sound.

Now consider the graph of $y = \sin x + 3$ (not to be confused with $y = \sin(x + 3)$). To compute a value of y for a given x in $y = \sin x + 3$, we first compute the value of $\sin x$ and then add 3 to this value. This means that for a given x, $\sin x + 3$ is 3 units greater than $\sin x$. Thus, if we compare the graphs of $y = \sin x$ and $y = \sin x + 3$, the second graph must be 3 units higher than the first, since to compute a y in the second equation we do the same thing as in the first (compute $\sin x$), but then add 3. This vertical shift is shown in figure 3–18.

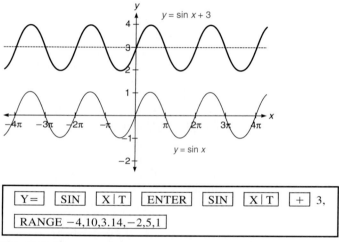

Figure 3–18

In general, the graph of $y = \sin x + D$ and $y = \cos x + D$, is the same as the graph of $y = \sin x$ and $y = \cos x$, respectively, but shifted up or down $|D|$ units. This shift is called a **vertical translation.**

■ *Example 3–3 A*

1. Graph $y = 4 \cos x$.

   This is the same as the graph of $y = \cos x$, except scaled vertically by a factor of 4. Thus, the amplitude is 4. This is shown in the figure.

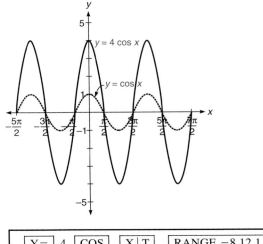

| Y= | 4 | COS | X|T | , | RANGE −8,12,1.57,−5,5,1 |

2. Graph $y = 2 \sin x - 3$.

   The 2 affects the amplitude of the graph, and the -3 causes a vertical translation down, because we are subtracting values from $2 \sin x$. In the first figure we draw a sine curve with amplitude 2.

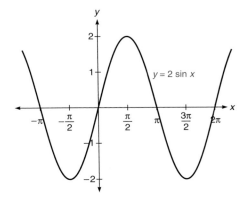

In the second figure we show the same curve translated down 3 units.

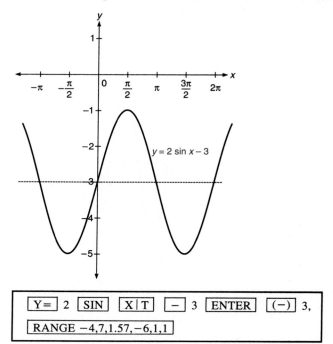

$$\boxed{Y=}\ 2\ \boxed{SIN}\ \boxed{X\,|\,T}\ \boxed{-}\ 3\ \boxed{ENTER}\ \boxed{(-)}\ 3,$$
$$\boxed{RANGE\ -4,7,1.57,-6,1,1}$$

3. Graph $y = -2 \cos x + 2.5$.

We first graph $y = -2 \cos x$; the amplitude is $\left| -2 \right| = 2$, and the -2 reflects the graph about the horizontal axis. See the first figure.

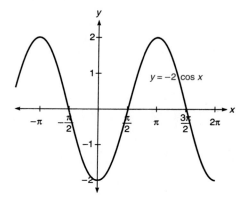

Now we shift this graph up 2.5 units. See the second figure.

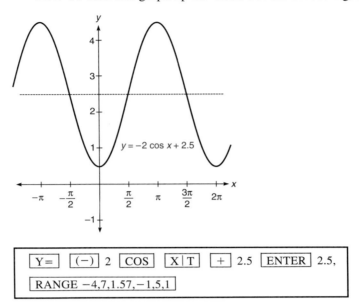

$$y = -2 \cos x + 2.5$$

```
Y=   (−)  2  COS   X|T   +  2.5  ENTER  2.5,
RANGE −4,7,1.57,−1,5,1
```

■

Horizontal scaling factors and translations

We have seen how to transform the graph of a sine or cosine function verti-cally. It is just as important to be able to do this horizontally.

The **argument** of a function is the expression to be used as the domain element when doing computations. In $y = \sin x$ or $y = \cos x$, the x is the argument of the function. In $y = \sin 3x$, the expression $3x$ is the argument. In $y = \cos(x - 4)$ the expression $x - 4$ is the argument. In $y = 2 \sin 4x - 3$, $4x$ is the argument. The argument is the quantity we ''take the sine or cosine of.''

Now consider what we know about the sine and cosine functions. As the argument goes from 0 to 2π, each of these functions produces the graph shown in figure 3–19. We call the portion of each graph shown in figure 3–19 the **basic sine cycle** and the **basic cosine cycle,** respectively. Each of these basic cycles is repeated over and over to get the final, complete graphs of $y = \sin x$ and $y = \cos x$. The important fact is that *as the argument takes on values from 0 to 2π, we get one basic cycle of the function*. Note that the basic sine cycle is 0 at its beginning, middle, and end points. The basic cosine function starts with $y = 1$, ends with $y = 1$, and $y = -1$ at the midpoint of the cycle.

Now consider what the graph of $y = \sin\left(x - \dfrac{\pi}{4}\right)$ should look like. We know that one basic cycle of the sine function is produced as the argument goes from 0 to 2π. In this case, the argument is the expression $x - \dfrac{\pi}{4}$. We

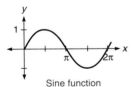

Sine function

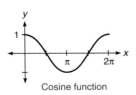

Cosine function

Figure 3–19

examine $x - \dfrac{\pi}{4}$ as it takes on all values from 0 to 2π to find out what values x takes on. We can do this algebraically, using

$$0 \le x - \frac{\pi}{4} \le 2\pi$$

This states that the argument runs (takes on values) from 0 to 2π. Now we can solve this statement for x by adding $\dfrac{\pi}{4}$ to each part.

$$\frac{\pi}{4} \le x \le 2\pi + \frac{\pi}{4}$$

$$\frac{\pi}{4} \le x \le \frac{9\pi}{4}$$

What we learn from this process is that for the expression $x - \dfrac{\pi}{4}$ to take on all values from 0 to 2π, x must take on all values from $\dfrac{\pi}{4}$ to $\dfrac{9\pi}{4}$. Now we can reason as follows:

1. We know that one basic cycle of the sine function is produced as the argument, in this case $x - \dfrac{\pi}{4}$, varies from 0 to 2π.

2. The expression $x - \dfrac{\pi}{4}$ varies from 0 to 2π as x varies from $\dfrac{\pi}{4}$ to $\dfrac{9\pi}{4}$.

3. Therefore, the expression $\sin\left(x - \dfrac{\pi}{4}\right)$ produces one basic cycle of the sine function as x varies from $\dfrac{\pi}{4}$ to $\dfrac{9\pi}{4}$.

Thus, our basic cycle does not start at 0 and end at 2π but starts at $\dfrac{\pi}{4}$ and ends at $\dfrac{9\pi}{4}$. See figure 3–20.

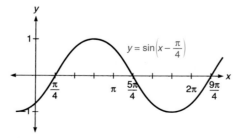

Figure 3–20

If we find the distance between $\dfrac{\pi}{4}$ and $\dfrac{9\pi}{4}$, it is $\dfrac{9\pi}{4} - \dfrac{\pi}{4} = \dfrac{8\pi}{4} = 2\pi$. This is the "length" of one basic cycle and is called the "period" of the function. We will define the period of the sine and cosine functions shortly. Right now, let us simply observe that a good rule for marking the x-axis is to divide it by using increments of one half of the period. To find this amount, divide the period by two (or multiply by one half). Thus, for convenience we marked the horizontal scale in increments of $\dfrac{2\pi}{2} = \pi$, starting at $\dfrac{\pi}{4}$. Note that the function crosses the x-axis halfway between the beginning and end of the cycle $\left(\text{at } \dfrac{5\pi}{4}\right)$ and has high and low points halfway between this point and the beginning and end points of the cycle.

Now, since we know that the sine function is periodic, and we have graphed one cycle, we repeat this cycle to obtain the complete graph. See figure 3–21.

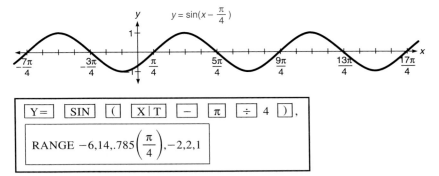

Figure 3–21

Although we looked at the previous function in some detail, we can state the process we used in just a few steps. To understand these steps, remember the underlying idea we used:

> We know what the graphs of the sine and cosine functions look like as their arguments take on values from 0 to 2π. We therefore find out what values x has to take on for the argument to take on all values from 0 to 2π. As x takes on these values, we get one basic cycle of the sine or cosine function.

We now state the procedure to graph sine and cosine functions where the argument is of the form $Bx + C$, $B > 0$.

> **Graphing**
>
> $$y = A \sin(Bx + C) + D \text{ and}$$
> $$y = A \cos(Bx + C) + D, \, B > 0$$
>
> 1. Solve $0 \le Bx + C \le 2\pi$ for x. This gives the left and right end points for one basic cycle.
> 2. Label the amplitude $|A|$. Use the left and right end points found in step 1, along with the amplitude, to draw one basic cycle. Reflect about the horizontal axis if $A < 0$.
> 3. Repeat this cycle to obtain as much of the graph as desired.
> 4. Apply a vertical shift D if necessary.

Note   We will discuss the case where $B < 0$ shortly.

We need to define the term period, used above, and another term, phase shift, before proceeding with more examples. To do this we perform step 1 for the general case. Solving $0 \le Bx + C \le 2\pi$ for x:

$$0 \le Bx + C \le 2\pi$$
$$-C \le Bx \le 2\pi - C \qquad \text{Subtract } C \text{ from each expression}$$
$$-\frac{C}{B} \le x \le \frac{2\pi - C}{B} \qquad \text{Divide each expression by } B$$

The expression $-\dfrac{C}{B}$ is called the **phase shift** of the sine or cosine function being examined. The difference between the left and right end points of the basic cycle,

$$\frac{2\pi - C}{B} - \left(-\frac{C}{B} \right) = \frac{2\pi - C}{B} + \frac{C}{B}$$
$$= \frac{2\pi - C + C}{B}$$
$$= \frac{2\pi}{B}$$

is called the **period** of the sine or cosine function. B is also the number of complete cycles in 2π units.

It is not necessary to memorize these general expressions since the method we are using will produce these results anyway. With these terms, however, we can now state a precise *guideline for marking off the x-axis* when we graph. Mark the axis in increments of one half of the period, starting at the phase shift.

■ *Example 3–3 B*

1. Graph $y = 2 \cos 4x$. Show three cycles. State the amplitude, period, and phase shift.

   Amplitude is 2, with no reflection about the x-axis.

   Step 1: Solve $0 \leq 4x \leq 2\pi$ for x.

   $$\frac{0}{4} \leq \frac{4x}{4} \leq \frac{2\pi}{4} \qquad \text{Divide by 4}$$

   $$0 \leq x \leq \frac{\pi}{2}$$

   We know that one basic cycle of the cosine function starts at 0 and ends at $\frac{\pi}{2}$. The period is $\frac{\pi}{2}$, and the phase shift is 0. The x-axis will be marked off in increments of one half of the period: $\frac{1}{2} \cdot \frac{\pi}{2} = \frac{\pi}{4}$.

   Step 2: Draw one basic cycle with amplitude 2. See part (a) of the figure.

   Step 3: We get two more basic cycles by marking off one more period to the right of $\frac{\pi}{2}$, and one more to the left of 0. We then draw in the basic cycles. See part (b) of the figure.

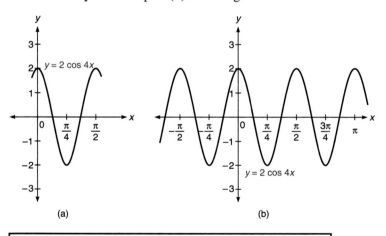

(a)   (b)

$$\boxed{\text{Y=}} \; 2 \; \boxed{\text{COS}} \; 4 \; \boxed{\text{X} | \text{T}}, \; \boxed{\text{RANGE } -2,4,.785,-3,3,1}$$

2. Graph $y = \cos(3x - \pi)$. Show three cycles. State the amplitude, period, and phase shift.

Step 1: $0 \le 3x - \pi \le 2\pi$

$\pi \le 3x \le 3\pi$ \qquad Add π to each expression

$\dfrac{\pi}{3} \le x \le \pi$ \qquad Divide each expression by 3

We know that we get one basic cycle of the cosine function as x varies from $\dfrac{\pi}{3}$ to π. The phase shift is $\dfrac{\pi}{3}$, and the period is $\pi - \dfrac{\pi}{3} = \dfrac{2\pi}{3}$. We mark the x-axis in increments of $\dfrac{1}{2} \cdot \dfrac{2\pi}{3} = \dfrac{\pi}{3}$, starting at $\dfrac{\pi}{3}$, the phase shift, because this is where one basic cycle will start.

Step 2: We mark the amplitude, 1, and draw one basic cycle. See part (a) of the figure.

Step 3: In part (b) of the figure we show one more cycle on each "side" of the basic cycle.

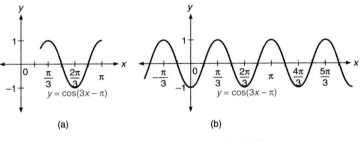

(a)   (b)

$$\boxed{\;\fbox{Y=}\;\; \fbox{COS}\;\; \fbox{(}\; 3\; \fbox{X|T}\;\; \fbox{$-$}\;\; \fbox{π}\;\; \fbox{)}\;, }$$

$$\boxed{\text{RANGE } -1.25, 6, .524\left(\dfrac{\pi}{6}\right), -2, 2, 1}$$

3. Graph $y = -3\sin\left(3x - \dfrac{\pi}{4}\right)$. Show three cycles. State the amplitude, period, and phase shift.

The amplitude will be $|-3| = 3$ for this function. Because $-3 < 0$, there will be a reflection of the graph about the horizontal axis.

Step 1: $0 \le 3x - \dfrac{\pi}{4} \le 2\pi$

$0 \le 12x - \pi \le 8\pi$ \qquad Multiply each expression by 4

$\pi \le 12x \le 9\pi$

$\dfrac{\pi}{12} \le x \le \dfrac{9\pi}{12}$ or $\dfrac{\pi}{12} \le x \le \dfrac{3\pi}{4}$

The phase shift is $\dfrac{\pi}{12}$, and the period is $\dfrac{9\pi}{12} - \dfrac{\pi}{12} = \dfrac{8\pi}{12} = \dfrac{2\pi}{3}$.

We mark the x-axis in increments of $\dfrac{1}{2} \cdot \dfrac{2\pi}{3} = \dfrac{\pi}{3}$, starting at $\dfrac{\pi}{12}$. Actually, we will use the value $\dfrac{4\pi}{12}$ instead of $\dfrac{\pi}{3}$ for convenience.

Step 2: We mark the x-axis in increments of $\dfrac{4\pi}{12}$ and draw a sine cycle between $\dfrac{\pi}{12}$ and $\dfrac{9\pi}{12}$ with amplitude 3. This is shown by the dashed lines in part (a) of the figure. Its reflection about the horizontal axis is shown in solid lines.

Step 3: We mark off more increments of $\dfrac{4\pi}{12}$ and draw two more cycles. See part (b) of the figure.

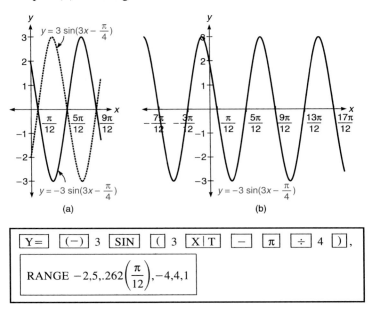

(a)   (b)

Y= (−) 3 SIN ((3 X|T − π ÷ 4)),

RANGE −2,5,.262$\left(\dfrac{\pi}{12}\right)$,−4,4,1

If B is negative in the argument $Bx + C$, we use the odd and even identities to get an equivalent expression with B positive. Recall these identities (section 3–1):

$$\sin(-x) = -(\sin x)$$
$$\cos(-x) = \cos x$$

> **Concept**
>
> We can change the sign of the argument of the sine function and still have an equivalent expression if we change the sign of the coefficient of the sine function itself. We can change the sign of the argument of the cosine function and still have an equivalent expression. We do *not* change the sign of the coefficient of the cosine function.

■ *Example 3–3 C*

1. Rewrite $y = 2 \cos(-3x)$ so that the coefficient of x is positive.

   Changing the sign of the argument, $-3x$, we get $3x$. We do not change the sign of the coefficient of the cosine function since it is an even function. Thus,

   $$y = 2 \cos(-3x) \text{ becomes}$$
   $$y = 2 \cos 3x$$

   These are equivalent functions, so they have the same graph.

2. Rewrite $y = 3 \sin(-2x + \pi)$ so that the coefficient of x is positive.

   The sine function is an odd function, so we change the sign of both the argument and the coefficient of the function. We change the sign of the coefficient of the function, 3, to -3.
   To change the sign of the argument, $-2x + \pi$, we must change the sign of both terms, giving $2x - \pi$. Thus,

   $$y = 3 \sin(-2x + \pi) \text{ becomes}$$
   $$y = -3 \sin(2x - \pi)$$

   These two functions have the same graph.

3. Rewrite $y = \cos\left(-\dfrac{x}{2} - 3\right)$ so that the coefficient of x is positive.

   We change the sign of each term of the argument, but we do not change the sign of the coefficient of the function itself. Thus,

   $$y = \cos\left(-\frac{x}{2} - 3\right) \text{ becomes}$$
   $$y = \cos\left(\frac{x}{2} + 3\right)$$

4. Rewrite $y = -\sin\left(-\dfrac{x}{3}\right)$ so that the coefficient of x is positive.

   Change the sign of $-\dfrac{x}{3}$ to $\dfrac{x}{3}$, and of the coefficient of the sine function, -1, to 1.

   $$y = -\sin\left(-\frac{x}{3}\right) \text{ becomes}$$
   $$y = \sin\frac{x}{3}$$

■

Example 3–3 D illustrates how to use the odd/even properties to help graph a function.

■ *Example 3–3 D*

Graph $y = -2 \sin\left(-\dfrac{2x}{3} + 1\right)$. Show three cycles, and state the amplitude, period, and phase shift.

Since the x term of the argument is negative, we use the odd property of the sine function to change both the sign of the argument and the sign of the coefficient of the function. This gives us the equivalent function

$$y = 2 \sin\left(\frac{2x}{3} - 1\right)$$

Step 1: $0 \le \dfrac{2x}{3} - 1 \le 2\pi$

$0 \le 2x - 3 \le 6\pi$

$3 \le 2x \le 6\pi + 3$

$\dfrac{3}{2} \le x \le \dfrac{6\pi + 3}{2}$

Phase shift is $\frac{3}{2}$, and period is $\dfrac{6\pi + 3}{2} - \dfrac{3}{2} = \dfrac{6\pi}{2} = 3\pi$. We mark the x-axis by using $\frac{3}{2}$ as our starting point and using increments of $\dfrac{3\pi}{2}$, which is one half of the period. In this case, we also compute decimal approximations to the results to make it easier to plot our points. Several of the computations are

$$\frac{3}{2} + \frac{3\pi}{2} = \frac{3 + 3\pi}{2} \approx 6.2$$

$$\frac{3 + 3\pi}{2} + \frac{3\pi}{2} = \frac{3 + 6\pi}{2} \approx 10.9$$

$$\frac{3 + 6\pi}{2} + \frac{3\pi}{2} = \frac{3 + 9\pi}{2} \approx 15.6$$

and

$$\frac{3}{2} - \frac{3\pi}{2} = \frac{3 - 3\pi}{2} \approx -3.2$$

$$\frac{3 - 3\pi}{2} - \frac{3\pi}{2} = \frac{3 - 6\pi}{2} \approx -7.9$$

Step 2: One basic cycle is shown in part (a) of the figure.

Step 3: Two more cycles are shown in part (b) of the figure.

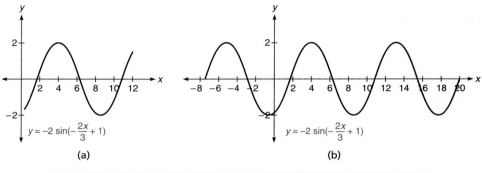

(a)   (b)

$$\boxed{\text{Y=} \quad \boxed{(-)} \; 2 \; \boxed{\text{SIN}} \; \boxed{(} \; \boxed{(-)} \; 2 \; \boxed{\text{X|T}} \; \boxed{\div} \; 3 \; \boxed{+} \; 1 \; \boxed{)} ,}$$
$$\boxed{\text{RANGE } -8,20,2,-3,3,1}$$

We can observe at this point that the method we have been using has given us both horizontal translations and scaling factors. Phase shift is a horizontal translation, and if we divide the period, $\dfrac{2\pi}{B}$, by 2π (the period of the basic sine or cosine function), we get $\dfrac{1}{B}$, a horizontal scale factor. Normally we do not actually compute the horizontal scale factor.

There are times when we will want to find the equation of a function, given some of its properties.

■ *Example 3–3 E*

1. Find the equation of the cosine function in the figure.

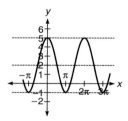

We know the equation is of the form

$$y = A \cos(Bx + C) + D$$

It is shifted up 2 units, so D is $+2$. The distance between the high and low points is 6. The amplitude is one half this value, or 3, so $|A| = 3$. Since a basic cycle starts at 0 and ends at 2π, we know the argument is simply x. Thus, the equation is $y = 3 \cos x + 2$.

2. Find an equation of the sine function in the figure.

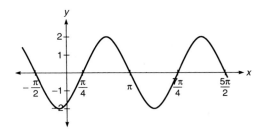

We know that the equation is of the form
$$y = A \sin(Bx + C) + D$$
Since the distance between the high and low points of the graph is 4, we know that A is 2. Also, there is no vertical shift, so D is 0.

We need to find the argument of the function. Note that a cycle of this function starts at $\dfrac{\pi}{4}$ and ends at $\dfrac{7\pi}{4}$. We can work backward from this information.

We know that we get one basic cycle as x takes on values between these two points; that is, $\dfrac{\pi}{4} \le x \le \dfrac{7\pi}{4}$.

Our objective is to arrange the values so that the left value is 0 and the right value is 2π. (Remember, we are working back to the argument of the function.)

First, we want the left value to be 0.

$$\pi \le 4x \le 7\pi \qquad \text{Multiply by 4}$$
$$0 \le 4x - \pi \le 6\pi \qquad \text{Subtract } \pi$$

Now we want the right point to be 2π. Dividing by 3 will do this.

$$\frac{0}{3} \le \frac{4x - \pi}{3} \le \frac{6\pi}{3}$$

$$0 \le \frac{4x}{3} - \frac{\pi}{3} \le 2\pi$$

We thus find the argument is $\dfrac{4x}{3} - \dfrac{\pi}{3}$. Thus, our final answer is

$$y = 2 \sin\left(\frac{4x}{3} - \frac{\pi}{3}\right). \qquad \blacksquare$$

In some applications we want to express values of x in degrees as opposed to radians. Our procedures are the same, except that our limits for the basic cycles are $0°$ and $360°$ instead of 0 and 2π.

■ *Example 3–3 F*

1. An AC (alternating current) signal with peak-to-peak voltage of 170 volts and phase shift of 120°, riding on a DC level of 100 volts, could be described by the function

$$y = 85 \sin(x + 120°) + 100$$

where y represents volts and x is in degrees. Graph one cycle of this function.

Amplitude is 85, and the 100 represents a vertical shift in the positive direction. To find period and phase shift we proceed as follows:

Step 1: $0° \le x + 120° \le 360°$

$-120° \le x \le 240°$

Phase shift is $-120°$ and period is $240° - (-120°) = 360°$. We mark the x-axis in increments of half the period, 180°, starting at $-120°$.

Step 2: We see that a basic cycle begins at $-120°$ and ends at 240°. See the figure.

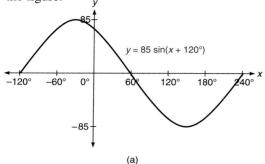

(a)

Step 3: We also label the amplitude, 85. We then shift the graph vertically by 100 units. See the figure.

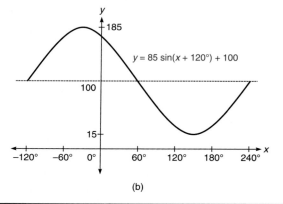

(b)

Put the calculator in DEGREE mode (use the ⬚MODE⬚ key).

⬚Y=⬚ 85 ⬚SIN⬚ ⬚(⬚ ⬚X|T⬚ ⬚+⬚ 120 ⬚)⬚ ⬚+⬚ 100 ⬚ENTER⬚ 100,

⬚RANGE $-130,250,60,-10,190,20$⬚

2. An electronic signal is to be modeled with the sine function. The peak-to-peak voltage is 340 volts (amplitude is 170 volts). There is a phase shift of 30°, and the period is 120°. The signal is at 200 volts above ground potential. (There is a vertical shift of 200.) Find the sine function that will model this signal.

We know that the function is of the form

$$y = A \sin(Bx + C) + D$$

and that $A = 170$ and $D = 200$. To find B and C we can proceed "backward." We know that we get one basic cycle as x varies between 30°, the phase shift, and 30° + 120°, or phase shift + period.

$$30° \leq x \leq 30° + 120°$$

Now adjust this so that phase shift is 0° and period is 360°.

$$30° \leq x \leq 150°$$

Subtract 30° from each expression to get 0° phase shift.

$$0° \leq x - 30° \leq 120°$$

Multiply each term by 3, since this will make the end point 360°.

$$0° \leq 3x - 90° \leq 360°$$

Thus, the argument of the function is $3x - 90°$, and the function we want is

$$y = 170 \sin(3x - 90°) + 200 \qquad \blacksquare$$

Mastery points

Can you
- Graph an equation of the form

$$y = A \sin(Bx + C) + D \text{ or}$$
$$y = A \cos(Bx + C) + D?$$

- Find a sine or cosine equation that is appropriate, given values of A and D and the initial and terminal points of a basic cycle?

Exercise 3–3

Graph three cycles of the following functions.

1. $y = 5 \sin x$

2. $y = 5 \cos x$

3. $y = \frac{2}{3} \cos x$

4. $y = \frac{1}{5} \sin x$

5. $y = -4 \cos x$

6. $y = -2 \sin x$

7. $y = -\frac{1}{3} \sin x$

8. $y = -\frac{5}{2} \sin x$

9. $y = 2 \sin x + 1$

10. $y = 3 \cos x - 2$

11. $y = -\frac{3}{4} \cos x - 2$

12. $y = -\frac{1}{2} \sin x + 3$

Graph three cycles of the following functions. State the amplitude, period, and phase shift of each.

13. $y = 2 \sin 4x$

14. $y = 3 \cos \dfrac{x}{2}$

15. $y = \cos\left(x - \dfrac{\pi}{2}\right)$

16. $y = 3 \sin(2x + \pi)$

17. $y = \frac{2}{3} \sin(3x + \pi)$

18. $y = \frac{5}{8} \cos 5x$

19. $y = -\cos 3x$

20. $y = -\sin x$

21. $y = -\cos\left(2x + \dfrac{\pi}{2}\right)$

22. $y = -\sin\left(3x - \dfrac{\pi}{3}\right)$

23. $y = \sin(3x + 2\pi)$

24. $y = \cos(2x - 3\pi)$

25. $y = \cos 2\pi x$

26. $y = \sin \pi x$

27. $y = 2 \sin 3x + 2$

28. $y = 3 \cos 2x - 3$

29. $y = -3 \cos x + 1$

30. $y = -\sin 4x + 1$

31. $y = 2 \sin(2x - \pi) + 1$

32. $y = 3 \sin(3x + \pi) - 3$

33. $y = \sin \pi x + 1$

34. $y = 2 \cos \dfrac{\pi x}{2} - 2$

Use the odd/even properties of the sine and cosine functions to rewrite each of the following functions as an equivalent function in which the coefficient of x is positive.

35. $y = \sin(-2x)$

36. $y = \cos(-x)$

37. $y = -\cos(-3x)$

38. $y = -\sin(-5x)$

39. $y = \sin(-x - 3)$

40. $y = \cos(-2x + 4)$

41. $y = \sin(-x) - 3$

42. $y = \cos(-2x) + 4$

43. $y = -3 \cos\left(-2x + \dfrac{\pi}{2}\right)$

44. $y = 2 \sin\left(-\dfrac{x}{3} - \pi\right)$

Use the odd/even properties of the sine and cosine functions to rewrite each of the following functions as an equivalent function in which the coefficient of x is positive. Then graph three cycles of the function.

45. $y = \sin(-x)$

46. $y = \cos(-2x)$

47. $y = \cos\left(-x - \dfrac{\pi}{3}\right)$

48. $y = 2 \sin(-2x + \pi)$

49. $y = -\sin(-2\pi x + \pi)$

50. $y = -\cos(-\pi x)$

51. $y = \sin(-\pi x + 1)$

52. $y = 2 \cos(-3\pi x - 2)$

Assume that each of the following graphs is the graph of a sine function of the form $y = A \sin(Bx + C) + D$. Find values of A, B, C, and D that would produce each graph.

53.

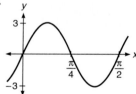

54.

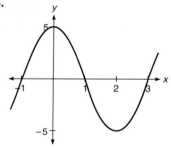

55.

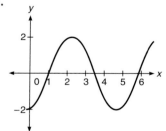

56.

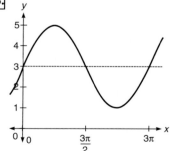

57. Do problem 53, assuming that the graph is a cosine function of the form $y = A \cos(Bx + C) + D$.

58. Do problem 54, assuming that the graph is a cosine function of the form $y = A \cos(Bx + C) + D$.

59. Do problem 55, assuming that the graph is a cosine function of the form $y = A \cos(Bx + C) + D$.

60. Do problem 56, assuming that the graph is a cosine function of the form $y = A \cos(Bx + C) + D$.

Graph one cycle of each of the following functions. Mark the horizontal axis in degrees.

61. $y = 3 \sin(x + 60°)$

62. $y = -50 \cos(x - 120°)$

63. $y = 25 \cos 3x$

64. $y = 10 \sin(2x - 180°)$

65. An electronic signal modeled with the sine function has a peak-to-peak voltage of 120 volts (amplitude is 60 volts), phase shift of 90°, and period of 54°. Find an equation of the sine function that will model this signal.

66. An ocean wave is being modeled with the sine function. Its amplitude is 6 feet and its phase shift (with respect to another wave) is −180°. If the period is 720°, find an equation of the sine function that will model this wave.

67. One of the components of a function that could describe the earth's ice ages for the last 500,000 years is described by a sine function with amplitude 0.5, period $\dfrac{360°}{43}$, 0° phase shift, and vertical translation 23.5. Find an equation for this component.

68. The activity of sunspots seems to follow an 11-year cycle. Assuming that this activity can be roughly modeled with a sine wave, construct a sine function with period $\dfrac{360°}{11}$, amplitude 1, phase shift 90°, and vertical translation 2.

69. Graph the following functions on the same set of axes:

$$y = \sin x; \ y = \sin 3x; \text{ and } y = \sin \frac{x}{3}.$$

70. Graph the following functions on the same set of axes:

$$y = \sin x; \ y = \sin\left(x + \frac{\pi}{2}\right); \text{ and } y = \sin x + \frac{\pi}{2}.$$

71. Graph the following functions on the same set of axes:

$$y = \cos\left(\frac{\pi}{2} - x\right) \text{ and } y = \sin x. \text{ Draw a conclusion from}$$

the graph. $\left[\textit{Hint:} \text{ Rewrite as } y = \cos\left(-x + \dfrac{\pi}{2}\right).\right]$

3–4 *Linear transformations of the tangent, cotangent, secant, and cosecant functions (optional)*

The tangent and cotangent functions

The tangent and cotangent functions are π-periodic, so the basic cycle for each is π units long instead of the 2π units for the sine and cosine functions. Figure 3–22 shows a basic cycle for the tangent and cotangent functions.

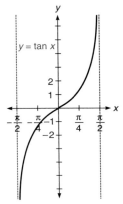
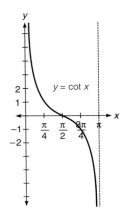

Figure 3–22

Note that the basic tangent cycle starts at $-\dfrac{\pi}{2}$ and ends at $\dfrac{\pi}{2}$. The basic cotangent cycle starts at 0 and ends at π. Also note that the functions are $+1$ or -1 at the points that are $\frac{1}{4}$ and $\frac{3}{4}$ of the distance between the cycle end points. We will call these the *one-quarter* and *three-quarter* points.

Graphing functions of the form $y = A \tan(Bx + C)$ and $y = A \cot(Bx + C)$ is done in a manner very similar to that for the sine and cosine functions. Although the concept of amplitude does not make sense for these functions, the vertical scaling factor A does affect the graph. In fact, these functions take on values of $\pm A$ at the one-quarter and three-quarter points (unless there is a vertical shift) instead of ± 1.

To graph functions of the form
$$y = A \tan(Bx + C) \text{ and}$$
$$y = A \cot(Bx + C)$$

1. For the tangent function, solve
$$-\frac{\pi}{2} < Bx + C < \frac{\pi}{2}$$

   for x.
   For the cotangent function, solve
$$0 < Bx + C < \pi$$

   for x.
2. Step 1 gives the left and right end points for one basic cycle. Draw this cycle. Label the "one-quarter" and "three-quarter" points with $y = A$ and $y = -A$, as appropriate. If $A < 0$, this cycle is reflected about the horizontal axis.
3. Repeat this cycle to obtain as much of the graph as desired.

We will not concern ourselves with defining the period and phase shift for the tangent and cotangent functions. A *guideline* for marking off the x-axis is to use increments of one fourth of the length of one basic cycle to locate the one-quarter and three-quarter points.

■ *Example 3–4 A*

1. Graph $y = \frac{1}{2} \tan 3x$. Show three cycles.

   Step 1: Solve $-\dfrac{\pi}{2} < 3x < \dfrac{\pi}{2}$ for x.

   $-\dfrac{\pi}{6} < x < \dfrac{\pi}{6}$. Divide by 3 (or multiply by $\frac{1}{3}$). The length of one basic cycle is $\dfrac{\pi}{6} - \left(-\dfrac{\pi}{6}\right) = \dfrac{\pi}{3}$. We use $\dfrac{1}{4} \cdot \dfrac{\pi}{3} = \dfrac{\pi}{12}$ increments on the x-axis.

Step 2: We now know that we get one basic tangent cycle starting at $-\frac{\pi}{6}$ and ending at $\frac{\pi}{6}$. We draw vertical asymptotes at these points and sketch one cycle of the tangent function. With the vertical scaling factor of $\frac{1}{2}$ we label the one-quarter and three-quarter points as shown in part (a) of the figure.

Step 3: Two more cycles are shown in part (b) of the figure.

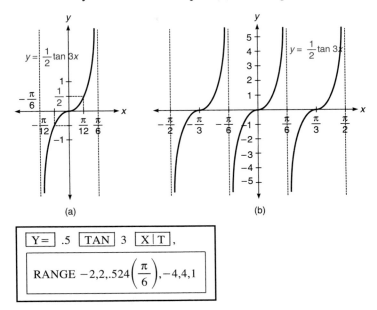

(a)   (b)

$$\boxed{\text{Y=}}\ .5\ \boxed{\text{TAN}}\ 3\ \boxed{\text{X}\,|\,\text{T}}\,,$$

$$\text{RANGE}\ -2,2,.524\left(\frac{\pi}{6}\right),-4,4,1$$

2. Graph $y = \cot\left(2x - \frac{\pi}{3}\right)$. Show three cycles.

Step 1: We put the argument between 0 and π and solve for x:

$$0 < 2x - \frac{\pi}{3} < \pi$$

$$0 < 6x - \pi < 3\pi \qquad \text{Multiply by 3}$$
$$\pi < 6x < 4\pi \qquad\quad \text{Add } \pi$$
$$\frac{\pi}{6} < x < \frac{4\pi}{6} \qquad\quad \text{Divide by 6}$$

or

$$\frac{\pi}{6} < x < \frac{2\pi}{3}$$

A basic cycle is $\dfrac{2\pi}{3} - \dfrac{\pi}{6} = \dfrac{\pi}{2}$ units long. We mark the x-axis by adding or subtracting increments of $\dfrac{\pi}{8}$ units from $\dfrac{\pi}{6}$.

Step 2: We have one basic cycle between $\dfrac{\pi}{6}$ and $\dfrac{2\pi}{3}$; the basic graph is shown in part (a) of the figure.

Step 3: The finished graph, including three cycles, is shown in part (b) of the figure.

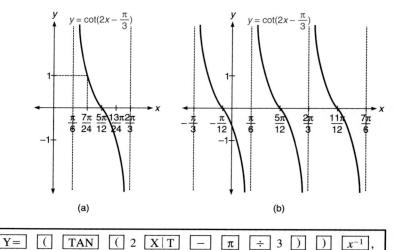

(a)   (b)

$$\boxed{\text{Y}=} \quad \boxed{(} \quad \boxed{\text{TAN}} \quad \boxed{(} \quad \boxed{2} \quad \boxed{\text{X}|\text{T}} \quad \boxed{-} \quad \boxed{\pi} \quad \boxed{\div} \quad \boxed{3} \quad \boxed{)} \quad \boxed{)} \quad \boxed{x^{-1}},$$

$$\boxed{\text{RANGE} \; -1.5, 4, 0.524, -3, 3, 1}$$

If the coefficient of x is negative, we use the fact that the tangent and cotangent functions are odd to rewrite the function with this coefficient positive.

■ *Example 3–4 B*

Graph $y = -\cot(-\pi x)$. Show three cycles.

Since the coefficient of x, $-\pi$, is negative, we rewrite this function as

$$y = \cot \pi x.$$

Step 1: $0 < \pi x < \pi$

$\quad\quad\quad 0 < x < 1$ Divide by π

A basic cycle is 1 unit long, and we use $\frac{1}{4}$ for an increment on the x-axis.

Step 2: One basic cycle is shown in part (a) of the figure.

Step 3: Two more cycles are shown in part (b) of the figure.

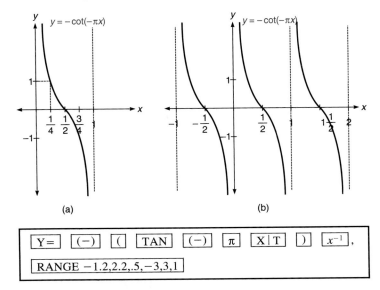

(a)   (b)

$$\boxed{Y=}\ \boxed{(-)}\ \boxed{(}\ \boxed{TAN}\ \boxed{(-)}\ \boxed{\pi}\ \boxed{X\,|\,T}\ \boxed{)}\ \boxed{x^{-1}},$$

$$\boxed{RANGE\ -1.2,2.2,.5,-3,3,1}$$

■

The secant and cosecant functions

To graph variations of the secant and cosecant functions, we use the fact that they are reciprocals of the cosine and sine functions, respectively. Figure 3–11 shows the graph of the cosecant function and figure 3–12 shows the graph of the secant function. Observe that the ranges are $|y| \geq 1$, and that they have vertical asymptotes where their reciprocal function, cosine or sine, is zero.

Consider the graph of a function of the form

$$y = A \csc(Bx + C)$$

We know it is a modification of the graph shown in figure 3–11. Since it is equivalent to the graph of

$$y = A\left(\frac{1}{\sin(Bx + C)}\right)$$

we can construct the graph of $y = \sin(Bx + C)$ and, graphically, form the reciprocal to get the graph we want.

For example, consider the graph of $y = 3 \csc 2x$. This will have the same graph as $y = 3\left(\dfrac{1}{\sin 2x}\right)$. Thus, we can first graph $y = \sin 2x$ and graphically form the reciprocal, as we did in section 3–3.

The graph of $y = \sin 2x$ is shown in figure 3–23. In figure 3–24 we show the graph of $y = \dfrac{1}{\sin 2x}$. We do this by drawing vertical asymptotes wherever $\sin 2x$ is zero, and letting the reciprocal graph go to infinity as $\sin 2x$ gets closer and closer to zero.

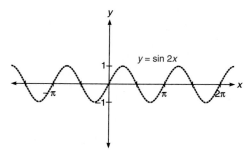

Figure 3–23

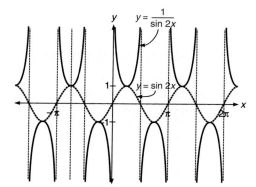

Figure 3–24

In figure 3–25 we show the graph of $y = 3\left(\dfrac{1}{\sin 2x}\right)$. Each point is three times higher or lower than each corresponding point on the graph in figure 3–25. This is also the graph we wanted originally.

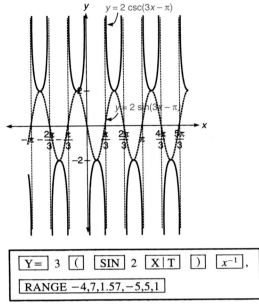

Figure 3–25

Observe that we could have originally graphed $y = 3 \sin 2x$ and used this as our guide, since in the graph of $y = 3 \sin 2x$, $|y| \leq 3$, while in the graph of $y = 3 \csc 2x$, $|y| \geq 3$.

Based on this example, and what we have done in the preceding sections of this chapter, we can state the following.

Procedure for graphing functions of the form

$$y = A \csc(Bx + C) \text{ and}$$
$$y = A \sec(Bx + C)$$

1. Graph $y = A \sin(Bx + C)$ or $y = A \cos(Bx + C)$, whichever is the appropriate reciprocal function.
2. Graphically form the reciprocal by drawing vertical asymptotes wherever the graph in step 1 is 0, and draw the graph getting larger and larger in absolute value wherever the reciprocal function approaches 0.

■ *Example 3–4 C*

Graph $y = 2 \csc(3x - \pi)$.

Step 1: Graph $y = 2 \sin(3x - \pi)$.

$$0 \le 3x - \pi \le 2\pi$$
$$\pi \le 3x \le 3\pi$$
$$\frac{\pi}{3} \le x \le \pi$$

Four cycles are shown in the first figure. We draw this graph using dashed lines, because it is not part of the graph we have been asked to show.

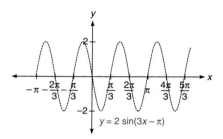

$y = 2 \sin(3x - \pi)$

Step 2: We draw vertical asymptotes wherever the graph of $y = 2 \sin(3x - \pi)$ is 0; that is, where it crosses the x-axis. We then form the reciprocal function, as shown in the next figure.

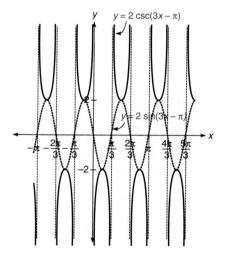

$y = 2 \csc(3x - \pi)$

$y = 2 \sin(3x - \pi)$

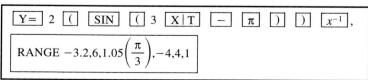

If the coefficient of x is negative, we use the odd/even properties of the sine and cosine functions as appropriate.

■ *Example 3–4 D*

Graph $y = 2 \csc\left(-\dfrac{2\pi x}{3}\right)$.

Step 1: Graph $y = 2 \sin\left(-\dfrac{2\pi x}{3}\right)$. Since the argument is negative, we use the

odd property of the sine function to rewrite this as $y = -2 \sin \dfrac{2\pi x}{3}$.

$$0 \le \frac{2\pi x}{3} \le 2\pi$$
$$0 \le 2\pi x \le 6\pi \qquad \text{Multiply by 3}$$
$$0 \le x \le 3 \qquad \text{Divide by } 2\pi$$

The graph of $y = -2 \sin \dfrac{2\pi x}{3}$ is shown in the figure, part (a).

Step 2: The reciprocal function is shown in part (b) of the figure.

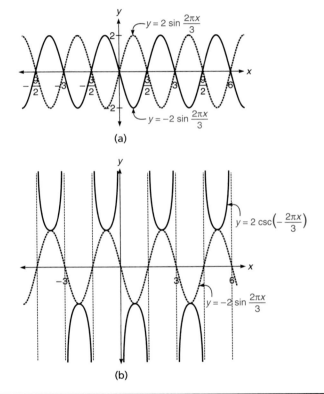

(a)

(b)

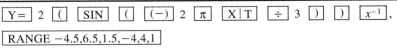

Y= 2 (SIN ((−) 2 π X|T ÷ 3)) x^{-1} ,

RANGE −4.5,6.5,1.5,−4,4,1

■

Mastery points

Can you
- Graph functions of the form

$$y = A \tan(Bx + C), \text{ and}$$
$$y = A \cot(Bx + C)?$$

- Graph functions of the form

$$y = A \sec(Bx + C) \text{ and}$$
$$y = A \csc(Bx + C)?$$

Exercise 3-4

Graph three cycles of the following functions.

1. $y = 5 \tan x$ **2.** $y = -4 \cot x$ **3.** $y = \tan 4x$ **4.** $y = \cot \dfrac{x}{2}$

5. $y = \cot\left(x - \dfrac{\pi}{2}\right)$ **6.** $y = 3 \tan(2x + \pi)$ **7.** $y = -\cot\left(2x + \dfrac{\pi}{2}\right)$ **8.** $y = -\tan\left(3x - \dfrac{\pi}{3}\right)$

9. $y = \cot 2\pi x$ **10.** $y = \tan \pi x$

Use the odd/even properties of the tangent and cotangent functions to rewrite each of the following functions as an equivalent function in which the coefficient of x is positive. Then graph three cycles of the function.

11. $y = \tan(-2x)$ **12.** $y = \cot(-x)$ **13.** $y = -\cot(-\pi x)$

14. $y = -\tan(-2\pi x)$ **15.** $y = \tan(-x - \pi)$ **16.** $y = \cot(-2x + 4\pi)$

Graph three cycles of the following functions.

17. $y = \frac{2}{3} \csc x$ **18.** $y = \frac{1}{5} \sec x$ **19.** $y = -4 \csc x$ **20.** $y = 2 \sec 4x$

21. $y = 3 \csc \dfrac{x}{2}$ **22.** $y = \csc\left(x - \dfrac{\pi}{2}\right)$ **23.** $y = 3 \sec(2x + \pi)$ **24.** $y = \frac{2}{3} \sec(3x + \pi)$

25. $y = \csc(2x - 3\pi)$ **26.** $y = \csc 2\pi x$ **27.** $y = \sec \pi x$

Use the odd/even properties of the sine and cosine functions to graph each of the following functions.

28. $y = \sec(-2x)$ **29.** $y = \csc(-x)$ **30.** $y = 3 \csc\left(-2x + \dfrac{\pi}{2}\right)$ **31.** $y = 2 \sec\left(-\dfrac{x}{3} - \pi\right)$

Chapter 3 summary

- **Basic graphs**
- Graph of the sine and cosine functions.

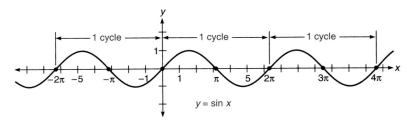

$$y = \sin x$$

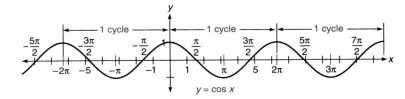

$$y = \cos x$$

- Graph of the tangent function.

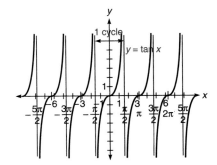

$$y = \tan x$$

- To graph sine and cosine functions of the form

  $$y = A \sin(Bx + C) + D \text{ and}$$
  $$y = A \cos(Bx + C) + D, \text{ where } B > 0$$

  1. Solve $0 \leq Bx + C \leq 2\pi$ so x is the middle member.
     - This gives the left and right end points for one basic cycle.
     - The left end point is the phase shift.
     - The difference between the end points is the period.

2. The amplitude is $|A|$.
   - This is the height of the basic graph above and below the x-axis.
   - The graph is shifted about the horizontal axis if $A < 0$.

   Draw one basic cycle with the information from steps 1 and 2.

3. Repeat the cycle obtained from steps 1 to 3 to obtain more of the graph.

4. Shift the graph vertically D units.

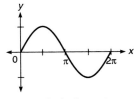
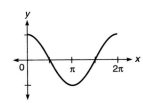

Basic sine cycle   Basic cosine cycle

- If the coefficient of x, B, is negative in the argument $Bx + C$ we first use the odd and even properties to get an equivalent expression with B positive.

- To graph functions of the form
$$y = A \tan(Bx + C) \text{ and}$$
$$y = A \cot(Bx + C), B > 0$$

1. For the tangent function, solve $-\dfrac{\pi}{2} < Bx + C$

$< \dfrac{\pi}{2}$ for x; for the cotangent function solve

$0 < Bx + C < \pi$ for x. This gives the left and right end points for one basic cycle. The difference between the end points is the period. The left end point is the phase shift.

2. Use the values from step 1 to draw one basic cycle. Label the one-quarter and three-quarter points with $y = A$ and $y = -A$ as appropriate. Repeat this cycle to obtain as much of the graph as desired.

Basic tangent cycle   Basic cotangent cycle

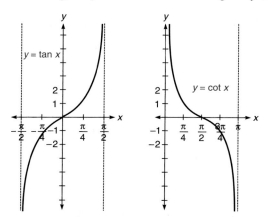

- To graph $y = A \csc(Bx + C)$ or $y = A \sec(Bx + C)$:
  1. Graph the appropriate reciprocal function,
  $$y = A \sin(Bx + C) \text{ or } y = A \cos(Bx + C)$$

  2. Sketch in vertical asymptotes wherever the sine or cosine function is zero.

3. Create the cosecant or secant graph by starting at the highest and lowest points of the sine or cosine graph and sketching values that increase in absolute value from that point as x approaches the vertical asymptotes. Note that these functions are not defined at the asymptotes.

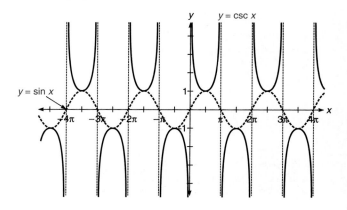

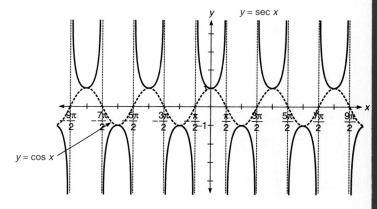

- Summary of the properties of the sine, cosine, and tangent functions (k an integer).

Function	Domain	Range	Period
$y = \sin x$	R	$-1 \le y \le 1$	2π
$y = \cos x$	R	$-1 \le y \le 1$	2π
$y = \tan x$	$x \ne \dfrac{\pi}{2} + k\pi$	R	π

$$\sin(-x) = -\sin x \quad \text{(odd)}$$
$$\cos(-x) = \cos x \quad \text{(even)}$$
$$\tan(-x) = -\tan x \quad \text{(odd)}$$

- Summary of the properties of the cosecant, secant, and cotangent functions (k an integer).

Function	Domain	Range	Period
$y = \csc x$	$x \ne k\pi$	$\lvert y \rvert \ge 1$	2π
$y = \sec x$	$x \ne \dfrac{\pi}{2} + k\pi$	$\lvert y \rvert \ge 1$	2π
$y = \cot x$	$x \ne k\pi$	R	π

$$\csc(-x) = -\csc x \quad \text{(odd)}$$
$$\sec(-x) = \sec x \quad \text{(even)}$$
$$\cot(-x) = -\cot x \quad \text{(odd)}$$

Chapter 3 review

[3–1]

1. Sketch the graph of the sine function; state the domain, range, and period of the sine function.
2. Using the graph of $y = \cos x$ as a guide, describe all values of x for which $\cos x$ is 1.

Use the appropriate property, even or odd, to calculate the exact function value.

3. $\cos\left(-\dfrac{\pi}{6}\right)$

4. $\tan\left(-\dfrac{4\pi}{3}\right)$

5. $\sin\left(-\dfrac{5\pi}{6}\right)$

6. $\sec\left(-\dfrac{\pi}{4}\right)$

Test the function for the even/odd property.

7. $f(x) = \dfrac{x^2 - 1}{x}$

8. $f(x) = x \sin x$

9. $f(x) = \tan x \cdot \cos x$

[3–2]

10. Sketch the graph of the cosecant function.
11. State the domain and range of the cotangent function.
12. Show that $f(x) = \dfrac{x}{\sec x}$ is an odd function.
13. Show that the function $f(x) = \sec x \cdot \sin^2 x + x^4$ is an even function.

[3–3] Graph three cycles of the following functions. State the amplitude, period, and phase shift of each.

14. $y = 2 \sin x$

15. $y = -\frac{2}{3} \cos x$

16. $y = 3 \sin x - 2$

17. $y = 2 \sin 3x$

18. $y = \cos\left(x + \dfrac{\pi}{3}\right)$

19. $y = 2 \sin\left(\dfrac{x}{2} + \dfrac{\pi}{3}\right)$

20. $y = \cos 3x\pi$

21. $y = 3 \cos 2x - 3$

Use the odd/even properties of the sine and cosine functions to rewrite each of the following functions as an equivalent function in which the coefficient of x is positive. Then graph three cycles of the function.

22. $y = \cos\left(-2x + \dfrac{\pi}{2}\right)$

23. $y = 3 \sin(-x + \pi)$

24. Graph three cycles of the function $y = 2 \sin(3x + 60°)$. Mark the horizontal axis in degrees.

25. Assume that the following graph is of a cosine function of the form $y = A \cos(Bx + C) + D$. Find the values of A, B, C, and D and rewrite the function using these values.

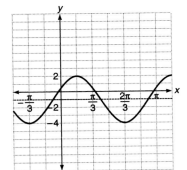

26. Most people have heard about the theory of biorhythms. This theory maintains that at birth three cycles are started—physical, emotional, and intellectual. The physical cycle has a period of 23 (days). Assuming an amplitude of 1, a phase shift of −10 (days), and no vertical translation, create an equation that describes the physical cycle in terms of the sine function.

[3–4] Graph three cycles of the following functions.

27. $y = \tan 4x$

28. $y = \tan(3x + \pi)$

29. $y = 2 \cot\left(x - \dfrac{\pi}{4}\right)$

30. $y = -2 \sec 3x$

31. $y = \csc \dfrac{x}{2}$

32. $y = \sec(2x - \pi)$

33. $y = \csc 3\pi x$

Chapter 3 test

1. Using the graph of $y = \sin x$ as a guide, describe all values of x for which $\sin x$ is -1.

2. Use the appropriate property, even or odd, to calculate the exact function value of $\tan\left(-\dfrac{5\pi}{3}\right)$.

3. Test the function $f(x) = x + \sin x$ for the even/odd property.

Graph three cycles of the following functions. State the amplitude, period, and phase shift of each.

4. $y = 2 \sin x + 2$

5. $y = 3 \cos 2x$

6. $y = 3 \sin\left(\dfrac{x}{3} + \dfrac{\pi}{2}\right)$

Graph three cycles of the following functions.

7. $y = 3 \tan \pi x$

8. $y = \sec(3x - \pi)$

9. $y = -\csc 4\pi x$

10. Assume that the graph is of the form $y = A \sin(Bx + C) + D$. Find values of A, B, C, and D that would produce the graph and write the corresponding equation.

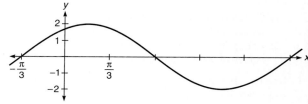

11. Sketch the graph of the secant function.

12. Show that the function $f(x) = \sec x \cdot \sin x + x^3$ is an odd function.

13. In the theory of biorhythms, the emotional cycle has a period of 28 (days). Assuming an amplitude of 1, a phase shift of 5 (days), and no vertical translation, create an equation that describes the emotional cycle in terms of the sine function.

14. An electronic signal is to be modeled with the sine function. Amplitude is 25 volts, phase shift is $-20°$, period is $150°$, and there is a vertical shift of 10 volts. Find a sine function that will model this signal.

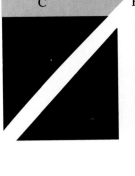

The Inverse Trigonometric Functions

In previous chapters we have used what we called the inverse trigonometric functions. For example, we stated that if $\sin \theta = 0.3$, then one value of θ is $\theta = \sin^{-1} 0.3$. In this chapter we examine these inverse trigonometric functions in complete detail.

We use these functions both to solve trigonometric equations like that in the last paragraph, to solve triangles, and to describe angles in terms of given information. These functions are also useful in advanced mathematics (calculus in particular) where they provide a means to simplify certain algebraic expressions.

We begin the chapter by examining the general topic of inverse functions, and then apply this topic to trigonometry.

4–1 The inverse of a function

In section 2–1 we introduced the idea of the inverse of a function. We stated that

- A function is a set of ordered pairs in which no first element is repeated.
- A one-to-one function is a function in which no second element is repeated.
- Reversing the elements of the ordered pairs of a function produces a function if, and only if, the function is one to one.

For example,

$$H = \{(1,5), (2,7), (-5,-5)\}$$

is a one-to-one function, and its inverse function is

$$H^{-1} = \{(5,1), (7,2), (-5,-5)\}$$

133

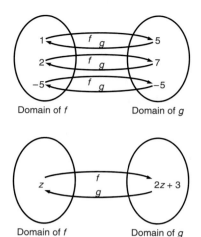

Domain of f   Domain of g

Domain of f   Domain of g

Figure 4–1

Showing that two given functions are inverses

Now consider the two functions $f(x) = 2x + 3$ and $g(x) = \dfrac{x - 3}{2}$. By computation we could determine the following facts.

$$f(1) = 5 \text{ and } g(5) = 1$$
$$f(2) = 7 \text{ and } g(7) = 2$$
$$f(-5) = -7 \text{ and } g(-7) = -5$$

(Compare to H and H^{-1} on page 133 and figure 4–1.)

Whatever value z we try, f sends z to some value z', and g sends z' back to z. In fact we can prove this; let z represent any real number. Then,

$$f(z) = 2z + 3 \text{ and}$$
$$g(2z + 3) = \frac{(2z + 3) - 3}{2} = z$$

Also

$$g(z) = \frac{z - 3}{2} \text{ and}$$
$$f\left(\frac{z - 3}{2}\right) = 2\left(\frac{z - 3}{2}\right) + 3 = z$$

When two functions f and g act this way we say they are inverse functions. This is because, whenever an ordered pair (a,b) is in f, the ordered pair formed by reversing its elements (b,a) is in g. The functions H and H^{-1}, and f and g, above, are examples of this.

The notation for the inverse of a function is the superscript -1, so using this notation, if $f(x) = 2x + 3$ (as above) we can say that $f^{-1}(x) = \dfrac{x - 3}{2}$. Note the superscript -1, when applied to the name of a function, is *not* an exponent; it does not indicate division, as it does if applied as an exponent of a real valued expression.

$$f^{-1}(x) \text{ does not mean } \frac{1}{f(x)}$$

> **To show that two functions *f* and *g* are inverses of each other**
> Show that
> [1]   If $f(x) = y$, then $g(y) = x$, and
> [2]   If $g(x) = y$, then $f(y) = x$.

Note   In practice "*y*" represents an expression in *x*.

■ *Example 4–1 A*

Show that f and g are the inverse functions of each other.

1. $f(x) = \frac{1}{3}x - 1$; $g(x) = 3x + 3$

  [1]   Assume $f(x) = y$, then $y = \frac{1}{3}x - 1$.   Replace $f(x)$ by y

     Show that $g(y) = x$:

$$g(y) = 3y + 3 \qquad\qquad \text{Replace } x \text{ by } y \text{ in } g(x) = 3x + 3$$
$$= 3(\tfrac{1}{3}x - 1) + 3 \qquad \text{Replace } y \text{ by } \tfrac{1}{3}x - 1$$
$$= x - 3 + 3$$
$$= x$$

  [2]   Assume $g(x) = y$, then $y = 3x + 3$.

     Show that $f(y) = x$:

$$f(y) = \tfrac{1}{3}y - 1 \qquad\qquad \text{Replace } x \text{ by } y \text{ in } f(x) = \tfrac{1}{3}x - 1$$
$$= \tfrac{1}{3}(3x + 3) - 1 \qquad \text{Replace } y \text{ by } 3x + 3$$
$$= x + 1 - 1$$
$$= x$$

Thus, we have shown conditions [1] and [2] above, so f and g are inverse functions.

2. $f(x) = \sqrt{x}$; $g(x) = x^2$, $x \geq 0$

  [1] $y = \sqrt{x}$ Let y represent $f(x)$

$$g(y) = y^2 \qquad\qquad \text{Determine } g(y)$$
$$= (\sqrt{x})^2$$
$$= x \qquad\qquad (\sqrt{a})^2 = a$$

  [2] $y = x^2$, $x \geq 0$ Let y represent $g(x)$

$$f(y) = \sqrt{y} \qquad\qquad \text{Determine } f(y)$$
$$= \sqrt{x^2}$$
$$= x \qquad\qquad \sqrt{a^2} = a \text{ if } a \geq 0$$

Thus, we have shown conditions [1] and [2], so f and g are inverse functions.   ■

Graphical analysis of relations for the function and one-to-one properties

The graph of a relation can be used to determine whether that relation is a function, and whether or not a function is one to one. This is done by the **vertical line test** and the **horizontal line test**.

> **Vertical line test for a function**
> If no vertical line crosses the graph of a relation in more than one place, the relation is a function.

The vertical line test works for the following reason. Assume a vertical line crosses a graph at more than one point. Since these two points are in a vertical line their first components (the *x*-values) are equal. Therefore, the function must have two points in which the first element repeats, and it is therefore not a function.

> **Horizontal line test for a one-to-one function**
> If no horizontal line crosses the graph of a function in more than one place, the function is one to one.

The horizontal line test works for reasons similar to those for the vertical line test. If a horizontal line crosses a function at two (or more) points, then these are different domain elements (first components) with the same range elements (second component). Therefore the function is not one to one.

■ *Example 4–1 B*

Tell which relations are functions, and which functions are one to one.

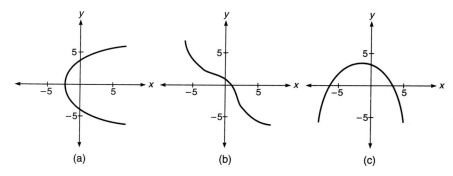

(a)   (b)   (c)

1. Relation (a) is not a function since there are clearly many vertical lines that would intersect the graph in at least two places.

2. Relation (b) is a function since no vertical line will intersect the graph in more than one place. It is also one to one since no horizontal line will intersect the graph in more than one place.

3. Relation (c) is a function by the vertical line test, but not a one-to-one function. ■

The graph of a function's inverse

The fact that the ordered pairs reverse in a function's inverse function means that *the graph of f^{-1} is a reflection of the graph of f about the line y = x.* By way of example, observe the graphs of the functions in example 4–1 A. These are shown in figure 4–2. To draw a graph that is symmetric about the line $y = x$ to a given graph, we draw lines perpendicular to the line $y = x$, as shown, and plot points at equal distances from this line, but on the other side of this line. Since the ordered pairs of f all reverse in f^{-1} *the domain of f is the range of f^{-1}, and the range of f is the domain of f^{-1}.*

$g(x) = 3x + 3$ (0,3) $y = x$
(−1,0) (3,0)
−4   4
(0,−1)
$f(x) = \frac{1}{3}x − 1$

$g(x) = x^2, x \geq 0$ (3,9) $y = x$
(2,4)
(4,2)
(9,3)
$f(x) = \sqrt{x}$
1   5   10

Figure 4–2

■ *Example 4–1 C*

Given the graph of the one-to-one function f, sketch the graph of its inverse function f^{-1}.

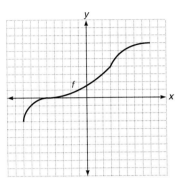

To graph f^{-1} we construct the line $y = x$, which is a straight line passing through the origin with a slope of 1. We then construct various straight lines perpendicular to this line, starting on the graph of the function, and extending an equal distance to the other side of the line $y = x$.

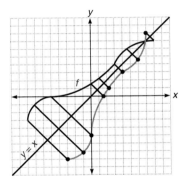

Connecting the points that result from this process gives the graph of f^{-1}.

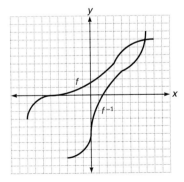

■

Mastery points

Can you
- Demonstrate that two functions are inverses of each other?
- Given a graph that represents a one-to-one function, graph its inverse function?

Exercise 4–1

Show that the following functions f and g are inverses of each other. Assume the domains as indicated are correct.

1. $f(x) = 2x - 7;\ g(x) = \frac{1}{2}x + 3\frac{1}{2}$

2. $f(x) = -\frac{1}{3}x + \frac{1}{2}\ ;\ g(x) = -3x + \frac{3}{2}$

3. $f(x) = \frac{1}{3}x + \frac{8}{3}\ ;\ g(x) = 3x - 8$

4. $f(x) = x - 1;\ g(x) = x + 1$

5. $f(x) = 2x - 5;\ g(x) = \frac{1}{2}(x + 5)$

6. $f(x) = \frac{x}{5} - 3;\ g(x) = 5(x + 3)$

7. $f(x) = \dfrac{2}{x - 3}\ ;\ g(x) = \dfrac{2}{x} + 3$

8. $f(x) = \dfrac{3}{x + 2}\ ;\ g(x) = \dfrac{3}{x} - 2$

9. $f(x) = 7 - \dfrac{3}{x}\ ;\ g(x) = \dfrac{3}{7 - x}$

10. $f(x) = 5 + \dfrac{3}{x - 1}\ ;\ g(x) = \dfrac{3}{x - 5} + 1$

11. $f(x) = \dfrac{x}{x - 1}\ ;\ g(x) = \dfrac{x}{x - 1}$

12. $f(x) = \dfrac{x + 1}{x - 5}\ ;\ g(x) = \dfrac{5x + 1}{x - 1}$

13. $f(x) = x^2 - 9,\ x \geq 0;\ g(x) = \sqrt{x + 9}$

14. $f(x) = \sqrt{4 - 2x};\ g(x) = 2 - \frac{1}{2}x^2,\ x \geq 0$

15. $f(x) = x^3;\ g(x) = \sqrt[3]{x}$

16. $f(x) = x^3 - 3;\ g(x) = \sqrt[3]{x + 3}$

17. $f(x) = x^2 - 2x + 3,\ x \geq 1;\ g(x) = \sqrt{x - 2} + 1$

18. $f(x) = \sqrt{x + 9} - 2;\ g(x) = x^2 + 4x - 5,\ x \geq -2$

19. $f(x) = \dfrac{2x}{x - 3}\ ;\ g(x) = \dfrac{3x}{x - 2}$

20. $f(x) = \dfrac{x - 3}{x - 2}\ ;\ g(x) = 2 - \dfrac{1}{x - 1}$

Tell which relation is a function, and which functions are one to one.

21.

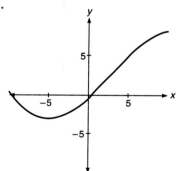

22.

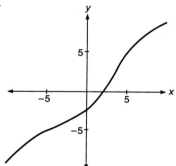

23.

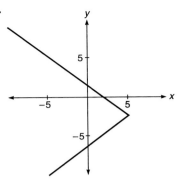

24.

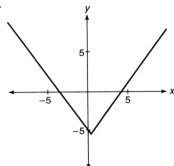

Sketch the graph of f^{-1}, given the graph of the one-to-one function f.

25.

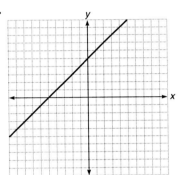

26.

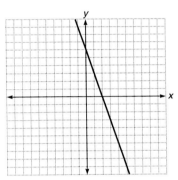

27.

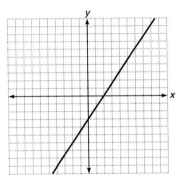

28.

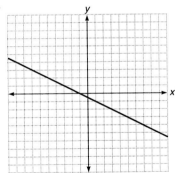

29.

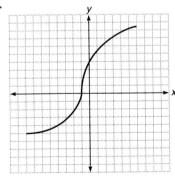

30.

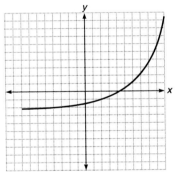

31.

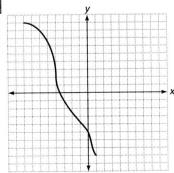

32.

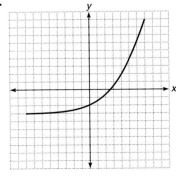

When a function is described by an algebraic expression involving polynomials and radicals, the inverse of the function can often be found by the following procedure, which is described in terms of the variables x and y, but could be in terms of any two variables:

1. Replace the $f(x)$ symbol by y.
2. Exchange the two variables; replace x by y and y by x.
3. Solve for y. The resulting expression in x describes the inverse function.

Example

Find the inverse of the function $f(x) = \dfrac{x + 1}{x}$.

1. Replace the $f(x)$ symbol by y:
$$y = \frac{x + 1}{x}$$
2. Exchange x and y variables:
$$x = \frac{y + 1}{y}$$
3. Solve for y:
$$xy = y + 1$$
$$xy - y = 1 \qquad \text{All } y \text{ terms on one side}$$
$$y(x - 1) = 1$$
$$y = \frac{1}{x - 1}$$

This is f^{-1}:
$$f^{-1}(x) = \frac{1}{x - 1}$$ ∎

33. The area of a rectangle with width 4 and length $x + 4$, $x \geq 0$, is $A(x) = 4(x + 4)$. Find the inverse of A, which would give the value of x for a given area.

34. A falling object with no initial vertical velocity falls a distance $d(t) = 16t^2$ feet in t seconds, $t > 0$. Find the inverse of this function, which would give the time necessary to fall a distance d.

35. In an electronic circuit in which two resistances are in parallel, and the value of the resistances are 20 ohms and x ohms, the total resistance is $R(x) = \dfrac{20x}{20 + x}$. Find the inverse of this function, which would give the value of x required for a total resistance R.

36. $C(t) = \frac{5}{9}(t - 32)$ gives the centigrade temperature for a given temperature t in degrees Fahrenheit. Find the inverse of this function, which would find the Fahrenheit temperature for a given temperature in degrees centigrade.

4–2 The inverse sine function

We have already encountered the inverse sine, cosine, and tangent functions in sections 1–3, 1–4, 2–3, 2–4, and 2–6. In these sections we solved for θ in equations such as $\sin \theta = 0.5$. We know that one solution is $\theta = 30°$, or $\theta = \dfrac{\pi}{6}$ (radians). Using the sine function in reverse in this way is really using the inverse sine function, which we will study in this section.

In section 2–1 we said that the inverse of a function is formed by interchanging the first and second components of all of the ordered pairs in the function and that a function has an inverse if and only if it is a one-to-one function. Since the sine function, like any other function, is a set of ordered pairs, we may ask if it has an inverse. Naturally, it does *only* if it is one to one. The sine function is, however, not one to one. We can see this by looking at its graph in figure 4–3. Note the horizontal line $y = \frac{1}{2}$. This line intersects with (crosses) the graph at many points: $\dfrac{\pi}{6}, \dfrac{5\pi}{6}, \dfrac{13\pi}{6}, \dfrac{17\pi}{6}$, etc. The points of intersection show all of the places where the sine function is $\frac{1}{2}$. Since there

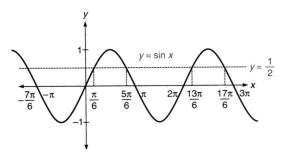

Figure 4–3

is more than one such point, there is more than one ordered pair in the sine function that has $\frac{1}{2}$ as its second element. Some of these ordered pairs are $\left(\frac{\pi}{6}, \frac{1}{2}\right)$, $\left(\frac{5\pi}{6}, \frac{1}{2}\right)$, $\left(\frac{13\pi}{6}, \frac{1}{2}\right)$, etc. Thus, there is a repetition in the second element of these ordered pairs, and the sine function is, therefore, not one to one.

In general, if we can find a horizontal line that intersects the graph of a function in more than one point, then the function cannot be one to one. This graphic test is the horizontal line test, presented in section 4–1.

Since we can quickly see from our knowledge of the graphs of the six trigonometric functions (see chapter 3) that they would all fail the horizontal line test, we know that none of these functions is one to one.

Experience has shown, however, that there is a real need for inverses of these functions. By compromising a little, we can indeed define inverse functions for the six trigonometric functions. The compromise we must make is to form the inverse of only a small part of each function. This part is chosen so that it will include the entire range of the given function but will be one to one. We do this by limiting the domain.

For the sine function we select that portion whose ordered pairs are defined for $-\frac{\pi}{2} \le x \le \frac{\pi}{2}$. See figure 4–4. Note that this new function is one to one, since there is no horizontal line that would intersect the graph in more than one point. Since it is one to one, it has an inverse function. This inverse function is denoted by $\sin^{-1}$, which is read "inverse sine function." The ordered pairs of this inverse sine function are the reversals of the ordered pairs of the one-to-one portion of the sine function we selected.

We know that if $y = \sin^{-1}x$, then the ordered pair (x,y) is in the inverse sine function. The ordered pair (y,x) is therefore in the selected one-to-one portion of the sine function. If (y,x) is in this part of the sine function, then

$$-\frac{\pi}{2} \le y \le \frac{\pi}{2} \text{ and } x = \sin y.$$

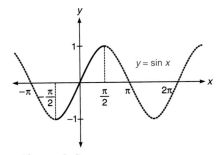

Figure 4–4

Note   Remember that if an ordered pair is in the sine function, then the second element of the pair is the sine of the first.

Using the previous statements as a guide, we make the following definition of the inverse sine function.

> ### The inverse sine function
>
> $y = \sin^{-1}x$ means
>
> 1. $\sin y = x$
> 2. $-\dfrac{\pi}{2} \le y \le \dfrac{\pi}{2}$
> 3. $|x| \le 1$
>
> #### Concept
> If we think of $\sin^{-1}x$ as representing an angle, and since we know that angles between $-\dfrac{\pi}{2}$ and $\dfrac{\pi}{2}$ are in the first and fourth quadrants, we can interpret $y = \sin^{-1}x$ in the following way: "$\sin^{-1}x$ is the angle in quadrant I or quadrant IV whose sine is x." (We are referring to negative angles in quadrant IV.)

The domain of the inverse sine function is $-1 \le x \le 1$, or $|x| \le 1$, which is the range of the sine function. The range of the inverse sine function is

$-\dfrac{\pi}{2} \le \sin^{-1}x \le \dfrac{\pi}{2}$, which is the domain of the one-to-one portion of the sine function that we selected. Note that these are parts 2 and 3 of the definition. More explicitly,

$$\text{Domain}_{\sin^{-1}}\colon |x| \le 1$$
$$\text{Range}_{\sin^{-1}}\colon -\frac{\pi}{2} \le y \le \frac{\pi}{2}$$

Another notation for $\sin^{-1}x$ is **arcsin** x. This is because an arc on the unit circle can represent an angle, and so arcsin x means "the arc (angle) whose sine is x, in quadrant I or quadrant IV." With the advent of the electronic calculator a third notation might be **invsin** x, since a key $\boxed{\text{INV}}$ is used on some calculators to find inverse sine values.

The graph of the inverse of any function can be found by reflecting each point in the graph of the function across the line $y = x$, as seen in section 4–1.

To graph $y = \sin^{-1}x$, we reflect the one-to-one portion of the graph of $y = \sin x$ (figure 4–4) across the line $y = x$. The reflecting process is illustrated in figure 4–5, and the final graph of $y = \sin^{-1}x$ is shown in figure 4–6.

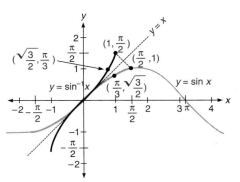

Figure 4–5

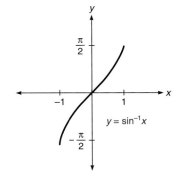

$Y_1 = \sin^{-1} X$
$\boxed{\text{RANGE } -3,3,.5,-2,2,.785}$

Figure 4–6

Although the inverse trigonometric functions are defined using radian measure, we often want the result in degrees. For the inverse sine function we therefore want angles between $-90°$ and $90°$, since these correspond to $-\dfrac{\pi}{2}$ and $\dfrac{\pi}{2}$ radians.

■ *Example 4–2 A*

1. Find $\sin^{-1}\frac{1}{2}$ in both radians and degrees.

   To use the definition, we write $y = \sin^{-1}\frac{1}{2}$. Then we know that

   $$\sin y = \tfrac{1}{2}$$

   and

   $$-\frac{\pi}{2} \le y \le \frac{\pi}{2}$$

   We know that $\sin \dfrac{\pi}{6} = \dfrac{1}{2}$, and $\dfrac{\pi}{6}$ is between $-\dfrac{\pi}{2}$ and $\dfrac{\pi}{2}$, so $y = \dfrac{\pi}{6} = \sin^{-1}\frac{1}{2}$.

   It is often easier to solve these problems if we restate them verbally. Remember that $\sin^{-1}\frac{1}{2}$ can be interpreted to mean "the angle in quadrant I or quadrant IV whose sine is $\frac{1}{2}$." We have memorized the fact that this is $\dfrac{\pi}{6}$.

   Thus, $\sin^{-1}\dfrac{1}{2} = \dfrac{\pi}{6}$. Note that this corresponds to $30°$.

2. Find $\arcsin\left(-\dfrac{\sqrt{2}}{2}\right)$ in both radians and degrees.

We are asked to find the angle in quadrant I or quadrant IV whose sine is $-\dfrac{\sqrt{2}}{2}$. Since the sine function is positive in quadrant I, we must look in quadrant IV. We know that $\sin\dfrac{\pi}{4} = \dfrac{\sqrt{2}}{2}$, so we use $\dfrac{\pi}{4}$ as a reference angle to find that the angle we want is $-\dfrac{\pi}{4}$.

Thus, $\arcsin\left(-\dfrac{\sqrt{2}}{2}\right) = -\dfrac{\pi}{4}$. This corresponds to $-45°$.   ■

We memorized the sine values for certain angles, such as $\dfrac{\pi}{6}$ (30°), $\dfrac{\pi}{4}$ (45°), and $\dfrac{\pi}{3}$ (60°). In most cases, however, we can obtain only decimal approximations. For this we use calculators, as shown below and in sections 1–3, 1–4, 2–4, and 2–6. We will round radian answers to two decimal places and degree answers to one decimal place.

■ *Example 4–2 B*

1. Find $\sin^{-1}0.5312$ in both radians and degrees.

Put the calculator in radian mode. Most calculators use either a $\boxed{\text{SIN}^{-1}}$ key or the $\boxed{\text{INV}}$ (or $\boxed{\text{ARC}}$ or $\boxed{\text{2nd}}$) before the $\boxed{\text{SIN}}$ key.

.5312 $\boxed{\text{INV}}$ $\boxed{\text{SIN}}$ or   Display: $\boxed{0.560016290}$

.5312 $\boxed{\text{SIN}^{-1}}$

$\boxed{\text{TI-81}}$ $\boxed{\text{2nd}}$ $\boxed{\text{SIN}}$ .5312 $\boxed{\text{ENTER}}$

Thus, $\sin^{-1}0.5312 \approx 0.56$.

To obtain the result in degrees, put the calculator in degree mode before performing the calculations. When we round to one decimal place, we get 32.1°.

2. Find $\arcsin(-0.9249)$ in both radians and degrees.

We want the arc (angle) whose sine is -0.9249 and is in quadrant I or quadrant IV. The negative value tells us we want an angle in quadrant IV.

Make sure the calculator is in radian mode.

.9249 $\boxed{+/-}$ $\boxed{\text{INV}}$ $\boxed{\text{SIN}}$ (or $\boxed{\text{SIN}^{-1}}$) Display: $\boxed{-1.180772498}$

$\boxed{\text{TI-81}}$ $\boxed{\text{2nd}}$ $\boxed{\text{SIN}}$ $\boxed{(-)}$ .9249 $\boxed{\text{ENTER}}$

and round to two decimal places, or -1.18. Thus, $\arcsin(-0.9249) \approx -1.18$.

Performing the same calculator steps in degree mode gives $-67.7°$.■

It is often important to be able to simplify expressions that involve combinations of the trigonometric and inverse trigonometric functions. This can often be done with the aid of the reference triangle we studied in section 2–4.

■ *Example 4–2 C*

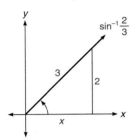

1. Simplify $\tan(\sin^{-1}\frac{2}{3})$.

   Since $\frac{2}{3}$ is positive, the angle represented by $\sin^{-1}\frac{2}{3}$ is in quadrant I. (Remember, the range of the $\sin^{-1}$ function is quadrant I and quadrant IV.) Since $\sin^{-1}\frac{2}{3}$ means the angle in quadrant I whose sine is $\frac{2}{3}$, we can draw a reference triangle (section 2–4) in quadrant I for this angle. See the figure. Using the Pythagorean theorem, we calculate the third side of the triangle to be $\sqrt{5}$. From this we can see that the tangent of this angle is $\dfrac{2}{\sqrt{5}} = \dfrac{2}{\sqrt{5}} \cdot \dfrac{\sqrt{5}}{\sqrt{5}} = \dfrac{2\sqrt{5}}{5}$. Thus, $\tan(\sin^{-1}\frac{2}{3}) = \dfrac{2\sqrt{5}}{5}$.

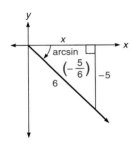

2. Simplify $\sec[\arcsin(-\frac{5}{6})]$.

   Arcsin$(-\frac{5}{6})$ represents an angle in quadrant IV whose sine is $-\frac{5}{6}$. A reference triangle for such an angle is shown in the figure.

   We compute the length of side x to be $\sqrt{11}$. Now we can compute the cosine of this angle to be $\dfrac{\sqrt{11}}{6}$, and the secant of this angle is then the reciprocal of the cosine. That is, $\dfrac{6}{\sqrt{11}} = \dfrac{6}{\sqrt{11}} \cdot \dfrac{\sqrt{11}}{\sqrt{11}} = \dfrac{6\sqrt{11}}{11}$. Thus, $\sec[\arcsin(-\frac{5}{6})] = \dfrac{6\sqrt{11}}{11}$.

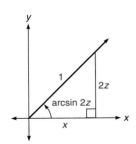

3. Simplify $\tan(\arcsin 2z)$, if $z > 0$.

   Since $z > 0$, then $2z$ is also positive, so $\arcsin 2z$ represents an angle in quadrant I whose sine is $2z$. A reference triangle for such an angle is shown in the figure.

   We find the horizontal side x by the Pythagorean theorem.

   $$1^2 = x^2 + (2z)^2$$
   $$x^2 = 1 - 4z^2$$
   $$x = \sqrt{1 - 4z^2}$$

   Since x is positive, we chose the positive solution when we took the square root.

   We can now find the tangent of this angle. We form the ratio of the side opposite the angle to the side adjacent to the angle to get $\dfrac{2z}{\sqrt{1 - 4z^2}}$.

   We will not rationalize this denominator.

   Thus, $\tan(\arcsin 2z) = \dfrac{2z}{\sqrt{1 - 4z^2}}$, if $z > 0$.

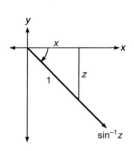

sin⁻¹z

4. Compute $\cos(\sin^{-1}z)$, $z < 0$.

Since $z < 0$, $\sin^{-1}z$ represents an angle in quadrant IV. A reference triangle for such an angle is shown in the figure. Note that we do not write $-z$, but simply z, for the directed vertical distance, since z already represents a negative quantity.

  We find the length x.

$$x^2 + z^2 = 1^2$$
$$x^2 = 1 - z^2$$
$$x = \sqrt{1 - z^2}$$

Now we compute the cosine of this angle. It is $\dfrac{\sqrt{1 - z^2}}{1}$ or $\sqrt{1 - z^2}$.

  Thus, $\cos(\sin^{-1}z) = \sqrt{1 - z^2}$ if $z < 0$.

5. Compute $\sin^{-1}\left(\sin\dfrac{7\pi}{6}\right)$.

We know that $\sin\dfrac{7\pi}{6} = -\dfrac{1}{2}$ since its reference angle is $\dfrac{\pi}{6}$ and it is in quadrant III. (See section 2–3.) Thus, $\sin^{-1}\left(\sin\dfrac{7\pi}{6}\right) = \sin^{-1}\left(-\dfrac{1}{2}\right)$.

Thus, we need the angle in quadrant I or quadrant IV whose sine is $-\tfrac{1}{2}$.

The angle is in quadrant IV since its sine is negative; therefore, it is $-\dfrac{\pi}{6}$ in radians or $-30°$.   ∎

  Part 5 of example 4–2 C shows that $\sin^{-1}(\sin x)$ is not necessarily x. If, however, x is an angle between $-\dfrac{\pi}{2}$ and $\dfrac{\pi}{2}$, then this is true (try a few examples). Thus, we note:

$$\sin^{-1}(\sin x) = x \text{ if and only if } -\frac{\pi}{2} \le x \le \frac{\pi}{2}$$

Also,

$$\sin(\sin^{-1}x) = x \text{ if and only if } -1 \le x \le 1$$

This last restriction applies simply because the domain of the inverse sine function is $-1 \le x \le 1$.

> ## Mastery points
>
> ### Can you
> - Compute exact and approximate values for the inverse of the sine function?
> - Simplify expressions that combine the trigonometric functions and the inverse sine function?
> - State the domain and range of the inverse sine function?

Exercise 4–2

1. Sketch the graph of the inverse sine function.

2. State the domain and range of the inverse sine function.

Find exact values for each of the following expressions. State the results in both radians and degrees.

3. $\sin^{-1}(-\frac{1}{2})$

4. $\arcsin \dfrac{\sqrt{3}}{2}$

5. $\sin^{-1}0$

6. $\arcsin\left(-\dfrac{\sqrt{2}}{2}\right)$

7. $\arcsin\left(-\dfrac{\sqrt{3}}{2}\right)$

8. $\sin^{-1}1$

Find approximate values for the following expressions in both radians and degrees. Round the values for radians to two decimal places and for degrees to one decimal place.

9. $\sin^{-1}0.8823$

10. $\arcsin 0.8253$

11. $\sin^{-1}0.9323$

12. $\sin^{-1}0.6442$

13. $\sin^{-1}(-0.9976)$

14. $\sin^{-1}(-0.2955)$

15. $\arcsin(-0.2571)$

16. $\arcsin(-0.9888)$

Simplify each of the following expressions.

17. $\tan(\arcsin \frac{5}{8})$

18. $\cos(\arcsin \frac{3}{5})$

19. $\sec[\sin^{-1}(-\frac{2}{3})]$

20. $\tan[\arcsin (-0.8)]$

21. $\cot\left(\sin^{-1}\dfrac{\sqrt{3}}{5}\right)$

22. $\csc\left(\sin^{-1}\dfrac{\sqrt{2}}{6}\right)$

23. $\cos(\arcsin 0.3)$

24. $\tan(\arcsin 0.4)$

25. $\cos(\sin^{-1}z), z > 0$

26. $\cos(\sin^{-1}3z), z < 0$

27. $\tan[\sin^{-1}(1 + z)], 1 + z < 0$

28. $\cos(\arcsin \sqrt{z})$

29. $\sec(\arcsin \sqrt{2z})$

30. $\cot(\sin^{-1} \sqrt{z - 1})$

31. $\sin^{-1}\left(\sin \dfrac{\pi}{6}\right)$

32. $\arcsin\left(\tan \dfrac{\pi}{4}\right)$

33. $\arcsin\left(\cos \dfrac{2\pi}{3}\right)$

34. $\sin^{-1}\left(\sin \dfrac{11\pi}{6}\right)$

35. $\sin^{-1}(\cos 0)$

36. $\arcsin\left(\sin \dfrac{5\pi}{6}\right)$

37. Recall that a function f is periodic if there is a number p, $p > 0$, such that $f(x) = f(x + p)$ for all x in the domain of the function. Can a periodic function be one to one? Give a reason for your answer.

4–3 The inverse cosine and inverse tangent functions

The inverse of the cosine function is formed in the same way as the inverse of the sine function. We first select a one-to-one portion. This is chosen to be between 0 and π. See figure 4–7.

The graph of $y = \cos^{-1}x$ is the reflection of this portion of the cosine function across the line $y = x$ (shown in figure 4–7 by a dashed line). The graph of the inverse cosine function is shown separately in figure 4–8.

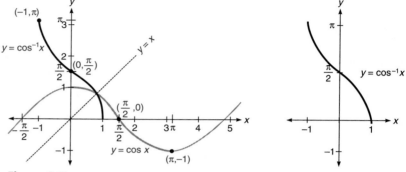

Figure 4–7

$Y_1 = \cos^{-1} X$
$\boxed{\text{RANGE } -3,3,.5,-.5,3.5,.785}$

Figure 4–8

We can see from the graph that

$$\text{Domain}_{\cos^{-1}}: \; |x| \leq 1$$
$$\text{Range}_{\cos^{-1}}: \; 0 \leq y \leq \pi$$

The inverse cosine function is defined as follows:

The inverse cosine function

$y = \cos^{-1}x$ means

1. $\cos y = x$
2. $0 \leq y \leq \pi$
3. $|x| \leq 1$

Concept

$\cos^{-1}x$ is the angle in quadrant I or quadrant II whose cosine is x.

Arccos x and **invcos** x mean the same thing as $\cos^{-1}x$. Note that in degrees the inverse cosine varies from 0° to 180°.

■ *Example 4–3 A*

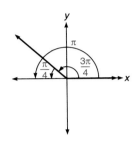

1. Find $\cos^{-1}\frac{1}{2}$ in both radians and degrees.

We want the angle in quadrant I or quadrant II whose cosine is $\frac{1}{2}$. Since this is a positive value, the angle is in quadrant I. We know cos $\frac{\pi}{3} = \frac{1}{2}$, so $\cos^{-1}\frac{1}{2} = \frac{\pi}{3}$. Note that this is equivalent to 60°.

2. Find $\arccos\left(-\frac{\sqrt{2}}{2}\right)$ in both radians and degrees.

We want the angle in quadrant I or quadrant II whose cosine is $-\frac{\sqrt{2}}{2}$.

Since this is a negative value, the angle is in quadrant II. We know cos $\frac{\pi}{4} = \frac{\sqrt{2}}{2}$, so we use $\frac{\pi}{4}$ as a reference angle in quadrant II. This gives us

$\pi - \frac{\pi}{4} = \frac{3\pi}{4}$ for our angle. See the figure.

Thus, $\arccos\left(-\frac{\sqrt{2}}{2}\right) = \frac{3\pi}{4}$, which is equivalent to 135°.   ■

As with the inverse sine function, we sometimes need approximate answers. This is illustrated in example 4–3 B.

■ *Example 4–3 B*

1. Find $\cos^{-1}0.9638$ in both radians and degrees.

We are looking for the angle in quadrant I or quadrant II whose cosine is 0.9638. Since this is a positive value, the angle is in quadrant I. Putting the calculator in radian mode,

.9638 [INV] [COS] (or [COS⁻¹])   Display: [0.269890866]

[TI-81] [2nd] [COS] .9638 [ENTER]

Thus, $\cos^{-1}0.9638 \approx 0.27$.

If the calculation is done with the calculator in degree mode the result is approximately 15.5°.

2. Find $\arccos(-0.5141)$ in both radians and degrees.

We are looking for the angle in quadrant I or quadrant II whose cosine is -0.5141. Since this value is negative, the angle is in quadrant II.

In radian mode,

.5141 [+/−] [INV] [COS]   Display: [2.110754365]

[TI-81] [2nd] [COS] [(−)] .5141 [ENTER]

Thus, $\arccos(-0.5141) \approx 2.11$. When calculated in degree mode the result is approximately 120.9°.   ■

The inverse of the tangent function is formed in the same way as the inverses of the sine and cosine functions. We first select a one-to-one portion. This is chosen to be between $-\dfrac{\pi}{2}$ and $\dfrac{\pi}{2}$. (In fact, this is the same as our basic tangent cycle from section 3–1.) The graph of $y = \tan^{-1}x$ is the reflection of this basic cycle across the line $y = x$. The graph of the basic cycle and its reflection are shown in figure 4–9 and the graph of the inverse tangent function is shown in figure 4–10.

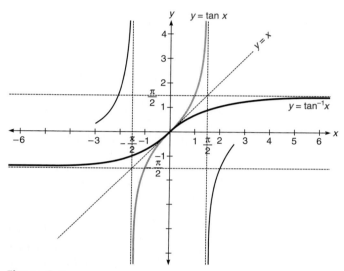

Figure 4–9

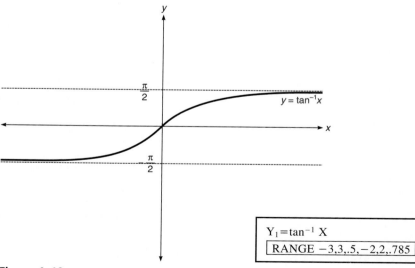

Figure 4–10

The domain of the inverse tangent function is all the reals, and the range is all values between $-\dfrac{\pi}{2}$ and $\dfrac{\pi}{2}$. Observe that the range is in quadrants I and IV, as is the range of the inverse sine function, except that the range of the inverse tangent function does not include the points $-\dfrac{\pi}{2}$ and $\dfrac{\pi}{2}$ themselves.

Thus,

$$\text{Domain}_{\tan^{-1}}: R$$

$$\text{Range}_{\tan^{-1}}: -\dfrac{\pi}{2} < y < \dfrac{\pi}{2}$$

The inverse tangent function

$y = \tan^{-1}x$ means

1. $\tan y = x$ and
2. $-\dfrac{\pi}{2} < y < \dfrac{\pi}{2}$

Concept

$\tan^{-1}x$ means the angle in quadrant I or quadrant IV whose tangent is x.

Note   Since x can take on any value, we do not restrict it in the definition as we did for the inverse sine and inverse cosine functions.

Arctan x and **invtan** x are other notations for $\tan^{-1}x$.

■ *Example 4–3 C*

1. Find $\tan^{-1}\sqrt{3}$ in both radians and degrees.

   We want the angle in quadrant I or quadrant IV whose tangent is $\sqrt{3}$. Since this is a positive value, the angle is in quadrant I. We know $\tan \dfrac{\pi}{3} = \sqrt{3}$, so $\tan^{-1}\sqrt{3} = \dfrac{\pi}{3}$. This is 60°, also.

2. Find $\arctan(-1)$ in both radians and degrees.

   We want the angle in quadrant I or quadrant IV whose tangent is -1. Since this is a negative value, the angle is in quadrant IV. We know $\tan \dfrac{\pi}{4} = 1$, so we use $\dfrac{\pi}{4}$ as a reference angle in quadrant IV. This gives us $-\dfrac{\pi}{4}$, or $-45°$, for our angle.

   Thus, $\arctan(-1) = -\dfrac{\pi}{4}$, or $-45°$.   ■

Example 4–3 D illustrates obtaining approximate values with the calculator.

■ *Example 4–3 D*

Find arctan(−1.9208) in both radians and degrees.

We are looking for the angle in quadrant I or quadrant IV whose tangent is −1.9208. Since this value is negative the angle is in quadrant IV.

1.9208 [+/−] [INV] [TAN] (or [TAN⁻¹]) Display: [−1.090791948]

[TI-81] [2nd] [TAN] [(−)] 1.9208 [ENTER]

Thus, the result is about −1.09 radians and −62.5°. ■

The domains and ranges of the inverses of the sine, cosine, and tangent functions are summarized in table 4–1. Also indicated are the quadrants to which the ranges correspond.

Function	Domain	Range	Quadrants
$y = \sin^{-1}x$	$|x| \le 1$	$-\dfrac{\pi}{2} \le y \le \dfrac{\pi}{2}$	I, IV
$y = \cos^{-1}x$	$|x| \le 1$	$0 \le y \le \pi$	I, II
$y = \tan^{-1}x$	R	$-\dfrac{\pi}{2} < y < \dfrac{\pi}{2}$	I, IV

Table 4–1

We can simplify expressions that involve combinations of the trigonometric and inverse trigonometric functions using the reference triangle, as we did in the previous section.

■ *Example 4–3 E*

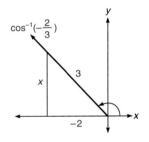

1. Simplify $\tan[\cos^{-1}(-\tfrac{2}{3})]$.

   Since $-\tfrac{2}{3}$ is negative, the angle represented by $\cos^{-1}(-\tfrac{2}{3})$ is in quadrant II. (Remember, the range of this function is quadrants I and II.) Since $\cos^{-1}(-\tfrac{2}{3})$ means the angle in quadrant II whose cosine is $-\tfrac{2}{3}$, we draw a reference triangle in quadrant II for this angle. See the figure.

   Using the Pythagorean theorem, we calculate the third side of the triangle to be $\sqrt{5}$. From this we can see that the tangent of this angle is $\dfrac{\sqrt{5}}{-2} = -\dfrac{\sqrt{5}}{2}$.

   $$\text{Thus, } \tan\left[\cos^{-1}\left(-\frac{2}{3}\right)\right] = -\frac{\sqrt{5}}{2}.$$

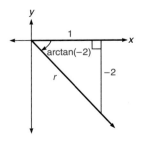

2. Simplify $\sec[\arctan(-2)]$.

   Arctan(−2) represents an angle in quadrant IV whose tangent is −2. A reference triangle for such an angle is shown in the figure.

   Using the Pythagorean theorem, we compute the length of the hypotenuse to be $\sqrt{5}$. From this triangle we can find the secant of this angle. We see that the cosine is $\dfrac{1}{\sqrt{5}}$, so the secant is the reciprocal, or $\sqrt{5}$.

   Thus, $\sec[\arctan(-2)] = \sqrt{5}$.

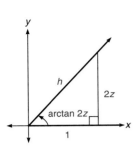

3. Simplify $\sin(\arctan 2z)$, if $z > 0$.

Since $z > 0$, then $2z$ is also positive, so $\arctan 2z$ represents an angle in quadrant I whose tangent is $2z$. A reference triangle for such an angle is shown in the figure.

We find the hypotenuse h using the Pythagorean theorem.

$$1^2 + (2z)^2 = h^2$$
$$1 + 4z^2 = h^2$$
$$\sqrt{1 + 4z^2} = h$$

We can now find the sine of this angle. We form the ratio of the side opposite the angle to the hypotenuse to get $\dfrac{2z}{\sqrt{1 + 4z^2}}$. We will not rationalize this denominator.

Thus, $\sin(\arctan 2z) = \dfrac{2z}{\sqrt{1 + 4z^2}}$ if $z > 0$.

4. Find $\tan^{-1}\left[\sin\left(-\dfrac{\pi}{2}\right)\right]$.

$$\tan^{-1}\left[\sin\left(-\dfrac{\pi}{2}\right)\right] = \tan^{-1}(-1)$$

$$= -\dfrac{\pi}{4} \text{ or } -45° \qquad \blacksquare$$

One application of the inverse trigonometric functions is to describe an angle in a given situation with a mathematical expression.

■ *Example 4–3 F*

1. Describe angle θ in the figure using an inverse trigonometric function.

We can see that the tangent of θ is $\dfrac{h}{d}$, so ''θ is an angle whose tangent is $\dfrac{h}{d}$.'' This is what $\tan^{-1}\dfrac{h}{d}$ means, so $\theta = \tan^{-1}\dfrac{h}{d}$.

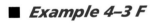

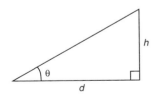

2. A jet aircraft is flying at 20,000 feet. If x represents the distance from a ground observer to the aircraft (also in feet), describe the angle of elevation from the observer to the aircraft in terms of an inverse trigonometric function.

If we represent the situation as shown in the figure, where θ indicates the angle of elevation, we see that θ is an angle whose sine is $\dfrac{20{,}000}{x}$. This is what the expression $\sin^{-1}\dfrac{20{,}000}{x}$ means.

Thus, since $\sin \theta = \dfrac{20{,}000}{x}$, $\theta = \sin^{-1}\dfrac{20{,}000}{x}$. $\qquad \blacksquare$

Another way in which the inverse trigonometric functions are used is to describe one of the solutions to a trigonometric equation in exact form.

■ *Example 4–3 G*

1. $\sin \theta = 0.7$. Describe one value of θ in exact form.

   Since the equation tells us that θ is an angle whose sine is 0.7, we write $\theta = \sin^{-1}0.7$. This expression is exact. We could approximate $\sin^{-1}0.7$ with a calculator, but the decimal number we obtained would only be an approximation.

   Thus, if $\sin \theta = 0.7$, one exact value of θ is $\sin^{-1}0.7$.

2. $\tan \theta = z$. Describe one value of θ in exact form.

   We see that $\theta = \tan^{-1}z$, so one value would be $\tan^{-1}z$.

3. $\cos 2\theta = 0.55$. Describe one value of θ in exact form.

   $2\theta = \cos^{-1}0.55$, so $\theta = \dfrac{\cos^{-1}0.55}{2}$ is one value of θ.

4. $3 \sin \theta = 0.69$. Describe one value of θ in exact form.

   If we divide both sides by 3, we see that $\sin \theta = 0.23$. Thus, $\theta = \sin^{-1}0.23$ gives one exact value of θ.

5. $A \sin Bx = C$. Describe one value of x in exact form.

   Dividing both sides by A:

   $$\sin Bx = \frac{C}{A}$$

   Then,

   $$Bx = \sin^{-1}\frac{C}{A}$$

   Dividing both sides by B:

   $$x = \frac{\sin^{-1}\dfrac{C}{A}}{B}$$

   Thus, one value of x that satisfies the equation $A \sin Bx = C$ is
   $\dfrac{\sin^{-1}\dfrac{C}{A}}{B}$. ■

Finally, it is not too hard to verify that the following identities are true:

$$\cos^{-1}(\cos x) = x \text{ if and only if } 0 \le x \le \pi$$
$$\cos(\cos^{-1}x) = x \text{ if and only if } -1 \le x \le 1$$
$$\tan^{-1}(\tan x) = x \text{ if and only if } -\frac{\pi}{2} < x < \frac{\pi}{2}$$
$$\tan(\tan^{-1}x) = x \text{ for all } x$$

Mastery points

Can you
- Compute exact and approximate values for the inverses of the cosine and tangent functions?
- Simplify expressions that combine the trigonometric functions and their inverses?
- State the domains and ranges of these inverse trigonometric functions?
- Apply these inverse trigonometric functions to describe angles in physical situations?
- Apply these inverse trigonometric functions to give one exact solution to trigonometric equations?

Exercise 4–3

1. Sketch the graph of each function.
   a. inverse sine
   b. inverse cosine
   c. inverse tangent

2. State the domain and range for each function.
   a. inverse sine
   b. inverse cosine
   c. inverse tangent

Find exact values for each of the following expressions in both radians and degrees.

3. $\cos^{-1}(-\frac{1}{2})$

4. $\arccos \dfrac{\sqrt{3}}{2}$

5. $\cos^{-1}0$

6. $\arccos\left(-\dfrac{\sqrt{2}}{2}\right)$

7. $\arcsin \dfrac{\sqrt{3}}{2}$

8. $\tan^{-1}1$

9. $\arctan(-\sqrt{3})$

10. $\cos^{-1}\dfrac{\sqrt{2}}{2}$

11. $\tan^{-1}\left(-\dfrac{\sqrt{3}}{3}\right)$

12. $\cos^{-1}\left(-\dfrac{\sqrt{3}}{2}\right)$

Find approximate values for the following expressions, in both degrees and radians. Round degrees to tenths and radians to hundredths.

13. $\sin^{-1}0.8823$

14. $\arctan 11.08$

15. $\arccos 0.8253$

16. $\arcsin 0.6131$

17. $\tan^{-1}0.9316$

18. $\cos^{-1}0.6442$

19. $\arcsin 0.7961$

20. $\sin^{-1}0.8776$

21. $\sin^{-1}(-0.9976)$

22. $\cos^{-1}(-0.2955)$

23. $\arctan(-0.2553)$

24. $\arccos(-0.9888)$

25. $\arccos(-0.9902)$

26. $\tan^{-1}(-3.4776)$

Simplify each of the following expressions.

27. $\cos(\tan^{-1}\frac{3}{5})$

28. $\sin(\cos^{-1}\frac{1}{4})$

29. $\sin(\arccos \frac{5}{8})$

30. $\cos(\arctan 2)$

31. $\tan[\cos^{-1}(-\frac{2}{3})]$

32. $\sin[\arccos(-0.8)]$

33. $\sin(\tan^{-1}\sqrt{5})$

34. $\csc\left(\cos^{-1}\dfrac{\sqrt{2}}{6}\right)$

35. $\cos(\arctan 0.3)$

36. $\sin(\arctan 0.4)$

37. $\sin(\cos^{-1}z),\ z > 0$

38. $\cos(\arccos z),\ z > 0$

39. $\tan(\arccos z),\ z > 0$

40. $\sin(\tan^{-1}z),\ z > 0$

41. $\cos(\arctan z),\ z < 0$

42. $\tan(\cos^{-1}z),\ z < 0$

43. $\sin(\cos^{-1}3z),\ z < 0$

44. $\cos(\arctan 2z),\ z > 0$

45. $\sec[\tan^{-1}(1 + z)],\ z > 0$

46. $\sin(\arccos \sqrt{z})$

47. $\cos(\arctan \sqrt{2z})$

48. $\tan(\cos^{-1}\sqrt{z - 1})$

49. $\tan^{-1}\left(\sin \dfrac{\pi}{2}\right)$

50. $\cos^{-1}\left(\sin \dfrac{7\pi}{6}\right)$

51. $\cos^{-1}\left(\cos \dfrac{11\pi}{6}\right)$

52. $\tan^{-1}(\cos 0)$

53. $\arccos\left(\tan \dfrac{5\pi}{4}\right)$

54. $\cos^{-1}\left(\cos \dfrac{3\pi}{2}\right)$

In the following problems state the angle θ shown in each diagram in terms of an inverse trigonometric function.

55.

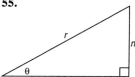

56.

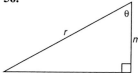

57.

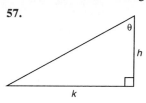

58.

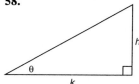

59. A picture hangs on a wall so that the bottom of the picture is 5 feet above the floor. The picture is 2 feet high. Describe the angle subtended by the picture at the eye of an observer, in terms of an inverse trigonometric function, if the observer's eye is also 5 feet above the floor and the observer is x feet away from the wall.

60. A radar antenna will track the launch of a rocket from a point 12,500 feet from the rocket. Both are at the same ground elevation at launch. If a represents the altitude of the rocket in feet, describe the angle of elevation of the rocket at the radar site in terms of an inverse trigonometric function.

61. An aircraft is flying toward an airport at an elevation of 3,500 feet above the airport. Describe the angle of depression of the airport at the aircraft in terms of the distance z from the aircraft directly to the airport, using an inverse trigonometric function.

In the following problems describe one value of θ, or x, in exact form, in terms of an inverse trigonometric function.

62. $\sin \theta = 0.75$

63. $\cos \theta = -0.8$

64. $\tan \theta = 3$

65. $\tan \theta = 4.1$

66. $2 \sin \theta = 1.6$

67. $3 \tan \theta = 5$

68. $\frac{1}{2} \sin \theta = -0.1$

69. $\dfrac{\tan \theta}{5} = 10$

70. $\sin 2\theta = 0.76$

71. $\tan 3\theta = 9$

72. $\cos \dfrac{\theta}{3} = -0.42$

73. $\sin \dfrac{3\theta}{2} = -0.56$

74. $4 \cos 3\theta = 3$

75. $2 \sin 4\theta = 1.5$

76. $\dfrac{3 \cos 2\theta}{8} = \dfrac{7}{40}$

77. $\dfrac{6 \sin 5\theta}{5} = \dfrac{10}{13}$

78. $\dfrac{A \cos Bx}{C} = D$

79. $A \tan(Bx + C) = D$

80. $\cos(x - 2) = 0.2$

81. $\sin(2x + 3) = 0.6$

82. Many computer languages only provide an arctangent function. In these situations we must program our own arcsine and arccosine functions. Use appropriate reference triangles to show that the following are identities.

a. $\arcsin(x) = \begin{cases} -\dfrac{\pi}{2} & \text{if } x = -1 \\[2mm] \arctan\left(\dfrac{x}{\sqrt{1 - x^2}}\right) & \text{if } |x| < 1 \\[2mm] \dfrac{\pi}{2} & \text{if } x = 1 \end{cases}$

b. $\arccos(x) = \begin{cases} \arctan\left(\dfrac{\sqrt{1 - x^2}}{x}\right) & \text{if } 0 < x \le 1 \\[2mm] \dfrac{\pi}{2} & \text{if } x = 0 \\[2mm] \arctan\left(\dfrac{\sqrt{1 - x^2}}{x}\right) + \pi & \text{if } -1 \le x < 0 \end{cases}$

4–4 *The inverse cotangent, secant, and cosecant functions*

The reciprocal trigonometric functions (cotangent, secant, cosecant) and their inverses were useful for computations before the advent of electronic calculating devices like calculators and computers; today they have no practical use in computation. This is why calculators do not have keys for the reciprocal functions, and why programming languages, such as FORTRAN, BASIC, or Pascal, do not support these functions. These functions still have value in expressing certain expressions in higher mathematics, however, and that is why we study them here.

The inverse cotangent function

We define the inverse cotangent function by reversing the ordered pairs in the basic cotangent cycle; that is, we restrict the domain to $0 < x < \pi$. Figure 4–11 shows the inverse cotangent function, $\cot^{-1}$. The domain is R, and the range is $0 < y < \pi$. As we might suspect **arccot** x also means $\cot^{-1} x$.

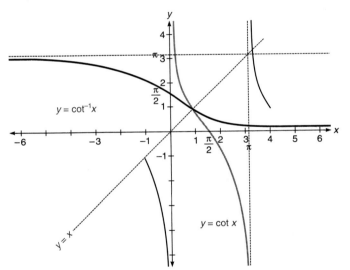

Figure 4–11

The inverse cotangent function
$y = \cot^{-1} x$ means

1. $\cot y = x$
2. $0 < y < \pi$

There are several ways to compute values of the inverse cotangent function. One way is to use the identity

$$\cot^{-1} x = \frac{\pi}{2} - \tan^{-1} x$$

This identity can be seen by considering the graphs of $y = \cot^{-1}x$ (figure 4–11) and $y = \tan^{-1}x$ (figure 4–12). Figure 4–12 shows the sequence of operations that will transform one graph into the other. Part (a) shows $y = \tan^{-1}x$. Part (b) shows the transformation caused by the scaling factor -1. Part (c) shows the vertical shift caused by adding $\dfrac{\pi}{2}$. This result is the same as the graph of the inverse cotangent function.

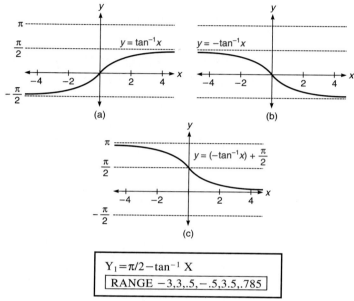

Figure 4–12

Note that this transformation of graphs does not absolutely guarantee that the identity $\cot^{-1}x = \dfrac{\pi}{2} - \tan^{-1}x$ is true. It should be proven algebraically. We will not prove it here.

The inverse secant function

Recall the identity $\sec\theta = \dfrac{1}{\cos\theta}$. We use this to define the inverse of the secant function. Suppose we stated that $y = \sec^{-1}x$. Then $\sec y = x$. We proceed as shown.

$$y = \sec^{-1}x \qquad \text{An expression we want to define}$$

$$\sec y = x \qquad \text{We expect the expression to have this property}$$

$$\frac{1}{\cos y} = x \qquad \sec \theta = \frac{1}{\cos \theta}$$

$$\cos y = \frac{1}{x} \qquad \frac{1}{\cos y} = x;\ 1 = x \cos y;\ \frac{1}{x} = \cos y$$

$$y = \cos^{-1}\frac{1}{x} \qquad \text{Since } y \text{ is the angle whose cosine is } \frac{1}{x}$$

$$\sec^{-1}x = \cos^{-1}\frac{1}{x}$$

We use this sequence of steps to motivate our definition. As expected, **arcsec** *x* also means $\sec^{-1}x$.

The inverse secant function

$$\sec^{-1}x = \cos^{-1}\frac{1}{x} \text{ if } |x| \geq 1$$

We require $|x| \geq 1$ so that $\left|\dfrac{1}{x}\right| \leq 1$, as required by the inverse cosine function. The range of the secant function is the range of the inverse cosine function since the latter defines the former, except that $\dfrac{\pi}{2}$ is not in the range.

This is because $\dfrac{\pi}{2} = \cos^{-1}0$, and there is no value of *x* such that $\dfrac{1}{x} = 0$.

Inverse cosecant function

The identity $\csc \theta = \dfrac{1}{\sin \theta}$, and reasoning similar to that above, leads to the following definition for the inverse cosecant (**arcsecant**) function.

The inverse cosecant function

$$\csc^{-1}x = \sin^{-1}\frac{1}{x} \text{ if } |x| \geq 1$$

For reasons similar to those stated earlier, the domain of the inverse cosecant function is $|x| \geq 1$, and the range is the same as that of the inverse sine function, except for 0, which is $\sin^{-1}0$, and $\dfrac{1}{x}$ can not take on the value 0.

Note   It is not worth the effort to study the graphs of the functions of this section. We presented the graph of the inverse cotangent function only to justify the identity presented earlier.

Summary of properties

Table 4–2 summarizes the domains and ranges of the functions introduced previously.

Function	Domain	Range	Quadrants
$y = \cot^{-1}x$	R	$0 < y < \pi$	I, II
$y = \sec^{-1}x$	$\lvert x \rvert \geq 1$	$0 \leq y \leq \pi,\ y \neq \dfrac{\pi}{2}$	I, II
$y = \csc^{-1}x$	$\lvert x \rvert \geq 1$	$-\dfrac{\pi}{2} \leq y \leq \dfrac{\pi}{2},\ y \neq 0$	I, IV

Table 4–2

Note in this table that quadrant I always corresponds to a nonnegative domain element (a nonnegative value of x), and quadrant II or IV corresponds to negative domain elements.

■ *Example 4–4 A*

Find the given values in both radians and degrees. Round radians to two decimal places and degrees to one decimal place where necessary.

1. $\cot^{-1}(-4)$

$$= \frac{\pi}{2} - \tan^{-1}(-4) \qquad \cot^{-1}x = \frac{\pi}{2} - \tan^{-1}x$$

$$\approx 2.90 \text{ (radians)} \qquad \text{Calculator in radian mode}$$

$$= 90° - \tan^{-1}(-4)$$

$$\approx 166.0° \qquad \text{Calculator in degree mode}$$

Thus, $\cot^{-1}(-4) \approx 166.0°$ or 2.90 (radians).

2. $\sec^{-1} 2$

$$= \cos^{-1}\tfrac{1}{2} \qquad \text{Definition of } \sec^{-1}\theta$$

$$= 60° \text{ or } \frac{\pi}{3}$$

Thus, $\sec^{-1}2 = 60°$ or $\dfrac{\pi}{3}$. ■

As we saw in section 4–3 some expressions that involve both the trigonometric and inverse trigonometric functions can be simplified by using a reference triangle.

■ *Example 4–4 B*

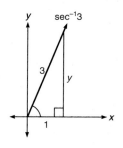

Simplify the expression.

1. $\sin(\sec^{-1}3)$

$\sec^{-1}3 = \cos^{-1}\tfrac{1}{3}$, by definition. This is a first quadrant angle. The figure shows a reference triangle in this quadrant in which the cosine of the angle is $\tfrac{1}{3}$.

$$y = \sqrt{3^2 - 1^2} = \sqrt{8} = 2\sqrt{2}$$

The sine of this angle is $\dfrac{\text{opposite}}{\text{hypotenuse}} = \dfrac{2\sqrt{2}}{3}$.

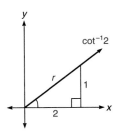

2. $\sec(\cot^{-1}2)$

$\cot^{-1}2$ is an angle in quadrant I. Since its cotangent is 2, its tangent is $\frac{1}{2}$. A reference triangle for a quadrant I angle with tangent $\frac{1}{2}$ is shown in the figure.

$$r = \sqrt{5} \text{ (Pythagorean theorem), so the cosine of the angle is } \frac{2}{\sqrt{5}},$$

and therefore the secant is $\dfrac{\sqrt{5}}{2}$. Thus, $\sec(\cot^{-1}2) = \dfrac{\sqrt{5}}{2}$.

Note The identity $\cot^{-1}x = \dfrac{\pi}{2} - \tan^{-1}x$ would not be helpful in simplifying this expression. It is used for computing values of $\cot^{-1}x$.

3. $\cos(\csc^{-1}(z + 2))$, $z > 0$

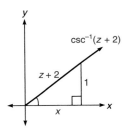

$\csc^{-1}(z + 2) = \sin^{-1}\dfrac{1}{z + 2}$ by definition. Since $\dfrac{1}{z + 2}$ is positive,

$\sin^{-1}\dfrac{1}{z + 2}$ is an angle in quadrant I (see the figure). We find y by the Pythagorean theorem.

$$(z + 2)^2 = 1^2 + y^2$$
$$z^2 + 4z + 4 - 1 = y^2$$
$$\sqrt{z^2 + 4z + 3} = y$$

The cosine of the angle is $\dfrac{\text{adjacent}}{\text{hypotenuse}} = \dfrac{y}{z + 2} = \dfrac{\sqrt{z^2 + 4z + 3}}{z + 2}$. ∎

Mastery points

Can you
- State the domain and range of the inverse cotangent, cosecant, and secant functions?
- Find exact values, in both radians and degrees, for expressions of the form $\cot^{-1}x$, $\csc^{-1}x$, and $\sec^{-1}x$, for appropriate values of x, using the definitions of these functions?
- Find approximate values, in both radians and degrees, for expressions of the form $\sin^{-1}x$, $\cos^{-1}x$, and $\tan^{-1}x$, using a calculator and the definitions of these functions?
- Simplify expressions that involve combinations of the trigonometric and inverse trigonometric functions, using a reference triangle where appropriate?

Exercise 4–4

Compute the exact value of the following expressions.

1. $\csc^{-1}2$

2. $\mathrm{arcsec}\left(-\dfrac{2\sqrt{3}}{3}\right)$

3. arccot 1

4. $\mathrm{arccsc}(-1)$

5. $\sec^{-1}(-2)$

6. $\cot^{-1}(-\sqrt{3})$

7. $\mathrm{arccsc}\dfrac{2\sqrt{3}}{3}$

8. $\csc^{-1}\sqrt{2}$

9. arccot 0

10. $\mathrm{arcsec}(-\sqrt{2})$

Compute approximate values of the following expressions in both radians (to hundredths) and degrees (to tenths).

11. $\csc^{-1}3.3534$

12. $\cot^{-1}0.5080$

13. $\mathrm{arcsec}(-2.9986)$

14. $\mathrm{arccsc}(-2.5087)$

15. arccot 5.1997

16. $\sec^{-1}(-2.0126)$

17. $\sec^{-1}(-11.1261)$

18. $\csc^{-1}(-3.8898)$

19. arccsc 3.1790

20. $\mathrm{arccot}(-8.3534)$

Simplify the following expressions.

21. $\sin(\csc^{-1}3)$

22. $\cos(\cot^{-1}2)$

23. cot(arcsec 4)

24. $\sin(\sec^{-1}1.5)$

25. csc(arccot 5)

26. $\sec(\mathrm{arccsc}\tfrac{7}{4})$

27. $\cos[\mathrm{arccsc}(-\tfrac{5}{4})]$

28. $\tan[\mathrm{arccsc}(-\tfrac{5}{3})]$

29. $\tan[\sec^{-1}(-\tfrac{6}{5})]$

30. $\csc[\sec^{-1}(-\tfrac{8}{7})]$

31. $\sin(\csc^{-1}z),\ z > 0$

32. $\cot(\sec^{-1}z),\ z > 0$

33. $\sec(\cot^{-1}z),\ z < 0$

34. $\tan(\mathrm{arcsec}\,z),\ z < 0$

35. $\cos(\mathrm{arcsec}\,2z),\ z > 0$

36. $\sin(\csc^{-1}3z),\ z < 0$

37. $\tan[\sec^{-1}(z + 1)],\ z + 1 > 0$

38. $\csc[\sec^{-1}(1 - z)],\ 1 - z > 0$

39. $\csc\left(\mathrm{arccsc}\dfrac{3}{z}\right),\ z > 0$

40. $\sec\left(\cot^{-1}\dfrac{2}{z + 1}\right),\ z + 1 > 0$

Chapter 4 summary

- To show that two functions f and g are inverses of each other

  Show that   [1] If $f(x) = y$, then $g(y) = x$, and

                [2] If $g(x) = y$, then $f(y) = x$.

- **Vertical line test for a function** If no vertical line crosses the graph of a relation in more than one place, the relation is a function.

- **Horizontal line test for a one-to-one function** If no horizontal line crosses the graph of a function in more than one place, the function is one to one.

- **Inverse sine function**

  $y = \sin^{-1}x$ means

  1. $\sin y = x$

  2. $-\dfrac{\pi}{2} \le y \le \dfrac{\pi}{2}$

  3. $-1 \le x \le 1$

- **Inverse cosine function**

  $y = \cos^{-1}x$ means

  1. $\cos y = x$

  2. $0 \le y \le \pi$

  3. $-1 \le x \le 1$

- **Inverse tangent function**

  $y = \tan^{-1}x$ means

  1. $\tan y = x$

  2. $-\dfrac{\pi}{2} < y < \dfrac{\pi}{2}$

- **Inverse cotangent function**

  $y = \cot^{-1}x$ means

  1. $\cot y = x$

  2. $0 < y < \pi$

- $\cot^{-1}x = \dfrac{\pi}{2} - \tan^{-1}x$

- **Inverse secant function** $\sec^{-1}x = \cos^{-1}\dfrac{1}{x}$ if $|x| \ge 1$

- **Inverse cosecant function** $\csc^{-1}x = \sin^{-1}\dfrac{1}{x}$ if $|x| \ge 1$

- Summary of the properties of the inverse sine, cosine, and tangent functions.

Function	Domain	Range	Quadrants
$y = \sin^{-1}x$	$\lvert x \rvert \le 1$	$-\dfrac{\pi}{2} \le y \le \dfrac{\pi}{2}$	I, IV
$y = \cos^{-1}x$	$\lvert x \rvert \le 1$	$0 \le y \le \pi$	I, II
$y = \tan^{-1}x$	R	$-\dfrac{\pi}{2} < y < \dfrac{\pi}{2}$	I, IV

- Summary of the properties of the inverse cotangent, secant, and cosecant functions.

Function	Domain	Range	Quadrants
$y = \cot^{-1}x$	R	$0 < y < \pi$	I, II
$y = \sec^{-1}x$	$\lvert x \rvert \ge 1$	$0 \le y \le \pi,\, y \ne \dfrac{\pi}{2}$	I, II
$y = \csc^{-1}x$	$\lvert x \rvert \ge 1$	$-\dfrac{\pi}{2} \le y \le \dfrac{\pi}{2},\, y \ne 0$	I, IV

Chapter 4 review

[4–1] Show that the following functions f and g are inverses of each other.

1. $f(x) = 3x - 5;\ g(x) = \dfrac{x + 5}{3}$

2. $f(x) = \dfrac{3x}{x + 1};\ g(x) = \dfrac{-x}{x - 3}$

Each of the following diagrams shows the graph of a function. Use the horizontal line test to determine if the function is or is not one to one.

3.   **4.**

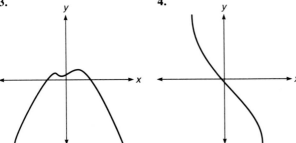

[4–2]

5. Sketch the graph of the inverse sine function.
6. State the domain and range of the inverse sine function.

Find exact values for each of the following expressions in both radians and degrees.

7. $\sin^{-1}(-\tfrac{1}{2})$ **8.** $\arcsin\dfrac{\sqrt{3}}{2}$

9. $\sin^{-1}\tfrac{1}{2}$ **10.** $\arcsin\left(-\dfrac{\sqrt{2}}{2}\right)$

11. $\arcsin 0$ **12.** $\sin^{-1}(-1)$

Find approximate values for the following expressions in both radians and degrees.

13. $\sin^{-1}0.9737$ **14.** $\arcsin(-0.4882)$

Simplify the following expressions.

15. $\cos(\sin^{-1}\tfrac{3}{5})$ **16.** $\tan(\sin^{-1}\tfrac{1}{4})$
17. $\sec[\sin^{-1}(-\tfrac{2}{3})]$ **18.** $\tan(\sin^{-1}z),\ z > 0$
19. $\cos[\arcsin(1 + z)],\ 1 + z > 0$

[4–3]

20. Sketch the graph of the inverse cosine function.
21. State the domain and range of the inverse tangent function.

Find exact values for each of the following expressions in both radians and degrees.

22. $\cos^{-1}(-\tfrac{1}{2})$ **23.** $\arccos\dfrac{\sqrt{3}}{2}$

24. $\cos^{-1}\tfrac{1}{2}$ **25.** $\arcsin\left(-\dfrac{\sqrt{2}}{2}\right)$

26. $\arctan\sqrt{3}$ **27.** $\tan^{-1}(-1)$

Find approximate values for the following expressions in both radians and degrees.

28. $\tan^{-1} 1.5601$ **29.** $\arccos 0.4882$

30. $\arccos(-0.3051)$

Simplify the following expressions.

31. $\cos(\tan^{-1}\frac{3}{5})$ **32.** $\sec(\cos^{-1}\frac{1}{4})$

33. $\tan[\cos^{-1}(-\frac{2}{3})]$ **34.** $\cos^{-1}\left(\sin\dfrac{7\pi}{6}\right)$

35. $\tan(\cos^{-1} z)$, $z > 0$

36. $\cos[\arctan(1 + z)]$, $1 + z > 0$

For the following diagrams state the angle θ in terms of an inverse trigonometric function.

37. 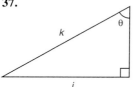   **38.**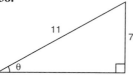

39. A camera is to be placed on the ground x feet from a flagpole that is 35 feet high. Describe the angle determined by the flagpole at the camera in terms of an inverse trigonometric function.

In the following problems describe one value of θ in exact form, in terms of an inverse trigonometric function.

40. $\cos\theta = 0.89$ **41.** $\sin\theta = -0.88$

42. $\frac{1}{2}\sin\theta = -0.1$ **43.** $2\tan\theta = 10$

44. $\sin 2\theta = 0.76$ **45.** $2\cos 3\theta = 1.4$

46. $\cos(2\theta + 3) = 0.6$ **47.** $\sin 2\theta + 3 = 3.6$

[4–4] Compute the exact value of the following expressions in both radians and degrees.

48. $\sec^{-1} 2$ **49.** $\operatorname{arccsc}\left(-\dfrac{2\sqrt{3}}{3}\right)$

50. $\operatorname{arccsc}(-2)$ **51.** $\cot^{-1}(-\sqrt{3})$

Compute approximate values of the following expressions in both radians and degrees.

52. $\csc^{-1} 4.3864$ **53.** $\cot^{-1} 1.5601$

54. $\operatorname{arcsec}(-4.0420)$ **55.** $\operatorname{arccsc}(-6.6917)$

Simplify the following expressions.

56. $\tan(\csc^{-1} 3)$ **57.** $\cot(\operatorname{arcsec} 4)$

58. $\sin(\operatorname{arccot} 5)$ **59.** $\csc[\operatorname{arcsec}(-\frac{7}{4})]$

60. $\sin(\cot^{-1} z)$, $z > 0$ **61.** $\cot(\csc^{-1} z)$, $z > 0$

62. $\tan[\sec^{-1}(z + 1)]$, $z + 1 > 0$

63. $\csc[\sec^{-1}(1 - z)]$, $1 - z > 0$

Chapter 4 test

1. Sketch the graph of the inverse tangent function.

2. State the domain and range of the inverse cosecant function.

Find exact values for each of the following expressions in both radians and degrees.

3. $\sec^{-1}(-2)$ **4.** $\arcsin\dfrac{\sqrt{2}}{2}$

5. $\csc^{-1} 2$ **6.** $\arctan\sqrt{3}$

Find approximate values for the following expressions in both radians and degrees.

7. $\tan^{-1} 1.4617$ **8.** $\arccos(-0.4169)$

9. $\operatorname{arcsec}(-1.4830)$ **10.** $\operatorname{arccsc} 3.4971$

Simplify the following expressions.

11. $\cot(\sin^{-1}\frac{3}{5})$ **12.** $\sin[\tan^{-1}(-4)]$

13. $\tan[\sec^{-1}(-3)]$ **14.** $\sec(\cos^{-1} z)$, $z > 0$

15. $\sin[\operatorname{arccot}(1 + z)]$, $1 + z > 0$

16. $\tan(\sec^{-1} 2z)$, $z > 0$

17. $\sec[\csc^{-1}(1 - z)]$, $1 - z > 0$

18. State the angle θ in terms of an inverse trigonometric function.

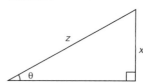

19. A taut line is connected to the top of a building that is 52 feet high and to a point on the ground some distance from the building. The length of the line is x. Let θ be the angle formed by the ground and by the line. Describe the angle θ in terms of an inverse trigonometric function.

In the following problems describe one value of θ in exact form in terms of an inverse trigonometric function.

20. $\sec\theta = 2.25$ **21.** $2\sin\theta = -1.88$

22. $\sin 3\theta = 0.75$ **23.** $4\cos(2\theta - 3) = 2.4$

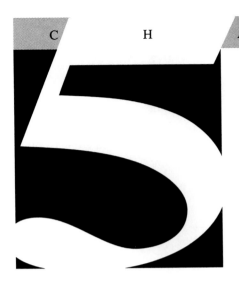

CHAPTER

Trigonometric Equations

Recall that trigonometric equations were introduced in section 1–4, and revisited in 2–6. In this chapter, we first study trigonometric identities; these are very important in the study of the calculus and certain engineering applications. We then examine conditional trigonometric equations in more depth than we did previously.

Section 5–0 reviews important facts about equations and equation solving. Some of this material has been covered in this text, and the rest should be known from previous mathematics courses.

5–0 Equation solving—review

Factoring

To factor means to write as a product. Several common types of factoring that we will need in this chapter to deal with equations are categorized as common factor, difference of two squares, and quadratic trinomial. It is assumed that the student is familiar with each topic. They are presented here both with familiar algebraic forms and with similar trigonometric forms.

	Expression	Factored form
Common factor		
Algebraic	$a^2b - ab^2$	$ab(a - b)$
Trigonometric	$\sin^2\theta \cos\theta - \sin\theta \cos^2\theta$	$\sin\theta \cos\theta(\sin\theta - \cos\theta)$
Difference of two squares		
Algebraic	$a^4 - b^4$	$(a^2 - b^2)(a^2 + b^2)$ or $(a - b)(a + b)(a^2 + b^2)$
Trigonometric	$\sin^4\theta - \cos^4\theta$	$(\sin^2\theta - \cos^2\theta)(\sin^2\theta + \cos^2\theta)$ which becomes $(\sin\theta - \cos\theta)(\sin\theta + \cos\theta)(1)$

	Expression	**Factored form**
Quadratic trinomial		
Algebraic	$2x^2 - x - 3$	$(2x - 3)(x + 1)$
Trigonometric	$2 \sin^2 x - \sin x - 3$	$(2 \sin x - 3)(\sin x + 1)$

When it is difficult to see how a particular trigonometric expression can be factored, a method called substitution may help. This is illustrated in example 5–0 A.

■ *Example 5–0 A*

Factor $6 \tan^2\theta - 11 \tan \theta + 3$
If this is difficult to factor, try substitution.
Let $u = \tan \theta$. Then $u^2 = \tan^2\theta$.
Thus, we can rewrite the equation as

$$6u^2 - 11u + 3$$

which factors into

$$(2u - 3)(3u - 1) \qquad \text{Quadratic trinomial}$$

Now replace u by $\tan \theta$:

$$(2 \tan \theta - 3)(3 \tan \theta - 1) \qquad ■$$

Equations

> An **equation** is a statement of equality of two expressions.

Examples of equations are

$$3x = 27$$
$$3x^2 = 27$$
$$\tan \theta = 1$$
$$x + 3x = 4x$$

An equation involving only one variable is called an equation in one variable.

> A **solution** to an equation in one variable is a real number that makes the statement of equality true when it replaces the variable.

For example, 9 is a solution to the equation $3x = 27$,

3 and -3 are both solutions to the equation $3x^2 = 27$

$\dfrac{\pi}{4}$ is a solution to the equation $\tan \theta = 1$

any number is a solution to the equation $x + 3x = 4x$

Identities and conditional equations

> An **identity** is an equation that is true for all valid replacement values of the variable.

> A **conditional equation** is an equation that is not true for all valid replacement values of the variable.

The equation

$$3x - 2(x + 5) = x - 10$$

is an identity, which can be seen by combining the terms in the left member, obtaining

$$x - 10 = x - 10$$

The left side will clearly equal the right side regardless of the value of x. We have seen that

$$\sin^2\theta + \cos^2\theta = 1$$

is an identity.

Most of this chapter is concerned with trigonometric identities.

Conditional linear equations

We have solved many linear trigonometric equations in previous sections, like the following.

1. $6 \sin x = 3$
$\sin x = \frac{1}{2}$
$x = \sin^{-1}\frac{1}{2}$

2. $3 \tan \theta - 1 = 1$
$3 \tan \theta = 2$
$\tan \theta = \frac{2}{3}$
$\theta = \tan^{-1}\frac{2}{3}$

Conditional quadratic equations

We have not previously discussed this type of equation. A quadratic equation is an equation of the form $ax^2 + bx + c = 0$, where $a \neq 0$. There are two common methods for solving these equations: factoring and the quadratic formula.

Factoring uses the zero product property introduced in section 2–6:

$$\text{If } ab = 0, \text{ then } a = 0 \text{ or } b = 0.$$

The quadratic formula is as follows.

> **Quadratic formula**
> If $ax^2 + bx + c = 0$, and $a \neq 0$, then
> $$x = \frac{-b + \sqrt{b^2 - 4ac}}{2a} \quad \text{and} \quad x = \frac{-b - \sqrt{b^2 - 4ac}}{2a}$$
> are both solutions to the equation.

The formula is usually abbreviated as $x = \dfrac{-b \pm \sqrt{b^2 - 4ac}}{2a}$.

Both methods for solving quadratic equations are illustrated in example 5–0 B.

■ *Example 5–0 B*

Solve each quadratic equation for $\sin x$, $\cos x$, or $\tan x$, as appropriate.

1. $6 \tan^2 x - 11 \tan x = -3$

$6 \tan^2 x - 11 \tan x + 3 = 0$	Add -3 to both members
$(2 \tan x - 3)(3 \tan x - 1) = 0$	Factor the left member
$2 \tan x - 3 = 0$ or $3 \tan x - 1 = 0$	Zero product property
$2 \tan x = 3$ or $3 \tan x = 1$	
$\tan x = \frac{3}{2}$ or $\tan x = \frac{1}{3}$	

2. $2 \cos^2 x - \cos x - 2 = 0$

This expression does not factor, so we use the quadratic formula.
$a = 2,\, b = -1,\, c = -2.$

$$\cos x = \frac{-(-1) + \sqrt{(-1)^2 - 4(2)(-2)}}{2(2)} \quad \text{or} \quad \frac{-(-1) - \sqrt{(-1)^2 - 4(2)(-2)}}{2(2)}$$

$$\cos x = \frac{1 + \sqrt{17}}{4} \quad \text{or} \quad \frac{1 - \sqrt{17}}{4}$$ ■

Equivalent equations using substitution

Consider the equation

$$(2x - 3)^2 - 3(2x - 3) - 10 = 0$$

If we replace $2x - 3$ by, say u, then we obtain the equation

$$u^2 - 3u - 10 = 0$$

which we solve as

$$(u - 5)(u + 2) = 0$$
$$u = -2 \text{ or } 5$$

We now replace u by $2x - 3$ to obtain

$$2x - 3 = -2 \text{ or } 2x - 3 = 5$$
$$2x = 1 \text{ or } 2x = 8$$
$$x = \tfrac{1}{2} \text{ or } x = 4$$

Anytime we can replace an expression by a variable like u we obtain an equivalent equation that may be easier to solve or otherwise manipulate.

■ *Example 5–0 C*

Use substitution to help solve each problem.

1. Solve the equation $2(5x + 3)^3 - (5x + 3)^2 = 0$.

Let $u = 5x + 3$. Then,

$$2u^3 - u^2 = 0$$
$$u^2(2u - 1) = 0$$
$$u^2 = 0 \text{ or } 2u - 1 = 0$$
$$u = 0 \text{ or } u = \tfrac{1}{2}$$
$$5x + 3 = 0 \text{ or } 5x + 3 = \tfrac{1}{2}$$
$$5x = -3 \text{ or } 5x = -\tfrac{5}{2}$$
$$x = -\tfrac{3}{5} \text{ or } x = \tfrac{1}{5}(-\tfrac{5}{2}) = -\tfrac{1}{2}$$

$\tfrac{1}{2} - 3 = \tfrac{1}{2} - \tfrac{6}{2}$

2. Simplify $\dfrac{\left(3\theta - \dfrac{\pi}{2}\right)^2 - 1}{1 - \left(3\theta - \dfrac{\pi}{2}\right)}$.

Let $u = 3\theta - \dfrac{\pi}{2}$. Then the expression is

$$\frac{u^2 - 1}{1 - u} = \frac{(u - 1)(u + 1)}{-(u - 1)} = \frac{u + 1}{-1} = -(u + 1) = -u - 1$$

Replace u by $3\theta - \dfrac{\pi}{2}$:

$$-u - 1 = -\left(3\theta - \frac{\pi}{2}\right) - 1 = -3\theta + \frac{\pi}{2} - 1$$ ■

Mastery points

Can you
- Factor trigonometric expressions?
- Solve quadratic equations for *x*, sin *x*, cos *x*, or tan *x?*
- Use substitution to help solve equations and simplify expressions?

Exercise 5–0

Note: The *solutions* to all of these exercises are given in appendix E. This section is not reviewed explicitly in the chapter review or the chapter test. It is designed to prepare for the rest of the chapter.

Factor each trigonometric expression.

1. $\sin^2\theta - \sin\theta$

2. $\cos^3\theta + 3\cos\theta$

3. $\cos^4\theta - \cos^2\theta$

4. $\sin^5\theta - \sin^3\theta$

5. $\cos^2 x + \cos x - 20$

6. $\tan^2 x + 2\tan x - 24$

7. $2\sin^2 x - 7\sin x + 3$

8. $9\cos^3\theta - 15\cos^2\theta - 6\cos\theta$

9. $6\csc^2\theta - 5\csc\theta + 1$

Solve each quadratic equation for sin θ, cos θ, tan θ, etc., as appropriate.

10. $\tan^2\theta - \tan\theta = 0$

11. $\tan^2\theta - \tan\theta = 2$

12. $6\sin^2\theta + 5\sin\theta + 1 = 0$

13. $\sec^4\theta - 5\sec^2\theta + 4 = 0$

14. $36\sin^4\theta - 13\sin^2\theta + 1 = 0$

15. $\dfrac{2}{3}\sin\theta + \dfrac{1}{3\sin\theta} = 1$

16. $\sin^2\theta - 3\sin\theta - 5 = 0$

17. $2\sec^2\theta + 3\sec\theta - 7 = 0$

Use substitution to help solve each equation.

18. $(2x - 6)^3 - (2x - 6)^2 = 0$

19. $12\left(\dfrac{x}{3} - 1\right)^2 - 5\left(\dfrac{x}{3} - 1\right) - 2 = 0$

Use substitution to help simplify each expression.

20. $5\left(\dfrac{\pi}{2} - 3\right) + 3\left[\left(\dfrac{\pi}{2} - 3\right) - 7\right] - \dfrac{\pi}{2} + 3$

21. $\dfrac{2(3x - \frac{1}{2})^2 - 3(3x - \frac{1}{2}) + 1}{(3x - \frac{1}{2})^2 - 1}$

5-1 *Basic trigonometric identities*

Review of some identities

Recall from section 1–4 and 5–0 that an identity is an equation that is true for every allowed value of its variable (or variables). We have seen the following identities in previous sections.

Reciprocal identities

$$\csc\theta = \frac{1}{\sin\theta}, \qquad \sec\theta = \frac{1}{\cos\theta}, \qquad \cot\theta = \frac{1}{\tan\theta}$$

$$\sin\theta = \frac{1}{\csc\theta}, \qquad \cos\theta = \frac{1}{\sec\theta}, \qquad \tan\theta = \frac{1}{\cot\theta}$$

Tangent/cotangent identities

$$\tan\theta = \frac{\sin\theta}{\cos\theta}, \qquad \cot\theta = \frac{\cos\theta}{\sin\theta}$$

Fundamental identity of trigonometry

$$\sin^2\theta + \cos^2\theta = 1$$

Two other forms of the fundamental identity are $\sin^2\theta = 1 - \cos^2\theta$ and $\cos^2\theta = 1 - \sin^2\theta$.

If each term in the fundamental identity is divided by $\cos^2\theta$ we obtain

$$\frac{\sin^2\theta}{\cos^2\theta} + \frac{\cos^2\theta}{\cos^2\theta} = \frac{1}{\cos^2\theta}$$

$$\left(\frac{\sin\theta}{\cos\theta}\right)^2 + 1 = \left(\frac{1}{\cos\theta}\right)^2$$

$$\tan^2\theta + 1 = \sec^2\theta$$

Similarly, if each term of the fundamental identity is divided by $\sin^2\theta$ we obtain the identity $\cot^2\theta + 1 = \csc^2\theta$. These two identities, along with the fundamental identity, are called the Pythagorean identities. They are summarized here.

Pythagorean identities

Useful forms

$$\sin^2\theta + \cos^2\theta = 1 \qquad \sin^2\theta = 1 - \cos^2\theta \qquad \cos^2\theta = 1 - \sin^2\theta$$
$$\tan^2\theta + 1 = \sec^2\theta \qquad \tan^2\theta = \sec^2\theta - 1 \qquad \sec^2\theta - \tan^2\theta = 1$$
$$\cot^2\theta + 1 = \csc^2\theta \qquad \cot^2\theta = \csc^2\theta - 1 \qquad \csc^2\theta - \cot^2\theta = 1$$

Preliminary notes on algebra

When working with trigonometric equations there are certain algebraic principles that are used over and over. It is a good idea to get used to these principles, and the associated notation, now—it will make the rest of this chapter much easier.

These principles are illustrated in example 5–1 A. We also use the principle that we *do not leave fractions in a final answer when possible.* For example, $\dfrac{1}{\cot\theta}$ can be rewritten as $\tan\theta$. Also we note that a binomial of the form $x + y$ is called the **conjugate** of the binomial $x - y$, and vice versa.

■ *Example 5–1 A*

Perform the algebra indicated, and note the category of algebraic manipulation for later reference. Do not leave a fraction for an answer when possible.

1. *Separating fractions:* $\dfrac{a + b}{c} = \dfrac{a}{c} + \dfrac{b}{c}$

Rewrite $\dfrac{1 - \sin\theta}{\sin\theta}$ as two fractions.

$$\frac{1 - \sin\theta}{\sin\theta} = \frac{1}{\sin\theta} - \frac{\sin\theta}{\sin\theta}$$
$$= \csc\theta - 1$$

2. *Multiplying binomial conjugates:* $(a + b)(a - b) = a^2 - b^2$
Multiply $(1 - \sin\theta)(1 + \sin\theta)$.

$$(1 - \sin\theta)(1 + \sin\theta) = 1^2 - (\sin\theta)^2$$
$$= 1 - \sin^2\theta$$
$$= \cos^2\theta \qquad \text{Pythagorean identity}$$

3. *Factoring quadratic binomials into conjugates:* $a^2 - b^2 = (a + b)(a - b)$

Factor the numerator of $\dfrac{\csc^2\theta - \cot^2\theta}{\csc\theta - \cot\theta}$.

$$\frac{\csc^2\theta - \cot^2\theta}{\csc\theta - \cot\theta} = \frac{(\csc\theta - \cot\theta)(\csc\theta + \cot\theta)}{\csc\theta - \cot\theta}$$
$$= \csc\theta + \cot\theta$$

4. *Multiplying numerator and denominator of a fraction by a conjugate of the numerator or denominator:*

Multiply the numerator and denominator of $\dfrac{1 - \cos\theta}{\sin\theta}$ by the conjugate of the numerator.

$$\frac{1 - \cos\theta}{\sin\theta} \cdot \frac{1 + \cos\theta}{1 + \cos\theta} = \frac{1 - \cos^2\theta}{\sin\theta(1 + \cos\theta)}$$

$$= \frac{\sin^2\theta}{\sin\theta(1 + \cos\theta)}$$

$$= \frac{\sin\theta}{1 + \cos\theta}$$

5. *Factoring the sign from a binomial:* $-(a - b) = b - a$

Simplify $\dfrac{\cos^2\theta - 1}{\sin\theta}$.

$$\frac{\cos^2\theta - 1}{\sin\theta} = \frac{-(1 - \cos^2\theta)}{\sin\theta}$$

$$= \frac{-\sin^2\theta}{\sin\theta}$$

$$= -\sin\theta \qquad\blacksquare$$

Transforming expressions

Identities and the principles illustrated above aid in simplifying and transforming trigonometric expressions. We proceed by replacing given parts of an expression by equivalent parts from the identities summarized above, as well as any other identities we have studied. *There is no single correct sequence of steps!* We proceed by trial and error, guided by past experience.

Although there are many ways to proceed in transforming an expression, we will note some guidelines for this process.

1. When functions appear raised to the second power, such as $\sin^2\theta$, $\tan^2\theta$, etc., look for expressions that appear in the Pythagorean identities.

   a. It may be possible to combine two terms into one.

   example: $\dfrac{\sec^2\theta - \tan^2\theta}{\sin\theta}$ becomes $\dfrac{1}{\sin\theta}$, which becomes $\csc\theta$.

   b. It is always possible to rewrite one second degree term as two.

   example: $\dfrac{\sec^2\theta}{\tan^2\theta + 1}$ becomes $\dfrac{\tan^2\theta + 1}{\tan^2\theta + 1}$, which becomes 1.

2. Sometimes it pays to rewrite all functions in terms of the sine and cosine functions.

Rewrite $\sec\theta$ as $\dfrac{1}{\cos\theta}$, $\csc\theta$ as $\dfrac{1}{\sin\theta}$, $\tan\theta$ as $\dfrac{\sin\theta}{\cos\theta}$, $\cot\theta$ as $\dfrac{\cos\theta}{\sin\theta}$.

3. Look for factors of the Pythagorean identities. These are things like $1 - \cos\theta$, which is a factor of $1 - \cos^2\theta$, and $\sec\theta + \tan\theta$, which is a factor of $\sec^2\theta - \tan^2\theta$. These can often be transformed as in part 4 of example 5–1 A.

Example 5–1 B illustrates these guidelines.

■ *Example 5–1 B*

Simplify each expression into one term.

1. $1 - \cos^2 4\alpha$
  $\sin^2 4\alpha$ $\sin^2 4\alpha + \cos^2 4\alpha = 1$, so $1 - \cos^2 4\alpha = \sin^2 4\alpha$

2. $(1 - \sec x)(1 + \sec x)$
  $1 - \sec^2 x$ $(a - b)(a + b) = a^2 - b^2$
  $-(\sec^2 x - 1)$
  $-\tan^2 x$

Simplify the expression into as few factors as possible.

3. $\cot\theta \, \sec\theta \, \sin\theta$

$\cot\theta \, \sec\theta \, \sin\theta$

$\dfrac{\cos\theta}{\sin\theta} \cdot \dfrac{1}{\cos\theta} \cdot \sin\theta$ Rewrite everything in terms of $\sin\theta$, $\cos\theta$

$\dfrac{\overset{1}{\cancel{\cos\theta}}}{\underset{1}{\cancel{\sin\theta}}} \cdot \dfrac{1}{\underset{1}{\cancel{\cos\theta}}} \cdot \overset{1}{\cancel{\sin\theta}}$ Divide out the common factors

1 ■

Verifying identities

If we can show that one member of an equation can be transformed into the other member by replacing expressions using identities and performing algebraic transformations, then we say we have *verified* the equation to be an identity.

Although there are many ways to proceed in verifying an identity, there are some guidelines for this process. The guidelines 1 through 3 apply to verifying identities as well as simplifying individual expressions. Example 5–1 C illustrates another guideline, which applies to verifying identities.

4. Begin with the more complicated member of an equation, and try to simplify it.

A fraction is almost always considered more complicated than a nonfraction.

■ *Example 5–1 C*

Verify that each equation is an identity by showing that one member of the identity can be transformed into the other member.

1. $\tan \theta \csc \theta = \sec \theta$

$\tan \theta \csc \theta$	Begin with the left member
$\dfrac{\sin \theta}{\cos \theta} \cdot \dfrac{1}{\sin \theta}$	Rewrite everything in terms of $\sin \theta$ and $\cos \theta$
$\dfrac{1}{\cos \theta}$	Reduce by a factor of $\sin \theta$
$\sec \theta$	$\sec \theta = \dfrac{1}{\cos \theta}$

2. $\dfrac{1}{\sin \beta - \csc \beta} = -\tan \beta \sec \beta$

$\dfrac{1}{\sin \beta - \csc \beta}$	Begin with the left member; it is more complicated
$\dfrac{1}{\sin \beta - \dfrac{1}{\sin \beta}}$	Rewrite everything in terms of $\sin \theta$ and $\cos \theta$; we arrive at a complex fraction
$\dfrac{1}{\sin \beta - \dfrac{1}{\sin \beta}} \cdot \dfrac{\sin \beta}{\sin \beta}$	Multiply numerator and denominator by $\sin \beta$; this is to simplify the complex fraction
$\dfrac{\sin \beta}{\sin^2\beta - 1}$	$\sin \beta \left(\sin \beta - \dfrac{1}{\sin \beta} \right) = \sin^2\beta - 1$
$\dfrac{\sin \beta}{-(1 - \sin^2\beta)}$	Factor the sign from the binomial denominator
$\dfrac{\sin \beta}{-\cos^2\beta}$	
$-\dfrac{\sin \beta}{\cos \beta} \cdot \dfrac{1}{\cos \beta}$	
$-\tan \beta \sec \beta$	

3. $\dfrac{\cos^2\alpha}{1 + \sin \alpha} = 1 - \sin \alpha$

$\dfrac{\cos^2\alpha}{1 + \sin \alpha}$	
$\dfrac{1 - \sin^2\alpha}{1 + \sin \alpha}$	$\cos^2\theta = 1 - \sin^2\theta$
$\dfrac{(1 - \sin \alpha)(1 + \sin \alpha)}{1 + \sin \alpha}$	$m^2 - n^2 = (m - n)(m + n)$
$1 - \sin \alpha$	

It is not absolutely necessary to transform just one side or the other of an identity. When both members of an identity are very complicated it is easier to transform both members, as in example 5–1 D.

■ *Example 5–1 D*

Verify the identity.

$$\sin^2\theta\,\tan^2\theta + 1 = \sec^2\theta - \cos^2\theta\,\sec^2\theta + \cos^2\theta$$

Left member	**Right member**
$\sin^2\theta\,\tan^2\theta + 1$	$\sec^2\theta - \cos^2\theta\,\sec^2\theta + \cos^2\theta$
$\sin^2\theta\,\tan^2\theta + \sin^2\theta + \cos^2\theta$	$\sec^2\theta(1 - \cos^2\theta) + \cos^2\theta$
$\sin^2\theta(\tan^2\theta + 1) + \cos^2\theta$	$\sec^2\theta\,\sin^2\theta + \cos^2\theta$
$\sin^2\theta\,\sec^2\theta + \cos^2\theta$	$\dfrac{1}{\cos^2\theta}\sin^2\theta + \cos^2\theta$
$\sin^2\theta\dfrac{1}{\cos^2\theta} + \cos^2\theta$	
$\tan^2\theta + \cos^2\theta$	$\tan^2\theta + \cos^2\theta$ ■

Since the left side and right side can be transformed into the same expression, they are equivalent. This is true because we could actually take the steps on one side and add them to the other side in reverse order, arriving at the required result.

Of course most equations are not identities. To show that an equation is not an identity we need to find a value for the variable for which each member of the equation is defined, but that produces different results in the two members. This value is called a **counter example;** it shows that the equation is *not* an identity.

■ *Example 5–1 E*

Show by counter example that $\cos x + \sin x \cot x = \sin x$ is not an identity.

Choose a value for which both the left and right members are defined; $x = \dfrac{\pi}{4}$ is such a value (most values would serve the purpose).

Left member	**Right member**	
$\cos x + \sin x \cot x$	$\sin x$	
$\cos \dfrac{\pi}{4} + \sin \dfrac{\pi}{4} \cot \dfrac{\pi}{4}$	$\sin \dfrac{\pi}{4}$	Replace x by $\dfrac{\pi}{4}$
$\dfrac{\sqrt{2}}{2} + \dfrac{\sqrt{2}}{2} \cdot 1$	$\dfrac{\sqrt{2}}{2}$	$\cos \dfrac{\pi}{4} = \sin \dfrac{\pi}{4} = \dfrac{\sqrt{2}}{2}$; $\cot \dfrac{\pi}{4} = 1$
$\dfrac{2\sqrt{2}}{2}$		
$\sqrt{2}$		

Since $\sqrt{2} \neq \dfrac{\sqrt{2}}{2}$ we have shown that the given equation is not an identity.   ■

As noted in example 5–1 E, most values will serve as a counter example for an equation that is not an identity. However, *avoid using zero,* since there are many equations that are not identities for which both sides evaluate to the same value when zero is used.

An example is $\sin \theta = 1 - \cos \theta$. This equation is *not* an identity, but observe that replacing θ by 0 produces $0 = 0$, which might lead one to believe that this equation is an identity.

Mastery points

Can you
- State the reciprocal identities, fundamental identity, and the remaining Pythagorean identities from memory?
- Recognize useful forms of the Pythagorean identities?
- Transform forms of the Pythagorean identities into simpler forms?
- Transform one side of an identity into the other side?
- Show that an equation is not an identity by a counter example?

Exercise 5–1

Each of the following expressions can be simplified into the form 1, -1, $\sin \theta$, $\cos \theta$, $\tan \theta$, $\cot \theta$, $\sec \theta$, $\csc \theta$, $\sin^2\theta$, $\cos^2\theta$, $\tan^2\theta$, $\cot^2\theta$, $\sec^2\theta$, or $\csc^2\theta$. Show the transformation of each expression into one of these forms.

1. $\dfrac{\sin \theta}{\tan \theta}$

2. $\dfrac{\cos \theta}{\cot \theta}$

3. $\tan \theta \csc \theta$

4. $\sec \theta \cot \theta$

5. $\cot^2\theta \sin^2\theta$

6. $\sin^2\theta \sec^2\theta$

7. $(\tan^2\theta + 1)(1 - \sin^2\theta)$

8. $(1 - \cos^2\theta)(1 + \cot^2\theta)$

9. $\dfrac{(\sec \theta - 1)(\sec \theta + 1)}{\sin^2\theta}$

10. $\dfrac{(\sec \theta + \tan \theta)(\sec \theta - \tan \theta)}{\cos^2\theta}$

11. $\dfrac{\csc \theta \sin \theta}{\cot \theta}$

12. $\dfrac{\tan \theta \cot \theta}{\sin \theta}$

13. $\cos \theta(\sec \theta - \cos \theta)$

14. $\cos^2\theta(1 + \cot^2\theta)$

15. $\csc^2\theta(1 - \cos^2\theta)$

16. $\sin^2\theta(\csc^2\theta - 1)$

17. $\cot^2\theta - \csc^2\theta$

18. $\tan^2\theta - \sec^2\theta$

19. $\tan^2\theta(\cot^2\theta + 1)$

20. $\dfrac{\cot x}{\sec x}$

21. $\sec^2\theta(\csc^2\theta - 1)$

22. $\dfrac{\sec \theta}{\tan \theta \csc \theta}$

23. $\dfrac{\cot \theta \sec \theta}{\csc \theta}$

24. $\dfrac{\csc^2\theta - 1}{\csc^2\theta}$

25. $\sin x + \cos x \cot x$

26. $\cos x + \sin x \tan x$

27. $\tan x \csc x \cos x$

28. $\dfrac{\csc x + \sec x}{\tan x + 1}$

29. $\sec x - \tan x \sin x$

30. $(\csc x + 1)(\sec x - \tan x)$

31. $(\csc x + \cot x)(1 - \cos x)$

32. $\dfrac{\sec^4 y - \tan^4 y}{\sec^2 y + \tan^2 y}$

Verify the following identities.

33. $\csc\theta + \cot\theta = \dfrac{1 + \cos\theta}{\sin\theta}$

34. $\tan\theta + \sec\theta = \dfrac{1 + \sin\theta}{\cos\theta}$

35. $\dfrac{\csc\theta}{\sec\theta + \tan\theta} = \dfrac{\cos\theta}{\sin\theta + \sin^2\theta}$

36. $\dfrac{\sec\theta}{\csc\theta + \cot\theta} = \dfrac{\tan\theta}{1 + \cos\theta}$

37. $\dfrac{1 + \csc\theta}{1 + \sec\theta} = \cot\theta\left(\dfrac{1 + \sin\theta}{1 + \cos\theta}\right)$

38. $\dfrac{\tan\theta + 1}{\tan\theta - 1} = \dfrac{\sin\theta + \cos\theta}{\sin\theta - \cos\theta}$

39. $\dfrac{\tan^2\theta + \sec^2\theta}{\sec^2\theta} = \sin^2\theta + 1$

40. $\dfrac{\cot^2\theta + \csc^2\theta}{\csc^2\theta} = 1 + \cos^2\theta$

41. $\tan y \sin y = \sec y - \cos y$

42. $\cot x \cos x = \csc x - \sin x$

43. $\dfrac{1 + \cot^2\theta}{\tan^2\theta} = \cot^2\theta\,\csc^2\theta$

44. $\dfrac{\cot^2\theta}{\csc\theta + 1} = 1 - \csc\theta$

45. $\dfrac{1}{\sec\theta - \cos\theta} = \cot\theta\,\csc\theta$

46. $\dfrac{1}{\cot\theta + \tan\theta} = \sin\theta\,\cos\theta$

47. $\dfrac{\tan\theta}{\csc\theta} = \sin\theta\,\tan\theta$

48. $\dfrac{\cot\theta}{\sec\theta} = \csc\theta - \sin\theta$

49. $\dfrac{\tan^2\theta}{\sec\theta - 1} = 1 + \sec\theta$

50. $\dfrac{1}{\sec x - \tan x} = \sec x + \tan x$

51. $\dfrac{\cot x + 1}{\cot x - 1} = \dfrac{\sin x + \cos x}{\cos x - \sin x}$

52. $\dfrac{1 + \sin y}{1 - \sin y} = \dfrac{\csc y + 1}{\csc y - 1}$

53. $\dfrac{\sin x}{1 + \cos x} = \dfrac{1 - \cos x}{\sin x}$

54. $\dfrac{1 + \sin y}{\cos y} = \dfrac{\cos y}{1 - \sin y}$

55. $\dfrac{\cos x}{\sec x - \tan x} = \dfrac{\cos^2 x}{1 - \sin x}$

56. $\dfrac{\cos x}{\cos x + \sin x} = \dfrac{\cot x}{1 + \cot x}$

57. $\dfrac{1}{1 - \sin x} + \dfrac{1}{1 + \sin x} = 2\sec^2 x$

58. $\dfrac{\cos y}{\csc y + 1} + \dfrac{\cos y}{\csc y - 1} = 2\tan y$

59. $\sin^4 x - \cos^4 x = 1 - 2\cos^2 x$

60. $(\tan^2 y + 1)(\cot^2 y + 1) = \sec^2 y + \csc^2 y$

61. $\cot^2 x - \cos^2 x = \cot^2 x \cos^2 x$

62. $\csc^2 y + \sec^2 y = \sec^2 y \csc^2 y$

63. $\dfrac{\tan y - \cot y}{\tan y + \cot y} = \dfrac{\tan^2 y - 1}{\sec^2 y}$

64. $\dfrac{\cot^2 x - 1}{\cot^2 x + 1} = 1 - 2\sin^2 x$

65. $\dfrac{1 - \sin x}{1 + \sin x} = (\tan x - \sec x)^2$

66. $\sec^4 x - 1 = \tan^2 x \sec^2 x + \tan^2 x$

67. $\sec^4 x - \sec^2 x = \tan^4 x + \tan^2 x$

68. $\tan x - \cot x = \dfrac{\sin^2 x - \cos^2 x}{\sin x \cos x}$

69. $2\cos^2 y - 1 = \cos^2 y - \sin^2 y$

70. $\cos^4 x - \sin^4 x = 1 - 2\sin^2 x$

In problems 71–80 show by counter example that each equation is not an identity.

71. $\sin\theta = 1 - \cos\theta$

72. $\tan^2\theta - \cot^2\theta = 1$

73. $\sec\theta = \dfrac{1}{\csc\theta}$

74. $\sin\theta = \dfrac{1}{\cos\theta}$

75. $\sin^2\theta - 2\cos\theta\sin\theta + \cos^2\theta = 2$

76. $\tan^2\theta - \tan\theta = 0$

77. $\csc\theta + \sec\theta\cot\theta = 2$

78. $\sin\theta + 2\sin\theta\cos\theta = 0$

79. $\dfrac{1 - \cos\theta}{1 + \cos\theta} = \sin^2\theta$

80. $\dfrac{1}{\tan\theta + \csc\theta} = \sec\theta$

81. Verify by calculation that $(1 - \csc^2\theta)(1 - \sec^2\theta) = 1$ for the values

a. $\theta = \dfrac{\pi}{6}$ **b.** $\theta = \dfrac{\pi}{4}$ **c.** Is this equation an identity?

82. Verify by calculation that $\dfrac{\sin\theta - \cos\theta}{\cos\theta} = \tan\theta - 1$ for the values

a. $\theta = \dfrac{\pi}{3}$ **b.** $\theta = \dfrac{3\pi}{4}$ **c.** Is this equation an identity?

83. Verify by calculation that $2\sin^2\theta + \sin\theta = 1$ for the values

a. $\theta = \dfrac{\pi}{6}$ **b.** $\theta = \dfrac{3\pi}{2}$ **c.** Is this equation an identity?

84. Verify by calculation that $\tan^4\theta - \tan^2\theta = 6$ for the values

a. $\theta = \dfrac{\pi}{3}$ **b.** $\theta = \dfrac{4\pi}{3}$ **c.** Is this equation an identity?

5–2 *The sum and difference identities*

Four important identities are called the sum and difference identities.

> **Sum and difference identities for sine and cosine**
> [1] $\cos(\alpha + \beta) = \cos \alpha \cos \beta - \sin \alpha \sin \beta$
> [2] $\cos(\alpha - \beta) = \cos \alpha \cos \beta + \sin \alpha \sin \beta$
> [3] $\sin(\alpha + \beta) = \sin \alpha \cos \beta + \cos \alpha \sin \beta$
> [4] $\sin(\alpha - \beta) = \sin \alpha \cos \beta - \cos \alpha \sin \beta$

The last three of these four identities can be developed using the first. Their verification is left as exercises. A demonstration that identity [1] is true is given in appendix B.

The sum and difference identities have several applications, illustrated in example 5–2 A.

■ *Example 5–2 A*

1. Use the fact that $\dfrac{7\pi}{12} = \dfrac{\pi}{4} + \dfrac{\pi}{3}$ to find the exact value of $\cos \dfrac{7\pi}{12}$.

$$\cos \frac{7\pi}{12} = \cos\left(\frac{\pi}{3} + \frac{\pi}{4}\right)$$

$$= \cos \frac{\pi}{3} \cos \frac{\pi}{4} - \sin \frac{\pi}{3} \sin \frac{\pi}{4} \qquad \cos(\alpha + \beta) = \cos \alpha \cos \beta - \sin \alpha \sin \beta$$

$$= \frac{1}{2} \cdot \frac{\sqrt{2}}{2} - \frac{\sqrt{3}}{2} \cdot \frac{\sqrt{2}}{2} = \frac{\sqrt{2}}{4} - \frac{\sqrt{6}}{4} = \frac{\sqrt{2} - \sqrt{6}}{4}$$

2. Show that $\cos(\pi - \theta) = -\cos \theta$ for any angle θ.

$$\cos(\pi - \theta) = \cos \pi \cos \theta + \sin \pi \sin \theta$$
$$= (-1) \cos \theta + 0 \sin \theta$$
$$= -\cos \theta$$ ■

Identity [1] can be used to prove the following identities (the proofs are left for the exercises). These identities are called the cofunction identities.

> **Cofunction identities**
>
> [5] $\sin\left(\dfrac{\pi}{2} - \theta\right) = \cos \theta$ [6] $\cos\left(\dfrac{\pi}{2} - \theta\right) = \sin \theta$
>
> [7] $\tan\left(\dfrac{\pi}{2} - \theta\right) = \cot \theta$ [8] $\cot\left(\dfrac{\pi}{2} - \theta\right) = \tan \theta$
>
> [9] $\sec\left(\dfrac{\pi}{2} - \theta\right) = \csc \theta$ [10] $\csc\left(\dfrac{\pi}{2} - \theta\right) = \sec \theta$

The reason for the name of these identities is as follows.

When the sum of two angles is 90°, or $\dfrac{\pi}{2}$ radians, the angles are said to be **complementary.** The angles $\dfrac{\pi}{2} - \theta$ and θ add up to $\dfrac{\pi}{2}$, so they are complementary angles. Each is said to be the complement of the other. The cofunction identities say, in effect,

trig function (angle) = ''co'' trig function (complement of angle)

Thus, the sine and ''co'' sine appear in one identity, the tangent and ''co'' tangent appear in another, and the secant and ''co'' secant in the third. Whenever the sum of two angles is $\dfrac{\pi}{2}$ (or 90°), a trigonometric function of one equals the ''co'' trigonometric function of the other. Thus for example, the following statements are true:

$$\sin 50° = \cos 40° \qquad\qquad 50° + 40° = 90°$$

$$\sec \frac{\pi}{6} = \csc \frac{\pi}{3} \qquad\qquad \frac{\pi}{6} + \frac{\pi}{3} = \frac{\pi}{2}$$

$$\cot 130° = \tan(-40°) \qquad\qquad 130° + (-40°) = 90°$$

■ *Example 5–2 B*

Rewrite each function value in terms of its cofunction.

1. $\sin 34°$

$$\sin 34° = \cos(90° - 34°) = \cos 56°$$

2. $\csc \dfrac{2\pi}{5}$

$$\csc \frac{2\pi}{5} = \sec\left(\frac{\pi}{2} - \frac{2\pi}{5}\right) = \sec \frac{\pi}{10}$$

Simplify each expression.

3. $\dfrac{\sin 10°}{\cos 80°}$

$$\frac{\sin 10°}{\cos 80°} = \frac{\cos 80°}{\cos 80°} = 1$$

4. $\sin^2 \dfrac{\pi}{6} + \sin^2 \dfrac{\pi}{3}$

$$\sin^2 \frac{\pi}{6} + \sin^2 \frac{\pi}{3} = \sin^2 \frac{\pi}{6} + \cos^2\left(\frac{\pi}{2} - \frac{\pi}{3}\right) = \sin^2 \frac{\pi}{6} + \cos^2 \frac{\pi}{6} = 1 \ ■$$

Two more important identities are the sum and difference formulas for the tangent function.

> ### Sum and difference identities for tangent
>
> [11] $\tan(\alpha + \beta) = \dfrac{\tan \alpha + \tan \beta}{1 - \tan \alpha \tan \beta}$
>
> [12] $\tan(\alpha - \beta) = \dfrac{\tan \alpha - \tan \beta}{1 + \tan \alpha \tan \beta}$

The derivation of the first identity is as follows.

$$\tan(\alpha + \beta) \;=\; \frac{\sin(\alpha + \beta)}{\cos(\alpha + \beta)} = \frac{\sin \alpha \cos \beta + \cos \alpha \sin \beta}{\cos \alpha \cos \beta - \sin \alpha \sin \beta}$$

$$= \frac{\dfrac{\sin \alpha \cos \beta + \cos \alpha \sin \beta}{\cos \alpha \cos \beta}}{\dfrac{\cos \alpha \cos \beta - \sin \alpha \sin \beta}{\cos \alpha \cos \beta}}$$

Divide numerator and denominator by

$\cos \alpha \cos \beta$

$$= \frac{\dfrac{\sin \alpha \cos \beta}{\cos \alpha \cos \beta} + \dfrac{\cos \alpha \sin \beta}{\cos \alpha \cos \beta}}{\dfrac{\cos \alpha \cos \beta}{\cos \alpha \cos \beta} - \dfrac{\sin \alpha \sin \beta}{\cos \alpha \cos \beta}}$$

$$= \frac{\dfrac{\sin \alpha}{\cos \alpha} + \dfrac{\sin \beta}{\cos \beta}}{1 - \dfrac{\sin \alpha}{\cos \alpha} \cdot \dfrac{\sin \beta}{\cos \beta}} = \frac{\tan \alpha + \tan \beta}{1 - \tan \alpha \tan \beta}$$

Example 5–2 C illustrates using this identity.

■ *Example 5–2 C*

Use the fact that $15° = 45° - 30°$ to find the exact value of $\tan 15°$.

$$\tan 15° = \tan(45° - 30°)$$

$$= \frac{\tan 45° - \tan 30°}{1 + \tan 45° \tan 30°} = \frac{1 - \dfrac{\sqrt{3}}{3}}{1 + 1\left(\dfrac{\sqrt{3}}{3}\right)}$$

$$= \frac{1 - \dfrac{\sqrt{3}}{3}}{1 + \dfrac{\sqrt{3}}{3}} \cdot \frac{3}{3} = \frac{3 - \sqrt{3}}{3 + \sqrt{3}} \cdot \frac{3 - \sqrt{3}}{3 - \sqrt{3}}$$

$$= \frac{9 - 6\sqrt{3} + 3}{9 - 3} = \frac{12 - 6\sqrt{3}}{6} = 2 - \sqrt{3}$$ ■

Some problems can be solved by using the identities above and reference triangles (section 2–4).

■ *Example 5–2 D* $\sin \alpha = \frac{2}{3}$, α in quadrant I; $\cos \beta = -\frac{4}{5}$, β in quadrant II. Find the exact value of $\cos(\alpha - \beta)$.

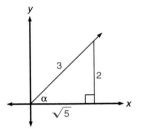 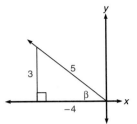

$$\cos \alpha = \frac{\sqrt{5}}{3}, \sin \beta = \frac{3}{5} \qquad \text{We find the necessary values from the reference triangles}$$

$$\cos(\alpha - \beta) = \cos \alpha \cos \beta + \sin \alpha \sin \beta$$

$$= \frac{\sqrt{5}}{3} \cdot \left(-\frac{4}{5}\right) + \frac{2}{3} \cdot \frac{3}{5}$$

$$= -\frac{4\sqrt{5}}{15} + \frac{6}{15}$$

$$= \frac{-4\sqrt{5} + 6}{15} \qquad ■$$

Mastery points

Can you
- State the sum and difference identities?
- State and apply the cofunction identities?
- Apply the sum and difference identities to find exact values of sine, cosine, and tangent for certain angles?
- Apply the sum and difference identities to find exact values of sine, cosine, and tangent for $\alpha + \beta$ and $\alpha - \beta$ given information about α and β?
- Verify identities using the sum and difference identities?

Exercise 5–2

Rewrite each function in terms of its cofunction.

1. $\sin 18°$ **2.** $\cos 42°$ **3.** $\tan 8°$ **4.** $\csc 100°$ **5.** $\sec \dfrac{\pi}{3}$

6. $\cot \dfrac{\pi}{6}$ **7.** $\cos \dfrac{5\pi}{6}$ **8.** $\sin\left(-\dfrac{\pi}{3}\right)$ **9.** $\sec\left(-\dfrac{3\pi}{4}\right)$ **10.** $\csc\left(-\dfrac{\pi}{4}\right)$

Simplify each expression.

11. $\dfrac{\cos 65°}{\sin 25°}$

12. $\tan \dfrac{\pi}{3} \tan \dfrac{\pi}{6}$

13. $\cos 20° \csc 70°$

14. $\dfrac{\sin^2 5°}{\cos^2 85°}$

15. $\sin \dfrac{\pi}{5} \sec \dfrac{3\pi}{10}$

16. $\cos^2 25° + \cos^2 65°$

17. $\tan^2 8° - \csc^2 82°$

18. $\dfrac{\cos^2 30°}{1 - \cos^2 60°}$

19. $\tan 40° \tan 50°$

20. $\tan 19° \tan 71°$

21. $\sec \dfrac{\pi}{6} \sin \dfrac{\pi}{3}$

22. $\cot \dfrac{\pi}{5} \cot \dfrac{3\pi}{10}$

23. $\sin^2 10° + \sin^2 80°$

24. $\tan^2 25° - \csc^2 65°$

25. $\sec^2 \dfrac{\pi}{3} - \cot^2 \dfrac{\pi}{6}$

26. $\cos^2 \dfrac{3\pi}{8} + \cos^2 \dfrac{\pi}{8}$

Use the sum and difference identities to find the exact value of each of the following. Observe that each value is the sum or difference of values chosen from $\dfrac{\pi}{6}(30°)$, $\dfrac{\pi}{4}(45°)$, and $\dfrac{\pi}{3}(60°)$.

27. $\cos \dfrac{\pi}{12}$ **28.** $\tan \dfrac{\pi}{12}$ **29.** $\sin \dfrac{5\pi}{12}$ **30.** $\cos \dfrac{5\pi}{12}$ **31.** $\sin \dfrac{7\pi}{12}$ **32.** $\tan \dfrac{7\pi}{12}$

33. $\sin 15°$ **34.** $\tan 15°$ **35.** $\cos 105°$ **36.** $\sin 105°$ **37.** $\tan 75°$ **38.** $\cos 15°$

Each of the following problems presents information about two angles, α and β, including the quadrant in which the angle terminates. Use the information to find the required value.

39. $\cos \alpha = \frac{1}{3}$, quadrant I; $\sin \beta = \frac{3}{4}$, quadrant I. Find $\sin(\alpha + \beta)$.

40. $\cos \alpha = -\frac{12}{13}$, quadrant II; $\sin \beta = \frac{1}{2}$, quadrant II. Find $\cos(\alpha - \beta)$.

41. $\sin \alpha = \frac{5}{13}$, quadrant II; $\cos \beta = -\frac{3}{4}$, quadrant III. Find $\tan(\alpha - \beta)$.

42. $\sin \alpha = -\frac{4}{5}$, quadrant IV; $\sin \beta = -\frac{1}{5}$, quadrant IV. Find $\sin(\alpha + \beta)$.

43. $\sin \alpha = -\frac{4}{5}$, quadrant IV; $\cos \beta = \frac{15}{17}$, quadrant IV. Find $\cos(\alpha + \beta)$.

44. $\cos \alpha = -\frac{3}{5}$, quadrant II; $\sin \beta = -\frac{8}{17}$, quadrant III. Find $\sin(\alpha - \beta)$.

45. $\sin \alpha = \frac{2}{3}$, quadrant I; $\cos \beta = -\frac{1}{3}$, quadrant III. Find $\cos(\alpha - \beta)$.

46. $\cos \alpha = \frac{\sqrt{2}}{2}$, quadrant IV; $\sin \beta = -\frac{\sqrt{3}}{2}$, quadrant III. Find $\tan(\alpha + \beta)$.

47. $\sin \alpha = \frac{2}{3}$, quadrant I; $\tan \beta = \frac{1}{4}$, quadrant I. Find $\sin(\alpha + \beta)$.

48. $\tan \alpha = \frac{3}{4}$, quadrant III; $\sin \beta = -\frac{4}{5}$, quadrant III. Find $\cos(\alpha - \beta)$.

49. $\cos \alpha = \frac{5}{13}$, quadrant IV; $\tan \beta = -\frac{5}{12}$, quadrant IV. Find $\tan(\alpha - \beta)$.

50. $\cos \alpha = \frac{1}{2}$, quadrant I; $\cos \beta = \frac{\sqrt{2}}{2}$, quadrant IV. Find $\sin(\alpha + \beta)$.

51. $\tan \alpha = 2$, quadrant III; $\cos \beta = -\frac{3}{5}$, quadrant II. Find $\cos(\alpha - \beta)$.

52. $\sin \alpha = -\frac{15}{17}$, quadrant III; $\tan \beta = -\frac{3}{4}$, quadrant IV. Find $\tan(\alpha + \beta)$.

53. $\sin \alpha = \frac{2}{3}$, quadrant I; $\sin \beta = -\frac{1}{5}$, quadrant III. Find $\sin(\alpha - \beta)$.

54. $\cos \alpha = -\frac{5}{13}$, quadrant III; $\cos \beta = -\frac{8}{17}$, quadrant III. Find $\cos(\alpha + \beta)$.

55. $\cos \alpha = -\dfrac{\sqrt{2}}{2}$, quadrant II; $\sin \beta = \dfrac{\sqrt{3}}{2}$, quadrant II. Find $\tan(\alpha + \beta)$.

56. $\cos \alpha = -\frac{3}{5}$, quadrant III; $\sin \beta = \frac{1}{3}$, quadrant II. Find $\tan(\alpha - \beta)$.

Use the sum and difference identities to verify the following identities.

57. $\sin(\pi - \theta) = \sin \theta$

58. $\sin(\pi + \theta) = -\sin \theta$

59. $\cos(\pi - \theta) = -\cos \theta$

60. $\cos(\pi + \theta) = -\cos \theta$

61. $\tan(\pi - \theta) = -\tan \theta$

62. $\tan(\pi + \theta) = \tan \theta$

63. Use the sum formula to show that the sine function is 2π-periodic; that is, that $\sin(\theta + 2\pi) = \sin \theta$.

64. Use the sum formula to show that the cosine function is 2π-periodic; that is, that $\cos(\theta + 2\pi) = \cos \theta$.

65. Use the sum formula to show that the tangent function is π-periodic; that is, that $\tan(\theta + \pi) = \tan \theta$.

The following identities are important because they express a product of factors as a sum of terms. Verify each identity.

66. $\sin \alpha \cos \beta = \frac{1}{2}[\sin(\alpha + \beta) + \sin(\alpha - \beta)]$

67. $\cos \alpha \sin \beta = \frac{1}{2}[\sin(\alpha + \beta) - \sin(\alpha - \beta)]$

68. $\cos \alpha \cos \beta = \frac{1}{2}[\cos(\alpha + \beta) + \cos(\alpha - \beta)]$

69. $\sin \alpha \sin \beta = \frac{1}{2}[\cos(\alpha - \beta) - \cos(\alpha + \beta)]$

70. A picture on a wall is 2 feet tall and 6 feet above eye level; see the diagram. Compute the exact value of $\sin(\alpha - \beta)$.

71. Referring to the figure, find (a) the exact value of $\tan \alpha$, and (b) use this to find the exact value of x. *Hint:* Compute $\tan(\alpha + 45°)$.

72. Use the identities for $\sin(\alpha + \beta)$ and $\cos(\alpha + \beta)$ to find $\sin \theta$ in the diagram.

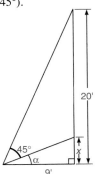

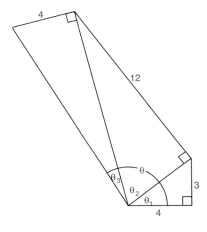

The following problems are designed to show that the sum and difference identities for sine and cosine [2], [3], and [4], and the cofunction identities, [5] through [10], are true, using the fact that identity [1] is true. The problems are in the necessary logical order.

73. Use identity [1], $\cos(\alpha + \beta) = \cos \alpha \cos \beta - \sin \alpha \sin \beta$, to verify identity [2], $\cos(\alpha - \beta) = \cos \alpha \cos \beta + \sin \alpha \sin \beta$. Do this by replacing β by $(-\beta)$ in the identity for $\cos(\alpha + \beta)$ and simplifying, using the even and odd properties for the sine and cosine functions.

74. Verify the identity [5], $\cos\left(\frac{\pi}{2} - \theta\right) = \sin \theta$, by using identity [2], letting $\alpha = \frac{\pi}{2}$ and $\beta = \theta$.

75. The identity [6], $\sin\left(\frac{\pi}{2} - \theta\right) = \cos \theta$, is really the same as identity [5]. Show this as follows. Let $\alpha = \frac{\pi}{2} - \theta$, so that $\theta = \frac{\pi}{2} - \alpha$. Replace $\frac{\pi}{2} - \theta$ by α in the left member of identity [5], then replace θ in the right member by $\frac{\pi}{2} - \alpha$. Then observe that α and θ are arbitrary values, so the result can be rewritten in terms of θ.

76. Verify identity [3], $\sin(\alpha + \beta) = \sin \alpha \cos \beta + \cos \alpha \sin \beta$, as follows.

$\sin \theta = \cos\left(\frac{\pi}{2} - \theta\right)$ This is identity [5], which we know is true

$\sin(\alpha + \beta) = \cos\left[\frac{\pi}{2} - (\alpha + \beta)\right]$ Replace θ by $\alpha + \beta$

$\sin(\alpha + \beta) = \cos\left[\left(\frac{\pi}{2} - \alpha\right) - \beta\right]$ Regroup $\frac{\pi}{2} - \alpha - \beta$

Now use identity [2] to expand the right member of this equation, then apply identities [5] and [6] to simplify the result and obtain identity [3].

77. Use the identity [3], $\sin(\alpha + \beta) = \sin \alpha \cos \beta + \cos \alpha \sin \beta$, to verify the identity [4], $\sin(\alpha - \beta) = \sin \alpha \cos \beta - \cos \alpha \sin \beta$. Do this by replacing β by $(-\beta)$ in identity [3].

78. Verify identity [7], $\tan\left(\frac{\pi}{2} - \theta\right) = \cot \theta$ using the fact that $\tan x = \frac{\sin x}{\cos x}$.

79. Verify identity [8], $\cot\left(\dfrac{\pi}{2} - \theta\right) = \tan\theta$. See problem 78 for guidance.

80. Verify identity [9], $\sec\left(\dfrac{\pi}{2} - \theta\right) = \csc\theta$ using the fact that $\sec x = \dfrac{1}{\cos x}$.

81. Verify identity [10], $\csc\left(\dfrac{\pi}{2} - \theta\right) = \sec\theta$. See problem 80 for guidance.

5–3 The double-angle and half-angle identities

Double-angle identities

Some more important identities are the **double-angle identities.** Recall that if we multiply a value by two we say we double the value.

> **Double-angle identities**
>
> [1] $\sin 2\alpha = 2\sin\alpha\cos\alpha$
>
> [3] $\tan 2\alpha = \dfrac{2\tan\alpha}{1 - \tan^2\alpha}$
>
> [2-a] $\cos 2\alpha = \cos^2\alpha - \sin^2\alpha$
>
> [2-b] $\cos 2\alpha = 1 - 2\sin^2\alpha$
>
> [2-c] $\cos 2\alpha = 2\cos^2\alpha - 1$

Observe that we present three identities for $\cos 2\alpha$. This is because identities [2-b] and [2-c] get so much use in the development of other identities.

The proof of [1] is as follows.

$\sin(\alpha + \beta) = \sin\alpha\cos\beta + \cos\alpha\sin\beta$ Sum identity from section 5–2

$\sin(\alpha + \alpha) = \sin\alpha\cos\alpha + \cos\alpha\sin\alpha$ Let $\beta = \alpha$

$\sin 2\alpha = 2\sin\alpha\cos\alpha$ $\alpha + \alpha = 2\alpha$

The verification of the remaining identities is left for the exercises. They are done in a similar way, starting with the identities for $\cos(\alpha + \beta)$ and $\tan(\alpha + \beta)$.

■ **Example 5–3 A**

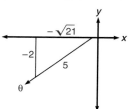

1. If $\sin\theta = -\frac{2}{5}$ and θ lies in quadrant III, find exact values of $\sin 2\theta$, $\cos 2\theta$, and $\tan 2\theta$.

First construct a reference triangle for θ to obtain any required trigonometric function values for that angle.

$$\sin 2\theta = 2\sin\theta\cos\theta$$
$$= 2\left(-\frac{2}{5}\right)\left(-\frac{\sqrt{21}}{5}\right) \qquad \sin\theta = -\frac{2}{5}\,;\ \cos\theta = -\frac{\sqrt{21}}{5}$$
$$= \frac{4\sqrt{21}}{25}$$
$$\cos 2\theta = \cos^2\theta - \sin^2\theta$$
$$= \left(-\frac{\sqrt{21}}{5}\right)^2 - \left(-\frac{2}{5}\right)^2 = \frac{21}{25} - \frac{4}{25} = \frac{17}{25}$$

$$\tan 2\theta = \frac{2 \tan \theta}{1 - \tan^2\theta}$$

$$= \frac{2\left(\dfrac{2}{\sqrt{21}}\right)}{1 - \left(\dfrac{2}{\sqrt{21}}\right)^2} = \frac{\dfrac{4}{\sqrt{21}}}{1 - \dfrac{4}{21}}$$

$$= \frac{\dfrac{4}{\sqrt{21}}}{\dfrac{17}{21}} = \frac{4}{\sqrt{21}} \cdot \frac{21}{17} = \frac{4\sqrt{21}}{17}$$

$\tan 2\theta$ could also be obtained from $\tan 2\theta = \dfrac{\sin 2\theta}{\cos 2\theta}$.

2. Find an identity for $\tan 3\theta$ in terms of $\tan \theta$.

$$\tan 3\theta = \tan(2\theta + \theta)$$

$3\theta = 2\theta + \theta$

$$= \frac{\tan 2\theta + \tan \theta}{1 - \tan 2\theta \tan \theta}$$

$\tan(\alpha + \beta) = \dfrac{\tan \alpha + \tan \beta}{1 - \tan \alpha \tan \beta}$

$$= \frac{\dfrac{2 \tan \theta}{1 - \tan^2\theta} + \tan \theta}{1 - \dfrac{2 \tan \theta}{1 - \tan^2\theta} \tan \theta}$$

Replace $\tan 2\theta$ by $\dfrac{2 \tan \theta}{1 - \tan^2\theta}$

$$= \frac{2 \tan \theta + \tan \theta(1 - \tan^2\theta)}{(1 - \tan^2\theta) - 2 \tan^2\theta}$$

Multiply numerator and denominator by $(1 - \tan^2\theta)$

$$= \frac{3 \tan \theta - \tan^3\theta}{1 - 3 \tan^2\theta}$$

Combine ■

Half-angle identities

A further set of important identities is the **half-angle identities.**

Half-angle identities

[4] $\sin \dfrac{\alpha}{2} = \pm\sqrt{\dfrac{1 - \cos \alpha}{2}}$

[6-a] $\tan \dfrac{\alpha}{2} = \pm\sqrt{\dfrac{1 - \cos \alpha}{1 + \cos \alpha}}$

[5] $\cos \dfrac{\alpha}{2} = \pm\sqrt{\dfrac{1 + \cos \alpha}{2}}$

[6-b] $\tan \dfrac{\alpha}{2} = \dfrac{\sin \alpha}{1 + \cos \alpha}$

[6-c] $\tan \dfrac{\alpha}{2} = \dfrac{1 - \cos \alpha}{\sin \alpha}$

We verify identity [5] as follows:

$$2 \cos^2\theta - 1 = \cos 2\theta \qquad \text{Identity [2-c] above}$$

$$2 \cos^2\theta = 1 + \cos 2\theta$$

$$\cos^2\theta = \frac{1 + \cos 2\theta}{2}$$

$$\cos^2\frac{\alpha}{2} = \frac{1 + \cos \alpha}{2} \qquad \text{Replace } \theta \text{ by } \frac{\alpha}{2}$$

$$\cos \frac{\alpha}{2} = \pm\sqrt{\frac{1 + \cos \alpha}{2}} \qquad \text{Take the square root of each member}$$

The verification of the remaining identities is left for the exercises.

The choice of plus or minus in identities [4], [5], and [6-a] depends on the quadrant in which the angle in question terminates (using the ASTC rule from section 2–3). It is only possible to determine the quadrant if we have information about the measure of the angle. To see why, consider figure 5–1.

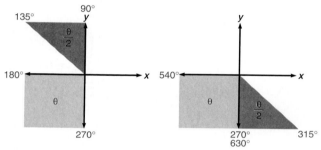

Figure 5–1

If $180° \le \theta \le 270°$ then $90° \le \dfrac{\theta}{2} \le 135°$; in this case, θ terminates in quadrant III and $\dfrac{\theta}{2}$ terminates in quadrant II. However, if $540° \le \theta \le 630°$, then $270° \le \dfrac{\theta}{2} \le 315°$. In this case, θ also terminates in quadrant III but $\dfrac{\theta}{2}$ terminates in quadrant IV.

These identities have applications such as those shown in example 5–3 B.

■ *Example 5–3 B*

1. Use the fact that 22.5° is one half of 45° to find the exact value of sin 22.5°.

$$\sin 22.5° = \sin \frac{45°}{2}$$

$$= \pm \sqrt{\frac{1 - \cos 45°}{2}} \qquad \sin \frac{\alpha}{2} = \pm \sqrt{\frac{1 - \cos \alpha}{2}};\ \alpha = 45°$$

We know sin 22.5° > 0, so choose plus

$$= \sqrt{\frac{1 - \frac{\sqrt{2}}{2}}{2}}$$

$$= \sqrt{\frac{2 - \sqrt{2}}{4}} \qquad \frac{1}{2}\left(1 - \frac{\sqrt{2}}{2}\right) = \frac{1}{2}\left(\frac{2 - \sqrt{2}}{2}\right).$$

$$= \frac{\sqrt{2 - \sqrt{2}}}{2}$$

2. $\cos \theta = \dfrac{3}{5}$ and $\dfrac{3\pi}{2} < \theta < 2\pi$. Find the exact value for $\cos \dfrac{\theta}{2}$.

Since $\dfrac{3\pi}{2} < \theta < 2\pi$, $\dfrac{3\pi}{4} < \dfrac{\theta}{2} < \pi$, so $\dfrac{\theta}{2}$ terminates in quadrant II, where the cosine function is negative.

$$\cos \frac{\theta}{2} = -\sqrt{\frac{1 + \cos \theta}{2}} \qquad \text{Choose minus since } \frac{\theta}{2} \text{ terminates in quadrant II}$$

where $\cos \dfrac{\theta}{2} < 0$

$$= -\sqrt{\frac{1 + \frac{3}{5}}{2}} \qquad \text{Replace } \cos \theta \text{ with } \frac{3}{5}$$

$$= -\sqrt{\frac{1}{2} \cdot \frac{8}{5}} = -\sqrt{\frac{4}{5}} = -\sqrt{\frac{20}{25}}$$

$$= -\frac{2\sqrt{5}}{5}$$

■

It is important to understand how to rewrite identities with different forms of the argument. For example, the following identities are all the same; the argument of each is shown in different forms.

[1] $\sin 2\alpha = 2 \sin \alpha \cos \alpha$ Identity [1] of the double-angle identities

$\sin 4\alpha = 2 \sin 2\alpha \cos 2\alpha$ Replace α in [1] by 2α

$\sin \alpha = 2 \sin \dfrac{\alpha}{2} \cos \dfrac{\alpha}{2}$ Replace α in [1] by $\dfrac{\alpha}{2}$

Example 5–3 C illustrates.

■ *Example 5–3 C*

Rewrite each expression as an expression of the form $a \sin x$, $a \cos x$, or $a \tan x$, for appropriate values of a and x.

1. $2 \sin 4\theta \cos 4\theta$
Compare

[1] $2 \sin \alpha \cos \alpha = \sin 2\alpha$
       $2 \sin 4\theta \cos 4\theta$

We can see that we should replace α by 4θ in identity [1] to obtain $2 \sin 4\theta \cos 4\theta$. Then,

$$2 \sin \alpha \cos \alpha = \sin 2\alpha \qquad \text{Identity [1]}$$
$$2 \sin 4\theta \cos 4\theta = \sin 2(4\theta) \qquad \text{Replace by } 4\theta$$
$$= \sin 8\theta$$

Thus, $2 \sin 4\theta \cos 4\theta = \sin 8\theta$.

2. $\dfrac{4 \tan 2\theta}{1 - \tan^2 2\theta}$

$$\dfrac{2 \tan \alpha}{1 - \tan^2 \alpha} = \tan 2\alpha \qquad \text{Identity [3]}$$

$$\dfrac{4 \tan \alpha}{1 - \tan^4 \alpha} = 2 \tan 2\alpha \qquad \text{Multiply each member by 2}$$

$$\dfrac{4 \tan 2\theta}{1 - \tan^2 2\theta} = 2 \tan 4\theta \qquad \text{Replace } \alpha \text{ by } 2\theta$$

3. $\cos^2 80° - \sin^2 80°$
Compare

$$\cos^2 \alpha - \sin^2 \alpha = \cos 2\alpha \qquad \text{Identity [2] of the double-angle identities}$$
$$\cos^2 80° - \sin^2 80°$$

Since $80°$ replaces α, we know that $\cos 2\alpha$ becomes $\cos 2(80)° = \cos 160°$. Thus, $\cos^2 80° - \sin^2 80° = \cos 160°$.   ■

A similar idea is illustrated in example 5–3 D.

■ *Example 5–3 D*

Find a value of θ for which the statement $\sin 110° = 2 \sin \theta \cos \theta$ is true, then rewrite the statement replacing θ by this value.

Compare

$$\sin 110° = 2 \sin \theta \cos \theta$$
$$\sin 2\theta = 2 \sin \theta \cos \theta$$

Let $2\theta = 110°$, so $\theta = 55°$.
The statement becomes $\sin 110° = 2 \sin 55° \cos 55°$.   ■

The identities of this and the previous sections may be combined to verify new identities.

■ *Example 5–3 E*

Verify the following identities.

1. $\sin 2\theta = \dfrac{2 \tan \theta}{1 + \tan^2\theta}$

It is best to work with the right member since it is more complicated.

$$\dfrac{2 \tan \theta}{1 + \tan^2\theta} = 2 \cdot \dfrac{\tan \theta}{\sec^2\theta} \qquad \tan^2\alpha + 1 = \sec^2\alpha$$

$$= 2 \cdot \tan \theta \cos^2\theta \qquad \cos \alpha = \dfrac{1}{\sec \alpha}$$

$$= 2 \cdot \dfrac{\sin \theta}{\cos \theta} \cos^2\theta$$

$$= 2 \sin \theta \cos \theta \qquad \dfrac{1}{\cos \theta} \cdot \cos^2\theta = \cos \theta$$

$$= \sin 2\theta \qquad \sin 2\alpha = 2 \sin \alpha \cos \alpha$$

2. $\sin 4\theta = 8 \sin \theta \cos^3\theta - 4 \sin \theta \cos \theta$

Although the right member is more complicated, it is easier to begin with $\sin 4\theta$ and expand this expression.

$$\sin 4\theta = \sin[2(2\theta)]$$

$$= 2 \sin 2\theta \cos 2\theta \qquad \text{Use } \sin 2\alpha = 2 \sin \alpha \cos \alpha, \text{ with } \alpha = 2\theta$$

$$= 2(2 \sin \theta \cos \theta)(2 \cos^2\theta - 1)$$

$$= 4 \sin \theta \cos \theta(2 \cos^2\theta - 1)$$

$$= 8 \sin \theta \cos^3\theta - 4 \sin \theta \cos \theta \qquad ■$$

Mastery points

Can you
- Write the double-angle and half-angle identities?
- Use the double-angle and half-angle identities to find exact values of

  $\sin 2\theta$, $\cos 2\theta$, $\tan 2\theta$, $\sin \dfrac{\theta}{2}$, $\cos \dfrac{\theta}{2}$, $\tan \dfrac{\theta}{2}$?

- Use the double-angle and half-angle identities to derive new identities and to verify given identities?
- Rewrite certain identities as a trigonometric function of $k\theta$, k an integer?

Exercise 5–3

Use the identities of this section to rewrite each expression as an expression of the form $a \sin x$, $a \cos x$, or $a \tan x$, for appropriate values of a and x.

1. $2 \sin \dfrac{\pi}{4} \cos \dfrac{\pi}{4}$

2. $2 \sin 52° \cos 52°$

3. $\cos^2 3\pi - \sin^2 3\pi$

4. $2 \cos^2 5\pi - 1$

5. $1 - 2 \sin^2 \dfrac{\pi}{10}$

6. $\dfrac{2 \tan \dfrac{\pi}{6}}{1 - \tan^2 \dfrac{\pi}{6}}$

7. $\dfrac{6 \tan 10°}{1 - \tan^2 10°}$

8. $8 \cos^2 \dfrac{\pi}{2} - 4$

9. $2 \sin 6\theta \cos 6\theta$

10. $4 \sin 2\theta \cos 2\theta$

11. $6 \cos^2 5\theta - 3$

12. $8 \cos^2 3\theta - 4$

13. $\dfrac{10 \tan 3\theta}{1 - \tan^2 3\theta}$

14. $\dfrac{8 \tan \dfrac{\theta}{2}}{1 - \tan^2 \dfrac{\theta}{2}}$

15. $2 - 4 \sin^2 7\theta$

16. $\frac{1}{2} - \sin^2 2\theta$

17. $3 \cos^2 3\theta - 3 \sin^2 3\theta$

18. $2 \cos^2 \dfrac{\theta}{2} - 2 \sin^2 \dfrac{\theta}{2}$

Find a value of θ for which each statement is true.

19. $\sin 140° = 2 \sin \theta \cos \theta$

20. $\sin \theta \cos \theta = \dfrac{1}{2} \sin \dfrac{\pi}{5}$

21. $\cos \dfrac{5\pi}{6} = \cos^2 \theta - \sin^2 \theta$

22. $2 \tan 86° = \dfrac{4 \tan \theta}{1 - \tan^2 \theta}$

23. $3 \cos 70° = 6 \cos^2 \theta - 3$

24. $\cos 560° = 1 - 2 \sin^2 \theta$

25. $\sin 10° = \sqrt{\dfrac{1 - \cos \theta}{2}}$

26. $\tan \theta = \sqrt{\dfrac{1 - \cos 46°}{1 + \cos 46°}}$

27. $\cos \theta = \sqrt{\dfrac{1}{2} \left(1 + \cos \dfrac{\pi}{4} \right)}$

28. $\sin \dfrac{\pi}{6} = \sqrt{\dfrac{1}{2}(1 - \cos \theta)}$

29. $\tan \dfrac{2\pi}{5} = \dfrac{1 - \cos \theta}{\sin \theta}$

30. $\cos 40° = \sqrt{\dfrac{1 + \cos \theta}{2}}$

Find the exact value of $\sin 2\theta$, $\cos 2\theta$, and $\tan 2\theta$ for each of the following.

31. $\sin \theta = \dfrac{3}{5}, 0 < \theta < \dfrac{\pi}{2}$

32. $\sin \theta = -\dfrac{12}{13}, \pi < \theta < \dfrac{3\pi}{2}$

33. $\cos \theta = -\dfrac{4}{5}, \dfrac{\pi}{2} < \theta < \pi$

34. $\tan \theta = -\dfrac{3}{4}, \dfrac{3\pi}{2} < \theta < 2\pi$

35. $\csc \theta = -\dfrac{8}{5}, \pi < \theta < \dfrac{3\pi}{2}$

36. $\tan \theta = \dfrac{5}{12}, \pi < \theta < \dfrac{3\pi}{2}$

Find the exact value of $\sin \dfrac{\theta}{2}$, $\cos \dfrac{\theta}{2}$, and $\tan \dfrac{\theta}{2}$ for each of the following.

37. $\sec \theta = -\dfrac{5}{2}, \pi < \theta < \dfrac{3\pi}{2}$

38. $\tan \theta = -\sqrt{15}, \dfrac{\pi}{2} < \theta < \pi$

39. $\cot \theta = -2, \dfrac{3\pi}{2} < \theta < 2\pi$

40. $\cos \theta = \dfrac{1}{4}, \dfrac{3\pi}{2} < \theta < 2\pi$

Use the half-angle identities to find the exact value of $\sin \theta$, $\cos \theta$, and $\tan \theta$ for the following values of θ.

41. $15°$, or $\dfrac{\pi}{12}$

42. $22.5°$, or $\dfrac{\pi}{8}$

43. $75°$, or $\dfrac{5\pi}{12}$

Use the sum/difference identities (from section 5–2) and the results of problems 41 and 42 to compute the exact value of the following. Observe that $37.5° = 15° + 22.5°$.

44. $\sin 37.5°$ **45.** $\cos 37.5°$ **46.** $\tan 37.5°$

47. Find $\sin 7.5°$; see problem 41.   **48.** Find $\cos 7.5°$; see problem 41.

Verify the following identities.

49. $\sin 2\theta + 1 = (\sin \theta + \cos \theta)^2$

50. $\cos 2\theta + 2 \sin^2\theta = 1$

51. $\cos^4\theta - \sin^4\theta = \cos 2\theta$

52. $\cot \theta = \dfrac{1 + \cos 2\theta}{\sin 2\theta}$

53. $\dfrac{1 + \cos 2\theta}{1 - \cos 2\theta} = \cot^2\theta$

54. $\tan 2\theta = \dfrac{2 \tan \theta}{2 - \sec^2\theta}$

55. $\cot \theta - \tan \theta = \dfrac{2 \cos 2\theta}{\sin 2\theta}$

56. $2 \csc 2\theta = \tan \theta + \cot \theta$

57. $\sin 2\theta - 4 \sin^3\theta \cos \theta = \sin 2\theta \cos 2\theta$

58. $\cos 4\theta = 1 - 8 \sin^2\theta \cos^2\theta$

59. $\csc^2\theta = \dfrac{2}{1 - \cos 2\theta}$

60. $\dfrac{2 \cos^3\theta}{1 - \sin \theta} = 2 \cos \theta + \sin 2\theta$

61. $\tan 2\theta = \dfrac{2(\tan \theta + \tan^3\theta)}{1 - \tan^4\theta}$

62. $\cot 4\theta = \dfrac{1 - \tan^2 2\theta}{2 \tan 2\theta}$

63. $2 \csc 2\theta \sin \theta \cos \theta = 1$

64. $\sec 2\theta = \dfrac{1}{1 - 2 \sin^2\theta}$

65. $\cos 2\theta = \dfrac{1 - \tan^2\theta}{1 + \tan^2\theta}$

66. $\dfrac{\csc \theta - \cot \theta}{1 + \cos \theta} = \csc \theta \tan^2 \dfrac{\theta}{2}$

67. $\cos^2 \dfrac{\theta}{2} = \dfrac{1 - \cos^2\theta}{2 - 2 \cos \theta}$

68. $\sec^2\theta - \cos^2 \dfrac{\theta}{2} = \tan^2\theta + \sin^2 \dfrac{\theta}{2}$

69. $\cos^2 \dfrac{\theta}{2} \sin^2 \dfrac{\theta}{2} = \dfrac{\sin^2\theta}{4}$

70. $\sin^2 \dfrac{\theta}{2} - \cos^2 \dfrac{\theta}{2} = -\cos \theta$

71. $\tan^2 \dfrac{\theta}{2} + \cos^2 \dfrac{\theta}{2} = \dfrac{\cos^2\theta + 3}{2 + 2 \cos \theta}$

72. $\tan^2 \dfrac{\theta}{2} = \dfrac{2}{1 + \cos \theta} - 1$

73. $\sin^2 \dfrac{\theta}{2} = \dfrac{\csc \theta - \cot \theta}{2 \csc \theta}$

74. $4 \sin^2 \dfrac{\theta}{2} \cos^2 \dfrac{\theta}{2} = \sin^2\theta$

75. $\dfrac{1 + \sec \theta}{\sec \theta} = 2 \cos^2 \dfrac{\theta}{2}$

76. $\tan \dfrac{\theta}{2} + \cot \dfrac{\theta}{2} = \dfrac{2}{\sin \theta}$

77. $2 \cos^2 \dfrac{\theta}{2} - \cos \theta = 1$

78. Show that $\sin 3\theta = 3 \sin \theta - 4 \sin^3\theta$.

79. ⬜ Find an identity for $\cos 3\theta$ in terms of $\cos \theta$. See problem 78.

80. ⬜ Find identities for (a) $\sin 4\theta$ in terms of $\sin \theta$ and $\cos \theta$ and for (b) $\cos 4\theta$ in terms of $\cos \theta$.

81. ⬜ Find identities for (a) $\sin 5\theta$ in terms of $\sin \theta$ and for (b) $\cos 5\theta$ in terms of $\cos \theta$.

82. Finding the center of gravity of a certain solid involves the expression $\frac{3}{16}a\left(\dfrac{1 - \cos 2\alpha}{1 - \cos \alpha}\right)$. Show that this is equivalent to $\frac{3}{8}a(1 + \cos \alpha)$.

83. Show that $\tan \dfrac{\alpha}{2} = \dfrac{1 - \cos \alpha}{\sin \alpha}$ (identity [6-c]). Do this as follows. Let $\dfrac{\alpha}{2} = \theta$, so that $\alpha = 2\theta$. Replace $\dfrac{\alpha}{2}$ and α in the identity. Then, simplify the right member; the most direct route will use $\cos 2\theta = 1 - 2 \sin^2\theta$.

84. Show that $\tan \dfrac{\alpha}{2} = \dfrac{\sin \alpha}{1 + \cos \alpha}$ (identity [6-b]). See the previous problem.

85. ⬜ **a.** Use the identity for $\sin \dfrac{\theta}{2}$ with $\theta = 30°$ to find the exact value of $\sin 15°$.
     b. Use $\alpha = 45°$, $\beta = 30°$ and $\sin(\alpha - \beta)$ to find the exact value of $\sin 15°$.
     c. Show that the values in (a) and (b) are the same. You may find useful the principle that if $a > 0$ and $b > 0$, then $a^2 = b^2$ implies that $a = b$.

86. **a.** Find $\tan 15°$ with the identity for $\tan \dfrac{\alpha}{2}$ (half-angle identity [6-a]), with $\alpha = 30°$.
     b. Rewrite $\tan 15°$ as $\dfrac{\sin 15°}{\cos 15°}$ and use identities [4] and [5], with $\alpha = 30°$ to compute $\tan 15°$.
     c. Show that the values in parts a and b are the same.

87. Verify half-angle identities [5] and [6-a].

88. Verify the double-angle identities [2-a], [2-b], [2-c], and [3].

89. In the figure, $\theta_1 = \theta_2$. Use the identity for $\cos \dfrac{\theta}{2}$ to find the length of side x.

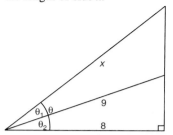

90. In the figure, $\theta_1 = \theta_2$. Use the identity for $\tan \dfrac{\theta}{2}$ to find the length of side x.

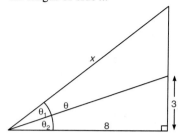

The following four identities are important in some situations because they relate the sums and differences of trigonometric expressions to the products of trigonometric expressions. Verify each identity.

91. $\sin 2\alpha + \sin 2\beta = 2 \sin(\alpha + \beta) \cdot \cos(\alpha - \beta)$

93. $\cos 2\alpha + \cos 2\beta = 2 \cos(\alpha + \beta) \cdot \cos(\alpha - \beta)$
(*Hint:* Convert everything to cosine.)

92. $\sin 2\alpha - \sin 2\beta = 2 \sin(\alpha - \beta) \cdot \cos(\alpha + \beta)$

94. $\cos 2\alpha - \cos 2\beta = -2 \sin(\alpha + \beta) \cdot \sin(\alpha - \beta)$
(*Hint:* Convert everything to cosine.)

95. Professor Gilbert Strang of the Massachusetts Institute of Technology has shown[1] an interesting relationship between the identity $\cot 2\theta = \dfrac{1}{2}\left(\cot \theta - \dfrac{1}{\cot \theta} \right)$ and the subject of chaotic behavior in iterative systems. Verify this identity.

[1]"A Chaotic Search for i," *The College Mathematics Journal*, Vol. 22, No. 1, January 1991.

5–4 Conditional trigonometric equations

Conditional trigonometric equations were introduced in section 1–4, and were revisited several times in chapter 2, as well as in section 5–0. In this section, we examine these equations in a more general way, and examine using the graphing calculator to find approximate solutions.

Remember that whenever we compute an inverse trigonometric function to solve an equation we *use the absolute value of the argument,* which gives us *the reference angle* of the answer.

Primary solutions

In this section we solve for values that are in both degree and radian measure. We determine all solutions that fall between $0° \leq x < 360°$ or, in radian measure, $0 \leq x < 2\pi$. We call such solutions **primary solutions.** Example 5–4 A illustrates.

■ *Example 5–4 A*

Find all primary solutions for the following trigonometric equations. Find the solutions in degrees (nearest tenth) and radians (four decimal places).

1. $5 \sin \alpha = -2$

$5 \sin \alpha = -2$

$\sin \alpha = -\frac{2}{5}$

Since $\sin \alpha < 0$ all solutions are in quadrants III and IV.

$\alpha' = \sin^{-1}\frac{2}{5}$ As noted earlier we use $\left|-\frac{2}{5}\right|$

$\alpha' \approx 23.6°$ or 0.4115 radians   Degree mode, radian mode

Degrees:

$$\alpha \approx 180° + 23.6° \text{ or } 360° - 23.6°$$

Radians:

$$\alpha \approx \pi + 0.4115 \text{ or } 2\pi - 0.4115$$

Thus, in degrees $\alpha \approx 203.6°$ or $336.4°$; in radians $\alpha \approx 3.5531$ or 5.8717.

2. $\cos \theta = -\frac{1}{2}$

$\cos \theta = -\frac{1}{2}$ $\cos \theta < 0$ so all solutions are in quadrants II and III

$\theta' = \cos^{-1}\frac{1}{2}$ Use the absolute value of $-\frac{1}{2}$

$\theta' = 60°$ or $\dfrac{\pi}{3}$ radians   Exact values, obtained from the unit circle, figure 2–18

$\theta = 180° \pm 60°$ or $\pi \pm \dfrac{\pi}{3}$ In quadrant II $\theta = 180° - \theta'$; in quadrant III $\theta = 180° + \theta'$

$\theta = 120°$ or $240°$ (degrees) or $\dfrac{2\pi}{3}$ or $\dfrac{4\pi}{3}$ (radians).

3. $2 \cos^2\theta - \cos \theta - 1 = 0$

The left member is quadratic in the variable $\cos \theta$. It can be factored. If this is difficult to see, try substitution as illustrated in section 5–0.

$2 \cos^2\theta - \cos \theta - 1 = 0$

$(2 \cos \theta + 1)(\cos \theta - 1) = 0$

$2 \cos \theta + 1 = 0$ or $\cos \theta - 1 = 0$ Zero factor property

$\cos \theta = -\frac{1}{2}$ $\cos \theta = 1$

$\theta' = \cos^{-1}\frac{1}{2}$ $\theta' = \cos^{-1}1$

$\theta' = 60°$ or $\dfrac{\pi}{3}$ $\theta' = 0°$ or 0 (radians)

$$\theta = 120° \text{ or } 240° \text{ (degrees)}$$

$$\theta = \frac{2\pi}{3} \text{ or } \frac{4\pi}{3} \text{ (radians)}; \theta = 0° \text{ or } 0.$$

In degrees, the solutions are $0°$, $120°$, and $240°$ and in radians they are 0, $\dfrac{2\pi}{3}$, and $\dfrac{4\pi}{3}$.

4. $\tan^2 x + 4 \tan x = 1$

$\qquad \tan^2 x + 4 \tan x - 1 = 0$

This is quadratic, but it will not factor. Solve it using the quadratic formula, as presented in section 5–0.

$$\tan x = \frac{-4 \pm \sqrt{4^2 - 4(1)(-1)}}{2(1)} \qquad \begin{array}{l} a = 1, b = 4, c = -1 \text{ in} \\ \dfrac{-b \pm \sqrt{b^2 - 4ac}}{2a} \end{array}$$

$$= \frac{-4 \pm \sqrt{20}}{2} = \frac{-4 \pm 2\sqrt{5}}{2} \qquad \sqrt{20} = \sqrt{4 \cdot 5} = 2\sqrt{5}$$

$$= -2 \pm \sqrt{5}$$

$\tan x = -2 + \sqrt{5}$	$\tan x = -2 - \sqrt{5}$
$x' = \tan^{-1}(-2 + \sqrt{5})$ $\approx 13.3°, 0.2318$ (radians) $\qquad x$ is in quadrants I or III since $\qquad -2 + \sqrt{5} > 0.$ $x \approx 13.3°$ or $180° + 13.3°$ $\qquad \approx 0.2318$ or $\pi + 0.2318$	$x' = \tan^{-1}\left\lvert -2 - \sqrt{5} \right\rvert$ $\quad = \tan^{-1}(2 + \sqrt{5})$ $\quad \approx 76.7°, 1.3390$ (radians) $\qquad x$ is in quadrants II or IV since $\qquad -2 - \sqrt{5} < 0.$ $x \approx 180° - 76.7°$ or $360° - 76.7°$ $\quad \approx \pi - 1.3390$ or $2\pi - 1.3390$

Thus, $x \approx 13.3°$, $193.3°$, $103.3°$, and $283.3°$ or 0.2318, 3.3734, 1.8026, and 4.9442. ∎

Using a graphing calculator to help solve an equation

How the solutions of an equation relate to its graph

To see the relationship between solving an equation and its graph, consider the equation $3 \sin x = 2$. This is equivalent to solving $3 \sin x - 2 = 0$. Now, consider the function $y = 3 \sin x - 2$. Solving $3 \sin x - 2 = 0$ is equivalent to finding all values of x that make $y = 0$ in the function $y = 3 \sin x - 2$. Figure 5–2 shows the graph of this function for the interval 0 to 2π (graphed with the calculator in radian mode).

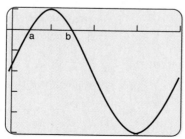

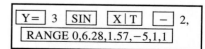

Y= 3 SIN X|T − 2,
RANGE 0,6.28,1.57,−5,1,1

Figure 5–2

The x-coordinates of the points where the curve crosses the x-axis, marked a and b, are $x \approx 0.7297$ or 2.4119. Because the value of y is zero at these values of x, we also refer to these x-values as **zeros** of the function.

Thus, if we are solving an equation in which one member is zero, the solutions correspond to the x-intercepts of the graph of the nonzero member of the equation. The graph in figure 5–2 shows that there are two primary solutions.

Using the TI-81 trace function to find approximations to solutions

The Trace function in the calculator can be used to find an approximate value of a solution. For example, graph the function as shown above, then select $\boxed{\text{TRACE}}$. A blinking box appears on the function toward the center of the screen. By using the left and right cursor keys $\boxed{\blacktriangleleft}$ and $\boxed{\blacktriangleright}$ we can cause the cursor to trace the function, all the while indicating its x- and y-coordinates at the bottom of the screen. By ''tracing'' to the point b we see that x is about 2.286 and y is about 0.057. Of course if we were at the exact solution, y would be zero.

By zooming in (using $\boxed{\text{ZOOM}}$ 2) and reselecting TRACE we can get a better approximation to the actual value, and by repeatedly zooming in again and tracing again we can obtain more and more accurate values for x.

This method of finding approximations to solutions is tedious and inefficient. We next show a much better way to find approximations to solutions.

The TI-81 and Newton's method

There are numeric methods for finding solutions to equations quickly and with great accuracy by using a programmable calculator. One can write a program that searches for a zero of a function. This is useful when the function is well behaved around the zero. For our purposes here, by well behaved we mean that one continuous, smooth line could be used to draw the graph of the function near the zero in question. A good method is called Newton's method. The Texas Instruments TI-81 calculator handbook presents a program called NEWTON that implements this method.

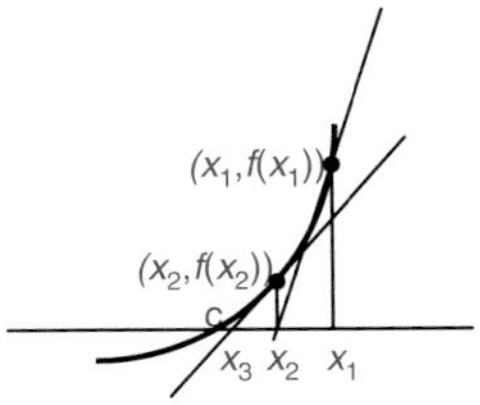

Figure 5–3 illustrates how Newton's method gets closer and closer to a root. Assume a function f has a zero at c in figure 5–3. Suppose x_1 is a value of x near c. The program uses the line that is tangent to (i.e., just touches) the function f at the point $(x_1, f(x_1))$ to locate the point x_2, which is closer to c. The program then uses the line that is tangent to the function f at the point $(x_2, f(x_2))$ to locate the point x_3, which is even closer to c. The program repeats this until the difference between the last x-value and the newest x-value is less than a predetermined error value.

Figure 5–3

The algebraic way in which the program discovers the tangent line at each step is left for a course in the calculus. With a little background in this subject, it is not hard to understand. The program NEWTON can be entered into the calculator as follows:

| PRGM | | ▶ | | ENTER | Program edit mode

| A-LOCK | | 2nd | | ALPHA | (Alpha lock)

Enter the keys that correspond to the word N E W T O N. For example, T is over the | 4 | key.

| ENTER | Use this after entering the name NEWTON.

Now type in the program as shown.

Program	**Keystroke guide**
:(Xmax − Xmin)/100→D	Xmax is in VARS RNG.
	Xmin is in VARS RNG.
	→D is | STO▶ | | x^{-1} |.
:Lbl 1	Lbl is in PRGM CTL.
:X-Y_1/NDeriv(Y_1,D)→R	Y_1 is in Y-VARS.
	NDeriv is | MATH | 8.
	'',D'' is | ALPHA | | . | | ALPHA |
	| x^{-1} |.
	→R is | STO▶ | | × |.
:If abs (X-R)≤abs (X/1E10)	If is in | PRGM | CTL.
	≤ is in TEST (| 2nd | | MATH |).
	1E10 is 1 | EE | 10.
:Goto 2	Goto is in | PRGM | CTL.
:R→X	Use | ALPHA | | × | | STO▶ |
	| X|T |.
:Goto 1	
:Lbl 2	
:Disp ''ROOT=''	Use | PRGM | I/O 1 | A-LOCK | | + |
	R O O T | TEST | 1 | + |
:Disp R	

Example 5–4 B illustrates using this program NEWTON to find approximate solutions to a trigonometric equation.

■ *Example 5–4 B*

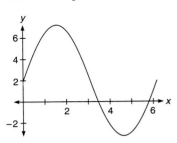

Solve the following problems using the programmable calculator.

1. $5 \sin \alpha = -2$

   This is equivalent to $5 \sin \alpha + 2 = 0$; find the zeros of the function $y = 5 \sin x + 2$.

   Graph $y = 5 \sin x + 2$. This is shown above, with Xmin=$-.1$, Xmax=6.3, Ymin=-3, Ymax=7. *The calculator is in radian mode.* Use the trace feature to position the cursor near the zero between 3 and 4. Now execute the program NEWTON. To do this, select ⎡PRGM⎤, select the number that corresponds to the NEWTON program, and use ⎡ENTER⎤ to execute the program. The value 3.5531095 appears. This is one of the zeros.

   Graph the function again, select trace, position the cursor near the second zero, and run the program NEWTON again. The value 5.871668461 appears. This is an approximation to the second zero.

   Repeating these steps in degree mode will find approximations to the zeros in degree mode. Of course Xmin should be something like $-10°$, and Xmax about 360°. The results displayed, in degrees, are 203.5781785° and 336.4218215°.

2. $\tan^2 x + 4 \tan x = 1$

   This is equivalent to $\tan^2 x + 4 \tan x - 1 = 0$. Graph $y = \tan^2 x + 4 \tan x - 1$ with Xmin=-0.1, Xmax=7, Ymin=-3, Ymax=6.3. This would be entered as $Y_1 = (\tan X)^2 + 4\tan X - 1$. The graph is shown in the figure.

   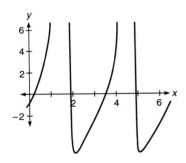

   Select trace, position the cursor near the first zero, and run the program NEWTON. The value 0.2318238045 appears. This is an approximation to the first zero.

   Regraph the function and repeat the first step at each zero. The values that appears are 1.802620131, 3.373416458, and 4.944212785.

   As in part 1 of the example, redo the problem in degree mode to obtain the results in degrees. The values displayed are 13.28252559°, 103.2825256°, 193.2825256°, and 283.2825256°.   ■

Using identities to help solve an equation

When an expression involves more than one trigonometric function we often use identities to rewrite the equation in terms of a single trigonometric function. This is illustrated in example 5–4 C.

■ *Example 5–4 C*

Find all primary solutions for the following trigonometric equations. Find the solutions in degrees (nearest tenth) and radians (four decimal places).

1. $\tan \theta - \cot \theta = 0$

$$\tan \theta - \cot \theta = 0$$

$$\tan \theta - \frac{1}{\tan \theta} = 0 \qquad \cot \theta = \frac{1}{\tan \theta} \text{ where } \tan \theta \neq 0$$

$$\tan^2\theta - 1 = 0 \qquad \text{Multiply each term by } \tan \theta$$

$$\tan^2\theta = 1$$

$$\tan \theta = \pm 1$$

When $\tan \theta = 1$, θ' is $45°$ or $\dfrac{\pi}{4}$ (see table 2–1), so using this fact and the ASTC rule for $\tan \theta > 0$ we obtain $\theta = 45°$ or $180° + 45°$, or $\dfrac{\pi}{4}$ or $\pi + \dfrac{\pi}{4}$.

When $\tan \theta = -1$, $\theta' = 45°$ or $\dfrac{\pi}{4}$, but $\theta = 180° - 45°$ or $360° - 45°$, or in radians $\pi - \dfrac{\pi}{4}$ or $2\pi - \dfrac{\pi}{4}$.

Thus, the primary solutions in degrees are $45°$, $135°$, $225°$, and $315°$ and in radians are $\dfrac{\pi}{4}$, $\dfrac{3\pi}{4}$, $\dfrac{5\pi}{4}$, and $\dfrac{7\pi}{4}$.

2. $2 \cos^2x - 3 \sin x - 3 = 0$

$$2 \cos^2x - 3 \sin x - 3 = 0$$

$$2(1 - \sin^2x) - 3 \sin x - 3 = 0 \qquad \cos^2\theta = 1 - \sin^2\theta$$

$$2 - 2 \sin^2x - 3 \sin x - 3 = 0$$

$$-2 \sin^2x - 3 \sin x - 1 = 0$$

$$2 \sin^2x + 3 \sin x + 1 = 0$$

$$(2 \sin x + 1)(\sin x + 1) = 0$$

$2 \sin x + 1 = 0$	$\sin x + 1 = 0$
$2 \sin x = -1$	$\sin x = -1$
$\sin x = -\frac{1}{2}$	$x = 270°$ or $\dfrac{3\pi}{2}$
$x = 210°, 330°,$ or $\dfrac{7\pi}{6}, \dfrac{11\pi}{6}$	

The primary solutions are $210°$, $270°$, $330°$ or $\dfrac{7\pi}{6}$, $\dfrac{3\pi}{2}$, $\dfrac{11\pi}{6}$.   ■

Finding all solutions to a trigonometric equation

We need to take note of the fact that there are an infinite number of solutions to the equations we solved in the preceding problems. Because the trigonometric functions are periodic the set of all solutions can be found by adding all integral values of the appropriate period (2π or π) to the solution.

This can be illustrated for part 3 of example 5–4 A, where we found that the primary solutions to $\cos \theta = -\frac{1}{2}$ are $\frac{2\pi}{3}$ and $\frac{4\pi}{3}$ (in radians). However, the cosine function is 2π-periodic, which means that $\cos(\theta + 2k\pi) = \cos \theta$ for any value of θ and for integer values of k. Thus, the actual set of all radian-valued solutions for this problem is $\frac{2\pi}{3} + 2k\pi$ and $\frac{4\pi}{3} + 2k\pi$, k any integer. This idea is illustrated in figure 5–4.

We use this periodicity for solving trigonometric equations where the coefficient of the argument is not 1. In this situation, it is easier to find all solutions than to find just the primary solutions. This is illustrated in example 5–4 D.

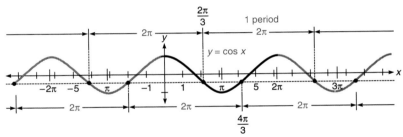

Figure 5–4

■ *Example 5–4 D*

Find *all* solutions for the following trigonometric equations. Find the solutions in degrees (nearest tenth) and radians (four decimal places).

1. $3 \sin 2x = -2$

$$3 \sin 2x = -2$$
$$\sin 2x = -\tfrac{2}{3}$$

Since $\sin 2x < 0$, $2x$ is in quadrants III or IV.

$$(2x)' = \sin^{-1}\tfrac{2}{3}$$
$$(2x)' \approx 41.8° \text{ or } 0.7297 \text{ radians}$$

Note   1. Do not divide both members by 2 at this point. It is necessary to find all solutions for $2x$ *before* dividing by 2.

2. Although we show the intermediate values above as 41.8° and 0.7297, it is important to keep the maximum accuracy of the calculator up to the last step of the problem. Thus, the calculations that follow are actually performed with the values $\boxed{41.8103149}$ and $\boxed{0.7297276562}$. All calculators have the capability to store at least one value in memory, which should be used to avoid tedious and error-prone reentry of values.

$$2x \approx \begin{cases} 180° + 41.8° \text{ or } 360° - 41.8° \text{ (degrees)} \\ \pi + 0.7297 \text{ or } 2\pi - 0.7297 \text{ (radians)} \end{cases}$$ $2x$ is an angle in quadrants III or IV

$$2x \approx \begin{cases} 221.8°, 318.2° \text{ (degrees)} \\ 3.8713, 5.5535 \text{ (radians)} \end{cases}$$ Primary solutions for $2x$

To describe all solutions we add multiples of the period of the sine function, 360° or 2π.

$$2x \approx \begin{cases} 221.8° + k \cdot 360°, 318.2° + k \cdot 360° \\ 3.8713 + 2k\pi, 5.5535 + 2k\pi \end{cases}$$

We now divide each solution by 2.

$$x \approx \begin{cases} 110.9° + k \cdot 180°, 159.1° + k \cdot 180° \\ 1.9357 + k\pi, 2.7768 + k\pi \end{cases}$$

This describes *all* solutions to the equation. To find primary solutions for x we would compute the values above for $k = 0$ and $k = 1$. If $k = 2$ the solutions are greater than 360° (2π), and if k is negative the solutions are negative.

2. $\tan \dfrac{x}{2} = \dfrac{\sqrt{3}}{3}$

$$\tan \frac{x}{2} = \frac{\sqrt{3}}{3}$$

$$\left(\frac{x}{2}\right)' = \tan^{-1}\frac{\sqrt{3}}{3}$$

$$\left(\frac{x}{2}\right)' = 30°, \frac{\pi}{6}$$

$$\frac{x}{2} = 30°, 210°, \text{ or } \frac{\pi}{6}, \frac{7\pi}{6}$$ These are the primary solutions for $\dfrac{x}{2}$

The tangent function is π-periodic. Thus, we add integer multiples of 180° (π) to obtain all solutions.

$$\frac{x}{2} = \begin{cases} 30° + k \cdot 180°, 210° + k \cdot 180° \text{ (degrees)} \\ \dfrac{\pi}{6} + k\pi, \dfrac{7\pi}{6} + k\pi \text{ (radians)} \end{cases}$$

This describes all solutions. However, $210° - 30° = 180°$, and similarly $\frac{7\pi}{6} - \frac{\pi}{6} = \pi$, so the solutions can be described more compactly.

$$\frac{x}{2} = 30° + k \cdot 180°, \text{ or } \frac{\pi}{6} + k\pi$$

$$x = 60° + k \cdot 360° \text{ or } \frac{\pi}{3} + 2k\pi \qquad \text{Multiply each member by 2}$$

All solutions for x are $x = 60° + k \cdot 360°$ or $\frac{\pi}{3} + 2k\pi$. ■

Equations involving more than one multiple of the angle

If an equation mixes multiples of values with the values themselves, such as θ and 2θ in example 5–4 E, we can eliminate the multiple value with an appropriate identity.

■ *Example 5–4 E*

Solve $\sin 2\theta - \sin \theta = 0$; find primary solutions.

$$\sin 2\theta - \sin \theta = 0$$
$$2 \sin \theta \cos \theta - \sin \theta = 0 \qquad \sin 2\alpha = 2 \sin \alpha \cos \alpha$$
$$\sin \theta (2 \cos \theta - 1) = 0$$
$$\sin \theta = 0 \text{ or } 2 \cos \theta - 1 = 0$$

$\sin \theta = 0$ | $2 \cos \theta - 1 = 0$
$\cos \theta = \frac{1}{2}$

$\theta = 0°, 180°, \text{ or } 0, \pi \text{ (radians)}$ | $\theta = 60°, 300°, \text{ or } \frac{\pi}{3}, \frac{5\pi}{3} \text{ (radians)}$

The solutions are $0°, 60°, 180°, 300°$ or $0, \frac{\pi}{3}, \pi, \frac{5\pi}{3}$ (radians). ■

Mastery points
Can you   • Solve linear and quadratic trigonometric equations?   • Solve trigonometric equations involving multiple angles?   • Solve trigonometric equations by applying an appropriate identity?

Exercise 5–4

Find all primary solutions to the following trigonometric equations. Leave answers in both degrees and radians. All answers should be exact.

1. $\tan \theta + 1 = 0$
2. $\sin \theta - 1 = 0$
3. $2 \cos \theta - 1 = 0$
4. $2 \cos \theta + 1 = 0$
5. $\sqrt{3} \tan \theta - 1 = 0$
6. $\cot \theta + \sqrt{3} = 0$
7. $\csc \theta + 2 = 0$
8. $\sec \theta - 2 = 0$
9. $3 \sin^2\theta - 3 = 0$
10. $3 \csc^2\theta = 3$
11. $\sec^2\theta = 1$
12. $\tan^2\theta - 1 = 0$

13. $(\cos\theta - 1)(\sin\theta + 1) = 0$

14. $(\sec\theta + 2)(\csc\theta - 2) = 0$

15. $(2\cos^2\theta - 1)(\cot\theta - 1) = 0$

16. $(3\tan^2\theta - 1)(\sqrt{3}\sec\theta - 2) = 0$

17. $\sin^2\theta - \sin\theta = 0$

18. $\cos^2\theta + \cos\theta = 0$

19. $\tan^2\theta - \sqrt{3}\tan\theta = 0$

20. $\cos^2\theta - \frac{1}{2}\cos\theta = 0$

21. $2\sin^2\theta + \sin\theta - 1 = 0$

22. $\cos^2\theta + 2\cos\theta + 1 = 0$

23. $2\sin^3\theta - \sin\theta = 0$

24. $2\cos^2\theta + 3\cos\theta = 2$

25. $2\sin\theta\cos\theta - \sin\theta = 0$

26. $2\sin\theta\cos\theta + \cos\theta = 0$

27. $\sqrt{3}\tan\theta\cot\theta + \cot\theta = 0$

28. $2\tan^2\theta\cos\theta - \tan^2\theta = 0$

29. $\tan x\cot x = 0$

30. $\sin x\cos x = 0$

31. $2\sin x - \csc x + 1 = 0$

32. $2\cos x + \sec x - 3 = 0$

33. $\tan x + \cot x = -2$

34. $2 - \sin x - \csc x = 0$

35. $2\sin^2 x - \cos x = 1$

36. $2\cos^2 x - 3\sin x = 3$

37. $4\tan^2 x = 3\sec^2 x$

38. $4\cot^2 x - 3\csc^2 x = 0$

39. $\sin^2 x - \cos^2 x = 0$

40. $\cot^2 x + \csc^2 x = 0$

41. $2\tan^2 x\sin x = \tan^2 x$

42. $\sin^2 x\cos x - \cos x = 0$

Solve the following equations using the quadratic formula if necessary and the calculator. Find the primary solutions in both radians and degrees. Round radian answers to hundredths, and degree answers to tenths.

43. $6\sin^2 x - 2\sin x - 1 = 0$

44. $3\cos^2 x + \cos x - 2 = 0$

45. $\cot^2 x - 3\cot x - 2 = 0$

46. $\tan^2 x + 5\tan x + 2 = 0$

47. $\sec^2 x - 2\sec x - 4 = 0$

48. $2\csc^2 x - \csc x - 5 = 0$

49. $\tan x + 2\sec x = 3$

50. $3\cot x - \csc x - 1 = 0$

Find all solutions to the following trigonometric equations, both in degrees and in radians.

51. $\cos x = \frac{1}{2}$

52. $\sin x = 1$

53. $\cot x = -\sqrt{3}$

54. $\cos x = -\dfrac{\sqrt{3}}{2}$

55. $\sin x = -\dfrac{\sqrt{2}}{2}$

56. $\tan x = -1$

57. $\tan x = 1$

58. $\sec x = \dfrac{2}{\sqrt{3}}$

59. $\csc x = 2$

60. $\tan\dfrac{x}{2} = 1$

61. $\sin\dfrac{x}{2} = \dfrac{\sqrt{3}}{2}$

62. $\sin 3x = 0$

63. $\cos 3x = -1$

64. $\sec\dfrac{x}{2} = 1$

65. $3\cot 2x = \sqrt{3}$

66. $2\sin 3x = -1$

67. $2\cos 4x = -1$

68. $-\sqrt{3}\tan 5x = 1$

69. $2\cos 2x + 1 = 0$

70. $\tan 2\theta - 1 = 0$

71. $\cot 2\theta - \sqrt{3} = 0$

72. $2\cos 3\theta = -1$

73. $2\sin 2\theta = 1$

74. $\sin\dfrac{\theta}{3} = \dfrac{\sqrt{3}}{2}$

75. $\sec 3\theta = 2$

76. $\csc 2\theta = -\dfrac{2\sqrt{3}}{3}$

77. $\sqrt{3}\tan\dfrac{\theta}{4} = 1$

78. $\cot\dfrac{\theta}{3} = \dfrac{\sqrt{3}}{3}$

Find the primary solutions to the following trigonometric equations, both in radians and degrees. Find solutions in radians to hundredths, and in degrees to the nearest tenth of a degree, where necessary.

79. $\cos 2\theta + \sin\theta = 0$

80. $\cos 2\theta - \cos\theta = 0$

81. $\sin 2\theta + \sin\theta = 0$

82. $\cos^2\theta - \sin^2\theta = 1$

83. $\cos 2\theta = 1 - \sin\theta$

84. $\cos 2\theta = \cos\theta - 1$

85. $\sin\dfrac{\theta}{2} = \tan\dfrac{\theta}{2}$

86. $\sin\dfrac{\theta}{2} = \cos\theta$

87. $2\sec\theta = \csc^2\dfrac{\theta}{2}$

88. $\sin^2\dfrac{\theta}{2} = \cos\theta$

89. $\tan\dfrac{\theta}{2} = \cos\theta - 1$

90. $\cot\theta - \tan\dfrac{\theta}{2} = 0$

91. $\sin 2\theta - \cos\theta = \cos^2\theta$

In the mathematical modeling of an aerodynamics problem the following equation arises:

$$y = x\cos A\cos B - x^2\cos A\sin B - x^3\sin A$$

Problems 92 and 93 use this equation.

92. If $A = 0.855$, $B = 1.052$, and $y = 0$, solve for x to the nearest 0.01.

93. If $B = 0.7$, $x = 2$, and $y = -8$, find A to the nearest 0.01. Find the least nonnegative solution(s).

A mechanical device is constructed as shown in the diagram. The arm OA moves through angle θ, from $0°$ to $90°$. Two positions are shown. Point A moves along a circle of radius 1.0 meters, and point B moves horizontally only. The distance AB is fixed by arm AB at 1.2 meters. The area of the shaded rectangle is the product of its length and width, $A = \ell w$.

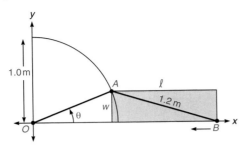
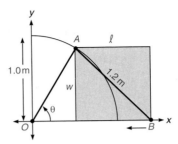

94. Show that $A = \sin \theta \sqrt{1.44 - \sin^2\theta}$. (The units are square meters.)

96. Find θ when $A = 0.5$ m². Round the answer to the nearest $0.1°$.

95. Find A, to the nearest 0.01 m², when $\theta = 0°$, $30°$, $45°$, $60°$, and $90°$.

Chapter 5 summary

- **A trigonometric identity** is a trigonometric equation that is true for all permissible replacements of the variable for which each member is defined.

- To verify that a trigonometric equation is an identity we must show that each member of the equation is equivalent to the same expression.

- To show that an equation is not an identity find a value for the variable for which the statement is not true. This value is called a counter example.

- **Reciprocal identities**

$$\csc \theta = \frac{1}{\sin \theta}, \quad \sec \theta = \frac{1}{\cos \theta}, \quad \cot \theta = \frac{1}{\tan \theta}$$

$$\sin \theta = \frac{1}{\csc \theta}, \quad \cos \theta = \frac{1}{\sec \theta}, \quad \tan \theta = \frac{1}{\cot \theta}$$

- **Tangent and cotangent identities**

$$\tan \theta = \frac{\sin \theta}{\cos \theta}, \quad \cot \theta = \frac{\cos \theta}{\sin \theta}$$

- **Fundamental identity of trigonometry**

$$\sin^2\theta + \cos^2\theta = 1$$

- **Pythagorean identities**

	Useful forms
$\sin^2\theta + \cos^2\theta = 1$	$\sin^2\theta = 1 - \cos^2\theta$
	$\cos^2\theta = 1 - \sin^2\theta$
$\sec^2\theta = \tan^2\theta + 1$	$\tan^2\theta = \sec^2\theta - 1$
	$\sec^2\theta - \tan^2\theta = 1$
$\csc^2\theta = \cot^2\theta + 1$	$\cot^2\theta = \csc^2\theta - 1$
	$\csc^2\theta - \cot^2\theta = 1$

- **Sum and difference identities for sine and cosine**

$$\cos(\alpha + \beta) = \cos \alpha \cos \beta - \sin \alpha \sin \beta$$
$$\cos(\alpha - \beta) = \cos \alpha \cos \beta + \sin \alpha \sin \beta$$
$$\sin(\alpha + \beta) = \sin \alpha \cos \beta + \cos \alpha \sin \beta$$
$$\sin(\alpha - \beta) = \sin \alpha \cos \beta - \cos \alpha \sin \beta$$
$$\tan(\alpha + \beta) = \frac{\tan \alpha + \tan \beta}{1 - \tan \alpha \tan \beta}$$
$$\tan(\alpha - \beta) = \frac{\tan \alpha - \tan \beta}{1 + \tan \alpha \tan \beta}$$

- When the sum of two angles is $90°$, or $\dfrac{\pi}{2}$ radians, the angles are said to be complementary.

- **Cofunction identities**

$$\sin\left(\frac{\pi}{2} - \theta\right) = \cos \theta \qquad \cot\left(\frac{\pi}{2} - \theta\right) = \tan \theta$$

$$\cos\left(\frac{\pi}{2} - \theta\right) = \sin \theta \qquad \sec\left(\frac{\pi}{2} - \theta\right) = \csc \theta$$

$$\tan\left(\frac{\pi}{2} - \theta\right) = \cot \theta \qquad \csc\left(\frac{\pi}{2} - \theta\right) = \sec \theta$$

- **Double-angle identities**

$$\sin 2\alpha = 2 \sin \alpha \cos \alpha \qquad \cos 2\alpha = \cos^2\alpha - \sin^2\alpha$$
$$\tan 2\alpha = \frac{2 \tan \alpha}{1 - \tan^2\alpha} \qquad \cos 2\alpha = 1 - 2 \sin^2\alpha$$
$$\cos 2\alpha = 2 \cos^2\alpha - 1$$

• **Half-angle identities**

$$\sin \frac{\alpha}{2} = \pm\sqrt{\frac{1 - \cos \alpha}{2}} \qquad \tan \frac{\alpha}{2} = \pm\sqrt{\frac{1 - \cos \alpha}{1 + \cos \alpha}}$$

$$\cos \frac{\alpha}{2} = \pm\sqrt{\frac{1 + \cos \alpha}{2}} \qquad \tan \frac{\alpha}{2} = \frac{\sin \alpha}{1 + \cos \alpha}$$

$$\tan \frac{\alpha}{2} = \frac{1 - \cos \alpha}{\sin \alpha}$$

• **Primary solutions** are solutions that fall between $0° \le x \le 360°$ or, in radian measure, $0 \le x < 2\pi$.

• The trigonometric functions are periodic, so the set of all solutions can be found by adding all integral values of the appropriate period (2π or π) to the solution.

Chapter 5 review

[5–1] Show that the trigonometric expression on the left is equivalent to the simplified expression on the right.

1. $\dfrac{\cot \theta}{\cos \theta}$; $\csc \theta$

2. $\sec \theta \tan \theta$; $\sec^2\theta \sin \theta$

3. $\dfrac{\tan^2\theta}{\sec^2\theta - 1}$; $\sin^4\theta \csc^4\theta$

4. $\dfrac{\csc^2\theta - 1}{\sec^2\theta - 1}$; $\cot^4\theta$

5. $\dfrac{\csc \theta \tan \theta}{\sin \theta}$; $\csc \theta \sec \theta$

6. $\sin^2\theta - \cos^2\theta$; $2 \sin^2\theta - 1$

Obtain an equivalent expression involving only the sine and cosine functions. Simplify the resulting expression.

7. $\csc \theta - \sec \theta$

8. $\tan \theta + \cot \theta$

9. $\dfrac{\sec \theta}{\tan \theta - \cot \theta}$

10. $\dfrac{1 - \cot \theta}{\csc \theta + 1}$

11. $\dfrac{\sec^2\theta - 1}{\sec^2\theta}$

12. $\dfrac{1 - \cot^2\theta}{\csc^2\theta - 1}$

Verify that each equation is an identity.

13. $\csc x - \tan x \cot x = \csc x - 1$

14. $\sin^2x + \sin^2x \cot^2x = 1$

15. $\csc^2x - \sec^2x = \csc^2x \sec^2x(\cos^2x - \sin^2x)$

16. $\dfrac{1}{\csc x - \cot x} = \dfrac{\sin x}{1 - \cos x}$

17. $\tan x - 1 = \sec x(\sin x - \cos x)$

18. $\dfrac{\csc^2x - 1}{\sin^2x} = \cos^2x \csc^4x$

19. $\dfrac{1}{1 + \csc x} + \dfrac{1}{1 - \csc x} = -2 \tan^2x$

20. $\sin^2x + \sin^2x \cos^2x = 1 - \cos^4x$

21. $\tan^4x + \tan^2x = \dfrac{\sec^2x}{\cot^2x}$

22. $\dfrac{1 - \cot x}{1 + \csc x} = \dfrac{\sin x - \cos x}{\sin x + 1}$

Show by counter example that the following equations are not identities.

23. $\sin \theta + \cos \theta = 1$

24. $\tan \theta - \sin \theta \cos \theta = 0$

25. $\dfrac{1}{\cot \theta - \csc \theta} = \sec \theta$

[5–2] Use the sum and difference formulas to find the exact value of the following.

26. $\cos \dfrac{\pi}{12}$

27. $\tan\left(-\dfrac{\pi}{12}\right)$

28. $\sin 105°$

29. $\tan(-15°)$

30. Given $\sin \alpha = \frac{3}{4}$ and $\cos \beta = -\frac{5}{6}$, α and β lie in quadrant II, find
   a. $\sin(\alpha - \beta)$ **b.** $\tan(\alpha + \beta)$

31. Given $\cos \alpha = -\dfrac{\sqrt{3}}{2}$ and $\sin \beta = -\dfrac{1}{4}$, α lies in quadrant II and β lies in quadrant III, find
   a. $\cos (\alpha + \beta)$ **b.** $\tan(\alpha - \beta)$

32. Given $\sin \alpha = -\frac{5}{12}$ and $\cos \beta = \frac{8}{17}$, α lies in quadrant IV and β lies in quadrant I, find
   a. $\sec(\alpha + \beta)$ **b.** $\cot(\alpha - \beta)$

Using the sum and difference formulas, verify each of the following identities.

33. $\dfrac{\sin(\alpha + \beta)}{\cos(\alpha - \beta)} = \dfrac{\cot \alpha + \cot \beta}{\cot \alpha \cot \beta + 1}$

34. $\cos\left(\dfrac{3\pi}{2} + \theta\right) = \sin \theta$

35. $\sin\left(\dfrac{\pi}{4} - \theta\right) = \dfrac{\sqrt{2}}{2}(\cos \theta - \sin \theta)$

36. $\dfrac{\cos(\alpha + \beta)}{\sin \alpha \cos \beta} = \cot \alpha - \tan \beta$

37. Using the identity $\cot \alpha = \dfrac{1}{\tan \alpha}$ and the identity

$\tan(\alpha + \beta)$, show that $\cot(\theta + \pi) = \cot \theta$.

[5–3] Using the double-angle identities, find angle θ that makes the following statements true.

38. $\cos \theta = \cos^2 62° - \sin^2 62°$
39. $\sin \theta = 2 \sin 5\pi \cos 5\pi$

40. $\tan \theta = \dfrac{2 \tan \dfrac{7\pi}{12}}{1 - \tan^2 \dfrac{7\pi}{12}}$ **41.** $\cos 24° = 1 - 2 \sin^2 \theta$

42. Express $6 \sin \dfrac{\theta}{2} \cos \dfrac{\theta}{2}$ as a single trigonometric function of a constant k times θ.

43. Express $\dfrac{4 \tan 4\theta}{1 - \tan^2 4\theta}$ as a single trigonometric function of a constant k times θ.

44. Given $\cos \theta = -\frac{5}{12}$, θ lies in quadrant III, find the exact value of **a.** $\tan 2\theta$ **b.** $\sin 2\theta$

45. Given $\sin \theta = \frac{4}{5}$, θ lies in quadrant II, find the exact value of **a.** $\cos 2\theta$ **b.** $\tan 2\theta$

46. Given $\tan \theta = -\frac{5}{4}$, θ lies in quadrant IV, find the exact value of **a.** $\csc 2\theta$ **b.** $\cot 2\theta$

Verify the following identities.

47. $\sin 2x - \cos x = \cos x(2 \sin x - 1)$
48. $1 + \cos 2x = 2 \cos^2 x$
49. $\dfrac{\cos 2x}{2 - 4 \sin^2 x} = \dfrac{1}{2}$ **50.** $\tan 2x = \dfrac{2 \cot x}{\cot^2 x - 1}$
51. $\sin 2x - \cos 2x = 2 \cos x(\sin x - \cos x) + 1$

Using the half-angle identities, find the exact value of the following.

52. $\tan 22.5°$ **53.** $\cos(-15°)$
54. $\sin \dfrac{5\pi}{12}$ **55.** $\cos \dfrac{3\pi}{8}$

56. Given $\cos x = \frac{12}{13}$, $0 < x < \dfrac{\pi}{2}$, find

   a. $\sin \dfrac{x}{2}$ **b.** $\tan \dfrac{x}{2}$

57. Given $\sin x = -\frac{2}{3}$, $\pi < x < \dfrac{3\pi}{2}$, find

   a. $\sec \dfrac{x}{2}$ **b.** $\cot \dfrac{x}{2}$

58. Find $\sin \dfrac{\theta}{2}$ if $\cos \theta = -\dfrac{7}{18}$ and $\pi < \theta < \dfrac{3\pi}{2}$.

Verify the following equations are identities.

59. $\cot \dfrac{\theta}{2} = \dfrac{1 + \cos \theta}{\sin \theta}$ **60.** $\sec^2 \dfrac{\theta}{2} - \tan^2 \dfrac{\theta}{2} = 1$

61. $\tan \dfrac{\theta}{2} \csc^2 \dfrac{\theta}{2} = \dfrac{2}{\sin \theta}$

[5–4] Solve the following conditional equations for $0 \le x \le \dfrac{\pi}{2}$.

62. $2 \sin x - 1 = 0$ **63.** $3 \cot^2 x - 1 = 0$
64. $(\sin x - 1)(2 \cos x - 1) = 0$
65. $(4 \sin^2 x - 1)(\sec x - 2) = 0$

Solve the following conditional equations for $0° \le \theta < 360°$.

66. $\cot^2 \theta - \cot \theta = 0$ **67.** $\sec^2 \theta - 4 = 0$
68. $2 \cos^2 \theta - \cos \theta - 1 = 0$
69. $2 \sin \theta - \csc \theta + 1 = 0$
70. $2 \cot \theta \cos \theta = \cot^2 \theta$ **71.** $2 \sin^2 \theta - 3 \cos \theta = 3$

Find all solutions in radians to the following equations. Use the quadratic formula and calculator where necessary (round such answers to the nearest hundredth).

72. $\cos^2 x - 1 = 0$ **73.** $\tan^2 x - 3 \tan x - 3 = 0$
74. $\sin x - 2 \csc x = 5$ **75.** $\sec^2 x - \sec x = 2$

Solve each of the following equations for $0 \le x < 2\pi$ (primary solutions, radians).

76. $2 \sin 4x = 1$ **77.** $2 \cos \dfrac{x}{2} - \sqrt{3} = 0$
78. $\sqrt{3} \tan \dfrac{x}{3} + 1 = 0$ **79.** $\sin^2 \dfrac{x}{4} = \dfrac{1}{2}$

Solve each of the following equations for $0° \le \theta < 360°$.

80. $2 \cos 5\theta = 1$ **81.** $3 \tan^2 \dfrac{\theta}{4} = 9$
82. $\tan 6\theta - \cot 6\theta = 0$ **83.** $\cos \theta + \sin 2\theta = 0$

Find all solutions in radians to the following equations. Find solutions to the nearest hundredth, where necessary.

84. $\cos \dfrac{x}{2} - \sin x = 0$
85. $(\cot 4x - \sqrt{3})(\csc 3x + 2) = 0$
86. $3 \sin^2 2x - \sin 2x - 2 = 0$

Chapter 5 test

1. Show that the expression $\csc^2 x \sin x \cos x$ is equivalent to $\cot x$.

2. Write the expression $\dfrac{\csc x - \sec x}{\tan x + \cot x}$ as an expression in sine and cosine and simplify.

3. Show by counter example that the equation $\cot x - 2 \tan x = 1$ is not an identity.

4. Given $\cos \alpha = -\frac{1}{2}$ and $\sin \beta = \frac{15}{17}$, α lies in quadrant III and β lies in quadrant II, find $\sin(\alpha + \beta)$.

5. Given $\cos x = -\frac{8}{17}$, x lies in quadrant II, find $\sin 2x$.

6. Given $\csc x = \frac{5}{3}$, $\dfrac{\pi}{2} < x < \pi$, find $\tan \dfrac{x}{2}$.

7. Using the appropriate half-angle formula, find $\sec 22.5°$.

8. Verify the following identities.

a. $\dfrac{1 + \cot \theta}{\csc \theta} = \sin \theta + \cos \theta$

b. $\dfrac{\cos^2 x - 1}{\sin^2 x} = -1$

c. $\cos\left(\theta - \dfrac{3\pi}{2}\right) = -\sin \theta$

d. $\cos 2x - \sin 2x = -1 + 2 \cos x(\cos x - \sin x)$

9. Solve the equation $4 \cos^2 x - 1 = 0$ for $0 \le x < 2\pi$.

10. Solve the equation $(\cot \theta - \sqrt{3})(\sec \theta + 2) = 0$ for $0° \le 0 < 360°$.

11. Find all primary solutions, in radians, to the equation $6 \sin^2 x + 5 \sin x - 1 = 0$. (Use the quadratic formula and the calculator if necessary.)

12. Solve the equation $\sin^2 5\theta - 1 = 0$ for $0° \le 0 < 360°$.

13. Find all primary solutions, in radians, to the equation

$$\sec^2 \dfrac{x}{4} - 2 = 0.$$

14. If $\sin^2 x = \dfrac{1 + \sqrt{1 - m^2}}{2}$, find $\sin 2x$. (*Hint:* Use $\sin^2 2x = 4 \sin^2 x \cos^2 x$.)

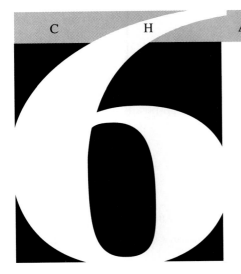

Oblique Triangles and Vectors

In this chapter we examine several applications of the trigonometric functions. We begin with the law of sines and the law of cosines. These are theorems that permit the solution of triangles which are not right triangles. (Recall that we examined the solution of right triangles in section 1–3.) We then introduce the subject of vectors, which has wide application in science and engineering, and which, in a generalized form called linear algebra, has applications in the social and economic sciences as well.

6–1 *The law of sines*

A triangle in which none of the angles is a right angle is called an **oblique triangle.** One method for solving certain oblique triangles is the **law of sines.** The following paragraphs develop this law.

First, we observe that *at least two of the angles in every triangle are acute.* If only one angle were acute (less than 90°) then the other two would be obtuse or right (greater than or equal to 90°). This is impossible since the sum of these two angles would be greater than or equal to 180°, and thus the sum of all three angles would be greater than 180°.

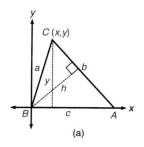

(a)

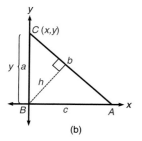

(b)

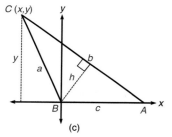

(c)

Figure 6–1

Now we consider any triangle ABC, and label two of the acute angles A and C. Angle B may be acute, obtuse, or right. We place the triangle in a coordinate system so that angle B is in standard position. Figure 6–1 shows sketches for the cases where B is (a) acute, (b) right, and (c) obtuse.

From vertex B we construct a line segment perpendicular to side AC and label this line h. From what we know about right triangles we can see that, in all three cases,

$$\sin A = \frac{h}{c} \quad \text{and} \quad \sin C = \frac{h}{a}$$

If we solve for h in each, we obtain

$$h = c \sin A \quad \text{and} \quad h = a \sin C$$

Since $c \sin A$ and $a \sin C$ equal the same quantity (h) they themselves must be equal. Thus,

$$c \sin A = a \sin C$$
$$\frac{c \sin A}{ac} = \frac{a \sin C}{ac} \qquad \text{Divide both members by } ac$$
$$\frac{\sin A}{a} = \frac{\sin C}{c} \qquad \text{Remove common factors}$$

We now extend the relation above to include angle B and side b. Let (x,y) be the coordinates of the vertex of angle C. From what we know about the trigonometric functions for any angle in standard position (chapter 2), we see that

$$\sin B = \frac{y}{a} \quad \text{or} \quad y = a \sin B$$

From what we know about right triangles,

$$\sin A = \frac{y}{b} \quad \text{or} \quad y = b \sin A$$

Thus, $a \sin B = y = b \sin A$, so

$$a \sin B = b \sin A$$
$$\frac{\sin A}{a} = \frac{\sin B}{b}$$

Putting these results together we have the law of sines.

The law of sines
In any triangle ABC,
$$\frac{\sin A}{a} = \frac{\sin B}{b} = \frac{\sin C}{c}$$

Concept
The ratio of the sine of an angle to the length of the side opposite that angle is the same for all angles in any triangle.

Note   We only use two of the three ratios at a time.

In the rest of this chapter we always assume side a is opposite angle A, side b is opposite angle B, and side c is opposite angle C.

■ *Example 6–1 A*

Solve the triangle ABC. Round off answers to tenths.

$a = 13.2, A = 21.3°, B = 61.4°$

It is a good idea to make a table of values:

a: 13.2 A: 21.3°
b: ? B: 61.4°
c: ? C: ?

We can find C first.

$$C = 180° - A - B$$

The sum of the measure of all three angles is 180°

$$= 180° - 21.3° - 61.4°$$
$$= 97.3°$$

Now we fill in the law of sines.

$$\frac{\sin A}{a} = \frac{\sin B}{b} = \frac{\sin C}{c}$$

$$\frac{\sin 21.3°}{13.2} = \frac{\sin 61.4°}{b} = \frac{\sin 97.3°}{c}$$

To use the law of sines we must always know one of the three ratios completely. In this case, we know the first ratio, so we use it to solve the other two. Using the first and second ratios:

$$\frac{\sin 21.3°}{13.2} = \frac{\sin 61.4°}{b}$$

$$b \sin 21.3° = 13.2 \sin 61.4° \quad \text{Multiply each member by } 13.2b$$

$$b = \frac{13.2 \sin 61.4°}{\sin 21.3°} \approx 31.9 \quad \text{Divide each member by } \sin 21.3°$$

Using the first and third ratios:

$$\frac{\sin 21.3°}{13.2} = \frac{\sin 97.3°}{c}$$

$$c \sin 21.3° = 13.2 \sin 97.3° \quad \text{Multiply each member by } 13.2c$$

$$c = \frac{13.2 \sin 97.3°}{\sin 21.3°} \approx 36.0 \quad \text{Divide each member by } \sin 21.3°$$

Thus we have solved the triangle:

a: 13.2 A: 21.3°
b: 31.9 B: 61.4°
c: 36.0 C: 97.3°.

■

The ambiguous case

If we are given only one of the two angles of a triangle it is possible to get two different solutions to the problem. The reason for this is shown in example 6–1 B. When we use the law of sines to solve a triangle *for which only one angle is known* we call this the **ambiguous case.**

■ *Example 6–1 B*

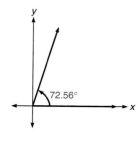

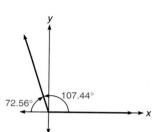

Solve each triangle. Round off answers to tenths.

1. $a = 28.5$, $b = 30.0$, $A = 65°$.

a: 28.5	*A:* 65°
b: 30.0	*B:* ?
c: ?	*C:* ?

Make a table of values

$$\frac{\sin 65°}{28.5} = \frac{\sin B}{30.0} = \frac{\sin C}{c}$$

Fill values into the law of sines

$$\frac{\sin 65°}{28.5} = \frac{\sin B}{30.0}$$

Use the first two ratios to find angle B

$$30.0 \sin 65° = 28.5 \sin B$$

$$\frac{30.0 \sin 65°}{28.5} = \sin B$$

A *reference angle* for angle B is found with the inverse sine function.

$$B' = \sin^{-1}\left(\frac{30.0 \sin 65°}{28.5}\right) \approx 72.56°$$

Since angle B is in a triangle, we know its measure is between 0° and 180°. Thus, using B' as a reference angle B could be either 72.56° or $180° - 72.56° = 107.44°$. See the figure.

At this point we must divide the problem into two cases: the case where $B \approx 72.56°$ and the one where $B \approx 107.44°$.

Case 1: $B \approx 72.56°$

a: 28.5	*A:* 65°
b: 30.0	*B:* 72.56°
c: ?	*C:* ?

$$C \approx 180° - 65° - 72.56° \approx 42.44°$$

We can use the value of angle C to find c.

$$\frac{\sin 65°}{28.5} \approx \frac{\sin 42.44°}{c}$$

$$c \sin 65° \approx 28.5 \sin 42.44°$$

$$c \approx \frac{28.5 \sin 42.44°}{\sin 65°} \approx 21.2$$

Thus, $C \approx 42.4°$, $c \approx 21.2$.

Case 2: $B \approx 107.44°$

a: 28.5 A: 65°

b: 30.0 B: 107.44°

c: ? C: ?

$$C \approx 180° - 65° - 107.44° \approx 7.56°$$

$$\frac{\sin 65°}{28.5} \approx \frac{\sin 7.56°}{c}$$

$$c \sin 65° \approx 28.5 \sin 7.56°$$

$$c \approx \frac{28.5 \sin 7.56°}{\sin 65°} \approx 4.1$$

Thus, $C \approx 7.6°$, $c \approx 4.1$.

We can summarize these two solutions in two tables.

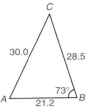

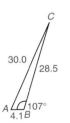

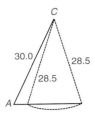

Figure 6–2

Case 1		Case 2	
a: 28.5 A: 65°		a: 28.5 A: 65°	
b: 30.0 B: 72.6°		b: 30.0 B: 107.4°	
c: 21.2 C: 42.4°		c: 4.1 C: 7.6°	

Figure 6–2 shows the two triangles. The last figure shows both triangles together, where we can see why the ambiguous case was possible—with the given information ($a = 28.5$, $b = 30.0$, $A = 65°$), side a could be in one of two positions, giving two possible triangles.

As a final check on our work, we observe that the sum of the angles in each case is 180°, and that in each case the longest side is opposite the largest angle and the shortest side is opposite the smallest angle. These are facts that should be true for any triangle.

2. $b = 51.2$, $c = 32.1$, $B = 6.1°$

a: ?	A: ?	Make a table of values
b: 51.2	B: 6.1°	
c: 32.1	C: ?	

$$\frac{\sin A}{a} = \frac{\sin 6.1°}{51.2} = \frac{\sin C}{32.1}$$ Fill values into the law of sines

$$\sin C = \frac{32.1 \sin 6.1°}{51.2}$$ Using the last two ratios

$C' \approx 3.82°$, which we will round to 3.8° in the final answer.
$C \approx 3.82°$ or $180° - 3.82° \approx 176.18°$.

Case 1: $C \approx 3.82°$

a: ?	A: ?
b: 51.2	B: 6.1°
c: 32.1	C: 3.82°

$$A \approx 180° - 3.82° - 6.1° = 170.08°$$

$$\frac{\sin 170.08°}{a} = \frac{\sin 6.1°}{51.2}$$ Use the first two ratios

$$a = \frac{51.2 \sin 170.08°}{\sin 6.1°} \approx 83.00$$

This finishes case 1: $A \approx 170.08°$, $a \approx 83.0$.

Case 2: $C \approx 176.18°$

a: ?	A: ?
b: 51.2	B: 6.1°
c: 32.1	C: 176.18°

$A \approx 180° - 176.18° - 6.1° = -2.28°$
Since an angle in a triangle cannot have negative measure this case does not produce a solution.

Thus, the solution to case 1 is the only solution.

a: 83.0	A: 170.1°
b: 51.2	B: 6.1°
c: 32.1	C: 3.8°

The law of sines is used in many applications of trigonometry.

■ *Example 6–1 C*

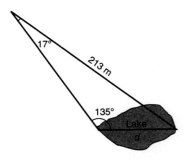

Solve the following problems using the law of sines.

1. A surveyor made the measurements shown in the figure to measure the distance *d* across a lake. Find the distance to the nearest meter.

Using the law of sines, we know that

$$\frac{\sin 135°}{213} = \frac{\sin 17°}{d}$$

$$\frac{213d}{1} \cdot \frac{\sin 135°}{213} = \frac{213d}{1} \cdot \frac{\sin 17°}{d}$$

$$d \sin 135° = 213 \sin 17°$$

$$d = \frac{213 \sin 17°}{\sin 135°} \approx 88.1 \text{ meters}$$

Thus, to the nearest meter the distance across the lake is 88 meters.

2. The figure illustrates the following situation. A hang glider is flying at 18.4 mph pointed due east, with the wind blowing at 17.9 mph in the direction shown. The result is that the hang glider travels in a direction 42.3° north of east, with a ground speed of *r* mph. Assuming that θ_1 is acute, find the ground speed *r* and the direction of the wind, θ_2.

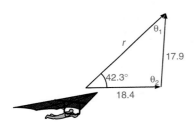

Using the law of sines, we know

$$\frac{\sin 42.3°}{17.9} = \frac{\sin \theta_1}{18.4} = \frac{\sin \theta_2}{r}$$

$$\sin \theta_1 = \frac{18.4 \sin 42.3°}{17.9}$$

$$\theta_1' \approx 43.77°$$

$$\theta_1 = \theta_1' \approx 43.77° \qquad\qquad \theta_1 \text{ is an acute angle}$$

$$\theta_2 \approx 180° - 42.3° - 43.77° = 93.93°$$

We can now find *r*.

$$\frac{\sin 42.3°}{17.9} = \frac{\sin 93.93°}{r}$$

$$r = \frac{17.9 \sin 93.93°}{\sin 42.3°} \approx 26.5$$

Thus, the hang glider is traveling with a ground speed of 26.5 mph, and the wind is blowing in the direction 93.9° north of west (or 3.9° east of north). ■

Mastery points

Can you
- State and use the law of sines to solve oblique triangles?
- Recognize and solve the ambiguous case when using the law of sines?

Exercise 6–1

In the following problems round answers to the same number of decimal places as the data, unless otherwise specified.
Solve the following oblique triangles using the law of sines.

1. $a = 12.5$, $A = 35°$, $B = 49°$
2. $b = 17.1$, $B = 100°$, $C = 10°$
3. $a = 1.25$, $B = 13.6°$, $C = 132°$
4. $c = 9.04$, $A = 51.6°$, $B = 40.0°$
5. $b = 92.5$, $A = 47°$, $B = 100°$
6. $c = 10.2$, $A = 16.7°$, $B = 89.2°$
7. $a = 0.452$, $A = 67.6°$, $C = 91.8°$
8. $b = 0.508$, $B = 13.1°$, $C = 5.2°$
9. $c = 5.00$, $A = 100°$, $B = 45°$
10. $a = 10.9$, $B = 76.9°$, $C = 100°$

Solve the following oblique triangles using the law of sines.

11. $a = 12.5$, $b = 13.2$, $B = 49°$
12. $b = 37.1$, $c = 21.3$, $B = 100°$
13. $a = 4.25$, $c = 2.86$, $A = 132°$
14. $c = 9.04$, $a = 21.3$, $C = 10.0°$
15. $b = 92.5$, $c = 98.6$, $B = 43.7°$
16. $c = 10.2$, $a = 16.7$, $A = 89.2°$
17. $a = 4$, $b = 22$, $A = 30°$
18. $a = 0.452$, $c = 0.606$, $C = 91.8°$
19. $b = 6.35$, $c = 4.29$, $C = 42.3°$
20. $b = 0.508$, $c = 1.09$, $C = 5.2°$
21. $c = 5.00$, $b = 8.00$, $B = 45.0°$
22. $a = 10.9$, $c = 16.9$, $C = 100.0°$

23. Ground-based radar at point A determines that the angle of elevation to an aircraft 42.9 miles away is 13.2°. Radar at point B is on a straight line between a point on the ground directly below the aircraft and the radar at A and determines that the same aircraft is 13.6 miles away from point B. To the nearest 0.1 mile, find the distance from A to B. (See the diagram.)

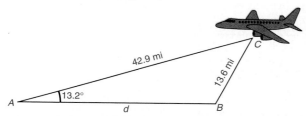

24. Two forest rangers sight a fire. Their reports are plotted on a map and yield the results shown in the diagram.

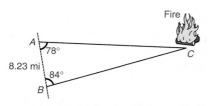

If the locations of the rangers are 8.23 miles apart, how far is the fire from Station A, to the nearest 0.1 mile?

25. The diagram shows a situation in which astronomers made measurements at two locations of a new, slow-moving asteroid. Using their measurements, find the distance d to the asteroid, to the nearest 100 miles.

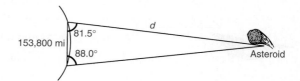

26. A surveyor made the measurements shown in the diagram. Find the distance across the lake, to the nearest foot.

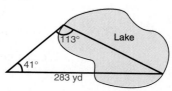

27. The diagram illustrates a situation in which a ship is moving at 12.6 knots heading due east. It is moving through a current moving east of north at 8.4 knots. The result is that the ship is moving at an angle of 58° east of north. Find the true speed S of the ship.

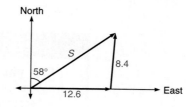

28. A ship travels due east to a point 8,000 meters from its starting point. It then turns toward the south through an angle of 65° and proceeds until it crosses a line of sight from the starting position to itself that is 35° south of east. At this point, how far is the ship from its starting point, to the nearest 10 meters?

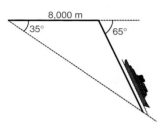

29. Two cities are 75 miles apart. An aircraft that is between the two cities is being tracked from radar in each city. City A's radar shows that the aircraft is at an angle of elevation of 40°; city B's radar shows that the slant distance of the plane to city B is 58 miles and that the angle of elevation there is less than 40°. What is the slant distance d from the plane to city A, to the nearest mile?

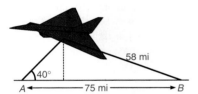

30. Find the height of the aircraft in problem 29, to the nearest 100 feet (1 mile = 5,280 feet). Use the diagram for help.

31. Show that in any oblique triangle ABC, if h is the altitude of the triangle relative to side b, then an expression for h is $h = \dfrac{b \cdot \tan A \cdot \tan C}{\tan A + \tan C}$. Use the diagrams for help.

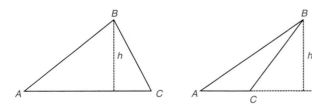

32. Quadrilateral $ABCD$ is shown in the diagram. $AB = 17.3$, $AD = 18.9$, angle $A = 110°$, angle $ABD = 52°$, angle $BDC = 41°$, angle $C = 93°$. Find the length of CD to the nearest 0.1. (*Hint:* Draw diagonal BD.)

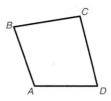

33. Show that in any triangle ABC, (1) $a = b \cos C + c \cos B$, (2) $b = c \cos A + a \cos C$, and (3) $c = a \cos B + b \cos A$. (*Hint:* The diagram shows angle A in standard position when the angle is acute, right, or obtuse.)

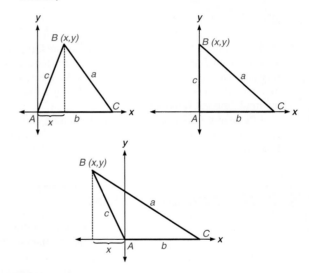

Show why the statements

$$\cos A = \frac{x}{c} \text{ and } \cos C = \frac{b - x}{a}$$

are true in each case, and then use them to show that (2) is true.

34. An Army observation point is 325 yards northeast (i.e., 45° north of east) of a second point. At this point a tank is sighted on a line of sight 37° south of east. The same tank is sighted at the second point along a line of sight 18° north of east. To the nearest yard, how far is the tank from the first observation point?

35. 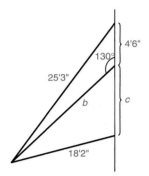 Recall that the formula for the area of a triangle is $\frac{1}{2}bh$ (one half the product of the base and height). Use the formula to show that the area of any triangle ABC is $\frac{1}{2}bc \sin A$.

36. The figure shows three wires that are attached from a common point to the side of a building. Find the lengths of b and c, to the nearest inch.

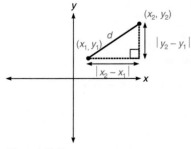

37. 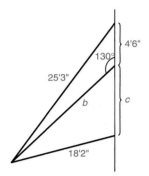 The Rhind Mathematical Papyrus is an Egyptian work on mathematics. It dates to the sixteenth century B.C., and contains material from the nineteenth century B.C. It contains 84 problems, including tables for manipulations of fractions.

Problems 51–53 of the Papyrus include the following formula for finding the area of a four-sided figure like $ABCD$ in the figure: $\frac{1}{2}(a + c) \times \frac{1}{2}(b + d)$. (Observe that $\frac{1}{2}(a + c)$ is the average length of the two sides a and c; the same is true for $\frac{1}{2}(b + d)$.) This formula is inaccurate. Except for rectangles, it gives an answer that is too large. It was used for the purpose of taxing land, which shows that there is not always an economic incentive to get the correct answer.

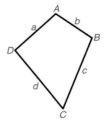

Problem 35 shows that the area of any triangle ABC is $\frac{1}{2}bc \sin A$. It is also $\frac{1}{2}ac \sin B$, or $\frac{1}{2}ab \sin C$. Geometrically, this is one-half the product of two sides and the sine of the angle between those two sides.

a. Use this result to show that the area of the four-sided figure can be described by

$$\tfrac{1}{4}(ab \sin A + ad \sin D + bc \sin B + cd \sin C)$$

b. Use the result of part a, along with the fact that for $0 < \theta < 180°$, $0 < \sin \theta < 1$ to show that the Egyptian formula is always too large, except for rectangles, when it is exact. (Assume angles A, B, C, and D are all less than $180°$.)

6–2 *The law of cosines*

There are some oblique triangles that cannot be solved using the law of sines. This happens when we do not know any of the three ratios completely. In these cases we use the *law of cosines*. To develop this law, we will use the **distance formula** of analytic geometry: If (x_1, y_1) and (x_2, y_2) are two points in the x-y coordinate plane, then the distance d between them is defined as

$$d = \sqrt{(x_2 - x_1)^2 + (y_2 - y_1)^2}$$

This definition is based on the Pythagorean theorem, since the value $|x_2 - x_1|$ is the length of one side of a right triangle of which the distance d is the hypotenuse, and $|y_2 - y_1|$ is the length of the second side. See figure 6–3.

Figure 6–3

■ Example 6–2 A

1. Find the distance between the points $(-4,7)$ and $(2,10)$.

   Using $(x_1,y_1) = (-4,7)$ and $(x_2,y_2) = (2,10)$, we have

   $$d = \sqrt{[2 - (-4)]^2 + (10 - 7)^2}$$
   $$= \sqrt{36 + 9}$$
   $$= \sqrt{45}$$
   $$= \sqrt{9 \cdot 5}$$
   $$= 3\sqrt{5}$$

   Note   The points could have been used in the reverse order with the same result. That is, $(x_1,y_1) = (2,10)$ and $(x_2,y_2) = (-4,7)$.

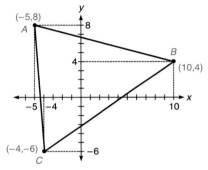

2. Assume that an optics table is coordinatized in the usual rectangular coordinate system. Three mirrors are located on the table at points $A(-5,8)$, $B(10,4)$, and $C(-4,-6)$. Find the distance traversed by a laser beam traveling from A to B to C and back to A, both exactly and to the nearest 0.1. See the figure.

   We use the distance formula: $d = \sqrt{(x_2 - x_1)^2 + (y_2 - y_1)^2}$. To find the distance from A to B, we can let A be the first point and B be the second. Then the formula becomes

   $$AB = \sqrt{(x_B - x_A)^2 + (y_B - y_A)^2}.$$

   We fill in the given values.

   $$AB = \sqrt{[10 - (-5)]^2 + (4 - 8)^2}$$
   $$= \sqrt{15^2 + (-4)^2}$$
   $$= \sqrt{241} \approx 15.52 \text{ (to two decimal places)}$$

   To find the distance from A to C, we can let A be the first point and C be the second.

   $$AC = \sqrt{(x_C - x_A)^2 + (y_C - y_A)^2}$$
   $$= \sqrt{[(-4) - (-5)]^2 + [(-6) - 8]^2}$$
   $$= \sqrt{1^2 + (-14)^2}$$
   $$= \sqrt{197} \approx 14.04$$

   To find the distance from B to C, we can let B be the first point and C be the second.

   $$BC = \sqrt{(x_C - x_B)^2 + (y_C - y_B)^2}$$
   $$= \sqrt{[(-4) - 10]^2 + [(-6) - 4]^2}$$
   $$= \sqrt{(-14)^2 + (-10)^2}$$
   $$= \sqrt{296} = \sqrt{4(74)} = 2\sqrt{74} \approx 17.20$$

   The exact total distance is

   $$AB + AC + BC = \sqrt{241} + \sqrt{197} + 2\sqrt{74} \text{ (exactly)}$$
   $$\approx 46.8$$ ■

We now use the distance formula in our development of the law of cosines.

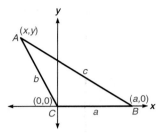

Figure 6–4

Let $\triangle ABC$ be any triangle. Put angle C in standard position, and call (x,y) the point at vertex A, as illustrated in figure 6–4.

Note   The figure shows C as an obtuse angle. The algebraic statements that follow do not use this fact, however. Thus, they would also apply if C were acute or right.

Now apply the distance formula to distance c.

$$d = \sqrt{(x_2 - x_1)^2 + (y_2 - y_1)^2}$$

Use $(x_2, y_2) = (a, 0)$ and $(x_1, y_1) = (x, y)$.

$$c = \sqrt{(a - x)^2 + (0 - y)^2}$$
$$c^2 = (a - x)^2 + (-y)^2$$
$$= a^2 - 2ax + x^2 + y^2$$

We know that $x^2 + y^2 = b^2$ (also by the distance formula), so we replace $x^2 + y^2$ in the above equation by b^2.

$$c^2 = a^2 - 2ax + b^2$$
$$= a^2 + b^2 - 2ax$$

We know that $\cos C = \dfrac{x}{b}$ by the definition of the cosine function (chapter 2).

Thus, $x = b \cos C$, and we replace x in the equation above by $b \cos C$.

$$c^2 = a^2 + b^2 - 2ab \cos C$$

The equation $c^2 = a^2 + b^2 - 2ab \cos C$ is called the **law of cosines** for angle C. If we had put angle A or angle B in standard position, we would have arrived at two other versions of this law. All three versions are:

The law of cosines

Law of cosines for angle A: $a^2 = b^2 + c^2 - 2bc \cos A$
Law of cosines for angle B: $b^2 = a^2 + c^2 - 2ac \cos B$
Law of cosines for angle C: $c^2 = a^2 + b^2 - 2ab \cos C$

Concept
The law of cosines states that in any triangle the square of the length of one side equals the sum of the squares of the lengths of the other two sides less twice the product of these lengths and the cosine of the angle opposite the first side.

When solving oblique triangles, the law of cosines should be used whenever the law of sines cannot be used.

■ *Example 6–2 B*

1. Solve oblique triangle *ABC* if *a* = 3.7, *c* = 4.8, and angle *B* = 43.9°. See the figure.

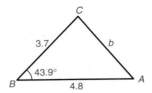

Observe that we do not know any of the three ratios of the law of sines completely: we know the length of side *a* but not the measure of angle *A*, the length of side *c* but not the measure of angle *C*, and the measure of angle *B* but not the length of side *b*. This indicates that we must use the law of cosines to help solve the problem.

Since we know angle *B*, we use the form of the law of cosines in which angle *B* appears:

$$b^2 = a^2 + c^2 - 2ac \cos B$$
$$= 3.7^2 + 4.8^2 - 2(3.7)(4.8)(\cos 43.9°)$$
$$b = \sqrt{3.7^2 + 4.8^2 - 2(3.7)(4.8)(\cos 43.9°)} \qquad \boxed{\text{CS 1}}$$
$$\approx 3.337068251 \dots$$

(which we will round off to 3.337 for now and to 3.3 in the final answer).

Now we use the law of sines to find one of the angles, either *A* or *C*. It is best to find angle *A* first, because we know angle *A* is not the largest angle in the triangle (angle *C* is) and, therefore, angle *A* must be acute. This will eliminate the ambiguous case.

$$\frac{3.7}{\sin A} \approx \frac{3.337}{\sin 43.9°}$$
$$3.337(\sin A) \approx 3.7(\sin 43.9°)$$
$$\sin A \approx \frac{3.7(\sin 43.9°)}{3.337}$$
$$A' \approx 50.2°$$

(remember, *A'* is the reference angle for angle *A*). We know that *A* is acute, so we do not have to worry about the supplement of *A* (which we normally do whenever we find an angle using the law of sines), so *A* ≈ 50.2°. Also, *C* = 180° − *A* − *B* ≈ 180° − 50.2° − 43.9° ≈ 85.9°. Since we now know all three angles and all three sides of the triangle, we are done.

$$A \approx 50.2°, B = 43.9°, C \approx 85.9°$$
$$a = 3.7, b = 3.3, c = 4.8$$

Note   As illustrated in the last example, it is never necessary to use the law of cosines more than once to solve a triangle. We complete the solution with the law of sines.

2. Solve oblique triangle ABC if $a = 0.915$, $b = 0.207$, and $c = 0.719$. See the figure.

We do not know any of the angles, so we cannot use the law of sines. (Without any angles, we cannot know any of the three ratios in the law of sines.) We use the law of cosines to find one of the angles.

It is best to find the largest angle first; this will be angle A since it is opposite the longest side a. The reason for finding the largest angle first is explained in the note below. We must use the form of the law of cosines that includes angle A.

$$a^2 = b^2 + c^2 - 2bc \cos A$$

We often solve for $\cos A$ before we use the law of cosines.

$$a^2 = b^2 + c^2 - 2bc \cos A$$
$$2bc \cos A = b^2 + c^2 - a^2$$
$$\cos A = \frac{b^2 + c^2 - a^2}{2bc}$$

Substituting values, we get

$$\cos A = \frac{0.207^2 + 0.719^2 - 0.915^2}{2(0.207)(0.719)}$$
$$\approx -0.9320.$$
$$A \approx 158.74°$$

$\boxed{\text{CS 2}}$

Now we know the measure of the largest angle: $A \approx 158.74°$. We can now use the law of sines to find another angle. We must use the ratio $\dfrac{a}{\sin A}$ since A is the only angle measure we know. To find angle B we use

$$\frac{0.915}{\sin 158.74°} \approx \frac{0.207}{\sin B}$$

to find that

$$B' \approx 4.70°.$$

Since we have already found the largest angle A, we know that the remaining two angles are acute, and so we do not have to worry about the supplement of B'; thus, $B \approx 4.70°$ and $C \approx 180° - 158.7° - 4.7° = 16.6°$. The triangle is solved because we now know all three sides (which were given) and all three angles. $A \approx 158.7°$, $B \approx 4.7°$, $C \approx 16.6°$.

Note   There is no ambiguous case for the law of cosines because the range of the inverse cosine function includes all angles from 0° to 180°. If an angle is not acute, its cosine will be negative (as above), and then we know the angle is between 90° and 180°. Thus, *when finding an angle of a triangle using the law of cosines* (as above), *it is best to find the largest angle first.* If the largest angle is obtuse we will find this out directly; either way, the remaining angles are acute and, therefore, easy to find with the law of sines.

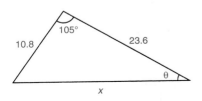

3. A sheet metal worker must make the triangular pattern shown in the figure. Find the angle of inclination θ and the length of side x.

   Using the law of cosines, we see that

   $$x^2 = 10.8^2 + 23.6^2 - 2(10.8)(23.6) \cos 105°$$
   $$\approx 805.54$$
   $$x \approx 28.38$$

   We can now use the law of sines to find θ.

   $$\frac{28.38}{\sin 105°} \approx \frac{10.8}{\sin \theta}$$
   $$28.38 \sin \theta \approx 10.8 \sin 105°$$
   $$\sin \theta \approx \frac{10.8 \sin 105°}{28.38} \approx 0.3676$$
   $$\theta' \approx 21.6°$$

   θ is acute because it is not the largest angle in the triangle, so $\theta = 21.6°$.

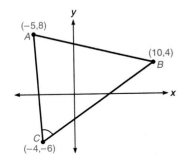

4. Find the measure of angle ACB in part 2 of example 6–2 A to the nearest 0.1°. Recall that we have a triangle whose vertices were the points A $(-5,8)$, B (10,4), and C $(-4,-6)$. See the figure.

   In part 2 of example 6–2 A we used the distance formula to establish

   $$AB = \sqrt{241} \approx 15.52$$
   $$AC = \sqrt{197} \approx 14.04$$
   $$BC = 2\sqrt{74} \approx 17.20$$

   To find angle ACB, we use the law of cosines with angle C.

   $$c^2 = a^2 + b^2 - 2ab \cos C$$
   $$\cos C = \frac{a^2 + b^2 - c^2}{2ab}$$
   $$= \frac{(2\sqrt{74})^2 + (\sqrt{197})^2 - (\sqrt{241})^2}{2(2\sqrt{74})(\sqrt{197})}$$
   $$= \frac{296 + 197 - 241}{4(\sqrt{74})(\sqrt{197})} \approx 0.5218$$
   $$C \approx 58.5° \qquad \boxed{\text{CS 3}}$$

■ *Example 6–2 C*

In triangle ABC, $a = 4$, $b = 6$, $c = 12$. Solve the triangle.

We must use the law of cosines to solve this triangle. If we wish to find the largest angle, which is C, we use

$$\cos C = \frac{a^2 + b^2 - c^2}{2ab}$$

$$= \frac{4^2 + 6^2 - 12^2}{2(4)(6)}$$

$$= \frac{-92}{48}$$

$$\approx -1.9167$$

Note that this result shows that there is no angle C, since $|\cos x| \leq 1$ for any value of x. Thus, there is no solution to this triangle.   ■

Example 6–2 C illustrates a situation in which the law of cosines shows us that there is no solution. There is no solution because $a + b < c$. It is a fact that any two sides of a triangle must have a total length greater than the third side. This is often called the **triangle inequality.** Any time we are given the lengths of three sides of a triangle, it is a good idea to check that the sum of the lengths of any two sides is greater than the length of the remaining side.

Mastery points

Can you
- State the three forms of the law of cosines?
- Use the law of cosines to solve triangles when the law of sines cannot be used?
- Use the distance formula?

Calculator steps

1.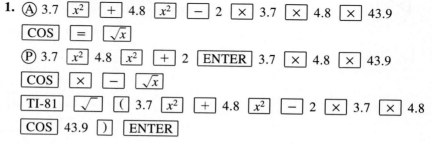

2. (A) .207 $\boxed{x^2}$ $\boxed{+}$ .719 $\boxed{x^2}$ $\boxed{-}$ .915 $\boxed{x^2}$ $\boxed{=}$ $\boxed{\div}$ 2 $\boxed{\div}$ .207

$\boxed{\div}$ .719 $\boxed{=}$ $\boxed{\text{INV}}$ $\boxed{\text{COS}}$

(P) .207 $\boxed{x^2}$ .719 $\boxed{x^2}$ $\boxed{+}$ .915 $\boxed{x^2}$ $\boxed{-}$ 2 $\boxed{\div}$ .207 $\boxed{\div}$ .719

$\boxed{\div}$ $\boxed{\text{COS}^{-1}}$

$\boxed{\text{TI-81}}$ $\boxed{\cos^{-1}}$ $\boxed{(}$ $\boxed{(}$ .207 $\boxed{x^2}$ $\boxed{+}$ .719 $\boxed{x^2}$ $\boxed{-}$ .915 $\boxed{x^2}$

$\boxed{)}$ $\boxed{\div}$ $\boxed{(}$ 2 $\boxed{\times}$ .207 $\boxed{\times}$ .719 $\boxed{)}$ $\boxed{)}$ $\boxed{\text{ENTER}}$

3. (A) 296 $\boxed{+}$ 197 $\boxed{-}$ 241 $\boxed{=}$ $\boxed{\div}$ 4 $\boxed{\div}$ 74 $\boxed{\sqrt{x}}$ $\boxed{\div}$ 197

$\boxed{\sqrt{x}}$ $\boxed{=}$ $\boxed{\text{INV}}$ $\boxed{\text{COS}}$

(P) 296 $\boxed{\text{ENTER}}$ 197 $\boxed{+}$ 241 $\boxed{-}$ 4 $\boxed{\div}$ 74 $\boxed{\sqrt{x}}$ $\boxed{\div}$ 197

$\boxed{\sqrt{x}}$ $\boxed{\div}$ $\boxed{\text{COS}^{-1}}$

$\boxed{\text{TI-81}}$ $\boxed{\cos^{-1}}$ $\boxed{(}$ $\boxed{(}$ 296 $\boxed{+}$ 197 $\boxed{-}$ 241 $\boxed{)}$ $\boxed{\div}$ $\boxed{(}$ 4

$\boxed{\sqrt{}}$ 74 $\boxed{\sqrt{}}$ 197 $\boxed{)}$ $\boxed{)}$ $\boxed{\text{ENTER}}$

Exercise 6–2

Find the distance between the following points.

1. $(3,-4)$, $(-2,6)$
2. $(3,-1)$, $(4,-8)$
3. $(-5,-2)$, $(10,-1)$
4. $(-2,-3)$, $(-4,-1)$
5. $(0,-3)$, $(-9,-12)$
6. $(10,-1)$, $(2,0)$

Solve the following oblique triangles. You will have to use the law of cosines as the first step. Round your answers to the same number of decimal places as the data.

7. $a = 3.2$, $b = 5.9$, $C = 39.4°$
8. $a = 4.9$, $b = 3.2$, $C = 78.2°$
9. $b = 61.3$, $c = 23.9$, $A = 124.0°$
10. $b = 123.0$, $c = 89.4$, $A = 19.5°$
11. $a = 31.4$, $c = 17.0$, $B = 100.3°$
12. $a = 67.25$, $c = 13.56$, $B = 76.30°$
13. $a = 23.5$, $b = 19.4$, $c = 35.0$
14. $a = 61.7$, $b = 80.0$, $c = 102.0$
15. $a = 0.214$, $b = 0.399$, $c = 0.500$
16. $a = 1.03$, $b = 0.98$, $c = 1.75$
17. $a = 13.2$, $b = 5.9$, $C = 139.4°$
18. $a = 14.9$, $b = 13.2$, $C = 45.0°$
19. $b = 61.3$, $c = 43.9$, $A = 24.5°$
20. $b = 23.9$, $c = 89.4$, $A = 79.5°$
21. $a = 30.0$, $c = 20.0$, $B = 112.0°$
22. $a = 6.72$, $c = 1.55$, $B = 76.35°$
23. $a = 235$, $b = 194$, $c = 354$
24. $a = 61.7$, $b = 80.0$, $c = 42.0$
25. $a = 0.21$, $b = 0.49$, $C = 1.50°$
26. $a = 10.0$, $b = 13.9$, $c = 17.5$

27. A surveyor made the measurements shown in the diagram to calculate the distance across a lake.

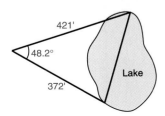

Compute the distance to the nearest 0.1 foot.

28. Calculate the measure of the smallest angle in a triangle whose sides have measure 22.1 cm, 32.6 cm, and 40.5 cm.

29. Calculate the measure of the largest angle in a triangle whose sides have measure 12.3 in., 16.2 in., and 19.0 in.

30. A numerically controlled laser cloth cutter is being set up to cut a triangular pattern. The vertices of the triangle are at A $(2,5)$, B $(4,8)$, and C $(5,12)$.
   a. Find the length of side AB.
   b. Determine the measure of the three angles to the nearest 0.1°.

31. In the same situation as in problem 30, the vertices of another piece of triangular cloth are determined to be at $A(0,5)$, $B(2,3)$, and $C(8,4)$. Determine the measure of the largest of the three angles A, B, or C, to the nearest 0.1°.

32. Two ships are being tracked by radar. One ship is determined to be 17.6 miles from the radar, while the second is 22.5 miles from the radar. The lines of sight from the radar to the two ships form an angle of 47.2°. (See the diagram.) Find the distance between the two ships to the nearest 0.1 mile.

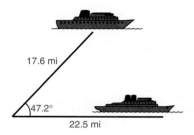

33. In the situation described in problem 32, what would be the angle formed by the two lines of sight to the ships if the ships were 31.5 miles apart?

34. A ship leaves a harbor heading due east and travels 17.3 km. It then turns north through a 33° angle and travels for another 22.0 km. How far is the ship from its starting point, to the nearest kilometer?

35. A plane takes off and travels southeast (45° south of east) for 27 miles, then turns due south and travels for 16 miles. How far is it from its starting position, to the nearest mile?

36. The points (5,3), (−2,1), and (1,−4) form a triangle. Find the measure of the smallest angle in this triangle, to the nearest 0.1°.

37. Find the measure of the largest angle in the triangle of problem 36, to the nearest 0.1°.

38. Two observers are 87 meters apart, and a range finder shows that a certain building is 111 meters from one observer and 114 meters from the other. What is the angle formed by the two lines of sight from the building to the observers, to the nearest degree?

39. The triangle in the diagram is a right triangle. Can the law of cosines be used to find the length of c? Compare using the law of cosines to using the Pythagorean theorem.

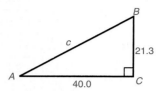

40. The diagram shows three triangles in which angle C is (a) acute, (b) right, and (c) obtuse.

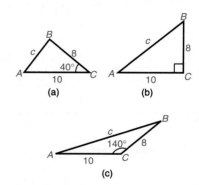

If we use the Pythagorean theorem and apply it to the right triangle in (b) and apply the law of cosines to angle C in all three situations, the resulting equations are

$$c^2 = a^2 + b^2 \text{ and}$$
$$c^2 = a^2 + b^2 - 2ab \cos C$$

We can view the expression $-2ab \cos C$ as a "correction factor" to the Pythagorean theorem that will give the correct result, even when angle C is not 90°.

Solve for side c in each case, using the law of cosines, and discuss how the correction factor "knows" when to increase the length of side c (as in [c]) and when to decrease it (as in [a]).

6–3 *Vectors*

If we know that a plane flying over a certain spot is flying at 100 mph, we cannot tell where it will be in 1 hour without also knowing its direction. This combination of speed and direction is called *velocity*. Many other natural phenomena are described by a magnitude and direction: forces of all types, accelerations, alternating voltage in electricity theory are all examples. A conceptual tool used to describe two such pieces of information is the **vector.** It is noteworthy that the concept of vectors extends into an area of mathematics called *linear algebra,* which has applications in every field of knowledge, from physics and economics to medicine and sociology.

We imagine a vector as a directed line segment. That is, a finite portion of a straight line that is considered to be pointing in one direction. Our representation of vectors would commonly be called ''arrows.'' Examples of vectors are shown in figure 6–5. Observe that we use the terms **head** and **tail** to describe the ''end'' and ''beginning'' of a vector, respectively, and that we often use capital letters, such as *A* and *B*, to name a vector.

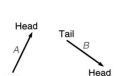

Figure 6–5

One way to describe a vector is by specifying its length and direction. The length is called the **magnitude** of the vector, and for a vector *A* we denote its magnitude by $|A|$ (the same notation as that for absolute value of a real number). The **direction** of a vector is specified by an angle, θ, usually specified in degrees, measured in the same way as angles in standard position. When we specify a vector this way we say it is in **polar form.**

Polar form of a vector
A vector *A* in polar form is the ordered pair $A = (|A|, \theta_A)$
$|A|$ is the magnitude of vector A; $|A| \geq 0$.
θ_A is the direction of vector A.

Note   The polar form of a vector is not unique; all coterminal values of θ_A are equivalent.

Figure 6–6 illustrates the vectors $(2, 45°)$ and $(3, -120°)$.

A vector can also be specified by using its *relative rectangular coordinates.* For a vector in standard position this is equivalent to specifying the coordinates of its head (see figure 6–8). If a vector is not in standard position, its relative rectangular coordinates are relative to the coordinates of the vector's tail. We refer to these coordinates as describing the **rectangular form** of a vector.

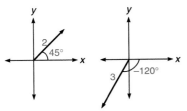

Figure 6–6

Rectangular form of a vector
A vector *A* in rectangular form is $A = (A_x, A_y)$, where A_x is called the **horizontal component** of the vector and A_y is called the **vertical component** of the vector.

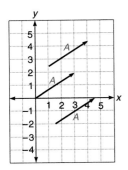

Figure 6–7

Figure 6–7 illustrates the vector $A(3,2)$, shown in three different positions.

Converting polar form to rectangular form

There is a useful relation for converting the polar form of a vector to its rectangular form. If we recall the definitions of section 2–2 for an angle in standard position, we can see the following.

To convert polar form to rectangular form
Given vector $A = (|A|, \theta_A) = (A_x, A_y)$,
$$A_x = |A| \cos \theta_A \quad \text{and} \quad A_y = |A| \sin \theta_A$$

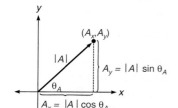

Figure 6–8

This is true because, by the definitions of section 5–2, $\cos \theta_A = \dfrac{A_x}{|A|}$ and $\sin \theta_A = \dfrac{A_y}{|A|}$. Figure 6–8 illustrates this relationship.

Example 6–3 A illustrates converting a vector in polar to form to its rectangular form.

■ *Example 6–3 A*

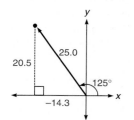

Convert from polar to rectangular form.

1. Convert the polar form of the vector to the rectangular form (approximate to the nearest tenth). $A = (25.0, 125°)$.
$$A_x = |A| \cos \theta_A = 25.0 \cos 125° \approx -14.3$$
$$A_y = |A| \sin \theta_A = 25.0 \sin 125° \approx 20.5$$

Thus, the rectangular form is $(-14.3, 20.5)$ (see the figure).

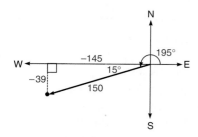

2. An aircraft is moving in the direction 15° south of west at 150 knots. Find the east-west and north-south components of its velocity V to the nearest knot and interpret the results.

As we see in the figure the aircraft's velocity is the vector $V = (150, 195°)$. The east-west component is
$$V_x = |V| \cos \theta_V$$
$$= 150 \cos 195° \approx -145$$

The north-south component is
$$V_y = |V| \sin \theta_V$$
$$= 150 \sin 195° \approx -39$$

Thus, the aircraft is moving west at 145 knots and south at 39 knots.   ■

Converting rectangular form to polar form

When we convert from rectangular to polar form we always give the direction of the vector θ_V so that it has the smallest possible absolute value. This means *we will choose θ_V so that $-180° < \theta_V \leq 180°$*. One reason for doing this is that this is the result obtained from electronic calculators (see the discussion following example 6–3 B).

Examining figure 6–8 shows that, for a given vector $V = (V_x, V_y) = (|V|, \theta_V)$, $|V| = \sqrt{V_x^2 + V_y^2}$, and $\tan\theta'_V = \dfrac{V_y}{V_x}$ if $V_x \neq 0$. The angle $\theta'_V = \tan^{-1}\dfrac{V_y}{V_x}$ is only the reference angle and θ_V depends on the quadrant in which the vector occurs.

Reference angles obtained with the inverse tangent function fall in the range $-90° < \theta' < 90°$ (quadrant I and quadrant IV). If $V_x > 0$ this is the value of θ_V, since that angle should be in quadrant I or quadrant IV.

If $V_x < 0$, θ_V can be obtained by adding or subtracting 180° to or from θ'_V. If $\theta'_V < 0$, add 180°, and if $\theta'_V > 0$, subtract 180°. This can be incorporated into a rule as follows.

To convert rectangular form to polar form

Given vector $V = (V_x, V_y) = (|V|, \theta_V)$. Then,

$$|V| = \sqrt{V_x^2 + V_y^2}, \quad \theta'_V = \tan^{-1}\frac{V_y}{V_x} \text{ if } V_x \neq 0, \text{ and}$$

$$\theta_V = \begin{cases} \theta'_V & \text{if } V_x > 0 \\ \theta'_V - 180° \text{ if } \theta'_V > 0 & \\ \theta'_V + 180° \text{ if } \theta'_V < 0 & \text{if } V_x < 0 \end{cases}$$

Note If $V_x = 0$ then θ_V is 90° if $V_y > 0$, and $-90°$ if $V_y < 0$. This is clear from a sketch of the vector.

The examples and the exercises will make clear why the rule works when $V_x < 0$. Example 6–3 B illustrates finding the polar form of a vector when its rectangular form is known.

■ *Example 6–3 B*

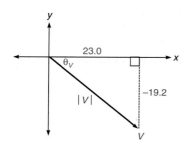

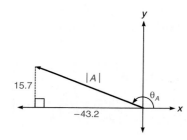

Convert to polar form.

1. The horizontal component of a force vector is 23.0 pounds to the right; its vertical component is 19.2 pounds down. Find the force vector V, to the nearest 0.1 pound.

The vector is $(23.0, -19.2)$ in rectangular form. We can find $|V|$ using the Pythagorean theorem:

$$|V|^2 = 23.0^2 + (-19.2)^2$$
$$|V| \approx 30.0$$

We now find θ'_V the reference angle for θ_V.

$$\theta'_V = \tan^{-1}\left(\frac{-19.2}{23.0}\right) \approx -39.9°$$
$$\theta_V = \theta'_V, \quad V_x > 0$$

Thus, $V \approx (30.0, -39.9°)$.

2. Vector $A = (-43.2, 15.7)$. Find the polar form of A.

$$|A| = \sqrt{A_x^2 + A_y^2}$$
$$= \sqrt{(-43.2)^2 + (-15.7)^2} \approx 46.0 \qquad \text{Nearest tenth}$$
$$\theta'_A = \tan^{-1}\left(\frac{15.7}{-43.2}\right) \approx -20.0°$$
$$\theta_A \approx -20.0° + 180° \approx 160.0° \qquad A_x < 0, \theta'_A < 0$$

Thus, $A \approx (46.0, 160.0°)$. ■

Using special calculator keys

Most engineering/scientific calculators are programmed to perform the conversions of examples 6–3 A and 6–3 B. These calculators have keys marked "R → P" or simply "→P" (rectangular to polar conversion) and "P → R" or "→ R" (polar to rectangular conversion), or something equivalent. The results are stored in locations referred to as x and y. Typical keystrokes are illustrated here. Part 1 of example 6–3 A would be done as follows. (The TI-81 is discussed below.)

$A = (25.0, 125°)$

25 $\boxed{P \to R}$ 125 $\boxed{=}$ Display: $\boxed{-14.33941091}$

$\boxed{x \leftrightarrow y}$ Display: $\boxed{20.47880111}$

Thus $A \approx (-14.3, 20.5)$.

Part 1 of example 6–3 B would be done in the following way.

$V = (23.0, -19.2)$

23 $\boxed{R \to P}$ 19.2 $\boxed{+/-}$ $\boxed{=}$ Display $\boxed{29.96064085}$

$\boxed{x \leftrightarrow y}$ Display: $\boxed{-39.855454183}$

Thus, $V \approx (30.0, -39.9°)$.

The TI-81 uses the values X, Y, R, θ. (Y, R, θ are $\boxed{\text{ALPHA}}$ 1, $\boxed{\times}$, and 3, respectively.) It also uses the two MATH functions "R ▶ P(" (Rectangular to polar) and "P ▶ R(" (Polar to rectangular).

Example 6–3 A, part 1:

$\boxed{\text{MODE}}$ Deg $\boxed{\text{ENTER}}$ Make sure the calculator is in degree mode.

$\boxed{\text{MATH}}$ 2 25 $\boxed{\text{ALPHA}}$ $\boxed{\text{.}}$ 125 $\boxed{)}$

$\boxed{\text{ENTER}}$ Display: $\boxed{-14.33941091}$

$\boxed{\text{ALPHA}}$ 1 $\boxed{\text{ENTER}}$ Display: $\boxed{20.47880111}$

Example 6–3 B, part 1:

$\boxed{\text{MATH}}$ 1 23 $\boxed{\text{ALPHA}}$ $\boxed{\text{.}}$ $\boxed{(-)}$ 19

$\boxed{\text{.}}$ 2 $\boxed{)}$ $\boxed{\text{ENTER}}$ Display: $\boxed{29.96064085}$

$\boxed{\text{ALPHA}}$ 3 $\boxed{\text{ENTER}}$ Display: $\boxed{-39.855454183}$

Addition of vectors

It has been shown experimentally that most natural phenomena that are described by vectors combine as if they were connected tail to head in a series. The result is a vector with its tail at the tail of the first vector in the series, and its head at the head of the last vector in the series. The resulting vector is called the **resultant vector.** This is illustrated in figure 6–9, where vectors A, B, and C combine into the resultant vector Z. This idea is the basis for the definition of addition of vectors which we develop here.

Example 6–3 C illustrates that this process is equivalent to summing all the horizontal components and, separately, the vertical components. This is the basis for the definition of the addition of two vectors.

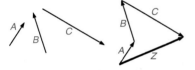

Figure 6–9

> **Vector sum**
> Let Z be the resultant (vector sum) of two vectors $A = (A_x, A_y)$ and $B = (B_x, B_y)$. Then we say $Z = A + B$, where
> $$Z_x = A_x + B_x \quad \text{and} \quad Z_y = A_y + B_y$$

Observe that this definition describes how to add two vectors whose rectangular form is known. When vectors are known in polar form they must first be converted to rectangular form. This is illustrated in example 6–3 C.

■ *Example 6–3 C*

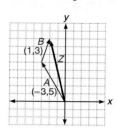

Find the vector sum of the given vectors.

1. $A = (-3,5)$ and $B = (1,3)$

$$Z_x = A_x + B_x = -3 + 1 = -2$$
$$Z_y = A_y + B_y = 5 + 3 = 8$$
$$Z = (-2,8)$$

This is illustrated in the figure.

2. $A = (2,-\frac{1}{2})$, $B = (-6,3\frac{1}{2})$, $C = (3,-2)$

$$Z_x = A_x + B_x + C_x = 2 + (-6) + 3 = -1$$
$$Z_y = A_y + B_y + C_y = -\frac{1}{2} + 3\frac{1}{2} + (-2) = 1$$
$$Z = (-1,1)$$

3. $V = (13.8,40.2°)$, $W = (20.9,164.6°)$

Note that these vectors are in polar form. See the figure.

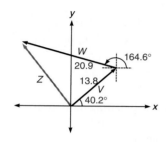

$$
\begin{aligned}
Z_x &= V_x + W_x \\
&= |V| \cos \theta_V + |W| \cos \theta_W \\
&= 13.8 \cos 40.2° + 20.9 \cos 164.6° \approx -9.6093 \\
Z_y &= V_y + W_y \\
&= |V| \sin \theta_V + |W| \sin \theta_W \\
&= 13.8 \sin 40.2° + 20.9 \sin 164.6° \approx 14.4574
\end{aligned}
$$

Thus, $Z \approx (-9.6,14.5)$ (to nearest tenth).

We should find Z in polar form, since V and W were given in this form.

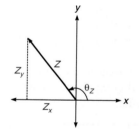

$$Z = \sqrt{Z_x^2 + Z_y^2} = \sqrt{(-9.6093)^2 + 14.4589^2} \approx 17.4 \quad \text{(nearest 0.1)}$$

$$\theta_Z' = \tan^{-1}\frac{Z_y}{Z_x} \approx \tan^{-1}\left(\frac{14.4589}{-9.6093}\right) \approx -56.4°$$

$$\theta_Z = \theta_Z' + 180° \approx 123.6° \quad \text{Since } Z_x < 0, \text{ and } \theta_z' \text{ is negative, we add } 180°$$

Thus, in polar form, $Z \approx (17.4,123.6°)$.

4. Three forces are acting on a point, where F_1 is 25 pounds acting in the direction 30°, F_2 is 40 points acting in the direction 100°, and F_3 is 50 pounds acting in the direction $-40°$. Find the resultant force acting on the point.

Find the resultant of the three vectors $A(25,30°)$, $B(40,100°)$, and $C(50,-40°)$.

$$
\begin{aligned}
Z_x &= F_{1x} + F_{2x} + F_{3x} \\
&= 25 \cos 30° + 40 \cos 100° + 50 \cos(-40°) \approx 53.01 \\
Z_y &= F_{1y} + F_{2y} + F_{3y} \\
&= 25 \sin 30° + 40 \sin 100° + 50 \sin(-40°) \approx 19.75 \\
|Z| &= \sqrt{Z_x^2 + Z_y^2} \\
&= \sqrt{53.01^2 + 19.75^2} \approx 56.6 \text{ pounds}
\end{aligned}
$$

$$\tan \theta_Z' = \frac{Z_y}{Z_x} = \frac{19.75}{53.01} \; ; \; \theta_Z' \approx 20.4°$$

Since Z_x and Z_y are both positive, the resultant is in the first quadrant, so
$\theta_Z = \theta'_Z \approx 20.4°$.
Thus, $Z \approx (56.6, 20.4°)$.   ∎

⌨ Problem 76 in the exercises presents a program that adds two or more vectors given in polar form.

Example 6–3 D illustrates a general principle of navigating aircraft (and, analogously, ships at sea). The speed of the aircraft relative to the air is called the airspeed, and the direction in which the aircraft is pointed is its heading. The airspeed and heading combine into the heading vector, H. The wind vector, W, is the speed and direction of the wind. If we add these two vectors we get the true course and ground speed of the plane, T = H + W. T is the speed and direction relative to the earth's surface.

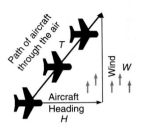

■ *Example 6–3 D*

An aircraft is flying with heading 5° north of east and airspeed 123 knots. The wind is blowing at 32 knots in the direction 10° west of south. Find the true course and ground speed of the aircraft (see the figure).

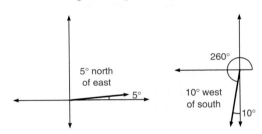

$H = (123, 5°); \; W = (32, 260°)$

$T = H + W$

$T_x = H_x + W_x$
$\quad = |H|\cos\theta_H + |W|\cos\theta_W$
$\quad = 123\cos 5° + 32\cos 260° \approx 116.98$

$T_y = H_y + W_y$
$\quad = |H|\sin\theta_H + |W|\sin\theta_W$
$\quad = 123\sin 5° + 32\sin 260° \approx -20.79$

$\theta'_T = \tan^{-1}\dfrac{T_y}{T_x} = \tan^{-1}\left(\dfrac{-20.79}{116.98}\right) \approx -10°$ To nearest degree

$\theta_T = \theta'_T$ since $T_x > 0$, $|T| = \sqrt{T_x^2 + T_y^2} = \sqrt{116.98^2 + (-20.79)^2} \approx 119$.

Thus, the ground speed of the aircraft is 119 knots and the true course is 10° south of east.   ∎

The zero vector and the opposite of a vector

It is useful to define a zero vector and the opposite of a vector. The zero vector is defined so its length is zero. The direction does not matter. The opposite of a vector is defined to have equal length but opposite direction. We do this by adding or subtracting 180°. Both definitions are in terms of polar form.

> **Zero vector**
> The vector $0 = (0,\theta)$, where θ is any angle, is the zero vector.
>
> **Opposite of a vector**
> Given a vector $V = (|V|,\theta_V)$, then $-V$ means its opposite, and $-V = (|V|,\theta_V \pm 180°)$.

In computing the opposite we generally choose whichever value, $\theta_V + 180°$ or $\theta_V - 180°$, has the smallest absolute value. It is easy to show that for any vector V,

$$V + (-V) = 0$$

Example 6–3 E illustrates uses of the zero vector and the opposite of a vector.

■ *Example 6–3 E*

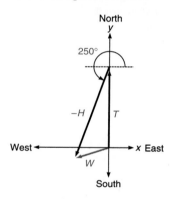

1. An aircraft's on-board inertial navigation computer shows that the aircraft is traveling due north at 200 knots with respect to the ground, and that the aircraft is headed 20° east of north with an airspeed of 225 knots. Using vector subtraction, find the wind vector W. Interpret this vector.

We know that true course and ground speed T are due north and 200 knots. Thus, $T = (200,90°)$. Heading and airspeed are 20° east of north and 225 knots. Thus, $H = (225,70°)$ (see the figure).

$$H + W = T \qquad \text{Aircraft heading + wind = true course}$$
$$W = T - H \qquad \text{Solve}^1 \text{ for } W$$
$$\quad = T + (-H)$$
$$W = (200,90°) + (225,250°) \qquad -H = (225,70° + 180°)$$
$$W_x = 200\cos 90° + 225\cos 250° \approx -76.95$$
$$W_y = 200\sin 90° + 225\sin 250° \approx -11.43$$
$$|W| = \sqrt{W_x^2 + W_y^2} \approx 77.80$$
$$\theta'_W \approx \tan^{-1}\left(\frac{-11.43}{-76.95}\right) \approx -8.4°$$
$$\theta_W = \theta'_W - 180° \approx -8.4° + 180° \qquad W_x < 0 \text{ and } \theta'_W > 0$$
$$\quad \approx -171.6°$$

Thus, $W \approx (77.8,-171.6°)$. This tells us that the wind is blowing in a direction 8.4° south of west at 77.8 knots.

---

[1]We are assuming we can solve a vector-valued equation as we solve real-valued equations. In fact, it can be proved that this is valid.

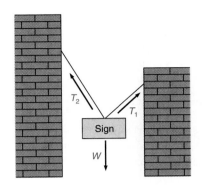

2. A large sign is suspended between two buildings by two wires, as in the figure. One wire acts at an angle of 45° above the horizontal and has a tension (force) T_1, of 400 pounds. If the sign weighs 800 pounds (vector W), compute a vector that describes T_2, the tension and direction of the second wire, to the nearest unit.

We use a fact from physics to describe the situation. Since the sign is motionless, all the forces acting on it must be balanced, or add to zero. Thus, we proceed as follows.

$T_1 + T_2 + W = 0$ All forces balanced

$T_2 = -T_1 - W$ Solve for T_2

$T_1 = (400, 45°)$, so $-T_1 = (400, 45° + 180°) = (400, 225°)$

$W = (800, 270°)$, so $-W = (800, 270° - 180°) = (800, 90°)$

$T_{2x} = -T_{1x} + (-W_x)$

$\quad = 400 \cos 225° + 800 \cos 90° \approx -282.84$

$T_{2y} = -T_{1y} + (-W_y)$

$\quad = 400 \sin 225° + 800 \sin 90° \approx 517.16$

$|T_2| = \sqrt{(-282.84)^2 + 517.16^2} \approx 589$ pounds.

$\theta'_{T_2} \approx \tan^{-1}\left(\dfrac{517.16}{-282.84}\right) \approx -61.3°$

$\theta_{T_2} = 180° + \theta'_{T_2}$ $T_{2x} < 0, \theta'_{T_2} < 0$

$\quad \approx 118.7°$

Thus, to the nearest unit $T_2 \approx (589, 119°)$.   ■

Mastery points

Can you
- Find the horizontal and vertical components of a vector?
- Find the magnitude and direction of a vector when given the horizontal and vertical components?
- Add or subtract vectors?
- Apply vectors to navigation and force problems?

Exercise 6–3

Convert each vector from its polar to its rectangular form. Leave all answers to the nearest tenth unless the reference angle is 30°, 45°, or 60°.

1. $(40, 30°)$ **2.** $(15.2, 33.6°)$ **3.** $(100.0, 122.3°)$ **4.** $(4.2, 97.3°)$

5. $(10.0, 200.0°)$ **6.** $(18, 120°)$ **7.** $(25, 300°)$ **8.** $(82.0, 341.9°)$

9. $(6, -45°)$ **10.** $(5.9, 59.2°)$ **11.** $(7.8, -264.3°)$ **12.** $(20.0, -333.0°)$

Convert each vector to polar form. Round to the nearest tenth unless an exact form is possible (if the reference angle is 30°, 45°, or 60°).

13. (3.0,4.0)   **14.** (31.2,6.9)   **15.** (−3.0,5.2)   **16.** (−12.5,31.0)
17. ($\sqrt{3}$,−2)   **18.** (3,−3)   **19.** (5,−10)   **20.** (−12.5,−20.3)
21. (−6.8,3.4)   **22.** (−8,4)   **23.** (−$\sqrt{2}$,−$\sqrt{8}$)   **24.** (−1,0.4)

Add the following vectors. Leave the resultant in rectangular form. Round the resultant to the nearest tenth.

25. (−3,8), (2,12)   **26.** (4,$3\frac{1}{2}$), (−1,−$2\frac{1}{2}$)
27. ($\sqrt{2}$,5), ($\sqrt{8}$,1), ($\sqrt{50}$,−6)   **28.** (5,−13), (−$\frac{1}{2}$,8), ($7\frac{1}{2}$,−1)

Add the following vectors. Leave the resultant in polar form. Round the resultant to the nearest tenth.

29. (30.0,30°), (15.2,33.6°)   **30.** (100,0°), (4.2,97.3°)
31. (10.0,200°), (29.3,250°)   **32.** (13.7,300.0°), (82.0,341.9°)
33. (3.2,−45.0°), (5.9,−59.2°)   **34.** (37.9,−100.5°), (69.2,−170.1°)
35. (41.9,−213.0°), (7.7,−264.3°)   **36.** (20.0,−333.0°), (39.2,−359.0°)
37. (3.5,19.2°), (2.7,83.1°), (4.3,145.7°)   **38.** (7.1,13.8°), (6.2,131°), (10.4,215°)
39. (15.3,311°), (20.9,117°), (13.2,83°)   **40.** (3.2,19.5°), (5.1,45.0°), (6.0,180°)
41. (3.5,−25°), (6.8,25°), (4.2,50°)   **42.** (25,−30°), (25,−60°), (25,−100°)

43. An aircraft is moving in the direction 25° north of west at 150 knots. Find the east-west and north-south components of its velocity to the nearest knot and interpret the results.

44. An aircraft is moving in the direction 35° east of south at 120 knots. Find the east-west and north-south components of its velocity to the nearest knot and interpret the results.

45. An aircraft is moving in the direction 15° north of east at 200 knots. Find the east-west and north-south components of its velocity to the nearest knot and interpret the results.

46. A rocket is climbing with a speed of 825 knots and an angle of climb of 58.6°. (The angle of climb is the angle measured from the ground to its flight path.) Find the horizontal and vertical components of the rocket's velocity, to the nearest knot.

47. An aircraft is traveling in a direction 30° west of north. Its speed is 456 knots. Find the east-west and north-south components of its velocity, to the nearest knot. (Remember that 30° west of north corresponds to the angle 120°.)

48. At the location of a ship, the Gulf Stream ocean current is moving to the northwest at a speed of 8.2 knots. Find the east-west and north-south components of its velocity, to the nearest knot.

49. A ship has left an east-coast harbor and has been sailing in a direction 32° north of east for 2.5 hours, at a speed of 18 knots. (a) How far north of the harbor has it gone, to the nearest nautical mile? (b) How far east of the harbor has it gone, to the nearest nautical mile?

50. A force is acting on a tree stump at a 40° angle of elevation. See the diagram. If the force is 2,500 pounds, find its vertical and horizontal components, to the nearest pound.

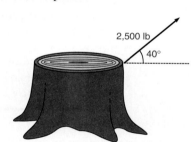

2,500 lb   40°

51. A 2,250 pound force is pulling on a sled loaded with lumber, at an angle of elevation of 33°. If the sled will not move until the horizontal component of the force exceeds 1,900 pounds, will the sled move?

52. A sled loaded with lumber will not move until the horizontal component of the applied force is 1,200 pounds or more. If a winch being used to move the sled can apply a maximum force of 1,700 pounds, what is the largest angle of elevation at which the winch can act on the sled and move it?

53. Consider a force of 1,000 pounds acting at an angle of elevation of 15° on a point.
    a. Compute the horizontal and vertical components of the force.
    b. Double the force to 2,000 pounds and recompute the horizontal and vertical components. Do they double also?
    c. Double the angle of elevation to 30° (keep the force at 1,000 pounds). Recompute the horizontal and vertical components. Do they double also?

54. A plane is flying over Minneapolis with a ground speed of 200 miles per hour and true course due east. After 1 hour it turns to a true course of 60° south of east, maintaining the same ground speed. After flying for an additional half-hour, the navigator notes its position on a map. How far and in what direction is the plane from Minneapolis, to the nearest unit?

55. A plane is flying over Orlando with ground speed 135 miles per hour, and true course 23° north of east. After 1 hour it turns to a true course of 40° south of west, maintaining the same ground speed. After flying for an additional hour the navigator notes its position on a map. How far and in what direction is the plane from Orlando, to the nearest unit?

56. Two forces are acting on a point, 12.6 pounds in the direction 123° and 15.8 pounds in the direction 211°. Compute the magnitude and direction of the resultant force to the nearest tenth.

57. Two forces are acting on a point, 2.6 newtons in the direction 18.3° and 15.8 newtons in the direction −86.2°. Compute the magnitude and direction of the resultant force, to the nearest tenth.

58. Three forces are acting on a point: 27.6 newtons in the direction 18.3°, 32.1 newtons at 223.0°, and 46.8 newtons at −30.0°. Find the resultant force acting on the point, to the nearest 0.1 newton.

59. Three forces are acting on a point: 199 pounds at 19.0°, 175 pounds at 131.0°, and 96 pounds at 130.0°. Find the resultant force acting on the point, to the nearest 0.1 pound.

60. A ship leaves its harbor traveling 10° north of east. After 1 hour it turns to the direction 40° south of east. After 2 more hours, it turns to the direction 15° west of south. The shop travels for 1 half hour more and then stops. The ship has maintained a steady speed of 16 knots (nautical miles per hour) for the entire trip. How many nautical miles, and in what direction, is the ship from its starting position, to the nearest knot?

61. A ship leaves its harbor traveling 15° west of south. After 1 hour it turns to the direction 34° south of west. After 2 more hours, it turns to the direction 10° north of west. The ship travels for 1 half hour more and then stops. The ship has maintained a steady speed of 20 knots for the entire trip. How many nautical miles, and in what direction, is the ship from its starting position, to the nearest knot?

62. An aircraft is flying with an airspeed of 123 knots and a heading of 30° west of north. The wind is blowing in the direction 15° south of west at 26 knots. Add the heading and wind vectors to find the aircraft's true course and ground speed, to the nearest integer.

63. If the wind in problem 62 now shifts to 35 knots in the direction 10° west of south, find the aircraft's new true course and ground speed, to the nearest integer.

64. A ship is traveling through an ocean current that flows in the direction 5° east of north at 7.2 knots. The ship's heading is 10° north of west, and its speed relative to the water is 19.6 knots. Add these two vectors to find the ship's true course and speed, to the nearest tenth.

65. A ship is traveling through an ocean current that flows in the direction 15° west of north at 7.2 knots. The ship's heading is 10° north of east, and its speed relative to the water is 26.1 knots. Add these two vectors to find the ship's true course and speed, to the nearest tenth.

66. The voltage in an alternating current circuit adds vectorially. If one voltage E_1 is 122 volts with phase angle 30° and a second voltage E_2 is 86 volts with phase angle 21°, find the magnitude and phase angle of the resultant voltage E_T to the nearest unit.

67. (Refer to problem 66.) In an AC circuit E_1 is 240 volts at −45° and E_2 is 115 volts at +45°. Find the resultant E_T to the nearest unit.

68. An aircraft has a ground speed of 135 knots and true course 35° east of north. If its heading is due north and airspeed is 120 knots, find the direction and speed of the wind, to the nearest unit.

69. An aircraft has a ground speed of 80 knots and true course 15° west of north. If the wind is directly from the northeast at 12 knots, find the plane's heading and airspeed, to the nearest unit.

70. A ship is traveling at 14 knots, relative to the water, with heading 20° south of west. If the true speed and direction of the ship is 12 knots due west, find the speed and direction of the ocean current, to the nearest tenth.

71. The ocean current in a certain area is 6.4 knots with direction 8° east of south. A ship in the area is traveling with true direction of 12 knots at 25° east of north. Find the ship's heading and speed relative to the water, to the nearest tenth.

72. Two cables support a 1-ton (2,000 pound) sign between two buildings. One of the cables has a tension of 1,500 pounds and acts at an angle of 33° above the horizontal. The other cable is attached to the other building. Find the tension in the other cable as well as its direction relative to the horizontal, to the nearest unit.

73. Two cables support a sign between two buildings. The tension and direction of one cable is 456 pounds at 63° above the horizontal. If the sign weighs 650 pounds, find the tension in the other cable, as well as its direction relative to the horizontal, to the nearest unit.

74. Prove that vector addition is commutative. That is, if A and B are vectors, then $A + B = B + A$. (*Hint:* Real number addition is commutative, and the horizontal and vertical components of a vector are real values.)

75. Prove that vector addition is associative. That is, if A, B, and C are vectors, then $(A + B) + C = A + (B + C)$. (*Hint:* Real number addition is associative, and the horizontal and vertical components of a vector are real values.)

76. Write a program for a computer or programmable calculator that will add two or more vectors when given in polar form.

Chapter 6 summary

- **The law of sines**
  In any triangle ABC, $\dfrac{\sin A}{a} = \dfrac{\sin B}{b} = \dfrac{\sin C}{c}$.

- **The ambiguous case** When the law of sines is applied to a situation in which only one of the two angles of a triangle is known, it is possible to get two different solutions to the problem. This is called the ambiguous case.

- **The law of cosines** For any triangle ABC,
  $a^2 = b^2 + c^2 - 2bc \cos A$
  $b^2 = a^2 + c^2 - 2ac \cos B$
  $c^2 = a^2 + b^2 - 2ab \cos C$

- **Polar form of a vector** A vector A in polar form is the ordered pair $A = (|A|, \theta_A)$.
  $|A|$ is the magnitude of vector A; $|A| \geq 0$.
  θ_A is the direction of vector A.

- **Rectangular form of a vector** A vector A in rectangular form is $A = (A_x, A_y)$, where A_x is the horizontal component of the vector and A_y is the vertical component of the vector.

- **To convert polar form to rectangular form**
  Given vector $A = (|A|, \theta_A) = (A_x, A_y)$,
  $$A_x = |A| \cos \theta_A$$
  $$A_y = |A| \sin \theta_A$$

- **To convert rectangular form to polar form**
  Given vector $V = (V_x, V_y) = (|V|, \theta_V)$. Then,
  $$|V| = \sqrt{V_x^2 + V_y^2}, \quad \theta_V' = \tan^{-1}\frac{V_y}{V_x} \text{ if } V_x \neq 0, \text{ and}$$
  $$\theta_V = \begin{cases} \theta_V' & \text{if } V_x > 0 \\ \theta_V' - 180° & \text{if } \theta_V' > 0 \\ \theta_V' + 180° & \text{if } \theta_V' < 0 \end{cases} \text{ if } V_x < 0$$

- **Vector sum** Let $Z = (Z_x, Z_y)$ be the resultant (vector sum) of two vectors $A = (A_x, A_y)$ and $B = (B_x, B_y)$. Then, $Z = A + B$, and $Z_x = A_x + B_x$ and $Z_y = A_y + B_y$.

- With regard to an aircraft, $T = H + W$, where
  T is the vector of ground speed and true course
  H is the vector of airspeed and aircraft heading
  W is the vector of the speed and direction of the wind.

- **Zero vector** The vector $0 = (0, \theta)$, where θ is any angle, is the zero vector.

- **Opposite of a vector** Given a vector $V = (|V|, \theta_V)$, then $-V = (|V|, \theta_V \pm 180°)$.

Chapter 6 review

[6–1] Solve the following oblique triangles using the law of sines. Round answers to the nearest tenth.

1. $a = 10.6$, $A = 47.9°$, $B = 10.3°$
2. $b = 3.55$, $B = 23.8°$, $C = 5.2°$
3. $a = 10.0$, $b = 13.0$, $B = 79.0°$
4. $a = 12.6$, $c = 7.0$, $C = 32.7°$
5. A lost pilot is given a position report by triangulation with two radar sites. The situation is shown in the diagram. Find the distance of the aircraft from radar site A, to the nearest mile.

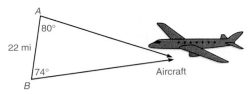

[6–2] Solve the following oblique triangles, to the nearest tenth. You will have to use the law of cosines as the first step.

6. $a = 4.1$, $b = 6.8$, $C = 29.4°$
7. $b = 60.0$, $c = 20.0$, $A = 92.1°$
8. $a = 21.4$, $c = 27.0$, $B = 112°$
9. $a = 43.5$, $b = 17.8$, $c = 35.0$
10. $a = 31.7$, $b = 80.0$, $c = 105$

11. A technician is setting up a numerically controlled grinding machine. A triangular pattern is to be ground and, therefore, must be coordinatized. The vertices of the triangle are at $A(-2,5)$, $B(4,7)$, and $C(5,-2)$. Solve the resulting triangle. Round answers to the nearest 0.1.

12. A ship leaves a harbor heading due west and travels 23.3 km. It then turns north through a 63° angle and travels for another 10.0 km. How far is the ship from its starting point, to the nearest kilometer?

[6–3]

13. Convert the vector (27.2,29.0°), to rectangular form. Round to the nearest 0.1.

14. The horizontal and vertical components of a vector are 19.6 and 30.5, respectively. Find the magnitude and direction of the vector.

15. A rocket climbs with a speed of 450 knots and an angle of climb of 34.6°. (The angle of climb is the angle measured from the ground to its flight path.) Find the horizontal and vertical components of the rocket's velocity, to the nearest knot.

16. A force is acting on a cart at a 13.5° angle of elevation (13.5° measured from the ground up to the force vector). If the force is 256 pounds, find the vertical and horizontal components, to the nearest pound.

Add the following vectors. Round the resultant to the nearest tenth.

17. (33.0,14.7°), (15.2,33.6°)
18. (10.2,112.3°), (4.2,19.3°)
19. (3.5,29.2°), (1.7,43.1°), (4.3,115.0°)
20. (7.1,13.8°), (6.6,142.0°), (11.9,215.0°)

21. Two forces are acting on a point, 126 pounds in the direction 223° and 158 pounds in the direction 311°. Compute the magnitude and direction of the resultant force, to the nearest unit.

22. A ship leaves its harbor traveling 15° south of east. After 1 hour it turns to the direction 40° south of east. After 2 more hours it turns to the direction 25° west of south. The ship travels for 1 half-hour more and then stops. The ship has maintained a steady speed of 18 knots for the entire trip. How many nautical miles and in what direction is the ship from its starting position, to the nearest integer?

23. An aircraft is flying with an airspeed of 195 knots and heading of 24° west of north. The wind is blowing in the direction 25° west of south at 19 knots. Add the heading and wind vectors to find the aircraft's true course and ground speed, to the nearest integer.

24. An aircraft's true course and ground speed are 120° at 225 knots. The wind is blowing in a direction 15° south of east at 30 knots. Find the heading and airspeed of the aircraft, to the nearest unit.

Chapter 6 test

1. In triangle *ABC*, $b = 22.6$, $A = 13.5°$, and $C = 82.1°$. Solve this triangle. Round answers to the nearest tenth.

2. In triangle *ABC*, $b = 22.6$, $c = 24.0$, and $C = 62.1°$. Solve this triangle. Round answers to the nearest tenth.

3. In triangle *ABC*, $a = 25.9$, $c = 16.2$, and $B = 100°$. Solve this triangle. Round answers to the nearest tenth.

4. In triangle *ABC*, $a = 2.55$, $b = 3.12$, and $c = 4.00$. Solve this triangle. Round answers to the nearest tenth.

5. The distance to a boat on a lake is being found by triangulation from two points on shore. The situation is shown in the diagram. Find the distance to the boat from site *B*, to the nearest yard.

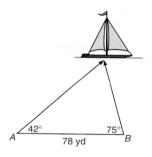

6. Given the three points $A(6,8)$, $B(-3,5)$, and $C(10,-4)$, find the angle formed by line segments *AB* and *BC*, to the nearest 0.1°.

7. Convert the vector $(2,30°)$ to rectangular form. Leave the answer in exact form.

8. The horizontal and vertical components of a vector are 4.0 and 5.0. Find the magnitude and direction of the vector, to the nearest tenth.

9. Add the vectors $(5.4,19.0°)$ and $(8.0,123°)$. Round the resultant to the nearest tenth.

10. A sign is suspended between two buildings. One cable from which the sign is suspended has a tension of 535 pounds and acts at an angle of elevation of 62°. If the weight of the sign is 1,000 pounds, find the tension and angle of elevation in the other cable, to the nearest unit.

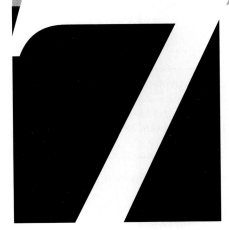

Complex Numbers and Polar Coordinates

In this chapter we examine more applications of the trigonometric functions. We first define complex numbers, and then show how trigonometry is useful in representing these numbers as well as computing with them.

We then introduce polar coordinates, a system of coordinates that is useful in describing many situations where periodic motion is involved.

7–1 Complex numbers

Complex numbers were developed hundreds of years ago, but they became much more important about 100 years ago when they began to be used to model physical phenomena, particularly in the study of electricity. Their development and use centers on the number i.

The i stands for the word *imaginary;* and represents $\sqrt{-1}$. We learned in the past that the square root of a negative number is not defined since, for example, if $i = \sqrt{-1}$, then $i^2 = -1$, and we know that the square of any real number is positive or zero. Nevertheless, equations like $x^2 = -1$ produce the "solution" $\sqrt{-1}$. To the mathematicians of the sixteenth and later centuries these numbers were bothersome. They keep occurring when solving equations, yet, to these people, such numbers could not exist. René Descartes coined the term "imaginary" to describe solutions to equations that involved the square roots of negative numbers, and this term has persisted to this day. (In fact, the term "real" number was coined in reaction to the word "imaginary.")

It turned out, however, that the study of certain physical laws almost demanded the existence of $\sqrt{-1}$, and today the existence of a number such as i is no longer doubted. Since the property $i^2 = -1$ is incompatible with the properties of the real number system, a new number system was introduced to incorporate these imaginary numbers. This system is the complex number system, and we now study its properties.

> **The square root of −1**
>
> $$i = \sqrt{-1}$$

> **Rectangular form of a complex number**
> A **complex number** is an expression of the form $a + bi$, where a and b are real numbers. a is called the *real part*, and b is called the *imaginary part* of the number. $a + bi$ is called the **rectangular form** of a complex number.

$2 + 3i$ is an example of a complex number; 2 is its real part and 3 is its imaginary part.

■ *Example 7–1 A*

Identify the real and imaginary parts of the following complex numbers:

a. $5 + 7i$ **b.** $2 - i$ **c.** 4 **d.** $-6i$

a. Real part: 5; imaginary part: 7.

b. Real part: 2; imaginary part: -1. $2 - i = 2 + (-1)i$

c. If we represent 4 as $4 + 0i$, we see that the real part is 4 and the imaginary part is 0.

d. Represent $-6i$ as $0 - 6i$ to see that the real part is 0 and the imaginary part is -6. A complex number in which the real part is zero is usually called a pure imaginary number. ■

> **Complex conjugate**
> $a - bi$ is called the **complex conjugate** of $a + bi$.

■ *Example 7–1 B*

Form the complex conjugate of each complex number.

1. $5 + 7i$
    $5 - 7i$ is the complex conjugate of $5 + 7i$.

2. $4 - 5i$
    $4 + 5i$ is the complex conjugate of $4 - 5i$.

3. 7
    We rewrite 7 as $7 + 0i$, whose complex conjugate is $7 - 0i$ or 7. Thus, 7 is the complex conjugate of 7.

4. $-9i$
    We rewrite $-9i$ as $0 - 9i$, whose complex conjugate is $0 + 9i$ or $9i$. Thus, $9i$ is the complex conjugate of $-9i$. ■

An algebra exists for the complex numbers. Rules have been established for the addition, subtraction, multiplication, and division of complex numbers. These operations obey the rules of the real number system if we treat i as a symbol having the property $i^2 = -1$. The definitions of these operations are given and illustrated in the following paragraphs. First, however, we must define what it means for two complex numbers to be equal.

Equality of complex numbers

The complex numbers $a + bi$ and $c + di$ are *equal* if and only if $a = c$ and $b = d$.

The complex numbers are not ordered; that is, a given complex number is never said to be greater than or less than another complex number.

We now define and illustrate addition and subtraction.

Addition and subtraction of complex numbers
$$(a + bi) + (c + di) = (a + c) + (b + d)i$$
$$(a + bi) - (c + di) = (a - c) + (b - d)i$$

Concept
To add or subtract two complex numbers, add or subtract the real parts and the imaginary parts separately.

■ *Example 7–1 C*

Perform the indicated operations and simplify.

1. $(5 + 4i) + (3 + 2i)$
$$(5 + 4i) + (3 + 2i) = 5 + 3 + 4i + 2i = 8 + 6i$$

2. $(5 + 4i) - (3 + 2i)$
$$(5 + 4i) - (3 + 2i) = 5 - 3 + 4i - 2i = 2 + 2i$$ ■

Multiplication of complex numbers
$$(a + bi)(c + di) = (ac - bd) + (ad + bc)i$$

Concept
This definition is equivalent to our usual rules for the multiplication of real number expressions if we replace i^2 by -1.

$(a + bi)(c + di)$	Multiply as if real expressions
$= ac + adi + bci + bdi^2$	
$= ac + adi + bci - bd$	Remember that $i^2 = -1$
$= (ac - bd) + (ad + bc)i$	

■ *Example 7–1 D*

Perform the indicated operations and simplify.

1. $(5 + 4i)(3 + 2i)$
$$(5 + 4i)(3 + 2i) = 15 + 10i + 12i + 8i^2$$
$$= 15 + 22i + 8(-1)$$
$$= 15 + 22i - 8$$
$$= 7 + 22i$$

2. $(-2 + 5i)(3 - 5i)$

$$(-2 + 5i)(3 - 5i) = -6 + 10i + 15i - 25i^2$$
$$= -6 + 25i - 25(-1)$$
$$= -6 + 25i + 25$$
$$= 19 + 25i$$

3. $5i(6 - 4i)$

$$5i(6 - 4i) = 30i - 20i^2$$
$$= 30i + 20$$
$$= 20 + 30i$$

Note   We always write the real part of a complex number first.   ■

Division of complex numbers

$$\frac{a + bi}{c + di} = \frac{ac + bd}{c^2 + d^2} + \frac{bc - ad}{c^2 + d^2}i$$

Concept

The above result is obtained by multiplying the numerator and denominator of the quotient by the conjugate of the denominator.

$$\frac{a + bi}{c + di} = \frac{a + bi}{c + di} \cdot \frac{c - di}{c - di}$$

$$= \frac{ac - adi + bci - bdi^2}{c^2 - cdi + cdi - d^2i^2}$$

$$= \frac{ac + bd + (bc - ad)i}{c^2 + d^2}$$

$$= \frac{ac + bd}{c^2 + d^2} + \frac{bc - ad}{c^2 + d^2}i$$

■ *Example 7–1 E*

Perform the indicated operations and simplify each expression.

1. $\dfrac{5 + 4i}{3 + 2i}$

$$\frac{5 + 4i}{3 + 2i} = \frac{5 + 4i}{3 + 2i} \cdot \frac{3 - 2i}{3 - 2i} = \frac{15 - 10i + 12i - 8i^2}{9 - 6i + 6i - 4i^2}$$

$$= \frac{15 + 2i + 8}{9 + 4}$$

$$= \frac{23 + 2i}{13}$$

$$= \tfrac{23}{13} + \tfrac{2}{13}i$$

Note   A complex number must have two parts, a real and an imaginary part. This is why we performed the last step in the previous part.

2. $\dfrac{-2 + 5i}{3 - 4i}$

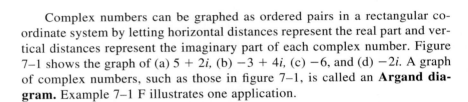

$$\frac{-2 + 5i}{3 - 4i} = \frac{-2 + 5i}{3 - 4i} \cdot \frac{3 + 4i}{3 + 4i} = \frac{-6 - 8i + 15i - 20}{9 + 12i - 12i + 16}$$

$$= \frac{-26 + 7i}{25}$$

$$= -\frac{26}{25} + \frac{7}{25}i$$

3. $\dfrac{5i}{6 - 4i}$

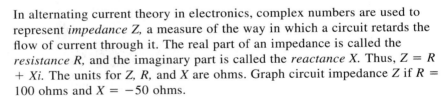

$$\frac{5i}{6 - 4i} = \frac{5i}{6 - 4i} \cdot \frac{6 + 4i}{6 + 4i} = \frac{30i - 20}{36 + 16} = -\frac{20}{52} + \frac{30}{52}i$$

$$= -\frac{5}{13} + \frac{15}{26}i \qquad\blacksquare$$

Complex numbers can be graphed as ordered pairs in a rectangular co-ordinate system by letting horizontal distances represent the real part and vertical distances represent the imaginary part of each complex number. Figure 7–1 shows the graph of (a) $5 + 2i$, (b) $-3 + 4i$, (c) -6, and (d) $-2i$. A graph of complex numbers, such as those in figure 7–1, is called an **Argand diagram.** Example 7–1 F illustrates one application.

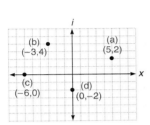

Figure 7–1

■ *Example 7–1 F*

In alternating current theory in electronics, complex numbers are used to represent *impedance Z,* a measure of the way in which a circuit retards the flow of current through it. The real part of an impedance is called the *resistance R,* and the imaginary part is called the *reactance X.* Thus, $Z = R + Xi$. The units for Z, R, and X are ohms. Graph circuit impedance Z if $R = 100$ ohms and $X = -50$ ohms.

$Z = R + Xi = 100 - 50i$. The graph is shown in the figure.

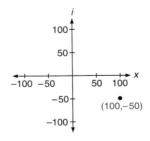

$\qquad\qquad\qquad\qquad\qquad\qquad\qquad\qquad\qquad\blacksquare$

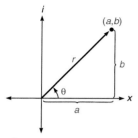

Figure 7-2

Polar form of a complex number

We can use the graph of a complex number as a guide to develop another way to represent a complex number. Given the complex number $a + bi$, let r represent the distance from the origin to the point (a,b) and let θ represent the angle in standard position determined by the ray containing the origin and (a,b). See figure 7-2. Using the definitions of section 2-2 we obtain $\cos \theta = \dfrac{a}{r}$ and $\sin \theta = \dfrac{b}{r}$. Thus, $a = r \cos \theta$ and $b = r \sin \theta$. This means we can rewrite $a + bi$ as $r \cos \theta + (r \sin \theta)i$, or $r(\cos \theta + i \sin \theta)$. The expression $\cos \theta + i \sin \theta$ occurs so often it is abbreviated as **cis** θ, so $a + bi = r$ cis θ. This form is called the **polar form** of a complex number.[1] Also, note that $r = \sqrt{a^2 + b^2}$ and that $\tan \theta = \dfrac{b}{a}$.

Polar form of a complex number

If $z = a + bi$ is a complex number that determines an angle θ, then

$$z = r \text{ cis } \theta$$

is its polar form, where cis θ means $\cos \theta + i \sin \theta$, and

$$r = \sqrt{a^2 + b^2}$$

The value r is called the **modulus** of z, which is also written $|z|$.

Note 1. The value of θ is not unique. All coterminal values produce the same rectangular form. Thus, 2 cis 10° is equivalent to 2 cis 370°.
2. The modulus is the distance from the origin to the complex coordinate (a,b).

Polar-rectangular conversions

As with vectors (section 6-3), we generally give a value of θ so that $-180° < \theta \leq 180°$. A method for converting from rectangular form to polar form is a paraphrase of the method for converting vectors from rectangular to polar form.

Given a complex number $z = a + bi = r$ cis θ. Then,

$$r = \sqrt{a^2 + b^2}, \quad \tan \theta = \tan^{-1}\frac{b}{a} \text{ (if } a \neq 0), \quad \text{and}$$

$$\theta = \begin{cases} \theta' & \text{if } a > 0 \\ \theta' - 180° \text{ if } \theta' > 0 \\ \theta' + 180° \text{ if } \theta' < 0 \end{cases} \text{if } a < 0$$

Note If $a = 0$ then θ is 90° if $b > 0$, and $-90°$ if $b < 0$. A sketch will make the choice clear.

---

[1]In 1893 Irving Stringham first used the notation cis $\beta = \cos \beta + i \sin \beta$.

■ *Example 7–1 G*

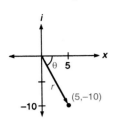

Convert between polar and rectangular form.

1. $5 - 10i$

The graph is shown in the figure.

$$r = \left|5 - 10i\right| = \sqrt{5^2 + (-10)^2} = \sqrt{125} = 5\sqrt{5}$$

$$\theta' = \tan^{-1}\frac{b}{a} = \tan^{-1}\left(\frac{-10}{5}\right) = \tan^{-1}(-2), \text{ so } \theta' \approx -63.4°$$

$$\theta = \theta' \approx -63.4°\quad a > 0$$

Thus, the polar form of $5 - 10i$ is $5\sqrt{5}\ \text{cis}(-63.4°)$ or about $(11.1, -63.4°)$.

2. $5\ \text{cis}\ 150°$

$$5\ \text{cis}\ 150° = 5(\cos 150° + i \sin 150°)$$

$$= 5\left(-\frac{\sqrt{3}}{2} + i \cdot \frac{1}{2}\right)$$

$$= -\frac{5\sqrt{3}}{2} + \frac{5}{2}i$$

Thus, $5\ \text{cis}\ 150° = -\dfrac{5\sqrt{3}}{2} + \dfrac{5}{2}i$ or about $-4.3 + 2.5i$. ■

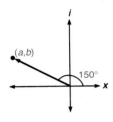

Polar-rectangular conversions on a calculator

As stated in the previous section, most calculators are programmed to perform polar/rectangular conversions. This conversion works equally well for vectors (section 6–3) and for complex numbers. The conversion is done with keys marked "R → P" or "→ P" and "P → R" or "→ R" or something equivalent. The results are stored in locations referred to as x and y. Typical keystrokes are illustrated here. (The TI-81 steps are shown below.)

Part 1 of example 7–1 G would be done as follows.

$z = 5 - 10i$

5   $\boxed{R \rightarrow P}$ 10 $\boxed{+/-}$ $\boxed{=}$ Display: $\boxed{11.18033989}$

     $\boxed{x \leftrightarrow y}$ Display: $\boxed{-63.43494882}$

Thus, $z \approx (11.1, -63.4°)$.

Part 2 of example 7–1 G would be done in the following way.

$z = 5\ \text{cis}\ 150°$

5   $\boxed{P \rightarrow R}$ 150 $\boxed{=}$ Display: $\boxed{-4.330127019}$

     $\boxed{x \leftrightarrow y}$ Display: $\boxed{2.5}$

Thus, $z \approx -4.3 + 2.5i$.

     The TI-81 uses the values X, Y, R, and θ. (Y, R, θ are $\boxed{\text{ALPHA}}$ 1, $\boxed{\times}$, and 3, respectively.) It also uses the two MATH functions "R ◆ P(" (rectangular to polar) and "P ◆ R(" (polar to rectangular).

| MODE | Deg | ENTER | Make sure the calculator is in degree mode.

Example 7–1 G, part 1:

| MATH | 1 5 | ALPHA | . | (−) | 10 |) |

| ENTER | Display: | 11.18033989 |

| ALPHA | 3 | ENTER | Display: | −63.43494882 |

Example 7–1 G, part 2:

| MATH | 2 5 | ALPHA | . | 150 |) |

| ENTER | Display: | −4.330127019 |

| ALPHA | 1 | ENTER | Display: | 2.5 |

Multiplication and division of complex numbers in polar form

Multiplication and division of complex numbers in rectangular form is quite complicated. The following theorems show that these procedures are quite simple when the complex numbers are in polar form.

Complex multiplication—polar form

$$(r_1 \text{ cis } \theta_1)(r_2 \text{ cis } \theta_2) = r_1 r_2 \text{ cis } (\theta_1 + \theta_2)$$

Complex division—polar form

$$\frac{r_1 \text{ cis } \theta_1}{r_2 \text{ cis } \theta_2} = \frac{r_1}{r_2} \text{ cis } (\theta_1 - \theta_2), r_2 \neq 0$$

Concept

To *multiply*, multiply the moduli and add the angles. To *divide*, divide the moduli and subtract the angles.

We can see that the first theorem is true by converting the complex numbers into rectangular form and performing the multiplication as defined earlier in this section.

$(r_1\text{cis}\theta_1)(r_2\text{cis}\theta_2)$

$= (r_1\cos\theta_1 + ir_1\sin\theta_1)(r_2\cos\theta_2 + ir_2\sin\theta_2)$

$= r_1r_2\cos\theta_1\cos\theta_2 + ir_1r_2\cos\theta_1\sin\theta_2 + ir_1r_2\sin\theta_1\cos\theta_2 + i^2r_1r_2\sin\theta_1\sin\theta_2$

$= r_1r_2\cos\theta_1\cos\theta_2 - r_1r_2\sin\theta_1\sin\theta_2 + ir_1r_2\cos\theta_1\sin\theta_2 + ir_1r_2\sin\theta_1\cos\theta_2$

Recall that $i^2 = -1$

$= r_1r_2[(\cos\theta_1\cos\theta_2 - \sin\theta_1\sin\theta_2) + i(\sin\theta_1\cos\theta_2 + \cos\theta_1\sin\theta_2)]$

Now use the identities for $\cos(\alpha + \beta)$ and $\sin(\alpha + \beta)$ from section 5–2.

$= r_1r_2[\cos(\theta_1 + \theta_2) + i \sin(\theta_1 + \theta_2)]$

$= r_1r_2\text{cis}(\theta_1 + \theta_2)$

The proof of the process for division in polar form is left as an exercise.

In electronics, Ohm's law states $V = IZ$, where V means voltage, I means current, and Z means impedance. The units are volts, amperes, and ohms, respectively. Often complex numbers are used to describe the values of volts, amperes, and ohms. The fact that the angles add in forming the product models the physical situation in an electronics circuit. This use is illustrated in example 7–1 H, part 2.

■ *Example 7–1 H*

Multiply or divide the complex numbers.

1. $(2 \text{ cis } 110°)(10 \text{ cis } 300°)$
$\qquad = 2 \cdot 10 \text{ cis}(110° + 300°)$
$\qquad = 20 \text{ cis } 410°$
$\qquad = 20 \text{ cis } 50° \qquad$ 410° and 50° are coterminal

2. In a certain electronic circuit current $I = 4 \text{ cis } 30°$ amperes and impedance $Z = 2 \text{ cis } 15°$. Use Ohm's law, $V = IZ$, to compute voltage V.

$$V = IZ$$
$$= (4 \text{ cis } 30°)(2 \text{ cis } 15°)$$
$$= 8 \text{ cis } 45° \text{ (volts)}$$

3. $\dfrac{15 \text{ cis } 30°}{18 \text{ cis } 80°}$
$\qquad = \frac{15}{18}\text{cis}(30° - 80°) = \frac{5}{6}\text{cis}(-50°)$ ■

De Moivre's theorem

Consider the following computations for successive powers of a complex number $r \text{ cis } \theta$.

$(r \text{ cis } \theta)^1 = r \text{ cis } \theta$
$(r \text{ cis } \theta)^2 = (r \text{ cis } \theta)(r \text{ cis } \theta) = r^2 \text{ cis } 2\theta$
$(r \text{ cis } \theta)^3 = (r \text{ cis } \theta)(r \text{ cis } \theta)^2 = (r \text{ cis } \theta)(r^2 \text{ cis } 2\theta) = r^3 \text{ cis } 3\theta$
$(r \text{ cis } \theta)^4 = (r \text{ cis } \theta)(r \text{ cis } \theta)^3 = (r \text{ cis } \theta)(r^3 \text{ cis } 3\theta) = r^4 \text{ cis } 4\theta$

It is logical to assume that the pattern above continues. This is true, and the result is called **De Moivre's theorem.** It actually turns out that the exponent can be any real number.

De Moivre's theorem
$(r \text{ cis } \theta)^n = r^n\text{cis } n\theta$ for any real number n.

This theorem is illustrated in example 7–1 I.

■ *Example 7–1 I*

Use De Moivre's theorem to compute the following.

1. $(5 \text{ cis } 137°)^3$; leave the answer in polar form.
$\qquad = 5^3 \text{ cis}(3 \cdot 137°)$
$\qquad = 125 \text{ cis } 411°$
$\qquad = 125 \text{ cis } 51°$

2. $(1 + 0.8i)^6$; leave the answer in rectangular form; round to the nearest tenth.

We could of course multiply $(1 + 0.8i)$ by itself five times to obtain the result. The amount of work is prohibitive. If we put the number in polar form we can use De Moivre's theorem.

$$|1 + 0.8i| = \sqrt{1^2 + 0.8^2} \approx 1.281; \ \theta = \tan^{-1}\frac{0.8}{1} \approx 38.66°$$

Then $1 + 0.8i \approx 1.281 \text{ cis } 38.66°$. Then

$$(1 + 0.8i)^6 \approx (1.281 \text{ cis } 38.66°)^6$$
$$= 1.281^6 \text{ cis}(6 \cdot 38.66°)$$
$$\approx 4.42 \text{ cis } 231.96°$$
$$= 4.42 \cos 231.96° + 4.42 \sin 231.96°i$$
$$\approx -2.7 - 3.5i$$

Thus, $(1 + 0.8i)^6 \approx -2.7 - 3.5i$, to the nearest tenth. ∎

De Moivre's theorem for roots

In the complex number system, every number except 0 has n nth roots; that is, two square roots, three cube roots, four fourth roots, etc. These can be expressed by De Moivre's theorem by replacing n by $\frac{1}{n}$; recall that $x^{\frac{1}{2}} = \sqrt{x}$, $x^{\frac{1}{3}} = \sqrt[3]{x}$, $x^{\frac{1}{4}} = \sqrt[4]{x}$, etc.

De Moivre's theorem for roots
The n nth roots of r cis θ are of the form

$$r^{\frac{1}{n}} \text{ cis}\left(\frac{\theta}{n} + \frac{k \cdot 360°}{n}\right), 0 \le k < n$$

where k and n are positive integers.

We can show that any number of the form above is an nth root of r cis θ by raising it to the nth power.

$$\left[r^{\frac{1}{n}}\text{cis}\left(\frac{\theta}{n} + \frac{k \cdot 360°}{n}\right)\right]^n = \left(r^{\frac{1}{n}}\right)^n \text{cis}\left[n\left(\frac{\theta}{n} + \frac{k \cdot 360°}{n}\right)\right]$$
$$= r \text{ cis}(\theta + k \cdot 360°)$$
$$= r \text{ cis } \theta \qquad \theta + k \cdot 360° \text{ is coterminal to } \theta$$

If $k \ge n$ we get a repetition of a previous root. The proof of this is left as an exercise. The proof of the fact that the roots are all distinct and that there are no other roots is beyond the scope of this text.

■ *Example 7–1 J*

Find the roots.

1. Find the three cube roots of 1.

$$1 = 1 \text{ cis } 0°$$

Evaluate $1^{\frac{1}{3}} \text{ cis}\left(\frac{0°}{3} + \frac{k \cdot 360°}{3}\right) = \text{cis}(k \cdot 120°)$ for $k = 0, 1, 2$.

$k = 0$:   cis $0° = \cos 0° + i \sin 0° = 1 + 0i = 1$

$k = 1$:   cis $120° = \cos 120° + i \sin 120° = -\dfrac{1}{2} + \dfrac{\sqrt{3}}{2}i$

$k = 2$:   cis $240° = \cos 240° + i \sin 240° = -\dfrac{1}{2} - \dfrac{\sqrt{3}}{2}i$

Thus, the three cube roots of 1 are $1, -\dfrac{1}{2} + \dfrac{\sqrt{3}}{2}i, -\dfrac{1}{2} - \dfrac{\sqrt{3}}{2}i$.

2. Find decimal approximations (to tenths) of the four fourth roots of $10 - 2\sqrt{39}i$.

$$10 - 2\sqrt{39}i \approx 16 \text{ cis } 308.68°$$

$$16^{\frac{1}{4}} \text{ cis}\left(\frac{308.68°}{4} + \frac{k \cdot 360°}{4}\right) \approx 2 \text{ cis}(77.17 + k \cdot 90°)$$

Evaluate $2 \text{ cis}(77.17 + k \cdot 90°)$ for $k = 0, 1, 2, 3$.

$k = 0$: $2 \text{ cis } 77.17° = 2(\cos 77.17° + i \sin 77.17°) = 0.4 + 2.0i$
$k = 1$: $2 \text{ cis } 167.17° = 2(\cos 167.17° + i \sin 167.17°) = -2.0 + 0.4i$
$k = 2$: $2 \text{ cis } 257.17° = 2(\cos 257.17° + i \sin 257.17°) = -0.4 - 2.0i$
$k = 3$: $2 \text{ cis } 347.17° = 2(\cos 347.17° + i \sin 347.17°) = 2.0 - 0.4i$

Thus, the four fourth roots of $10 - 2\sqrt{39}i$ are approximately $0.4 + 2.0i$, $-2.0 + 0.4i$, $-0.4 - 2.0i$, and $2.0 - 0.4i$.

3. In electronics apparent power P can be determined by $P = I^2Z$. If we solve this for current I we get $I = \pm\sqrt{\dfrac{P}{Z}}$. Use $I = \sqrt{\dfrac{P}{Z}}$ to determine I to the nearest tenth if $P = 10 - 2i$ and $Z = 1 + 3i$.

$$P = 10 - 2i \approx 10.2 \text{ cis } 348.69°$$
$$Z = 1 + 3i \approx 3.16 \text{ cis } 71.57°$$
$$\frac{P}{Z} \approx \frac{10.2 \text{ cis } 348.69°}{3.16 \text{ cis } 71.57°} \approx 3.23 \text{ cis } 277.12°$$

We evaluate the expression $3.23^{\frac{1}{2}} \text{ cis}\left(\dfrac{277.12°}{2} + \dfrac{k \cdot 360°}{2}\right)$ for $k = 0, 1$.

$k = 0$: $\sqrt{3.23} \text{ cis } 138.56° \approx -1.3 + 1.2i$
$k = 1$: $\sqrt{3.23} \text{ cis } 318.56° \approx 1.3 - 1.2i$

Thus, the current I is about $-1.3 + 1.2i$ or $1.3 - 1.2i$ (amperes).   ■

Mastery points

Can you
- Identify the real and imaginary parts of a complex number?
- Form the conjugate of a complex number?
- Evaluate complex expressions involving addition, subtraction, multiplication, and division?
- Graph a complex number when given in rectangular or polar form?
- Convert between the rectangular and polar forms of complex numbers?
- Multiply and divide complex numbers in polar form?
- State and use De Moivre's theorem for integral powers?
- State and use De Moivre's theorem for roots?

Exercise 7–1

Identify the real and imaginary parts of the following complex numbers.

1. $4 - 5i$ **2.** $3 + 11i$ **3.** $-4 + i$ **4.** $3i$
5. 12 **6.** $-i$ **7.** $-10 + 2i$ **8.** $-9 - i$

For each problem (a) find the complex conjugate and (b) graph the number and its conjugate in the same graph.

9. $4 - 5i$ **10.** $3 + 11i$ **11.** $-4 + i$ **12.** $3i$
13. 12 **14.** $-i$ **15.** $-10 + 2i$ **16.** $-9 - i$

Simplify each expression by performing the indicated operations. Do all operations in rectangular form (do not convert to polar form).

17. $(5 + 4i) + (-3 + 2i)$ **18.** $(-11 + 3i) - (-1 + 4i)$
19. $(3 + 2i) + (-6i) - (2 + 3i) - 10$ **20.** $(7 + 4i) - (-13 + 4i)$
21. $13 - 7i + 3i - 4$ **22.** $-8 - (4 + 3i) + 2i - (-6 - i)$
23. $(15 + 4i)(3 + 12i)$ **24.** $(-2 + 5i)(-3 - 5i)$
25. $-5i(6 - 4i)$ **26.** $(4 - 3i)^2$ **27.** $(2 - 3i)^3$ **28.** $i(2i)(3i)(-i)$
29. $\dfrac{5 + 4i}{5 + 2i}$ **30.** $\dfrac{-2 + i}{2 + 4i}$ **31.** $\dfrac{3 + 6i}{-2 - i}$ **32.** $\dfrac{5 + i}{5i}$

Write the polar form of each complex number. Round the results to the nearest tenth.

33. $5 - 2i$ **34.** $\sqrt{2} + 3i$ **35.** $-1 + 3i$ **36.** $\sqrt{3} - 2i$ **37.** $-3 + 4i$ **38.** $13 - 9i$

Write the polar form of each complex number. Leave the result in exact form.

39. $\sqrt{3} + i$ **40.** $1 - \sqrt{3}i$ **41.** $3 + 3i$ **42.** $-1 + \sqrt{3}i$
43. $-1 - i$ **44.** $\sqrt{5} - \sqrt{5}i$ **45.** $5i$ **46.** $-3i$

Write the rectangular form of the following numbers. Round the results to the nearest tenth.

47. 3 cis 15°   **48.** 5 cis 20°   **49.** 4.5 cis 35°   **50.** 10 cis 40°
51. $\sqrt{2}$ cis 315°   **52.** 200 cis 8°   **53.** 13.6 cis(−25°)   **54.** 12 cis(−6°)

Write the rectangular form of the following numbers. Leave the result in exact form.

55. $\sqrt{3}$ cis 30°   **56.** 4 cis 210°   **57.** 10 cis 300°   **58.** 6 cis 135°
59. $\sqrt{10}$ cis 180°   **60.** 2 cis 90°   **61.** $\sqrt{8}$ cis 315°   **62.** 5 cis 240°

Multiply or divide the following complex numbers. Leave the result in polar form.

63. (5 cis 30°)(3 cis 45°)   **64.** (2 cis 18°)(4.5 cis 100°)   **65.** (5.4 cis 300°)(2 cis 300°)

66. (0.5 cis 230°)(80 cis 200°)   **67.** $\dfrac{20 \text{ cis } 100°}{5 \text{ cis } 20°}$ **68.** $\dfrac{100 \text{ cis } 45°}{200 \text{ cis } 15°}$

69. $\dfrac{40 \text{ cis } 80°}{18 \text{ cis } 160°}$ **70.** $\dfrac{90 \text{ cis } 300°}{50 \text{ cis } 100°}$

Use De Moivre's theorem to compute the power indicated. Leave the answer in the form in which the problem is stated (polar or rectangular).

71. (8 cis 100°)³   **72.** (5 cis 10°)⁴   **73.** (3 cis 200°)³   **74.** (2 cis 300°)⁵

75. $(0.5 - 1.2i)^8$ (round to nearest tenth)   **76.** $(0.8 + 0.6i)^{10}$ (round to nearest tenth)

77. Find the 3 cube roots of 8 in exact form.
78. Find the 4 fourth roots of −1 in exact form.
79. Find the 4 fourth roots of 81 in exact form.
80. Find the 6 sixth roots of −64 in exact form.
81. Find the 3 cube roots of $75 - 100i$ to the nearest tenth.
82. Find the 4 fourth roots of $\sqrt{3} + 3i$ to the nearest tenth.

83. In electronics, one version of Ohm's law says that $I = \dfrac{V}{Z}$, where I is current, V is voltage, and Z is impedance. Find I in a circuit in which V is 125 cis 25° and Z is 50 cis 45°.

84. Find I in a circuit in which $V = 200$ cis 40° and $Z = 4$ cis 50°. See problem 83.

85. Find V in a circuit where $I = 10$ cis 15° and $Z = 5$ cis 30°. See problem 83.

86. Find Z in a circuit where $I = 40$ cis 200° and $V = 10$ cis 125°. See problem 83.

87. In a parallel electronics circuit with two legs, total impedance Z_T is $\dfrac{Z_1 Z_2}{Z_1 + Z_2}$. Find Z_T in a circuit in which $Z_1 = 2 + i$ and $Z_2 = 3 - 5i$. Leave the answer in polar form.

88. Find Z_T in a parallel circuit in which $Z_1 = 12 + 3i$ and $Z_2 = 4 - 2i$. Leave the answer in polar form. See problem 87.

89. Use $I = \sqrt{\dfrac{P}{Z}}$ to determine I if $P = 5 + 2i$ and $Z = 1 - 4i$. Leave the result in rectangular form, to the nearest hundredth. Use the first square root ($k = 0$ in De Moivre's theorem).

90. Use $I = \sqrt{\dfrac{P}{Z}}$ to determine I if $P = -2 + 2i$ and $Z = 2 - i$. Leave the result in rectangular form, to the nearest hundredth. Use the first square root ($k = 0$ in De Moivre's theorem).

91. Is the following an identity: a cis$(-\theta) = -a$ cis θ? Show why or why not.

Multiplication by i can be interpreted as a 90° rotation. If z represents the complex number given in each of the following problems, compute and graph (a) z, (b) iz, (c) i^2z, (d) i^3z.

92. $4 + 2i$ **93.** $-3 + i$ **94.** $5i$ **95.** 6   **96.** $1 - i$ **97.** $-1 - i$

98. Let $z_1 = -2 + 2i$, $z_2 = 1 - \sqrt{3}i$. Form the product in two ways: (a) by multiplication in rectangular form and (b) by changing each value into polar form (in exact form) and performing the multiplication in polar form. Then (c) convert the answer to (b) back to rectangular form and verify that the answers to (a) and (b) are the same.

99. A numerically controlled machine is programmed to rotate a laser beam according to mathematical rules. The laser initially points to the point $1 + i$.
   a. Find the rectangular form of a complex number z such that the angle of the product $z(1 + i)$ is 30° greater than the angle of $1 + i$, without changing the modulus of $1 + i$.
   b. Give the rectangular form of the point to which the laser points after this rotation. Round the answer to two decimal places.
   c. Give the rectangular form of the point to which the laser points after eight such rotations, starting at the point $1 + i$. Round the answer to two decimal places.

100. In this section we stated that $\dfrac{r_1 \operatorname{cis} \theta_1}{r_2 \operatorname{cis} \theta_2} = \dfrac{r_1}{r_2} \operatorname{cis}(\theta_1 - \theta_2)$.
Prove that this is true. Use the proof in the text that $(r_1 \operatorname{cis} \theta_1)(r_2 \operatorname{cis} \theta_2) = r_1 r_2 \operatorname{cis}(\theta_1 + \theta_2)$ as a guide.

101. *Warning:* This problem requires a *great* deal of algebraic manipulation. De Moivre's theorem for roots states that the n nth roots of $r \operatorname{cis} \theta$ are of the form
$$(r \operatorname{cis} \theta)^{\frac{1}{n}} = r^{\frac{1}{n}} \operatorname{cis}\left(\frac{\theta}{n} + \frac{k \cdot 360°}{n}\right), \quad 0 \leq k < n,$$
where k and n are positive integers. Show that if $k \geq n$, then the expression is a repetition of another root. That is, it is the same as the expression for some value of $k < n$. Do this in the following manner.

First, if $k \geq n$, then $\dfrac{k}{n} = a + \dfrac{b}{n}$, where $b < n$. (Think of the example $22 \geq 5$, so $\frac{22}{5} = 4 + \frac{2}{5}$.) This means $k = an + b$, $b < n$.
Next, show that the following steps are true:

$$r^{\frac{1}{n}} \operatorname{cis}\left(\frac{\theta}{n} + \frac{k \cdot 360°}{n}\right)$$

$$= r^{\frac{1}{n}} \operatorname{cis}\left[\frac{\theta}{n} + \frac{(an + b) \cdot 360°}{n}\right] \qquad \text{Why?}$$

$$= r^{\frac{1}{n}} \operatorname{cis}\left[\left(\frac{\theta}{n} + \frac{b \cdot 360°}{n}\right) + a \cdot 360°\right].$$

Show the algebra for this step

Finally, now expand this last expression into terms of sine and cosine (i.e., expand "cis α"), and then apply the identities for the cosine and sine of a sum (section 5–2.).

7–2 *Polar coordinates*

Some natural phenomena, such as the motion of the planets, the contour of a cam on an automobile camshaft, the path traveled by a client on many of the rides in an amusement park, or the field strength around a radio transmitter, can be described most simply by describing the motion in terms of distance from some point as a line moves in a circle. The polar coordinate system is a coordinate system that is better suited to describing these phenomena than are rectangular coordinates. James Bernoulli is often credited with the creation of polar coordinates in 1691, although Isaac Newton used them earlier. A polar coordinate system is a series of concentric circles and an angle reference line (see figure 7–3). The common center of the circles is called the **pole.**

Basic definitions

Polar coordinates

The polar coordinates of a point is an ordered pair of the form (r, θ), where r is the *radius,* and θ is an angle, often measured in radians.

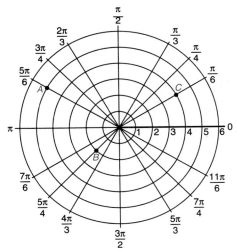

Figure 7–3

A point in polar form is located by finding the radius line corresponding to the angle θ, often stated in radians, and moving r units from the center along this line. Figure 7–3 shows the graphs[2] of the points $\left(5, \dfrac{5\pi}{6}\right)$ (A), $\left(2, \dfrac{5\pi}{4}\right)$ (B), and $\left(4, \dfrac{\pi}{6}\right)$ (C). In each of these cases $r > 0$.

If two points have equal radii and coterminal angles they will have the same graph. For this reason we define such points to be equivalent. If $r < 0$ we interpret this to mean a change of direction by π radians (the opposite direction).

Equivalence of points
1. $(r, \alpha) = (r, \beta)$ if α and β are coterminal angles.
2. $(-r, \theta) = (r, \theta + \pi)$.

Note $(-r, \theta) = (r, \theta - \pi)$ is also true.

This definition means that $(1, 0)$, $(1, 2\pi)$, $(1, 4\pi)$, $(1, -2\pi)$, $(1, -4\pi)$, $(-1, \pi)$, $(-1, 3\pi)$, $(-1, -\pi)$, etc. all describe the same point! This can occasionally lead to some confusion.

Example 7–2 A illustrates the basic definitions.

---

[2]Polar coordinate paper is widely available.

■ *Example 7–2 A*

1. List 3 other coordinates for the point $\left(2,\dfrac{3\pi}{4}\right)$, with at least one so that $r < 0$.

$$\left(2,\frac{3\pi}{4}\right) = \left(2,\frac{3\pi}{4} + 2\pi\right)$$ Adding 2π gives a coterminal angle

$$= \left(2,\frac{11\pi}{4}\right)$$

$$\left(2,\frac{3\pi}{4}\right) = \left(2,\frac{3\pi}{4} + 4\pi\right)$$ Adding 4π gives a coterminal angle

$$= \left(2,\frac{19\pi}{4}\right)$$

$$\left(2,\frac{3\pi}{4}\right) = \left(-2,\frac{3\pi}{4} + \pi\right)$$ Adding or subtracting π gives a coterminal angle in which r changes sign

$$= \left(-2,\frac{7\pi}{4}\right)$$

2. Plot the point $\left(-5,\dfrac{11\pi}{6}\right)$.

$$\left(-5,\frac{11\pi}{6}\right) = \left(5,\frac{11\pi}{6} - \pi\right) = \left(5,\frac{5\pi}{6}\right),$$ which is plotted at A in figure 7–3. ■

Polar-rectangular coordinate conversions

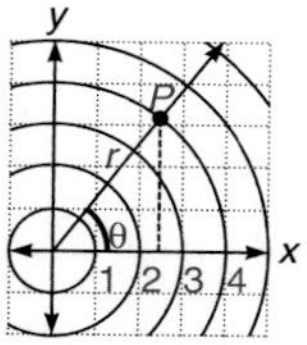

There is a way to relate polar and rectangular coordinates. Figure 7–4 shows polar and rectangular coordinates superimposed. From the definitions of section 2–2 we know that if $P = (x,y) = (r,\theta)$, $r > 0$, then $\cos\theta = \dfrac{x}{r}$ and $\sin\theta = \dfrac{y}{r}$.

Figure 7–4

Thus, *to convert from polar to rectangular coordinates* we have only to use

$$x = r\cos\theta$$
$$y = r\sin\theta$$

In fact, it will be an exercise to show that we can use the same relations when $r < 0$. Example 7–2 B illustrates a polar to rectangular conversion.

■ *Example 7–2 B*

Convert the polar coordinates $\left(2,\dfrac{\pi}{3}\right)$ to rectangular coordinates.

$$x = r\cos\theta = 2\cos\frac{\pi}{3} = 2 \cdot \frac{1}{2} = 1$$

$$y = r\sin\theta = 2\sin\frac{\pi}{3} = 2 \cdot \frac{\sqrt{3}}{2} = \sqrt{3}$$

Thus, the rectangular coordinates are $(1,\sqrt{3})$. ■

To convert from rectangular to polar coordinates we use the fact that $r^2 = x^2 + y^2$ and $\tan\theta = \dfrac{y}{x}$ if $x \neq 0$. This also means $\theta' = \tan^{-1}\dfrac{y}{x}$.

As with vectors and complex numbers (sections 6–3 and 7–1) we always leave the angle θ so that it is the smallest possible absolute value. In this case, using radian measure, we always choose θ so that $-\pi < \theta \leq \pi$.

A rule for finding θ is essentially the same as that for finding θ_V for vectors, and θ for complex numbers.

Given polar coordinates for point P, $P = (x, y) = (r, \theta)$,

$$r = \sqrt{x^2 + y^2}, \quad \tan\theta' = \tan^{-1}\frac{y}{x} \text{ if } x \neq 0, \text{ and}$$

$$\theta = \begin{cases} \theta' & \text{if } x > 0 \\ \theta' - \pi \text{ if } \theta' > 0 & \\ \theta' + \pi \text{ if } \theta' < 0 & \text{if } x < 0 \end{cases}$$

Note If $x = 0$ then θ is π if $y > 0$, and $-\pi$ if $y < 0$. This is clear from a sketch.

■ **Example 7–2 C**

Convert the rectangular coordinates into polar coordinates.

1. $(-2\sqrt{3}, 2)$

$$r^2 = (-2\sqrt{3})^2 + 2^2 = 16, \; r = 4$$

$$\theta' = \tan^{-1}\frac{2}{-2\sqrt{3}} = \tan^{-1}\left(-\frac{\sqrt{3}}{3}\right) = -\tan^{-1}\frac{\sqrt{3}}{3} \qquad \begin{array}{l} \tan^{-1} \text{ is an odd function,} \\ \text{so } \tan^{-1}(-x) = -\tan^{-1}x \end{array}$$

so $\theta' = -\dfrac{\pi}{6}$. $x < 0$, $\theta' < 0$, so $\theta = \theta' + \pi = -\dfrac{\pi}{6} + \pi = \dfrac{5\pi}{6}$.

Therefore, the required polar coordinates are $\left(4, \dfrac{5\pi}{6}\right)$.

2. $(-2, -5)$

$$r^2 = (-2)^2 + (-5)^2 = 29, \; r = \sqrt{29} \approx 5.39$$
$$\theta' = \tan^{-1}\tfrac{5}{2} \approx 1.19 \text{ (radians)}$$

$x < 0$, $\theta' > 0$, so $\theta = \theta' - \pi = \tan^{-1}\tfrac{5}{2} - \pi$ (exactly), or approximately $1.19 - \pi \approx -1.95$. Thus, the polar coordinates are $(\sqrt{29}, \tan^{-1}2.5 - \pi)$ exactly, or approximately $(5.39, -1.95)$. ■

Conversions with a calculator

Engineering/scientific calculators are programmed to perform the conversions of example 7–2 C, using the same method and keys shown in section 6–3 for vectors and in section 7–1 for complex numbers. These calculators have keys marked R → P and P → R, or something equivalent. The results are stored in locations referred to as x and y. Typical keystrokes are illustrated here. For these examples we want the *calculator in radian mode.* The steps for the TI-81 are shown below.

Example 7–2 B would be done as follows:

$$\left(2, \frac{\pi}{3}\right) \text{ (polar)}$$

2 | P → R | | (| | π | | ÷ | 3 |) | | = | Display: | 1 |

| x ↔ y | Display: | 1.732050808 |

Thus, $\left(2, \dfrac{\pi}{3}\right) \approx (1, 1.73)$.

Example 7–2 C, part 2, would be done in the following way:

$(-2, -5)$ (rectangular)

2 | ± | | R → P | 5 | +/− | | = | Display: | 5.385164807 |

| x ↔ y | Display: | −1.951302704 |

Thus, $(-2, -5)$ (rectangular) $\approx (5.39, -1.95)$ (polar).

The TI-81 uses the values X, Y, R, and θ. (Y, R, θ are | ALPHA | 1, | × |, and 3, respectively.) It also uses the two MATH functions "R ♦ P(" (rectangular to polar) and "P ♦ R(" (polar to rectangular).

Example 7–2 B:

| MODE | Rad | ENTER | Make sure the calculator is in radian mode.

| MATH | 2 2 | ALPHA | | . | | (| π | ÷ | 3 |) |

|) | | ENTER | Display: | 1 |

| ALPHA | 1 | ENTER | Display: | 1.732050808 |

Example 7–2 C, part 2:

| MATH | 1 | (−) | 2 | ALPHA | | . | | (−) | 5

|) | | ENTER | Display: | 5.385164807 |

| ALPHA | 3 | ENTER | Display: | −1.951302704 |

Conversion of equations between rectangular and polar form

Analytic geometry is the modeling of geometry in the language of algebra. Thus, a nonvertical line in analytic geometry is an equation of the form $y = mx + b$, and a circle with center at the origin and radius r is an equation of the form $x^2 + y^2 = r^2$.

Equations can also be written using polar coordinates. Examples are

$$r = 3 \cos \theta$$
$$r^2 = \sec \theta$$
$$r = 2$$
$$\cos \theta = 1$$

It is often useful to discover the polar coordinate version of a rectangular coordinate equation. We say that *a rectangular equation and a polar equation are equivalent if they describe the same set of points*, assuming the appropriate rectangular/polar conversions of the points themselves.

> ### Conversion of equations from rectangular to polar form
> To convert an equation in rectangular form into an equivalent equation in polar form, use the relations used to convert a point from rectangular to polar form:
> $$x = r \cos \theta, \quad y = r \sin \theta, \quad \text{and} \quad r^2 = x^2 + y^2.$$

When possible we customarily write a polar equation in which r is described as a function of θ. That is, to the extent possible, we put all terms with r in one member of the equation, and all other terms in the other member.

Example 7–2 D illustrates conversions from rectangular to polar form.

■ *Example 7–2 D*

Convert each rectangular equation into polar form.

1. The line $y = 3x - 2$.

$$y = 3x - 2$$
$$r \sin \theta = 3(r \cos \theta) - 2 \qquad x = r \cos \theta, \, y = r \sin \theta$$
$$2 = 3r \cos \theta - r \sin \theta \qquad \text{It is customary to solve a polar equation for } r \text{ if possible}$$
$$2 = r(3 \cos \theta - \sin \theta)$$
$$r = \frac{2}{3 \cos \theta - \sin \theta}$$

2. The line $y = -2x$.

$$y = -2x$$
$$r \sin \theta = -2r \cos \theta \qquad x = r \cos \theta, \, y = r \sin \theta$$
$$\sin \theta = -2 \cos \theta \qquad \text{Divide both members by } r, \text{ this assumes } r \neq 0 \text{ (see below)}$$
$$\frac{\sin \theta}{\cos \theta} = -2 \qquad \text{Divide both members by } \cos \theta; \text{ this assumes } \cos \theta \neq 0 \text{ (see below)}$$
$$\tan \theta = -2$$

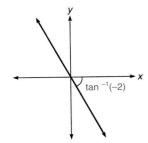

This equation is equivalent to the equation $y = -2x$. To see this, first observe that it does not mention r. This means r can be any value. The values of θ for which $\tan \theta = -2$ are in quadrants II and IV, where the tangent function takes on negative values. All points (r, θ) for which $\tan \theta = -2$ and r takes on any value are shown in the figure. This is the line $y = -2x$.

It was all right to assume $r \neq 0$ above because the resulting solution includes the pole as a solution (this is where $r = 0$).

It was also valid to assume $\cos \theta \neq 0$, for two reasons. One is that we arrive at an equation that satisfies the requirements and thus we do not need to consider the case where $\cos \theta = 0$. Second, when $\cos \theta = 0$, $\sin \theta$ is ± 1. These values do not solve the equation $\sin \theta = -2 \cos \theta$, so that $\cos \theta = 0$ cannot occur in this situation.

3. The circle $x^2 + y^2 = 1$.

$$x^2 + y^2 = 1$$
$$r^2 = 1 \qquad\qquad x^2 + y^2 = r^2$$
$$r = \pm 1$$

Either $r = 1$ or $r = -1$ describes a circle with radius one, since θ is not restricted but may take on any value. Thus, either equation is valid.

4. The hyperbola $x^2 - y^2 = 2$. (See footnote[3].)

$$x^2 - y^2 = 2$$
$$(r\cos\theta)^2 - (r\sin\theta)^2 = 2$$
$$r^2\cos^2\theta - r^2\sin^2\theta = 2$$
$$r^2(\cos^2\theta - \sin^2\theta) = 2$$
$$r^2\cos 2\theta = 2 \qquad\qquad \cos 2\theta = \cos^2\theta - \sin^2\theta$$
$$r^2 = \frac{2}{\cos 2\theta}$$
$$r^2 = 2\sec 2\theta$$

Thus, either $r^2\cos 2\theta = 2$ or $r^2 = 2\sec 2\theta$ are valid equations of the given rectangular equation.   ■

> ### Conversion of equations from polar to rectangular form
>
> To convert from polar to rectangular coordinates we use the relations
>
> $$\sin\theta = \frac{y}{r}, \quad \cos\theta = \frac{x}{r}, \quad r^2 = x^2 + y^2$$

Example 7–2 E illustrates converting polar equations into rectangular form.

■ *Example 7–2 E*

Convert the polar equation into rectangular form.

1. $r = 5\sec\theta$

$$r = \frac{5}{\cos\theta}$$
$$r\cos\theta = 5$$
$$r \cdot \frac{x}{r} = 5 \qquad\qquad \cos\theta = \frac{x}{r}$$
$$x = 5$$

---

[3]Hyperbolas are not covered in this text. Any equation of the form $ax^2 - by^2 = c$, $a, b, c \neq 0$, and a and b have the same sign, is a hyperbola.

2. $r^2 = \cos 2\theta$

We do not have any relation for $\cos 2\theta$, so we use an identity to replace it.

$$r^2 = \cos^2\theta - \sin^2\theta$$

$$\cos 2\theta = \cos^2\theta - \sin^2\theta$$

$$r^2 = \left(\frac{x}{r}\right)^2 - \left(\frac{y}{r}\right)^2$$

$$\cos\theta = \frac{x}{r}, \sin\theta = \frac{y}{r}$$

$$r^2 = \frac{x^2}{r^2} - \frac{y^2}{r^2}$$

$$r^4 = x^2 - y^2$$

$$(x^2 + y^2)^2 = x^2 - y^2$$

$$r^4 = (r^2)^2 = (x^2 + y^2)^2$$

3. $r = 1 + \cos\theta$

$$r = 1 + \frac{x}{r}$$

$$r^2 = r + x$$

Multiply each member by r

$$x^2 + y^2 = r + x$$

$$x^2 + y^2 - x = r$$

$$(x^2 + y^2 - x)^2 = r^2$$

Square both members to obtain r^2

$$(x^2 + y^2 - x)^2 = x^2 + y^2$$

Now replace r^2 by $x^2 + y^2$

$$x^4 - 2x^3 + y^4 + 2x^2y^2 - 2xy^2 - y^2 = 0$$

Expand the left member and combine terms ∎

Note   Observe that r can be replaced by squaring both members as necessary to obtain r^2, or any even power of r.

In example 7–2 E we used the identities $\sin\theta = \dfrac{y}{r}$ and $\cos\theta = \dfrac{x}{r}$. This is only valid if $r \neq 0$. The value of r is zero only if the pole is a solution to the given polar equation. Thus, when the pole is a solution to the polar equation we must verify that the point $(0,0)$ is a solution to the resulting rectangular equation.

In example 7–2 E, part 1, the pole is not a solution, since if $r = 0$, $0 = 5$ $\sec\theta = \dfrac{5}{\cos\theta}$. The equation $0 = \dfrac{5}{\cos\theta}$ has no solution. (The rectangular equation $x = 5$ does not pass through the origin either.)

In example 7–2 E, part 2, r can take on the value 0: $0 = \cos 2\theta$ has solutions. Thus, the pole is part of this equation. Observe that the point $(0,0)$ is also a solution to the equation $(x^2 + y^2)^2 = x^2 - y^2$.

Mastery points
Can you
• Graph points in the polar coordinate system?
• Give alternate polar coordinates for a given point?
• Convert between polar and rectangular coordinates?
• Convert equations between polar and rectangular form?

Exercise 7–2

Graph the following points in polar coordinates.

1. $(3,0)$

2. $(4,\pi)$

3. $\left(2,\dfrac{\pi}{6}\right)$

4. $\left(1,\dfrac{\pi}{3}\right)$

5. $\left(2,\dfrac{3\pi}{4}\right)$

6. $\left(3,\dfrac{7\pi}{6}\right)$

7. $\left(6,\dfrac{11\pi}{6}\right)$

8. $\left(5,\dfrac{\pi}{2}\right)$

9. $(-2,\pi)$

10. $\left(-4,\dfrac{5\pi}{3}\right)$

11. $\left(-1,\dfrac{\pi}{3}\right)$

12. $\left(-5,\dfrac{\pi}{6}\right)$

13. $(4,2)$

14. $(3,5)$

15. $(-4,6)$

16. $\left(-4,\dfrac{\pi}{2}\right)$

17. $\left(5,\dfrac{4\pi}{3}\right)$

18. $\left(4,\dfrac{5\pi}{6}\right)$

List three other coordinates for the point, with two points having $r > 0$ and one point having $r < 0$.

19. $\left(2,\dfrac{\pi}{6}\right)$

20. $\left(1,\dfrac{\pi}{3}\right)$

21. $\left(6,\dfrac{11\pi}{6}\right)$

22. $\left(-5,\dfrac{\pi}{6}\right)$

23. $(2,2)$

24. $\left(4,\dfrac{17\pi}{6}\right)$

Convert the following polar coordinates into rectangular coordinates. Leave the result in exact form.

25. $\left(4,\dfrac{\pi}{2}\right)$

26. $\left(2,\dfrac{\pi}{3}\right)$

27. $\left(5,\dfrac{5\pi}{6}\right)$

28. $\left(1,\dfrac{11\pi}{6}\right)$

29. $\left(4,\dfrac{4\pi}{3}\right)$

30. $\left(2,\dfrac{5\pi}{3}\right)$

Convert the following polar coordinates into rectangular coordinates to two-decimal place accuracy.

31. $(2,1)$

32. $(5,1.2)$

33. $(3,0.82)$

34. $(3,5)$

35. $(4,4)$

36. $(1,6)$

Convert the following rectangular coordinates into polar coordinates. Leave the result in exact form.

37. $(-2\sqrt{3},-2)$

38. $(3,-3)$

39. $(-2,0)$

40. $(-1,\sqrt{3})$

41. $(-4,-4)$

42. $(0,1)$

Convert the following rectangular coordinates into polar coordinates to two-decimal place accuracy.

43. $(2,3)$

44. $(-5,2)$

45. $(1,-4)$

46. $(-4,-3)$

47. $(5,4)$

48. $(-3,5)$

Convert the following rectangular equations into polar equations.

49. $y = 4x$

50. $y = -2x$

51. $y = -3x + 2$

52. $y = 5x - 3$

53. $y = mx + b, b \neq 0$

54. $y = 2$

55. $y^2 - 2x^2 = 5$

56. $y^2 - x = 4$

57. $3x^2 + 2y^2 = 1$

58. $x^2 + y^2 = 3$

Convert the following polar equations into rectangular equations.

59. $r = \sin\theta$

60. $2r = \cos\theta$

61. $r = 2\sec\theta$

62. $r = 3\csc\theta$

63. $r = 3\sin 2\theta$

64. $r = 2\cos\theta$

65. $r^2 = \sin 2\theta$

66. $r = \cos 2\theta$

67. $r^2 = \tan\theta$

68. $r\sin\theta = 5$

69. $r = \dfrac{3}{1 - 2\sin\theta}$

70. $r = \dfrac{5}{4 - \cos\theta}$

71. Show that a polar equation of $2xy = 5$ is $r^2 = 5 \csc 2\theta$.

72. In the text we noted that $x = r \cos \theta$ if $r > 0$. Show that this is also true for a point given in polar coordinates where $r < 0$. (*Hint:* Consider a point $P = (r,\theta)$, where $r < 0$. Then $P = (-r, \theta + \pi)$, where $-r > 0$. Therefore, since $-r > 0$, $x = -r \cos(\theta + \pi)$ is true. Proceed from here.)

73. In the text we noted that $y = r \sin \theta$ if $r > 0$. Show that this is also true for a point given in polar coordinates where $r < 0$. See the hint in problem 72.

74. The shape of a cam that drives a certain sewing machine needle is described by the polar equation $r = 3 - 2 \cos \theta$. Convert this equation into rectangular form.

75. The path that an industrial robot must follow to paint a pattern on a part being manufactured is described by the curve $r = 1 - 2 \sin \theta$. Convert this equation into rectangular form.

76. The pattern of strongest radiation of a certain bidirectional radio antenna is described by the curve $r = 1 + \sin 2\theta$. Convert this equation into rectangular form.

77. The pattern of strongest radiation of a certain radio antenna is described by the equation $r = 1 + 2 \sin 2\theta$. This pattern is said to have side lobes. Convert this equation into rectangular form.

In the October 1983 issue of *Scientific American,* Jearl Walker described several rides, the Scrambler and the Calypso, at the Geauga Lake Amusement Park near Cleveland, Ohio.

78. Assume the path taken by the Scrambler is described by the polar equation $r = 2 \cos 3\theta$. Convert this equation into rectangular form. It will be necessary to rewrite cos 3θ in terms of cos θ. See problem 79 in section 5–3.

79. Assume the path of the Calypso is described by the equation $r = 1 - 3 \cos \theta$. Convert this equation into rectangular form.

7–3 *Graphs of polar equations*

There are several ways to graph polar equations. The graphing calculator can be used, or one can sketch a graph by hand. We illustrate how to obtain polar graphs with the TI-81 graphing calculator. To achieve a sketch of a graph by hand we employ three methods:

1. plotting points,

2. putting a polar equation into rectangular form, and

3. using the corresponding rectangular graph as a guide.

The examples show how to create polar graphs both by hand and by graphing calculator.

Graphing polar equations with the graphing calculator

The TI-81 uses a mode called Parametric Mode to graph polar equations. Parametric mode uses two functions to produce rectangular coordinates. The first produces the x-coordinates, and the second produces the y-coordinates. We illustrate how to use the process by graphing the polar equation $r = \sin^2\theta$.

The polar equation $r = \sin^2\theta$ generates a collection of polar coordinates (r,θ). In this case, r is $\sin^2\theta$, so the polar coordinates generated are $(\sin^2\theta,\theta)$. To convert a polar coordinate to a rectangular coordinate we map (r,θ) to $(x,y) = (r \cos \theta, r \sin \theta)$ (section 7–2), so for this function we map $(\sin^2\theta,\theta)$ to the point $(x,y) = (\sin^2\theta \cdot \cos \theta, \sin^2\theta \cdot \sin \theta)$.

As stated above, in parametric mode a point (x,y) is calculated from two separate equations that depend on a third variable, usually called t (the TI-81 uses T). Thus, we graph the set of rectangular coordinates $(\sin^2 t \cdot \cos t, \sin^2 t \cdot \sin t)$, which of course is the same as $(\sin^2 t \cdot \cos t, \sin^3 t)$. We usually let t take on the values from 0 to 2π to obtain the graph, but this may need to be adjusted depending on the functions in question.

As illustrated above, to graph a polar function of the form $r = f(\theta)$, put the calculator in parametric mode and graph

$$X_{1T} = f(T) \cdot \cos T$$
$$Y_{1T} = f(T) \cdot \sin T$$

To create the graph of the polar equation $r = \sin^2\theta$ do the following:

| MODE | Select Param instead of Function. Do this by positioning the blinking square over Param and using ENTER. Also select Polar instead of Rect. This has no effect except when using the trace feature. Then the values T, R and θ are shown instead of T, X and Y. |

Y=	The display now shows the variables X_{1T} and Y_{1T} (as well as others). Enter the equations shown above. Note that in parametric mode the X T key is used to enter T. The display should look like $:X_{1T} = (\sin T)^2 * \cos T$
	$:Y_{1T} = (\sin T)^3$.
	Remember, the exponent 3 is MATH 3.

| RANGE | The range display is different in parametric mode. Set the following values: Tmin=0 |

$$\text{Tmax}=6.28 \quad {\scriptstyle (2\pi)}$$

$$\text{Tstep}=.105 \quad \left(\frac{\pi}{30}\right)$$

Xmin$=-1$
Xmax$=1$
Xscl$=.5$
Ymin$=-1$
Ymax$=1$
Yscl$=.5$

ZOOM 5   We want the display to be square.

The graph is drawn as shown in figure 7–5.

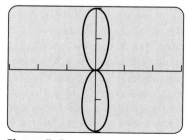

Figure 7–5

We show the range settings in the rest of this section in the order shown above. Thus, for the graph above we show

$$X_{1T}=(\sin T)^2*\cos T, \; Y_{1T}=(\sin T)^3,$$
RANGE   0,6.28,0.105,−1,1,.5,−1,1,.5,   ZOOM   5

Graphing polar equations by plotting points

Of course any graph can be obtained by plotting enough points. Example 7–3 A shows a case where this might be done without plotting too many points.

■ *Example 7–3 A*

Graph the polar equation $r = \dfrac{\theta}{2}$, $\theta \geq 0$.

We observe that r increases at half the rate of θ. A table of values is given in table 7–1, and these values are plotted in the figure.

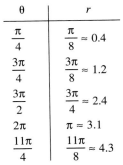

θ	r
$\dfrac{\pi}{4}$	$\dfrac{\pi}{8} \approx 0.4$
$\dfrac{3\pi}{4}$	$\dfrac{3\pi}{8} \approx 1.2$
$\dfrac{3\pi}{2}$	$\dfrac{3\pi}{4} \approx 2.4$
2π	$\pi \approx 3.1$
$\dfrac{11\pi}{4}$	$\dfrac{11\pi}{8} \approx 4.3$

Table 7–1

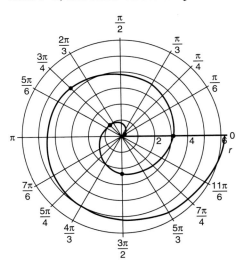

The graph shows points (r,θ) for $0 \leq \theta \leq 4\pi$, but the graph, a spiral, continues on forever.

$$X_{1T}=T/2*\cos T, \; Y_{1T}=T/2*\sin T,$$
RANGE   0,20,0.105,−6,6,1,−6,6,1,   ZOOM   5   ■

The next two methods presented can save the time required to calculate the many points that are often required to graph an equation by plotting points.

Graphing polar equations by putting in rectangular form

■ Example 7–3 B

Graph the polar equation $\theta = 2$.

An angle of 2 (radians) is shown in part (a) of the figure. Any point $(r,2)$, $r > 0$, lies on the terminal side of this angle.

Recall that $(-r,\theta) = (r,\theta + \pi)$. Therefore $(-r,2) = (r,2 + \pi)$. Thus, when r is negative, its graph is along the line containing the terminal side of the angle $\theta = 2 + \pi$. Thus, the graph of $\theta = 2$ is the line shown in part (b) of the figure.

Another way to see the shape of this graph is to *rewrite the equation in rectangular form.*

$$\tan \theta = \frac{y}{x}$$

$$\tan 2 = \frac{y}{x} \qquad \theta = 2$$

$$y = (\tan 2)x \qquad \text{Straight line, slope} = \tan 2$$

$$y \approx -2.2x \qquad \tan 2 \approx -2.2$$

Thus, the graph is the line $y \approx -2.2x$.

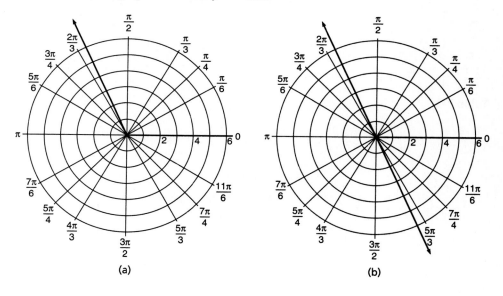

(a)   (b)

The equation $\theta = 2$ does not describe r as a function of θ, since r is not even mentioned! This means that r can take on any value. Thus, any point in the graph is of the form $(r, 2)$. Parametrically we let $r = T$ and $\theta = 2$.

$$X_{1T} = T*\cos 2, \quad Y_{1T} = T*\sin 2,$$

$\boxed{\text{RANGE}}$ $\quad -7, 7, 0.105, -6, 6, 1, -6, 6, 1, \quad$ $\boxed{\text{ZOOM}}$ 5

Graphing polar equations using the rectangular form as a guide

The rectangular form of an equation can provide guidance for drawing the polar form of an equation. This is especially true when the rectangular form is periodic. There are two principles involved in this process. To discuss this we define the term "positive lobe." A *positive lobe* is a portion of a graph in *rectangular* coordinates that starts and ends on the x-axis, and is continuous (it has no breaks, such as a vertical asymptote). Figure 7–6 (a) shows two positive lobes, at A and at B.

Every positive lobe corresponds to a lobe in a polar graph. A lobe (in a polar graph) is a closed figure that starts and ends at the pole. Figure 7–6 shows the correspondence between two positive lobes A and B in a rectangular graph (a), and the corresponding lobes in a polar graph (b).

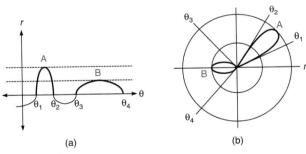

(a)   (b)

Figure 7–6

Another important point uses the fact that $(-r, \theta)$ has the same graph as $(r, \theta \pm \pi)$. This means that negative lobes in a rectangular graph may be redrawn as positive lobes by shifting their graphs $\pm\pi$ units, before graphing in polar coordinates. Although this method sometimes seems complicated, with a little practice it is much easier than having to plot many points. Example 7–3 C illustrates this method.

■ *Example 7–3 C*

Graph the polar equation, using the rectangular form as a guide.

1. $r = 2 \sin \theta$

Part (a) of the figure is the graph of $r = 2 \sin \theta$, $0 \le \theta \le 2\pi$, in rectangular coordinates (as done in chapter 3). We observe that there is a positive lobe from $0 \le \theta \le \pi$. This lobe is graphed in part (b) of the figure. Table 7–2 shows values plotted in both graphs. The negative lobe from π to 2π gives the same graph in polar form as the positive lobe. This is because if we shifted the negative lobe π units to the left and made it positive, it would be the same as the positive lobe.

θ	$2 \sin \theta$
0	0
$\dfrac{\pi}{6}$	1
$\dfrac{\pi}{3}$	1.7
$\dfrac{\pi}{2}$	2
$\dfrac{2\pi}{3}$	1.7
$\dfrac{5\pi}{6}$	1
π	0

Table 7–2

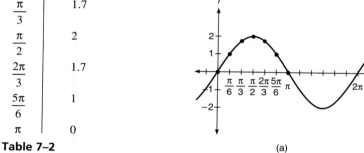

(a)

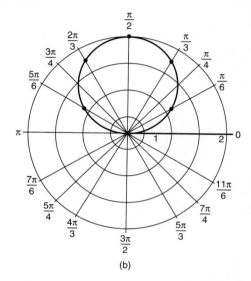

(b)

The lobe in the polar graph is a circle with center at the polar point $\left(\dfrac{\pi}{2}, 1 \right)$. We will not prove the fact that the graph is actually a circle.

$X_{1T} = 2*\sin T*\cos T$, $Y_{1T} = 2*\sin T*\sin T$,
RANGE $0, 3.14, 0.105, -2, 2, 1, -2, 2, 1$, ZOOM 5

2. $r = 3 \cos 2\theta$

First graph in rectangular coordinates (as in section 3–3).

$$0 \le 2\theta \le 2\pi$$
$$0 \le \theta \le \pi \qquad \text{Divide each member by 2}$$

We get one basic cosine cycle, with amplitude 3, as θ takes on values from 0 to π. There are thus two basic cycles from 0 to 2π. Part (a) of the figure shows this graph.

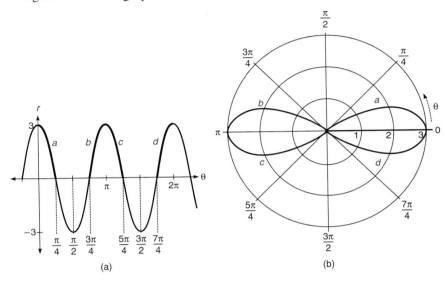

(a)   (b)

Part (b) of the figure is obtained from part (a) in the following manner. Part (a) shows that as θ goes from 0 to $\dfrac{\pi}{4}$, r goes from 3 down to 0. In part (b), $r = 3$ when $\theta = 0$. As θ increases to $\dfrac{\pi}{4}$, r moves down to 0. This produces the half of a lobe labeled a.

Part (a) also shows that as θ goes from $\dfrac{3\pi}{4}$ to π, r goes from 0 to 3. This produces the half lobe b in part (b) of the figure. As θ continues from π to $\dfrac{5\pi}{4}$ (part (a)), r goes from 3 back down to 0. This produces the effect at c in part (b).

The half lobe at d (part (b)) is produced from what r is doing at d in part (a).

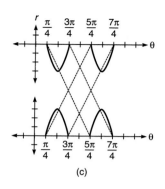

(c)

Part (c) of the figure shows one way to handle negative lobes in the rectangular graph. Shifting θ by π or $-\pi$ units causes r to change its sign; thus, we can shift the negative lobe between $\dfrac{\pi}{4}$ and $\dfrac{3\pi}{4}$, by adding π, to the interval $\dfrac{5\pi}{4}$ to $\dfrac{7\pi}{4}$, and in the process the negative lobe becomes positive.

Similarly, the negative lobe between $\dfrac{5\pi}{4}$ and $\dfrac{7\pi}{4}$ is shifted $-\pi$ units to lie on the interval $\dfrac{\pi}{4}$ to $\dfrac{3\pi}{4}$, and becomes a positive lobe. These positive lobes in the rectangular graph in part (c) produce the lobes shown in part (d) of the figure.

Part (e) of the figure shows the complete graph produced by combining the graphs of parts (b) and (d).

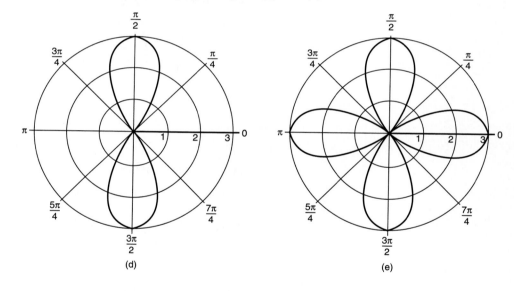

(d)   (e)

$$X_{1T}=3*\cos 2T*\cos T,\quad Y_{1T}=3*\cos 2T*\sin T,$$
$\boxed{\text{RANGE}}$ $\;0,6.3,0.105,-3,3,1,-3,3,1,\;$ $\boxed{\text{ZOOM}}$ $\;5$

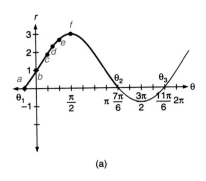

(a)

3. $r = 1 + 2 \sin \theta$

The graph of $r = 1 + 2 \sin \theta$ in rectangular coordinates is shown in part (a) of the figure. It is the graph of $y = 2 \sin \theta$, shifted up by one unit.

Note that r goes from 0 up to 3 and back to 0 between angles θ_1 and θ_2. It would help to find these two angles. They occur where $r = 0$, so we solve for θ where $r = 0$.

$$r = 1 + 2 \sin \theta$$
$$0 = 1 + 2 \sin \theta$$
$$-1 = 2 \sin \theta$$
$$-\tfrac{1}{2} = \sin \theta$$
$$\theta' = \sin^{-1}\tfrac{1}{2}$$
$$\theta' = \frac{\pi}{6}(30°)$$

θ is an angle in quadrant III or IV, since $\sin \theta < 0$. Thus, θ is

$\pi + \dfrac{\pi}{6} = \dfrac{7\pi}{6}$ and $2\pi - \dfrac{\pi}{6} = \dfrac{11\pi}{6}$. By subtracting the period, 2π,

from $\dfrac{11\pi}{6}$ we can see that θ_1 is $-\dfrac{\pi}{6}$.

Now, referring to part (a) of the figure, we see that as θ goes from

$-\dfrac{\pi}{6}$ to $\dfrac{\pi}{2}$, r goes from 0 to 3. This is shown in part (b) of the figure.

Similarly, as θ goes from $\dfrac{\pi}{2}$ to $\dfrac{7\pi}{6}$, r goes from 3 back down to 0. This

is shown in part (c).

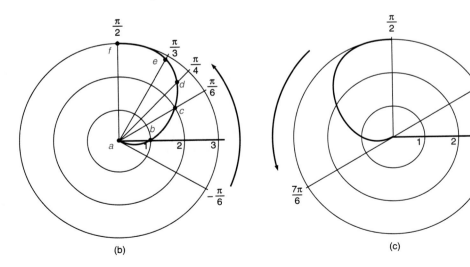

(b)

(c)

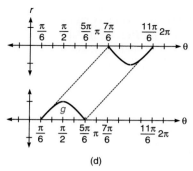

(d)

In part (a) of the figure we see that $r < 0$ for $\dfrac{7\pi}{6} \leq \theta \leq \dfrac{11\pi}{6}$. By adding or subtracting π, r becomes positive. Here it is easier to subtract π from each of these values, giving $\dfrac{\pi}{6} \leq \theta \leq \dfrac{5\pi}{6}$. The result is shown in rectangular coordinates in part (d), where we see that r varies from 0 to 1 and back to 0 as θ moves over this interval. The graph of the positive lobe g, in polar coordinates, is shown in part (e) of the figure. The final graph of $r = 1 + 2 \sin \theta$ is a combination of parts (b), (c) and (e). It is shown in part (f) of the figure.

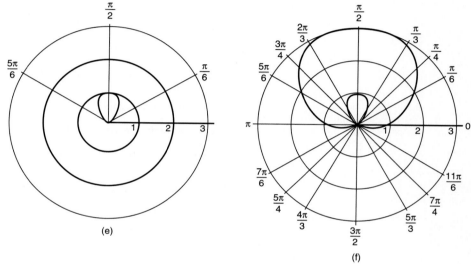

(e)

(f)

$$X_{1T}=(1+2\sin T)*\cos T,\ Y_{1T}=(1+2\sin T)*\sin T,$$
$\boxed{\text{RANGE}}$ $0,6.3,0.105,-3,3,1,-3,3,1,$ $\boxed{\text{ZOOM}}$ 5

■

Classification of the graphs of equations in polar coordinates

Some classification of the graphs of polar equations has been done. In the following, k represents a constant.

1. An equation of the form $r = k\theta$ produces a *spiral* (example 7–3 A).

2. An equation of the form $r \sin \theta = k$ or $r \cos \theta = k$ produces a *horizontal or vertical straight line* for its graph. When graphing these, it is easiest to put the equation in rectangular form. For example, $r \sin \theta = 2$ can be transformed, using $\sin \theta = \dfrac{y}{r}$.

$$r \sin \theta = 2$$
$$r \cdot \frac{y}{r} = 2$$
$$y = 2$$

This is a horizontal straight line.

3. Equations of the form $\theta = k$ also produce *straight lines* (example 7–3 B).

4. Equations of the form $r = k$ produce *circles with center at the pole.*

5. Equations of the form $r = k \cos \theta$ or $r = k \sin \theta$ also produce *circles, which pass through the pole, but have centers elsewhere* (example 7–3 C, part 1).

6. The graph of an equation of the form $r = k \cos n\theta$ or $r = k \sin n\theta$ is called a *rose*. It has *n* leaves if *n* is odd, and *2n* leaves if *n* is even. Example 7–3 C, part 2, is a four-leafed rose.

7. Equations of the form $r = a + b \cos \theta$ or $r = a + b \sin \theta$ produce a figure called the *limaçon*. Example 7–3 C, part 3, is an example. If $|a| = |b|$, the graph is heart shaped and is called a *cardioid*.

Mastery points

Can you
- Graph a polar equation by plotting points?
- Graph a polar equation by using its rectangular graph as a guide?

Exercise 7–3

Graph the polar equation.

1. $r = 6$

2. $r = 2$

3. $r = -3$

4. $r = -1$

5. $\theta = 1$

6. $\theta = 3$

7. $\theta = \dfrac{\pi}{3}$

8. $\theta = -1$

9. $r \sin \theta = 6$

10. $r \cos \theta = 1$

11. $r \cos \theta - 2 = 0$

12. $r \sin \theta = -3$

13. $r = 3 \sin \theta$

14. $r = 2 \cos \theta$

15. $r = 4 \cos \theta$

16. $r = \sin \theta$

17. $r = 3 \sin 2\theta$

18. $r = 2 \cos 3\theta$

19. $r = 3 \cos 4\theta$

20. $r = \sin 3\theta$

21. $r = 1 + \sin \theta$

22. $r = 1 - \sin \theta$

23. $r = 1 - 2 \cos \theta$

24. $r = 2 - 3 \sin \theta$

25. $r = 2 - 2 \sin 2\theta$

26. $r = 1 - \cos 2\theta$

27. $r = 1 + \cos 3\theta$

28. $r = 2 + \sin 2\theta$

29. $r = \theta, \theta < 0$

30. $r = 1 + \theta, \theta > 0$

31. $r = \dfrac{\theta}{4}, \theta > 0$

32. $r = 1 + \dfrac{\theta}{2}, \theta > 0$

33. The shape of a cam that drives a certain sewing machine needle is described by the polar equation $r = 3 - 2 \cos \theta$. Draw the cam by graphing this equation.

34. The path an industrial robot must follow to paint a pattern on a part being manufactured is described by the curve $r = 1 - 2 \sin \theta$. Graph this equation.

35. The pattern of strongest radiation of a certain bidirectional radio antenna is described by the curve $r = 1 + \sin 2\theta$. Graph this pattern.

36. The pattern of strongest radiation of a certain radio antenna is described by the equation $r = 1 + 2 \sin 2\theta$. This pattern is said to have side lobes. Graph the pattern.

As noted in section 7–2, in the October 1983 issue of *Scientific American,* Jearl Walker described several rides at the Geauga Lake Amusement Park near Cleveland, Ohio. The Scrambler is a ride whose motion could be described as a three-leafed rose, and the motion of the Calypso could be described as a limaçon.

37. Graph the path taken by the Scrambler, assuming that its motion is described by the polar equation $r = 2 \cos 3\theta$.

38. Graph the path of the Calypso, assuming that its motion is described by the equation $r = 1 - 3 \cos \theta$.

Chapter 7 summary

- **Imaginary unit** $i = \sqrt{-1}$
- **Complex number (rectangular form)** A number of the form $a + bi$, a and b both real numbers.
- **Complex conjugate** The complex conjugate of $a + bi$ is $a - bi$.
- **Equality of complex numbers** $a + bi = c + di$ if and only if $a = c$ and $b = d$.
- **Polar form of a complex number** If $z = a + bi$ is a complex number that determines an angle θ, then r cis θ is its polar form, where cis θ means $\cos \theta + i \sin \theta$. The value r is called the modulus of z, which is also written $|z|$, and

$$r = \sqrt{a^2 + b^2}, \quad \tan \theta' = \tan^{-1}\frac{b}{a}, \text{ and}$$

$$\theta = \begin{cases} \theta' & \text{if } a > 0 \\ \theta' - 180° \text{ if } \theta' > 0 \\ \theta' + 180° \text{ if } \theta' < 0 \end{cases} \text{if } a < 0$$

- **Complex multiplication—polar form**
  $(r_1 \text{ cis } \theta_1)(r_2 \text{ cis } \theta_2) = r_1 r_2 \text{ cis}(\theta_1 + \theta_2)$.
- **Complex division—polar form**
  $\dfrac{r_1 \text{ cis } \theta_1}{r_2 \text{ cis } \theta_2} = \dfrac{r_1}{r_2} \text{ cis}(\theta_1 - \theta_2)$, $r_2 \neq 0$.
- **De Moivre's theorem** $(r \text{ cis } \theta)^n = r^n \text{ cis } n\theta$ for any real number n.

- **De Moivre's theorem for roots** The n nth roots of r cis θ are of the form $(r \text{ cis } \theta)^{\frac{1}{n}} = r^{\frac{1}{n}} \text{ cis}\left(\dfrac{\theta}{n} + \dfrac{k \cdot 360°}{n}\right)$, $0 \leq k < n$, where k and n are positive integers.
- The polar coordinates of a point is an ordered pair of the form (r, θ), where r is the radius and θ is an angle.
- **Equivalence of points in polar coordinates**
  1. $(r, \alpha) = (r, \beta)$ if α and β are coterminal angles.
  2. $(-r, \theta) = (r, \theta \pm \pi)$.
- **Relation between polar and rectangular coordinates** If $P = (x, y) = (r, \theta)$, $r > 0$, then $\cos \theta = \dfrac{x}{r}$ and $\sin \theta = \dfrac{y}{r}$. Thus, $x = r \cos \theta$ and $y = r \sin \theta$. Also,

$$r = \sqrt{x^2 + y^2}, \quad \tan \theta' = \tan^{-1}\frac{y}{x}, \text{ and}$$

$$\theta = \begin{cases} \theta' & \text{if } x > 0 \\ \theta' - \pi \text{ if } \theta' > 0 \\ \theta' + \pi \text{ if } \theta' < 0 \end{cases} \text{if } x < 0$$

- To convert a rectangular equation into a polar equation use the relations $x = r \cos \theta$, $y = r \sin \theta$, and $r^2 = x^2 + y^2$.
- To convert a polar equation into a rectangular equation use the relations $\sin \theta = \dfrac{y}{r}$, $\cos \theta = \dfrac{x}{r}$, and $r^2 = x^2 + y^2$.

Chapter 7 review

[7–1] Identify the real and imaginary parts of the following complex numbers.

1. $3 - i$ **2.** $3i$ **3.** 12 **4.** $-i$

Simplify each expression by performing the indicated operations.

5. $(2 - 4i) + (-3 + 2i)$ **6.** $(-7 + 4i) - (-13 + 3i)$
7. $(5 - 4i)(3 + 12i)$ **8.** $(-2 + 5i)(3 - 6i)$
9. $4i(2 - 3i)$ **10.** $(4 - i)(2 - 3i)(5 + 2i)$
11. $\dfrac{10 - 4i}{5 + 2i}$ **12.** $\dfrac{-2 + i}{2 - 4i}$ **13.** $\dfrac{8 + 6i}{14i}$

If $z_1 = 2 + i$ and $z_2 = 3 - 2i$, evaluate the following expressions.

14. $2z_1 - z_2$ **15.** $z_1(3 - z_2)$
16. $\dfrac{z_1 + z_2}{z_1 - z_2}$ **17.** $\dfrac{z_1(z_1 - z_2)}{2z_2}$

In each of the following problems, (a) find the complex conjugate of the given number and (b) graph both the number and its complex conjugate in the same graph.

18. $-4 + 3i$ **19.** $-4 + i$ **20.** $3i$ **21.** 17

Write the polar forms of the following numbers (to the nearest tenth).

22. $3 - 2i$ **23.** $\sqrt{3} + 3i$ **24.** $-1 - 2i$

Write the polar forms of the following complex numbers. Leave the result in exact form.

25. $\sqrt{3} - i$ **26.** $3 + 3i$ **27.** $-4i$

Write the rectangular forms of the following complex numbers (to the nearest tenth).

28. $3 \text{ cis } 35°$ **29.** $3 \text{ cis } 243°$

Write the rectangular forms of the following complex numbers. Leave the result in exact form.

30. $3 \text{ cis } 240°$ **31.** $10 \text{ cis } 330°$

Multiply the following complex numbers.

32. $(2 \text{ cis } 25°)(3 \text{ cis } 45°)$
33. $(2 \text{ cis } 18°)(6.5 \text{ cis } 122°)$

Divide the following complex numbers.

34. $\dfrac{40 \text{ cis } 120°}{5 \text{ cis } 20°}$ **35.** $\dfrac{50 \text{ cis } 45°}{100 \text{ cis } 9°}$

36. Compute the cube of $2 \text{ cis } 130°$.
37. Compute the fourth power of $2 \text{ cis } 150°$.

38. Compute an approximation to $(0.8 + 0.6i)^8$ (to the nearest tenth).
39. Find the 4 fourth roots of 16 in exact form.
40. Find the 3 cube roots of -27 in exact form.
41. In electronics one version of Ohm's law says that $I = \dfrac{V}{Z}$, where I is current, V is voltage, and Z is impedance. Find I in a circuit in which $V = 130 \text{ cis } 25°$ and Z is $30 \text{ cis } 75°$.

[7–2] Graph the following points in polar coordinates.

42. $(2,0)$ **43.** $(2,\pi)$ **44.** $\left(3,\dfrac{5\pi}{6}\right)$
45. $\left(-6,\dfrac{11\pi}{6}\right)$ **46.** $\left(1,\dfrac{\pi}{2}\right)$ **47.** $(-3,\pi)$
48. $(2,1)$ **49.** $(3,4)$ **50.** $(-4,1)$

Convert the following polar coordinates into rectangular coordinates. Leave the result in exact form.

51. $\left(3,\dfrac{11\pi}{6}\right)$ **52.** $\left(4,\dfrac{2\pi}{3}\right)$ **53.** $\left(-2,\dfrac{5\pi}{3}\right)$

Convert the following polar coordinates into rectangular coordinates to two-decimal-place accuracy.

54. $(2,1)$ **55.** $(5,2)$ **56.** $(1,0.5)$

Convert the following rectangular coordinates into polar coordinates to two-decimal-place accuracy.

57. $(2,1)$ **58.** $(-5,3)$ **59.** $(-1,-4)$

Convert the following rectangular equations into polar equations.

60. $y = -3x$ **61.** $y = 4x + 2$
62. $2y^2 - x^2 = 5$ **63.** $y^2 - 3x = 0$

Convert the following polar equations into rectangular equations.

64. $r = \sin \theta$ **65.** $r = 2 \sec \theta$
66. $r^2 = \sin 2\theta$ **67.** $r^2 = \tan \theta$
68. $r \sin \theta = 2$ **69.** $r = \dfrac{3}{2 - \sin \theta}$

[7–3] Graph the polar equations.

70. $r = -2$ **71.** $\theta = \dfrac{5\pi}{6}$
72. $2r \sin \theta = 8$ **73.** $r = 3 \cos \theta$
74. $r = \sin 2\theta$ **75.** $r = 3 \cos 3\theta$
76. $r = 1 + 2 \cos \theta$ **77.** $r = 2 - \sin \theta$

Chapter 7 test

Simplify each expression by performing the indicated operations.

1. $(12 - 4i) - (-3 + 2i)$ **2.** $(1 - 4i)(2 + 8i)$

3. $\dfrac{2 - 5i}{2 - 3i}$

4. If $z = 1 + 2i$, evaluate $3z^2 - 2z + 5$.

5. Write the polar form of the number $4 - 5i$ (to the nearest tenth).

6. Write the rectangular form of the number 2 cis 120°. Leave the result in exact form.

7. Multiply (2 cis 325°)(7 cis 145°). Leave the result in polar form.

8. Divide $\dfrac{6 \text{ cis } 140°}{2 \text{ cis } 20°}$. Leave the result in polar form.

9. Compute the cube of 3 cis 150°.

10. Find the 4 fourth roots of -16 in exact form.

Graph the following points in polar coordinates.

11. $\left(2, \dfrac{11\pi}{6}\right)$ **12.** $\left(2, \dfrac{\pi}{3}\right)$ **13.** $(-2, 1)$

Convert the following polar coordinates into rectangular coordinates to two-decimal-place accuracy.

14. $(3, 0.8)$ **15.** $(-5, 2)$

Convert the following rectangular coordinates into polar coordinates. Leave the result in exact form.

16. $(-\sqrt{3}, -1)$ **17.** $(-5, 5)$

Convert the following rectangular equations into polar equations.

18. $y = -3x + 5$ **19.** $2y^2 - x = 5$

Convert the following polar equations into rectangular equations.

20. $r = 2 \csc \theta$ **21.** $r^2 = \cos 2\theta$

Graph the polar equations.

22. $r = -\theta, \theta > 0$ **23.** $r = 2 \csc \theta$

24. $r = 3 \cos 2\theta$

Appendix A

Graphing—Addition of Ordinates

Although the advent of desktop computers and calculators with graphics capabilities has given many users of trigonometry the ability to graph a function without putting pencil to paper, there are often instances where it is useful to be able to obtain a quick sketch of a function by hand. The method we examine in this section, **addition of ordinates,** can be very helpful in this regard. Also, studying this method leads to a fuller understanding of functions, and this understanding will aid even the person using a computer's graphing capabilities. We assume a thorough knowledge of section 3–3.

We learned in section 2–1 that a function is a set of ordered pairs in which no first element repeats. When we graph a function in a rectangular coordinate system, we use two perpendicular axes. We use horizontal distances to represent domain elements, or values of the argument of the function. Vertical distances are used to represent range elements, or values of the function for a given value of the argument. In this way, each ordered pair represents a domain element and the corresponding range element. In an ordered pair, the first element is sometimes called the **abscissa;** the second element is then called the **ordinate.** For example, consider the graph of a function f, shown in figure A–1. Although we do not know the "formula" for f (i.e., an expression that defines f), or even whether such a formula exists, we can still see that $f(1) = 2$ and $f(2) = 4$. We know that $f(1) = 2$, because if we go a horizontal distance of 1, corresponding to domain element 1, or an abscissa of 1, we see that the associated vertical distance is 2, representing a range element, or ordinate, of 2.

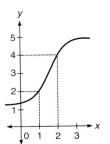

Figure A–1

> *In general, if we go a horizontal distance x, the corresponding vertical distance represents f(x).*

Since we use the y-axis to plot values of $f(x)$, we often write $y = f(x)$, or replace $f(x)$ by y in a formula.

The graph of a linear function is relatively simple. A linear function is a function of the form $f(x) = mx + b$. (We often simply write $y = mx + b$.) The graph of such a function is a straight line. This means that if we can find two points on the line (i.e., that satisfy the function) we know the graph is a straight line which must pass through them.

Thus, to graph a linear function, we find two points that lie on the line and draw a straight line through them. Usually these two points are the x- and y-intercepts.

■ *Example A*

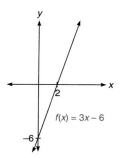

1. Graph the linear function $f(x) = 3x - 6$.

   It is easier to do the necessary algebra if we replace $f(x)$ by y, giving $y = 3x - 6$.

   To find the x-intercept we replace y by 0, since for any point on the x-axis, y is 0.

   $$y = 3x - 6$$
   $$0 = 3x - 6$$
   $$2 = x$$

   Therefore, the x-intercept is $(2,0)$.

   To find the y-intercept we replace x by 0.

   $$y = 3x - 6$$
   $$y = 3(0) - 6$$
   $$y = -6$$

   Therefore, the y-intercept is $(0,-6)$.

   In the figure we plot these two points and draw the straight line through them.

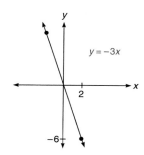

2. Graph the linear function $f(x) = -3x$.

   First we write $y = -3x$. Replacing x by 0 or y by 0 gives the same result, $(0,0)$. The origin is, therefore, the only intercept. Since one point is not enough to determine a straight line, we find another. Replace x by some value other than 0, say 2.

   $$y = -3x$$
   $$y = -3(2)$$
   $$y = -6$$

   Therefore, a second point that lies on the line is $(2,-6)$. In the figure, we plot both points and draw the line that passes through them. ■

Now, consider the graph of $f(x) = x + 2$. First, we shall relabel this as $y = x + 2$. Its graph is shown in figure A–2. If we graph the equation $y = x$, shown in dashed lines in figure A–2, we see that every point in the graph of $y = x + 2$ is two units above every point in the graph of $y = x$. Another way to view this is that the graph of $y = x + 2$ is the sum of the graphs of $y = x$ and $y = 2$. This summing is done vertically. (We are adding the ordinates.) That is, to graph $y = x + 2$ for a given value of x, we take the vertical distance in the graph of $y = x$ and add the vertical distance in $y = 2$. This process is shown for $x = 3$ and for $x = -5$ in figure A–3. Note that we treat each distance as a directed distance. If the function is positive, we move up; if negative, we move down.

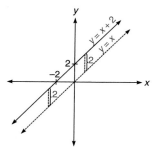

Figure A–2

For example, at the point $x = 3$, we move up three units and then two more units. The length 3 represents the value of the equation $y = x$ when x is 3. The length 2 represents the value of the equation $y = 2$ when x is 3.

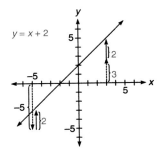

$y = x + 2$

Figure A–3

At the point $x = -5$, we add vertical lengths -5 and 2. The length -5 (5 in the downward direction) represents the value of the equation $y = x$ when x is -5, and the length 2 represents the value of the equation $y = 2$ when x is -5.

Figure A–4 illustrates the process of addition of ordinates in general. We assume that we have a function h described by an expression that is the sum of the expressions for two functions f and g. That is, $h(x) = f(x) + g(x)$. For the purpose of illustration, $f(x)$ might be the expression $0.25 + \sin x$, and $g(x)$ might be the expression $\cos(x + 0.5)$. Then, $h(x)$ would be

$$h(x) = f(x) + g(x)$$
$$= (0.25 + \sin x) + [\cos (x + 0.5)]$$
$$= \sin x + \cos(x + 0.5) + 0.25$$

In figure A–4 we see the graphs of the two functions, f and g, and the addition of ordinates at x_1, x_2, x_3, x_4, and x_5.

Figure A–4(a) shows the process at x_1. $f(x_1)$ and $g(x_1)$ are both positive, so the value of $h(x_1)$ is represented by the combined heights of f and g at this point.

Figure A–4(b) shows the case where $f(x_2) = g(x_2)$. Since these values are equal, the combined value $f(x_2) + g(x_2)$ is twice the height of either f or g at this point.

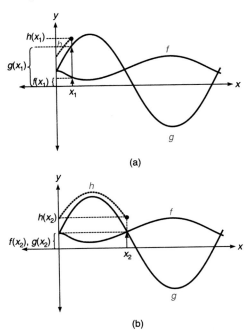

(a)

(b)

Figure A–4

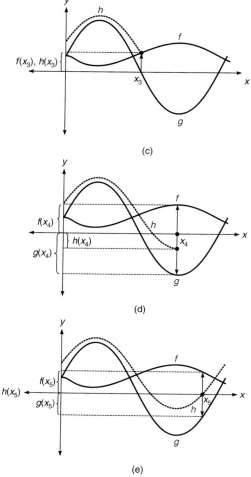

Figure A–4 *(continued)*

Figure A–4(c) illustrates the situation where one function is 0 at a point. Here, $g(x_3) = 0$; thus, the sum of $f(x_3) + g(x_3)$ is just $f(x_3)$. In other words, at x_3, the functions h and f take on equal values.

Figure A–4(d) illustrates a situation where the functions have opposite signs. $f(x_4)$ is positive and $g(x_4)$ is negative. Thus, to form the value of $h(x_4)$ we go up to $f(x_4)$ and come back down a distance corresponding to the height of $g(x_4)$.

Figure A–4(e) is like the situation at x_4, except that $f(x_5)$ and $g(x_5)$ have equal absolute values. Thus, their sum is 0, so that $h(x_5) = 0$.

This discussion can provide *guidelines for finding the graph of a sum of two functions using addition of ordinates.*

1. Wherever the two functions cross, the result is twice the height of the functions (as in figure A–4 (b)).

2. Wherever one function is zero the result is the same as the other function (figure A–4 (c)).

3. Wherever the functions have opposite signs but equal absolute values the result is 0 (figure A–4 (e)).

Using these guidelines we can often obtain quite a few points in the result. We must then graph enough intermediate points (as in figure A–4 (a) and (d)) to get a good idea of what the result looks like.

The function $f(x) = x + \sin x$ provides a concrete example. First we rewrite $y = x + \sin x$ for convenience. We view this as the sum of the graphs of $y = x$ and $y = \sin x$. See figure A–5, where the graph of each of these functions is shown.

To obtain the graph of $y = x + \sin x$, we proceed in the following way. We select an abscissa (moving a given horizontal distance along the x-axis) and then add the ordinate of $y = x$ and $y = \sin x$. This is shown for several abscissas in figure A–6. Observe that wherever the function $y = \sin x$ is zero, the result is the other function, $y = x$. This is guideline 2, above. Many other points in the graph of $y = x + \sin x$ are also shown in figure A–6, on the dotted line. We graph only enough points to see what the finished graph looks like. Actually, with a little experience, we often require only a few points to see the result. The graph of $y = x + \sin x$ is shown in figure A–7. We can view this as the function $y = \sin x$ "riding on" the function $y = x$.

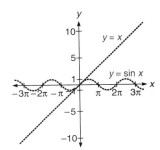

Figure A–5

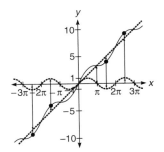

Figure A–6

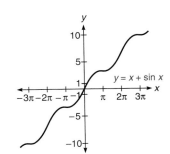

Figure A–7

■ *Example B*

1. Graph the equation $y = \sin x + \cos x$ for $0 \le x \le 2\pi$.

The figure shows the graphs of $y = \sin x$ and $y = \cos x$ in dashed lines, along with the additions of ordinates for several values of x. In particular, at x_1 the functions have equal values and so the result is twice the height of either. At x_2 one function is zero, so the result is the same as the nonzero function. At x_3 both functions are negative, but there is nothing special about either (i.e., none of the three guidelines apply). We must add the signed distances here. At x_4 the functions have equal absolute values but opposite signs. Thus, the result is 0 at this point.

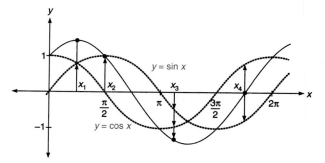

The result is shown at many other points also, on the solid line. The graph of $y = \sin x + \cos x$ is shown in the next figure.

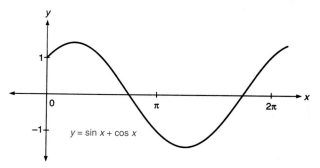

Note   It can be shown that $\sin x + \cos x = \sqrt{2} \sin\left(x + \dfrac{\pi}{4}\right)$.

2. Graph the equation $y = \sin x + \sin 2x$ for $0 \le x \le 2\pi$.

The figure shows the graphs of $y = \sin x$ and $y = \sin 2x$ in dashed lines, along with the additions of ordinates for several values of x, and the result at many other points (solid line).

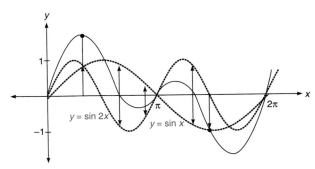

The result is shown in the next figure.

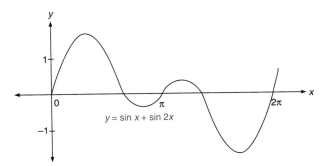

If the expression includes subtraction, we rewrite it in terms of addition.

■ *Example C*

Graph the equation $y = \sin x - \cos x$ for $0 \le x \le 2\pi$.

Since it is easier to picture addition of ordinates than to picture subtraction, we rewrite the equation as

$$y = \sin x + (-\cos x)$$

We now graph $y = \sin x$ and $y = -\cos x$. These are shown in the first figure with the additions of ordinates for several values of x and the result on the solid line.

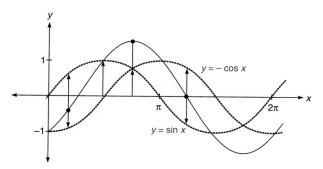

The result is shown in the second figure.

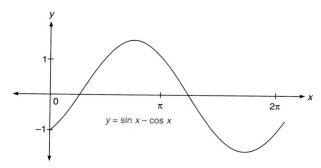

Note   It can be shown that $\sin x - \cos x = \sqrt{2} \sin\left(x - \dfrac{\pi}{4}\right)$.   ■

■ *Example D*

1. An electronic signal that is described by the equation $y = 2 \sin x - 1$ is serving as a carrier for another signal described by $y = \frac{1}{2} \sin 2x$. That is, the finished signal is described by $y = 2 \sin x - 1 + \frac{1}{2} \sin 2x$. Graph this signal for $0 \le x \le 2\pi$.
   We will graph $y = 2 \sin x - 1$ and $y = \frac{1}{2} \sin 2x$ in dashed lines. Although we could graph $y = 2 \sin x - 1$ itself by the method of addition of ordinates, we should recall that this is just the graph of $y = 2 \sin x$ shifted down by one unit (section 3–3). The graphs of these two signal components are shown in the first figure, as well as the addition of several ordinates. The results are shown for many points on the solid line.

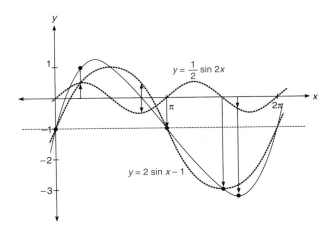

The result is shown in the second figure.

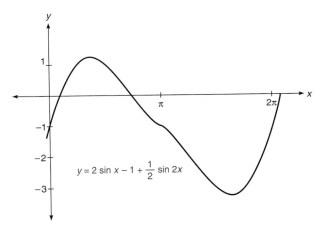

2. Assume a pure musical tone is being represented by $y = \sin x$. Its second harmonic is then $y = \frac{1}{2} \sin 2x$, and $y = \frac{1}{3} \sin 3x$ represents the third harmonic. Assume that all three tones are present and describe the result graphically.

We graph the three functions separately and then add the ordinates of all three. The three graphs are shown in the first figure, as are the addition of ordinates for several values of x and the result for many points on the dotted line.

There are some points that can be of help in a complicated case like this.

Wherever one of the functions is zero, the result is the sum of the other two functions. Thus, good selections for x are values where any of the three functions cross the x-axis (points x_2, x_4, x_5, x_6, x_7, x_8, x_{10}, and x_{11}).

Also, wherever two of the functions have equal absolute values but opposite signs, the result is the third function (points x_3 and x_9).

At other points we must simply compute the sum for three values (point x_1).

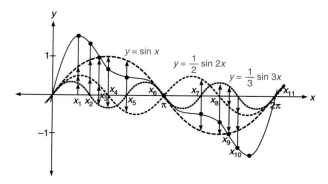

The result is shown in the second figure.

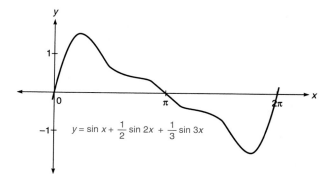

Mastery points

Can you
- Graph a function using addition of ordinates?

Exercise A

Graph the following linear functions.

1. $f(x) = 5x - 3$
2. $f(x) = -2x + 7$
3. $f(x) = -x + 3$
4. $f(x) = \frac{1}{2}x + 2$
5. $f(x) = \frac{2}{3}x - 1$
6. $f(x) = -2x$

Graph the following functions, using addition of ordinates, for $0 \leq x \leq 2\pi$.

7. $y = x + 2 \sin x$ **8.** $y = -x + \sin x$ **9.** $y = 2x + 2 \sin x$ **10.** $y = 2x + \sin 2x$

11. $y = \sin x + \sin 3x$ **12.** $y = \sin 2x + \cos x$ **13.** $y = \sin 2x + \cos 3x$ **14.** $y = 2x - \sin x$

15. $y = -x - \sin x$ **16.** $y = 2x - 2 \sin x$ **17.** $y = \sin x - \sin 3x$ **18.** $y = \sin x - \cos x$

19. $y = \sin 2x - \cos x$

20. The equation of time combines the effects of the inclination of the earth in its orbit about the sun, and the eccentricity of the orbit. It gives the difference between mean solar time and actual solar time throughout the year. The function that describes the effect of the eccentricity of the earth's orbit can be approximately described by $y = 7.5 \sin \frac{\pi}{6}x$, and the function that describes the effect of the inclination of the earth is approximately $y = 10 \sin \frac{\pi}{3}x$. The amplitudes tell the number of degrees of deviation between mean and actual solar time.

To find the combined effects, we graph the sum of the two functions, $y = 7.5 \sin \frac{\pi}{6}x + 10 \sin \frac{\pi}{3}x$. Graph this equation of time for $0 \leq x \leq 12$ (for 12 months).

21. The electric voltage supplied to United States homes has a frequency of 60 cycles per second (cps), or a period of $\frac{1}{60}$ of one second. It can be described by the function $y = 180 \sin 120\pi x$, where the amplitude is instantaneous voltage and x is in seconds.

a. Graph this function. Use divisions of $\frac{1}{240}$ of one second, and graph two complete cycles.

b. Suppose that a wind-driven home generator is generating electricity, but due to a fault in its speed governor it is generating at 50 cps and is only producing 25 volts. Assuming that these sources are in phase at some point and that they are tied together (electrically speaking), the resulting voltage can be described by $y = 180 \sin 120\pi x + 25 \sin 100\pi x$ (until a fuse blows). Graph this resultant voltage for $0 \leq x \leq \frac{1}{25}$.

22. Most people have heard about the theory of biorhythms. First stated by Dr. Wilhelm Fliess in Germany at the beginning of the century, this theory maintains that at birth three cycles are started—physical, emotional, and intellectual. These have periods of 23, 28, and 33 days, respectively, and can be (presumably) described by sinusoidal waves. With a time axis in days, we compute the equation for the physical as follows:

$$0 \leq x \leq 23$$
$$\frac{2\pi}{23}(0) \leq \frac{2\pi}{23}x \leq \frac{2\pi}{23}(23)$$
$$0 \leq \frac{2\pi}{23}x \leq 2\pi$$

Thus, the equation for the physical state is $y = \sin \frac{2\pi}{23}x$.

a. Find the equations for the emotional and intellectual cycles.

b. Graph the function that is the sum of these three cycles using addition of ordinates. Graph it for the first 33 days of life. (All three functions start together, or are in phase, at birth.)

c. Find the period of the resulting function, in both days and years.

Appendix B

Further Uses for Graphing Calculators and Computers

The use of a scientific calculator has been assumed throughout this text. We have also shown the use of graphing calculators. This appendix presents problems that are best done *only* with a graphing calculator.

Specific examples refer to the Texas Instruments *TI-81* programmable, graphing calculator and a Casio *fx*-7000G programmable, graphing calculator. It is assumed that the user has read at least the introductory material in the handbook for the calculator.

Finding zeros of functions

This topic was introduced in section 5–4. We revisit it here with examples that are difficult to solve algebraically. We also show how to accomplish these same tasks with the Casio and Texas Instruments calculators.

Estimating zeros from the graph

The approximate zeros of a function can be found by graphing the function. This is because a zero of a function is an *x*-intercept of the function's graph.

■ *Example A*

Find approximate zeros to the function $f(x) = 2 \sin(\sqrt{2x}) - \frac{1}{2}$ for $0 \le x < 2\pi$ by graphing.

Texas Instruments TI-81 Calculator

The following steps would produce a graph similar to that shown in the upper screen in the figure. It is essential that the $\boxed{\text{MODE}}$ key be used to set the calculator to radian (Rad) mode. As can be seen in the graph the function has

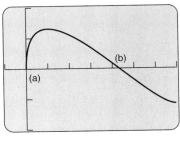

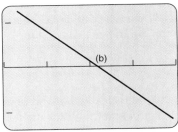

Steps	Explanation
$\boxed{\text{Range}}$	Enter the *x*- and *y*-axis limits.
0 $\boxed{\text{ENTER}}$	Xmin becomes 0.
7.5 $\boxed{\text{ENTER}}$	Xmax becomes 7.5.
1 $\boxed{\text{ENTER}}$	Xscl becomes 1.
$\boxed{(-)}$ 2.5 $\boxed{\text{ENTER}}$	Ymin becomes -2.5.
2.5 $\boxed{\text{ENTER}}$	Ymax becomes 2.5.
1 $\boxed{\text{ENTER}}$	Yscl becomes 1.
$\boxed{\text{2nd}}$ $\boxed{\text{CLEAR}}$	Quit

Enter the function into Y_1.

$\boxed{Y=}$ 2 $\boxed{\sin}$ $\boxed{(}$ $\boxed{\text{2nd}}$ $\boxed{x^2}$ $\boxed{(}$ 2 $\boxed{\text{X|T}}$ $\boxed{)}$ $\boxed{)}$
$\boxed{-}$ 0.5 $\boxed{\text{GRAPH}}$

zeros at approximate x-values of 0.1 and 4.1. It would be possible to obtain a better estimate by using the trace feature. For example, select ⬚TRACE⬚ and use the ⬚▷⬚ and ⬚◁⬚ keys to move the blinking dot as close to the point (b) as possible. Then use ⬚ZOOM⬚ 2 ⬚ENTER⬚ to expand the display. It will then look like the lower screen. Using the ⬚TRACE⬚ feature again will show that point (b) is between the values 4.16 and 4.20. The trace feature shows the current value of x and y in the display. By noting the values of x when the value of y changes sign we can find estimates of the value of x at the zero at (b). By repeating the zoom and trace features we could find a better and better estimate of the zero at (b). By resetting the range and zooming we could repeat the process for the zero at (a).

Casio *fx*-7000G Calculator

The following steps will produce a graph similar to that shown in the previous figure. As can be seen in the graph the function has zeros at approximate x-values of 0.1 and 4.1

Steps	Explanation
⬚Range⬚	Enter the x- and y-axis limits.
0 ⬚EXE⬚	Xmin becomes 0.
7.5 ⬚EXE⬚	Xmax becomes 7.5.
1 ⬚EXE⬚	Xscl becomes 1.
⬚(−)⬚ 2.5 ⬚EXE⬚	Ymin becomes −2.5.
2.5 ⬚EXE⬚	Ymax becomes 2.5.
1 ⬚EXE⬚	Yscl becomes 1.

We are back at the execution level at this point. If not, use the ⬚Range⬚ key again.

| ⬚Graph⬚ | "Y =" appears |
| 2 ⬚sin⬚ ⬚(⬚ ⬚√⬚ ⬚(⬚ 2 ⬚ALPHA⬚ ⬚+⬚ ⬚)⬚ ⬚)⬚ ⬚−⬚ 0.5 ⬚EXE⬚ | |

It is possible to obtain a better estimate by using the *Trace* feature. For example, select ⬚SHIFT⬚ ⬚Graph⬚ (trace) and use the ⬚→⬚ and ⬚←⬚ keys to move the blinking dot as close to the point (b) as possible. Then use ⬚SHIFT⬚ ⬚×⬚ (multiply) to expand the display. It will then look like the lower screen in the preceding figure. Using the trace feature again will show that point (b) is approximately 4.149. (The trace feature shows the current value of x in the display.) By repeating the trace feature we could find a better and better estimate of the zero at (b). By resetting the range and zooming we could repeat the process for the zero at (a). ∎

The TI-81 and Newton's Method

Section 5–4 presented solving equations using Newton's method on the TI-81 calculator. The next example solves the previous problem using this method.

■ *Example B*

Find the zeros of $y = 2\sin(\sqrt{2x}) - \frac{1}{2}$ for $0 \le x < 2\pi$ (from example A) using Newton's method.

We assume the function is entered into Y_1 as described in example A, and use the trace function to position the cursor near the point (a) in the figure there. Then select $\boxed{\text{PRGM}}$ 1 (assumes the program NEWTON is stored as the first program). The display shows Prgm1 in the display. Use $\boxed{\text{ENTER}}$ to run the program and find the approximate value of x at the point (a) to be 0.0319236557 when the program is finished.

Note   *The zoom feature must be used several times before the root at (a) can be found by the program NEWTON.* Not zooming produces an error. This is because the program calculates a value D $= \dfrac{\text{XMAX} - \text{XMIN}}{100}$. This value D is used to compute new values of x. Using XMAX of 7.5 and XMIN of 0 produces a value of D that causes the program to try to use a negative value of x. The value $\sqrt{2x}$ causes a problem when this happens. Rerun the program by resetting the range to its initial values, then selecting $\boxed{\text{GRAPH}}$ and then $\boxed{\text{TRACE}}$ again, placing the cursor near (b). This will show that the zero at (b) is approximately 4.172907423.   ■

Newton's method, used in example B, cannot be conveniently programmed into the Casio calculator. This is because the Texas Instruments calculator has a built-in function called NDeriv that is not available in the Casio. For the Casio, we illustrate another method for approximating zeros of functions—the method of bisection. This method is also suitable for programming on a computer. At the end of this appendix is a Pascal language program for this method.

The Casio *fx*-7000G and the method of bisection

Figure B–1 illustrates the method of bisection[1] for some hypothetical function. We let z mean zero, L mean lower, U mean upper, and A mean average. Suppose we know there is exactly one zero of the function, at z in the figure, between two values, L and U (part 1 of figure B–1). We can see that $f(L) < 0$ and $f(U) > 0$.

If we let $A = \dfrac{L + U}{2}$ be the average of L and U, A divides the interval between L and U in half. We calculate $f(A)$ and discover that $f(A) < 0$. This means the zero z must be between A and U. This is because the function must go from a negative value at A to a positive value at U, thus taking on the value 0 somewhere in between. Thus, change L to mean the value at c, and repeat the process (part 2 of figure B–1).

Figure B–1

[1]To "bisect" means to cut in half.

We now consider the new smaller interval from L to U, and compute the midpoint of this interval, $A = \dfrac{L + U}{2}$. Since $f(A) > 0$ the zero is between L and A. We therefore let U represent this value of c (part 3 of figure B–1) and repeat the process, obtaining the new point A. We repeat this process until we find a value x so that $f(x) = 0$, or until the interval is so short that its midpoint is a good enough approximation to the zero.

To simplify the program we require $f(L) < 0$ and $f(U) > 0$, as in figure B–1. If this is not true, we interchange the values of L and U. This does not affect the procedure.

An algorithm for this procedure is described below. A program for a Casio *fx*-7000G calculator and a Pascal language program are given at the end of this appendix.

Finding a root of a function by bisection

Assumptions
1. The function has exactly one zero between two values L and U, $L < U$.
2. The function is continuous for all values from L to U inclusive.
3. $f(L) \neq 0$ and $f(U) \neq 0$.
4. $f(L)$ and $f(U)$ have different signs (the root is not of even multiplicity).

Algorithm   {Comments are enclosed in braces.}
Start: Read in the values L and U.
          If $f(L) > 0$ then   {We want $f(L) < 0$, $f(U) > 0$}
              interchange L and U.
Loop: Let $A = \dfrac{L + U}{2}$.   {A is the average of L and U}
          If $f(A) = 0$ then
              go to Finish.   {A is the zero and we are done}
          If $|L - U| <$ some_predetermined_value then
              go to Finish.
          If $f(A) < 0$ then   {See figure B–1}
              Let $L = A$ {Part 1 of the figure.}
          otherwise {$f(A) > 0$ so}
              let $U = A$.   {Part 2 of the figure.}
          go to Loop.
Finish: Print out the value of A.

The program for the Casio given at the end of this appendix requires two input values of x, which provide an upper (U) and lower (L) bound for an interval that contains a single zero of an equation. These values might easily be found by graphing the equation. The program is stored in, say program 8.

The function for which the zeros are to be calculated is stored as program 9. It must be an expression in the variable X and its last statement must be →Y.

Example C illustrates using this program.

■ *Example C*

Find the zeros of $y = 2 \sin(\sqrt{2x}) - 0.5$ (from example A) using the method of bisection, programmed into program 8 on a Casio *fx*-7000G. (We assume the Casio program that implements the method of bisection has been entered into program 8.)

To enter the equation $y = 2 \sin(\sqrt{2x}) - 0.5$ into memory as program 9 proceed as follows.

Key strokes	Comments
MODE 2	Enter WRT (Program WRITE) mode.
Use the → key to select Program 9.	
Then EXE .	
2 sin ((√ ((2 ALPHA	
+)) − 0.5 →	
ALPHA −	
MODE 1	Go back to run mode.

To run the program to find the zero proceed as follows. Based on figure B–1 we use $L = 0$, $U = 1$.

Key strokes	Comments
Prog 8 EXE	Execute program 8.
?	The ? in the display means to enter a value.
0 EXE	Enter the value 0. This is L.
?	
1 EXE	Enter the value 1. This is U.

0.03192365567 appears when the program is finished.

The zero at (a) in figure B–1 is thus approximately 0.03192365567. Re-running the program with suitable values for L and U shows that the zero at (b) is approximately 4.172907423.   ■

Note that the program in 8 can be used with any expression that is entered into program 9. The only requirement is that the expression end with ''→y.''

Note   If the graph of a function does not cross the *x* axis at a zero, the zero is said to have even multiplicity. For example, $f(x) = (\sin x - \frac{1}{2})^2$ has a zero at $\dfrac{\pi}{6}$, but neither the method of bisection nor Newton's method will find it. Figure B–2 shows the graph of this function.

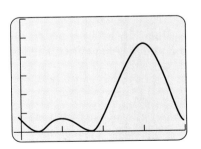

Figure B–2

Solving systems of two equations in two variables

A system of two equations in two variables is a collection of two equations, each of which is described in terms of the same two variables, usually x and y. To solve a system of two equations in two variables is to find all ordered pairs (x,y) that satisfy both equations. Graphically, these points are where the graphs intersect. Example D shows two methods to solve these systems with the graphing, programmable calculator.

■ *Example D*

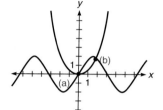

Solve the system of equations $y = 2 \sin x$ and $y = \frac{1}{2}x^2$.

Method 1: Graph both equations in the same coordinate system. The point(s) of intersection of the graphs are the solutions. In the figure, there are two such points. One is the origin (a) (0,0); the second appears to be approximately (1.9,1.9) (b).

By expanding the graph near this second point we might get a better estimate. A TI-81 displays both the x- and y-values when tracing. On the Casio fx-7000G, use the $\boxed{X \leftrightarrow Y}$ feature to see both the x- and y-values.

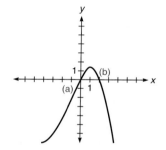

Method 2: A second method, which will obtain just the x-value, is to graph the difference of the two x-expressions, in this case $y = (2 \sin x) - (\frac{1}{2}x^2)$.

The points in which we are interested are zeros of this new function. The graph is shown in the figure, where we estimate the x-value of the point at (b) to be 1.9. Using Newton's method or bisection we can quickly find that $x \approx 1.933753763$.

The y-values can be found by evaluating either of the two equations $y = 2 \sin x$ or $y = \frac{1}{2}x^2$ for y using $x = 1.933753763$.

Doing this gives $y \approx 1.869701808$.   ■

The advantage of method 2 is that the x-values can be more accurately estimated, since they fall on the x-axis. They can also be accurately calculated using the methods cited earlier.

Verifying identities

An identity states that two expressions are equal for all values of x (for which each is defined) (chapter 5). If this is the case, then *each expression should have the same graph.*

■ *Example E*

Show that $\dfrac{\cos x}{\cos x + \sin x} = \dfrac{\cot x}{1 + \cot x}$ is probably an identity by graphing each member of the equation.

(This is an identity from section 5–1.)

Graph both $y = \dfrac{\cos x}{\cos x + \sin x}$ and $y = \dfrac{\cot x}{1 + \cot x}$. The figure is the graph of both, which indicates that it is probably an identity.

Note Most calculators and computers do not have the cotangent function built in. Thus, each instance of cot x must be replaced by $\dfrac{1}{\tan x}$ to graph the expression.

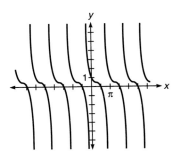

The fact that two graphs look the same is not *proof* that two expressions are identical. A graph is finite and constructed by a machine. For example, on a Casio fx-7000G the graphs of $y = \sin(6x)$ and $y = \sin(100x)$ are the same! This phenomenon is explored in the exercises.

Exercises for Appendix B

a. Graph the following equations for $0 \le x \le 4$.
b. Using the graph, estimate the value of all zeros of the equation for $0 \le x \le 4$.
c. Using the method of bisection or Newton's method find the value of each zero to at least six decimal places.

1. $y = \sin\left(\dfrac{x^2}{2}\right)$

2. $y = \sin(\sqrt{3x}) - \frac{1}{2}$

3. $y = \sin x - \sin 2x$

4. $y = \sin 3x + \sin 2x$

5. $y = 2 \sin x - \dfrac{x}{2}$

6. $y = \cos 3x + \sin 2x$

Solve the following systems of equations by (a) estimating the solutions from their graphs and then (b) using Newton's method or the method of bisection to find the value of each solution to at least six decimal places.

7. $y = \sin x;\ y = \dfrac{x}{2}$

8. $y = \sin 3x;\ y = \sqrt{x}$

9. $y = \cos \dfrac{x}{2};\ y = \dfrac{x}{2}$

10. $y = x;\ y = \sqrt{x}$

Show that the following are probably identities by graphing the left and right members and observing that the graphs look the same. Use $-2\pi \le x \le 2\pi$ for the domain of the graph.

11. $\csc \theta + \cot \theta = \dfrac{1 + \cos \theta}{\sin \theta}$

12. $\tan \theta + \sec \theta = \dfrac{1 + \sin \theta}{\cos \theta}$

13. $\dfrac{\csc \theta}{\sec \theta + \tan \theta} = \dfrac{\cos \theta}{\sin \theta + \sin^2 \theta}$

14. $\dfrac{\sec \theta}{\csc \theta + \cot \theta} = \dfrac{\tan \theta}{1 + \cos \theta}$

15. $\dfrac{1}{\sec \theta - \cos \theta} = \cot \theta \csc \theta$

16. $\dfrac{\cot \theta}{\sec \theta} = \csc \theta - \sin \theta$

17. Problems 7 through 19 in appendix A are problems for which a calculator is well suited. Do some of these problems. The results obtained with a calculator should be the same as the answers obtained in the method discussed in appendix A, addition of ordinates.

18. Do problem 20 in appendix A.

19. Do problem 21 in appendix A.

20. Do problem 22 in appendix A.

21. *Fourier series* are functions defined as a sum of an infinite number of terms of the form $a \sin(bx)$ or $a \cos(bx)$. They are used extensively in electronics, music, linguistics, and other areas to analyze wave forms. It turns out that any periodic wave form can be described by an appropriate Fourier series. The four examples in this problem describe "sawtooth" and square-wave forms.

   Graph an approximation to each of the following Fourier series by entering at least the first five terms into the calculator. Use the values $-\pi \le x \le \pi$ for the graphs. (As more and more terms are used the graphs become more accurate.)

   a. $f(x) = \sin x + \frac{1}{2}\sin(2x) + \frac{1}{3}\sin(3x) + \frac{1}{4}\sin(4x) + \cdots$.

   b. $f(x) = \sin x + \frac{1}{3}\sin(3x) + \frac{1}{5}\sin(5x) + \frac{1}{7}\sin(7x) + \cdots$.

   c. $f(x) = \frac{1}{2}\sin(2x) + \frac{1}{4}\sin(4x) + \frac{1}{6}\sin(6x) + \frac{1}{8}\sin(8x) + \cdots$.

   d. $f(x) = \sin x - \frac{1}{2}\sin(2x) + \frac{1}{3}\sin(3x) - \frac{1}{4}\sin(4x) + \cdots$.

22. As stated in this section, on a Casio graphing calculator the graphs of $y = \sin 6x$ and of $y = \sin 100x$ are the same. (At the range settings used for graphing the sine function: Xmin $= -6.2831853$, Xmax $= 6.2831853$.) The same phenomenon can occur with any graphing calculator or computer.

   To see why this sort of thing can happen, one must realize that the plotting area of most graphing devices is broken down into a grid of points, called pixels,[2] which are either darkened in or left light. The number of these pixels is insufficient for some purposes.

   By way of example, assume a situation where pixels represent 0.5 units. (Range settings for which this might occur in the TI-81 and the Casio *fx*-7000G are given below.) This situation is shown in figure B–3. To graph a function we compute values for the function for each value of the domain in increments of 0.5.

[2]Pixel means "picture element."

Table B–1 constructs a set of values for the two functions $y = \sin(x)$ and $y = \sin[(4\pi + 1)x]$, in x-increments of 0.5. These ordered pairs are plotted in figure B–3. Observe that the ordered pairs at the values of x shown have the same y-values, although for other values of x the two functions are not the same. The calculator can only darken complete 0.5 by 0.5 unit squares. When this is done we have the graph in figure B–4. We can see that *either function would produce the graph shown in figure B–4*.

x	$\sin(x)$	$\sin[(4\pi + 1)x]$
0	0.00	0.00
0.5	0.48	0.48
1	0.84	0.84
1.5	1.00	1.00
2	0.91	0.91
2.5	0.60	0.60
3	0.14	0.14
3.5	−0.35	−0.35
4	−0.76	−0.76
4.5	−0.98	−0.98
5	−0.96	−0.96
5.5	−0.71	−0.71
6	−0.28	−0.28
6.5	0.22	0.22

Table B–1

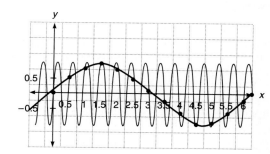

Figure B–3

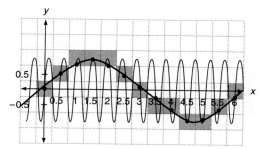

Figure B–4

To investigate this further, consider the following problems.

a. Make a table of values for the following four functions, letting x take on the values 0, 0.5, 1, 1.5, etc., up to 6.0. This is just an extension of table B–1, where the values for the first two functions are already done.

$$y = \sin(x)$$
$$y = \sin[(4\pi + 1)x]$$
$$y = \sin[(8\pi + 1)x]$$
$$y = \sin[(12\pi + 1)x]$$

Try to make a generalization from the results.

Note The four functions will give identical values for a given x, but this does not mean the functions are identical! Just reconsider figure B–3 to see that the first two functions are not identical.

b. Make a table of values for the following four functions, letting x take on the values 0, 0.25, 0.5, 0.75, etc., up to 3. This corresponds to a calculator display with pixels 0.25 units wide.

$$y = \sin(x)$$
$$y = \sin[(8\pi + 1)x]$$
$$y = \sin[(16\pi + 1)x]$$
$$y = \sin[(24\pi + 1)x]$$

Again, look for a pattern.

c. Make a table of values for the following four functions, letting x take on the values 0, 0.1, 0.2, 0.3, etc., up to 1.2. This corresponds to a calculator display 0.1 units wide.

$$\sin(x)$$
$$\sin[(20\pi + 1)x]$$
$$\sin[(40\pi + 1)x]$$
$$\sin[(60\pi + 1)x]$$

Try to find a pattern.

Note On a TI-81 the following settings create pixels of 0.1 units wide:

$$\text{Xmin} = -4.8, \text{Xmax} = 4.7, \text{Xres} = 1.$$

There are 96 pixels on this calculator, and

$$\frac{4.7 - (-4.8) + 0.1}{96} = 0.1.$$

For pixels 0.25 wide, find values so that

$$\frac{\text{Xmas} - \text{Xmin} + 0.25}{96} = 0.25. \text{ A similar}$$

calculation can be used to obtain pixels 0.5 units wide.

The Casio *fx*-7000G has 95 pixels, so the settings for creating pixels 0.1 units wide are Xmin = -4.7, Xmax = 4.7. Of course the division shown above then has the value 95 in the denominator.

d. Consider the results of the previous parts of this problem, and try to predict some values β so that $\sin(x)$ and $\sin(\beta x)$ have the same graph on a device that has pixels 0.01 units wide. (That is, that the functions $y = \sin x$ and $y = \sin(\beta x)$ have the same values for $x = 0, 0.01, 0.02, 0.03$, etc.)

e. Show why the generalizations of parts a, b, and c are true (use identities from section 5–2).

Program for the Casio *fx*-7000G calculator to calculate zeros of a function using the method of bisection. It is assumed the function to be solved is defined in program 9.

Generic program	Casio program	Casio key strokes/comments	
		MODE 2	Enter WRT (Program) mode.
Prepare the calculator to accept a program.		Use the ⇒ key to select Program 8.	Actually any program location will do.
		EXE	Ready to enter program 8.
Input the lower value L and the upper value U.	?→L:?→U	SHIFT → → ALPHA ˣ√ :	
		SHIFT → → ALPHA 1 EXE	

Generic program	Casio program	Casio key strokes/comments	
Let $x = L$. Compute $f(L)$. Store the result in A.	L→X:Prog 9:Y→A	ALPHA $^x\!\!\sqrt{}$ → ALPHA + : Prog 9 : ALPHA − → ALPHA x^{-1} EXE	
If $f(L) < 0$ then go to 1	A<0→Goto 1	ALPHA x^{-1} SHIFT 3 0 SHIFT 7 SHIFT Prog 1 EXE	

else
    switch the values
    in U and L.
	U→T:L→U:T→L	ALPHA 1 → ALPHA ÷ : ALPHA
		 $^x\!\!\sqrt{}$ → ALPHA 1 : ALPHA ÷ →
		 ALPHA $^x\!\!\sqrt{}$ EXE	

1:	Lbl 1	SHIFT ⇐ 1 EXE	
Let $X = \dfrac{L + U}{2}$	(L+U)÷2→X	(ALPHA $^x\!\!\sqrt{}$ + ALPHA 1) ÷ 2 → ALPHA + EXE	
Compute $f(x)$; store result in Y.	Prog 9	Prog 9 EXE	Assumes the equation to be solved will be in 9.
If $f(A) = 0$ then go to 3	Y=0→Goto 3	ALPHA − SHIFT 8 0 SHIFT 7 SHIFT Prog 3 EXE	
If $|U - L| \le$ error then go to 3	Abs (U−L)≤1 E−11 →Goto 3	SHIFT x^y (ALPHA 1 − ALPHA $^x\!\!\sqrt{}$) SHIFT 6 1 EXP (−) 1 1 SHIFT 7 SHIFT Prog 3 EXE	
If $Y > 0$ go to 2	Y>0→Goto 2	ALPHA − SHIFT 2 0 SHIFT 7 SHIFT Prog 2 EXE	

else
    let $L = x$
    go to 1
	X→L:Goto 1	ALPHA + → ALPHA $^x\!\!\sqrt{}$: SHIFT
		 Prog 1 EXE	

2:	Lbl 2	SHIFT ⇐ 2 EXE	
let $U = x$ go to 1	X→U:Goto 1	ALPHA + → ALPHA 1 : SHIFT Prog 1 EXE	
3:	Lbl 3	SHIFT ⇐ 3 EXE	
Display the final value, x.	X	ALPHA +	
Stop the program.		MODE 1	Go back to run mode.

Pascal language program that implements the method of bisection for finding approximations to zeros of functions.

```
program     BISECTION (input,output);
const       ERROR = 1.0E-6;                      { Practical smallest difference of
                                                   two real data values in Pascal. }

var         Lower, Upper, Average : real;
            Done : boolean;
{ ********** The function for which we want to approximate zeros. ********* }
function    F (x : real) : real;
            begin
                F := 2*sin(sqrt(2 * x)) − 0.5          { DEFINE FUNCTION HERE }
            end { F };
{ *********************************************************** }
procedure   Read_in (var L, U : real);
            begin
                Write('Enter Lower bound, then Upper bound: ');
                ReadLn(L, U);
            end { Read_in };
procedure   Interchange (var L, U : real);
            var temp : real;
            begin
                temp := L;
                L := U;
                U := temp
            end { Interchange };
begin    { BISECTION }
    Done := FALSE;
    Read_in(Lower, Upper);
    If F(Lower) > 0 then Interchange(Lower, Upper);
    While not Done do begin
        Average := (Lower + Upper) / 2;
        If (f(Average) = 0) or (abs(Upper–Lower) < ERROR) then
            Done := TRUE
        else { Average is not a zero and is not within ERROR units of a zero }
            If f(Average) < 0 then Lower := Average
            else { f(Average) > 0 } Upper := Average
    end { while };
    WriteLn(Average);
end { BISECTION }.
```

Appendix C

Development of the Identity
$\cos(\alpha + \beta) = \cos \alpha \cos \beta - \sin \alpha \sin \beta$

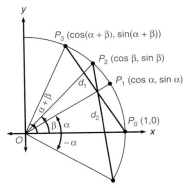

Figure C–1

A proof that this identity is true is beyond the scope of this text, but an argument for its correctness can be obtained in the following way.

Let α and β be two angles in standard position (see figure C.1). Let P_1 be the point where the terminal side of α intersects the unit circle, and P_2 be the point where angle β intersects the unit circle. Let P_3 be the point where the angle $\alpha + \beta$ (the sum of the angles α and β) intersects the circle. Let P_0 be the point $(1,0)$. Finally, let P_4 be the point where the terminal side of angle $-\alpha$ intersects the unit circle.

On the unit circle the x- and y-coordinates of a point are the cosine and sine values for the appropriate angle. Thus, the point P_1 has coordinates $(\cos \alpha, \sin \alpha)$. The coordinates for the other points are shown in the figure.

Angle $\alpha + \beta$, or angle P_0OP_3 in standard position, has the same measure as angle P_4OP_2. It is a geometric property that central angles of a circle having equal measure will have chords of equal length. Thus, the chords P_3P_0 and P_2P_4 have the same length. The length of a line segment with end points (x_1,y_1) and (x_2,y_2) is given by the distance formula

$$d = \sqrt{(x_2 - x_1)^2 + (y_2 - y_1)^2}$$

We apply this to the chords mentioned above.
Let $d_1 = $ length of P_3P_0, and $d_2 = $ length of P_2P_4.

$$d_1 = d_2$$
$$\sqrt{(\cos(\alpha + \beta) - 1)^2 + (\sin(\alpha + \beta) - 0)^2}$$
$$= \sqrt{(\cos \beta - \cos \alpha)^2 + (\sin \beta - (-\sin \alpha))^2}$$

We now square both sides.

$$[\cos(\alpha + \beta) - 1]^2 + [\sin(\alpha + \beta) - 0]^2 = (\cos \beta - \cos \alpha)^2 + [\sin \beta - (-\sin \alpha)]^2$$

Performing the indicated operations we obtain

$$\cos^2(\alpha + \beta) - 2 \cos(\alpha + \beta) + 1 + \sin^2(\alpha + \beta)$$
$$= \cos^2\beta - 2 \cos \alpha \cos \beta + \cos^2\alpha + \sin^2\beta + 2 \sin \alpha \sin \beta + \sin^2\alpha$$

Then

$$[\cos^2(\alpha + \beta) + \sin^2(\alpha + \beta)] - 2 \cos(\alpha + \beta) + 1$$
$$= (\cos^2\beta + \sin^2\beta) + (\cos^2\alpha + \sin^2\alpha) + 2 \sin \alpha \sin \beta - 2 \cos \alpha \cos \beta$$

Using the fundamental identity $\sin^2\theta + \cos^2\theta = 1$, we obtain

$$1 - 2 \cos(\alpha + \beta) + 1 = 1 + 1 + 2 \sin \alpha \sin \beta - 2 \cos \alpha \cos \beta$$
$$-2 \cos(\alpha + \beta) = 2 \sin \alpha \sin \beta - 2 \cos \alpha \cos \beta$$
$$\cos(\alpha + \beta) = \cos \alpha \cos \beta - \sin \alpha \sin \beta \qquad \text{Divide each member by } -2$$

Appendix D

Useful Templates

This appendix includes items that it might prove useful to reproduce in quantity and have handy. Note that rectangular coordinate graph paper and polar coordinate paper are both widely available in book stores.

The Unit Circle

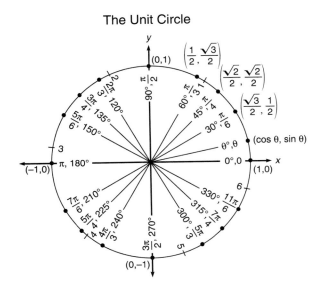

Reference Angles

$$0 < \theta < 360°$$
$$0 < \theta < 2\pi$$

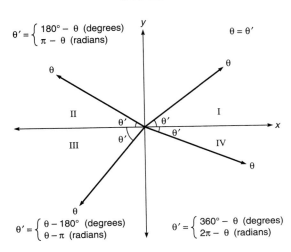

Templates Useful for Graphing Many Trigonometric Functions

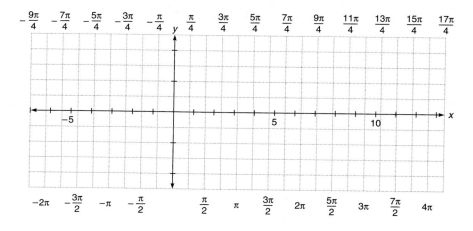

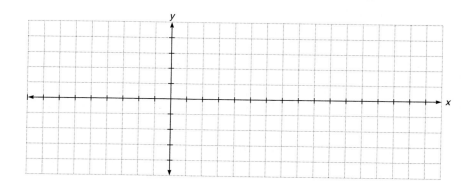

Rectangular Coordinates

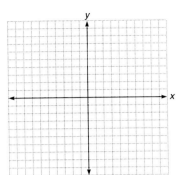
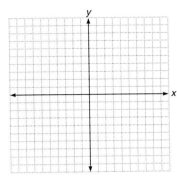

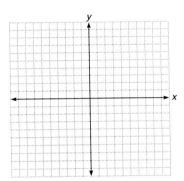
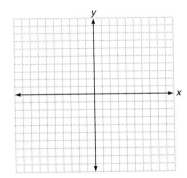

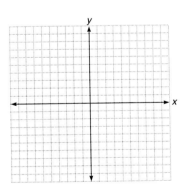
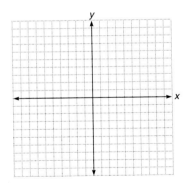

Polar Coordinates

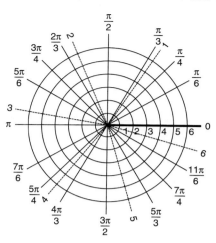
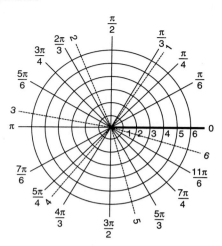

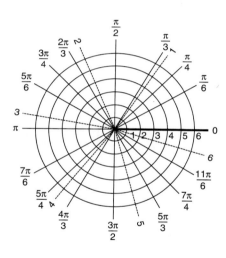
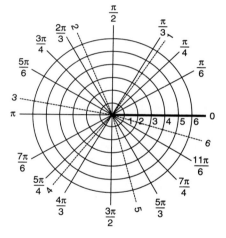

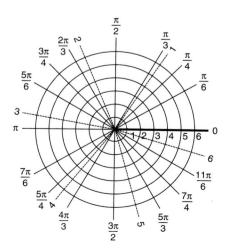
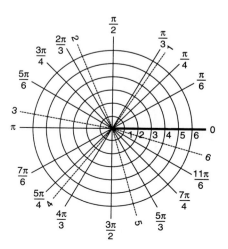

Appendix E

Answers and Solutions

Chapter 1

Exercise 1–1

Answers to odd-numbered problems

1. 13.417°, acute   **3.** 0.2°, acute
5. 25.555°, acute   **7.** 165.783°, obtuse
9. 33.099°, acute   **11.** 159.983°, obtuse

13.

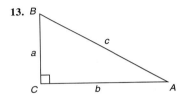

15. 48.2°   **17.** 71°48′   **19.** 106°
21. right triangle, hypotenuse = 0.5
23. right triangle, hypotenuse = $2\sqrt{5}$
25. right triangle, hypotenuse = 2.57
27. $c = 15$ **29.** $a = 6$
31. $b = 6\sqrt{5} \approx 13$ **33.** $c = \sqrt{14} \approx 4$
35. $c = 50\sqrt{13} \approx 180$ **37.** $c = 4$
39. $b = \sqrt{185.31} \approx 13.6$
41. $c = 7\sqrt{2} \approx 9.9$ **43.** $a = 3\sqrt{47} \approx 21$
45. $c = \sqrt{2} \approx 1$ **47.** 61 ft   **49.** 90.1 ft
51. 20.07 ohms   **53.** 3,770 ohms
55. Not accurate, measurements do not satisfy Pythagorean theorem
57. 23 minutes   **59.** no, 1.1 ft
61. 107 knots   **63.** 17 knots
65. 27 units

Solutions to trial exercise problems

6. $87°2′13″ = \left(87 + \dfrac{2}{60} + \dfrac{13}{3,600}\right)°$
$= (87 + 0.0333 + 0.0036)°$
$= 87.037°$
This angle is acute since it is less than 90°.

18.
$$
\begin{array}{rr}
28° & 17′ \\
+ \; 28° & 52′ \\
\hline
56° & 69′ \\
56° \; 60′ & + \; 9′ \\
57° & 9′
\end{array}
$$

$$
\begin{array}{rr}
180° & \\
- \; 57° & 9′ \\
\hline
179° & 60′ \\
- \; 57° & 9′ \\
\hline
122° & 51′
\end{array}
$$
The angle is 122°51′.

20.
$$
\begin{array}{rrr}
90° & & \\
-72° & 19′ & 51″ \\
\hline
89° & 60′ & \\
-72° & 19′ & 51″ \\
\hline
89° & 59′ & 60″ \\
-72° & 19′ & 51″ \\
\hline
17° & 40′ & 9″
\end{array}
$$

23. $(2\sqrt{5})^2 = 2^2(\sqrt{5})^2 = 4(5) = 20$;
$2^2 + 4^2 = 4 + 16 = 20$.
Since $(2\sqrt{5})^2 = 2^2 + 4^2$, the triangle is a right triangle; the hypotenuse is the longest side, with length $2\sqrt{5}$.

29. $a^2 + b^2 = c^2$, so $a^2 + 8^2 = 10^2$
$$
\begin{aligned}
a^2 + 64 &= 100 \\
a^2 &= 36 \\
a &= 6
\end{aligned}
$$

41. $c^2 = a^2 + b^2$
$c^2 = (3\sqrt{2})^2 + (4\sqrt{5})^2$
$= 9(2) + 16(5) = 98$
$c = \sqrt{98} = \sqrt{2 \cdot 49} = 7\sqrt{2}$

54. The sum of the angles is 110°0′ + 33°28′ + 28°32′ = 172°. Since the sum of the angles of a triangle is 180°, we can see that there is quite a bit of inaccuracy in these measurements. Although in practice we would not expect the three measurements to add exactly to 180° (they are approximations, as are any measurements), an error of 8° out of 180° (more than 4% error) probably indicates an error in a measurement.

---

57. The diagonal is $\sqrt{15^2 + 10.5^2} \approx 18.31$ inches. (See the diagram.) Divide 18.31 inches by 0.8 inch per minute to get 23 minutes.

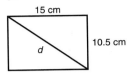

61. The headings of the aircraft and the wind form the wind triangle shown.

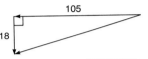

Ground speed = $\sqrt{105^2 + 18^2} \approx 107$ knots

Exercise 1–2

Answers to odd-numbered problems

1.

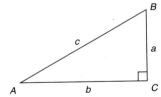

$\sin A = \dfrac{a}{c}$, $\cos A = \dfrac{b}{c}$, $\tan A = \dfrac{a}{b}$,
$\cot A = \dfrac{b}{a}$, $\sec A = \dfrac{c}{b}$, $\csc A = \dfrac{c}{a}$,
$\sin B = \dfrac{b}{c}$, $\cos B = \dfrac{a}{c}$, $\tan B = \dfrac{b}{a}$,
$\cot B = \dfrac{a}{b}$, $\sec B = \dfrac{c}{a}$, $\csc B = \dfrac{c}{b}$

3. $c = 5$, $\sin B = \frac{4}{5}$, $\cos B = \frac{3}{5}$, $\tan B = \frac{4}{3}$, $\csc B = \frac{5}{4}$, $\sec B = \frac{5}{3}$, $\cot B = \frac{3}{4}$

5. $c = \sqrt{10}$, $\sin B = \frac{3\sqrt{10}}{10}$, $\cos B = \frac{\sqrt{10}}{10}$, $\tan B = 3$, $\csc B = \frac{\sqrt{10}}{3}$, $\sec B = \sqrt{10}$, $\cot B = \frac{1}{3}$ **7.** $c = 4\sqrt{2}$, $\sin B = \frac{\sqrt{14}}{8}$, $\cos B = \frac{5\sqrt{2}}{8}$, $\tan B = \frac{\sqrt{7}}{5}$, $\csc B = \frac{4\sqrt{14}}{7}$, $\sec B = \frac{4\sqrt{2}}{5}$, $\cot B = \frac{5\sqrt{7}}{7}$

9. $b = 1$, $\sin B = \frac{\sqrt{5}}{5}$, $\cos B = \frac{2\sqrt{5}}{5}$, $\tan B = \frac{1}{2}$, $\csc B = \sqrt{5}$, $\sec B = \frac{\sqrt{5}}{2}$, $\cot B = 2$

11. $c = \sqrt{313}$, $\sin B = \frac{13\sqrt{313}}{313}$, $\cos B = \frac{12\sqrt{313}}{313}$, $\tan B = \frac{13}{12}$, $\csc B = \frac{\sqrt{313}}{13}$, $\sec B = \frac{\sqrt{313}}{12}$, $\cot B = \frac{12}{13}$

13. $b = 8$, $\sin A = \frac{3}{5}$, $\cos A = \frac{4}{5}$, $\tan A = \frac{3}{4}$, $\csc A = \frac{5}{3}$, $\sec A = \frac{5}{4}$, $\cot A = \frac{4}{3}$

15. $c = \sqrt{19}$, $\sin A = \frac{\sqrt{57}}{19}$, $\cos A = \frac{4\sqrt{19}}{19}$, $\tan A = \frac{\sqrt{3}}{4}$, $\csc A = \frac{\sqrt{57}}{3}$, $\sec A = \frac{\sqrt{19}}{4}$, $\cot A = \frac{4\sqrt{3}}{3}$

17. $b = \sqrt{z^2 - x^2}$, $\sin B = \frac{\sqrt{z^2 - x^2}}{z}$, $\cos B = \frac{x}{z}$, $\tan B = \frac{\sqrt{z^2 - x^2}}{x}$, $\csc B = \frac{z}{\sqrt{z^2 - x^2}}$, $\sec B = \frac{z}{x}$, $\cot B = \frac{x}{\sqrt{z^2 - x^2}}$

19. $b = \sqrt{3}$, $\sin B = \frac{\sqrt{3}}{2}$, $\cos B = \frac{1}{2}$, $\tan B = \sqrt{3}$, $\csc B = \frac{2\sqrt{3}}{3}$, $\sec B = 2$, $\cot B = \frac{\sqrt{3}}{3}$

21. $c = \sqrt{106}$, $\sin B = \frac{5\sqrt{106}}{106}$, $\cos B = \frac{9\sqrt{106}}{106}$, $\tan B = \frac{5}{9}$, $\csc B = \frac{\sqrt{106}}{5}$, $\sec B = \frac{\sqrt{106}}{9}$, $\cot B = \frac{9}{5}$

23. $\cos A = \frac{3}{5}$, $\tan A = \frac{4}{3}$, $\cot A = \frac{3}{4}$, $\sec A = \frac{5}{3}$, $\csc A = \frac{5}{4}$

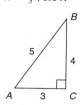

25. $\sin A = \frac{\sqrt{3}}{2}$, $\tan A = \sqrt{3}$, $\cot A = \frac{\sqrt{3}}{3}$, $\sec A = 2$, $\csc A = \frac{2\sqrt{3}}{3}$

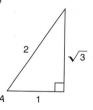

27. $\sin A = \frac{2\sqrt{2}}{3}$, $\cos A = \frac{1}{3}$, $\tan A = 2\sqrt{2}$, $\cot A = \frac{\sqrt{2}}{4}$, $\csc A = \frac{3\sqrt{2}}{4}$

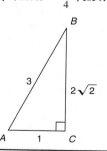

29. $\cos A = \frac{12}{13}$, $\tan A = \frac{5}{12}$, $\cot A = \frac{12}{5}$, $\sec A = \frac{13}{12}$, $\csc A = \frac{13}{5}$

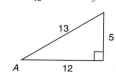

31. $\sin A = \frac{\sqrt{19}}{10}$, $\tan A = \frac{\sqrt{19}}{9}$, $\cot A = \frac{9\sqrt{19}}{19}$, $\sec A = \frac{10}{9}$, $\csc A = \frac{10\sqrt{19}}{19}$

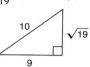

33. $\left(\frac{b}{c}\right)^2 + \left(\frac{a}{c}\right)^2$

$\frac{b^2}{c^2} + \frac{a^2}{c^2}$

$\frac{b^2 + a^2}{c^2}$

$\frac{c^2}{c^2} = 1$

35. 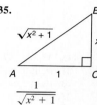 $\frac{1}{\sqrt{x^2 + 1}}$

37.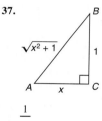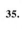

$\frac{1}{x}$

Solutions to trial exercise problems

15. $a = \sqrt{3}$, $b = 4$. Find ratios for angle A.

$c^2 = a^2 + b^2$

$c^2 = (\sqrt{3})^2 + 4^2$

$c^2 = 3 + 16 = 19$

$c = \sqrt{19}$

$\sin A = \frac{a}{c} = \frac{\sqrt{3}}{\sqrt{19}} = \frac{\sqrt{3}}{\sqrt{19}} \cdot \frac{\sqrt{19}}{\sqrt{19}} = \frac{\sqrt{57}}{19}$;

$\cos A = \frac{b}{c} = \frac{4}{\sqrt{19}} = \frac{4}{\sqrt{19}} \cdot \frac{\sqrt{19}}{\sqrt{19}} = \frac{4\sqrt{19}}{19}$;

$\tan A = \frac{a}{b} = \frac{\sqrt{3}}{4}$; $\csc A = \frac{1}{\sin A} = \frac{1}{\frac{\sqrt{3}}{\sqrt{19}}} = \frac{\sqrt{19}}{\sqrt{3}}$

$= \frac{\sqrt{19}}{\sqrt{3}} \cdot \frac{\sqrt{3}}{\sqrt{3}} = \frac{\sqrt{57}}{3}$; $\sec A = \frac{1}{\cos A} = \frac{1}{\frac{4}{\sqrt{19}}} = \frac{\sqrt{19}}{4}$;

$\cot A = \frac{1}{\tan A} = \frac{1}{\frac{\sqrt{3}}{4}} = \frac{4}{\sqrt{3}} = \frac{4}{\sqrt{3}} \cdot \frac{\sqrt{3}}{\sqrt{3}} = \frac{4\sqrt{3}}{3}$

19. $a = 1$, $c = 2$. Find ratios for angle B.

$a^2 + b^2 = c^2$, so

$1 + b^2 = 4$

$b^2 = 3$

$b = \sqrt{3}$

$\sin B = \dfrac{\text{opp}}{\text{hyp}} = \dfrac{b}{c} = \dfrac{\sqrt{3}}{2}$;

$\cos B = \dfrac{\text{adj}}{\text{hyp}} = \dfrac{a}{c} = \dfrac{1}{2}$;

$\tan B = \dfrac{\text{opp}}{\text{adj}} = \dfrac{b}{a} = \dfrac{\sqrt{3}}{1} = \sqrt{3}$;

$\cot B = \dfrac{1}{\tan B} = \dfrac{1}{\sqrt{3}} = \dfrac{\sqrt{3}}{3}$;

$\sec B = \dfrac{1}{\cos B} = \dfrac{1}{\frac{1}{2}} = 2$;

$\csc B = \dfrac{1}{\sin B} = \dfrac{1}{\frac{\sqrt{3}}{2}} = \dfrac{2\sqrt{3}}{3}$

31. $\cos A = 0.9$

$\cos A = \dfrac{9}{10} = \dfrac{b}{c}$, so a triangle in which $b = 9$ and $c = 10$ would work. This is shown in the diagram.

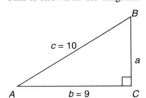

Using the Pythagorean theorem, we find a.

$c^2 = a^2 + b^2$

$100 = a^2 + 81$

$\sqrt{19} = a$

With this we can now compute the five remaining ratios.

$\sin A = \dfrac{a}{c} = \dfrac{\sqrt{19}}{10}$;

$\tan A = \dfrac{a}{b} = \dfrac{\sqrt{19}}{9}$;

$\cot A = \dfrac{1}{\tan A} = \dfrac{9\sqrt{19}}{19}$;

$\csc A = \dfrac{1}{\sin A} = \dfrac{1}{\frac{\sqrt{19}}{10}} = \dfrac{10\sqrt{19}}{19}$;

$\sec A = \dfrac{1}{\cos A} = \dfrac{1}{\frac{9}{10}} = \dfrac{10}{9}$

37. $\tan B = x$; if we think of x as $\dfrac{x}{1}$ we can use the triangle shown in the diagram, since $\tan B = \dfrac{b}{a} = \dfrac{x}{1}$.

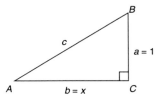

From the Pythagorean theorem we find c.

$c^2 = a^2 + b^2$

$c^2 = 1^2 + x^2$ so

$c = \sqrt{x^2 + 1}$

Now we find $\tan A$:

$\tan A = \dfrac{a}{b} = \dfrac{1}{x}$. (Note that we did not actually need c.)

Exercise 1–3

Answers to odd-numbered problems

1. 0.5192   **3.** 0.2116   **5.** 1.8137

7. 0.6465   **9.** 2.5048   **11.** 0.9793

13. 0.9801   **15.** 0.0790   **17.** 0.7037

19. 0.5534   **21.** 0.7447   **23.** 15.7801

25. 971.40   **27.** 0.47   **29.** 742.5 watts

31. 11.8 inches

33. $c^2 = 1^2 + 1^2$

$= 1 + 1$

$= 2$

$c = \sqrt{2}$

$\sin 45° = \dfrac{1}{\sqrt{2}} = \dfrac{\sqrt{2}}{2}$

$\cos 45° = \dfrac{1}{\sqrt{2}} = \dfrac{\sqrt{2}}{2}$

$\tan 45° = \dfrac{1}{1} = 1$

35. 53.2°   **37.** 62.0°   **39.** 31.6°

41. 31.7°   **43.** 63.4°   **45.** 78.00°

47. 68.63°   **49.** $A = 51.7°$, $b \approx 12.0$, $c \approx 19.4$ **51.** $B = 76.3°$, $b \approx 45.5$, $c \approx 46.9$ **53.** $B = 60.6°$, $a \approx 0.379$, $c \approx 0.771$ **55.** $A = 12°$, $a \approx 4.6$, $c \approx 22.3$ **57.** $B = 75°$, $a \approx 2.6$, $b \approx 9.7$

59. $A = 24.5°$, $a \approx 51$, $b \approx 111$

61. $c \approx 20.4$, $A \approx 40.0°$, $B \approx 50.0°$

63. $c \approx 1.36$, $A \approx 9.3°$, $B \approx 80.7°$

65. $b \approx 17.8$, $A \approx 44.9°$, $B \approx 45.1°$

67. $a \approx 98.4$, $A \approx 62.5°$, $B \approx 27.5°$

69. $b \approx 5$, $A \approx 67.4°$, $B \approx 22.6°$

71. $a \approx 32.6$, $A \approx 21.2°$, $B \approx 68.8°$

73. 55.1 ohms   **75.** 34°   **77.** 18.6 volts

79. 32,800 ft   **81.** 217 mm

83. 2.3°   **85.** 265.8

87. $A = 30°$, $a = \dfrac{8\sqrt{3}}{3}$, $c = \dfrac{16\sqrt{3}}{3}$

Solutions to trial exercise problems

9. $\sec 66.47° = \dfrac{1}{\cos 66.47°}$

66.47 $\boxed{\cos}$ $\boxed{1/x}$

$\boxed{\text{TI-81}}$ $\boxed{(}$ $\boxed{\text{COS}}$ 66.47 $\boxed{)}$ $\boxed{x^{-1}}$ $\boxed{\text{ENTER}}$

≈ 2.5048 Display: $\boxed{2.50482689}$

Make sure calculator is in degree mode.

11. $\sin 78.33°$

78.33 $\boxed{\sin}$

$\boxed{\text{TI-81}}$ $\boxed{\text{SIN}}$ 78.33 $\boxed{\text{ENTER}}$

≈ 0.9793 Display: $\boxed{0.9793288556}$

Make sure calculator is in degree mode.

13. $\sin 78°33'$

Ⓐ 78 $\boxed{+}$ 33 $\boxed{\div}$ 60 $\boxed{=}$ $\boxed{\sin}$

Ⓟ 78 $\boxed{\text{ENTER}}$ 33 $\boxed{\text{ENTER}}$ 60 $\boxed{\div}$ $\boxed{+}$ $\boxed{\sin}$

$\boxed{\text{TI-81}}$ $\boxed{\text{SIN}}$ $\boxed{(}$ 78 $\boxed{+}$ 33 $\boxed{\div}$ 60 $\boxed{)}$ $\boxed{\text{ENTER}}$

≈ 0.9801 Display: $\boxed{0.9800983128}$

Make sure calculator is in degree mode.

25. $R = \dfrac{LC}{2 \sin I}$, $LC = 611.1$ meters, $I = 18°20'$.

$$R = \frac{611.1}{2 \sin 18°20'} \approx \frac{611.1}{2(0.3145)} \approx \frac{611.1}{0.6290} \approx 971.40$$

27. $y = x \cos A \cos B - x^2 \cos A \sin B - x^3 \sin A$
   $= 1.2 \cos 10° \cos 15° - 1.2^2 \cos 10° \sin 15° - 1.2^3 \sin 10°$
   ≈ 0.47 (to two decimal places)

Ⓐ   1.2 $\boxed{\times}$ 10 $\boxed{\text{COS}}$ $\boxed{\times}$ 15 $\boxed{\text{COS}}$ $\boxed{-}$

     1.2 $\boxed{x^2}$ $\boxed{\times}$ 10 $\boxed{\text{COS}}$ $\boxed{\times}$ 15 $\boxed{\text{SIN}}$ $\boxed{-}$

     1.2 $\boxed{y^x}$ 3 $\boxed{\times}$ 10 $\boxed{\text{SIN}}$ $\boxed{=}$

Ⓟ   1.2 $\boxed{\text{ENTER}}$ 10 $\boxed{\text{COS}}$ $\boxed{\times}$ 15 $\boxed{\text{COS}}$ $\boxed{\times}$

     1.2 $\boxed{x^2}$ 10 $\boxed{\text{COS}}$ $\boxed{\times}$ 15 $\boxed{\text{SIN}}$ $\boxed{\times}$ $\boxed{-}$

     1.2 $\boxed{\text{ENTER}}$ 3 $\boxed{y^x}$ 10 $\boxed{\text{SIN}}$ $\boxed{\times}$ $\boxed{-}$

$\boxed{\text{TI-81}}$ 1.2 $\boxed{\text{STO}\blacktriangleright}$ $\boxed{\text{X}|\text{T}}$ $\boxed{\text{ENTER}}$ 10 $\boxed{\text{STO}\blacktriangleright}$
     $\boxed{\text{MATH}}$ $\boxed{\text{ENTER}}$ 15 $\boxed{\text{STO}\blacktriangleright}$ $\boxed{\text{MATRX}}$
     $\boxed{\text{ENTER}}$ $\boxed{\text{X}|\text{T}}$ $\boxed{\text{COS}}$ $\boxed{\text{ALPHA}}$
     $\boxed{\text{MATH}}$ $\boxed{\text{COS}}$ $\boxed{\text{ALPHA}}$ $\boxed{\text{MATRX}}$
     $\boxed{-}$ $\boxed{\text{X}|\text{T}}$ $\boxed{x^2}$ $\boxed{\text{COS}}$ $\boxed{\text{ALPHA}}$
     $\boxed{\text{MATH}}$ $\boxed{\text{SIN}}$ $\boxed{\text{ALPHA}}$ $\boxed{\text{MATRX}}$ $\boxed{-}$
     $\boxed{\text{X}|\text{T}}$ $\boxed{\text{MATH}}$ 3 $\boxed{\text{SIN}}$ $\boxed{\text{ALPHA}}$ $\boxed{\text{MATH}}$
     $\boxed{\text{ENTER}}$

31. $r = \dfrac{f}{2 \cos \theta} = \dfrac{21.4}{2 \cos 25°} \approx \dfrac{21.4}{1.8126} \approx 11.8$ inches

47. $\sec \theta = \dfrac{6.45}{2.35}$

$\cos \theta = \dfrac{2.35}{6.45}$

$\theta = \cos^{-1} \dfrac{2.35}{6.45}$

$\theta \approx 68.63°$ Display: $\boxed{68.6329624}$

     2.35 $\boxed{\div}$ 6.45 $\boxed{=}$ $\boxed{\cos^{-1}}$

$\boxed{\text{TI-81}}$ $\boxed{\text{COS}^{-1}}$ $\boxed{(\!(}$ 2.35 $\boxed{\div}$ 6.45 $\boxed{)}$ $\boxed{\text{ENTER}}$
Make sure calculator is in degree mode.
Remember, $\boxed{\cos^{-1}}$ is $\boxed{\text{SHIFT}}$ $\boxed{\cos}$ or $\boxed{\text{2nd}}$ $\boxed{\cos}$
on most calculators.

48. $\sin \theta = \dfrac{1}{\sqrt{10.8}}$

$\theta = \sin^{-1} \dfrac{1}{\sqrt{10.8}}$

$\theta \approx 17.72°$ Display: $\boxed{17.71547234}$

     10.8 $\boxed{\sqrt{x}}$ $\boxed{1/x}$ $\boxed{\sin^{-1}}$

$\boxed{\text{TI-81}}$ $\boxed{\text{SIN}^{-1}}$ $\boxed{(\!(}$ $\boxed{\sqrt{}}$ 10.8 $\boxed{)}$ $\boxed{x^{-1}}$
$\boxed{\text{ENTER}}$
Make sure calculator is in degree mode.
Remember, $\boxed{\sin^{-1}}$ is $\boxed{\text{SHIFT}}$ $\boxed{\sin}$ or $\boxed{\text{2nd}}$ $\boxed{\sin}$ on
most calculators.

49. $a = 15.2$, $B = 38.3°$
   $A = 90° - 38.3° = 51.7°$

Using angle B: $\sin B = \dfrac{b}{c}$, $\cos B = \dfrac{a}{c}$, $\tan B = \dfrac{b}{a}$

$\sin 38.3° = \dfrac{b}{c}$, $\cos 38.3° = \dfrac{15.2}{c}$, $\tan 38.3° = \dfrac{b}{15.2}$

Use the cosine and tangent ratios:

$\cos 38.3° = \dfrac{15.2}{c}$, $\tan 38.3° = \dfrac{b}{15.2}$; $c = \dfrac{15.2}{\cos 38.3°}$,

$15.2(\tan 38.3°) = b$; $c \approx 19.4$, $12.0 \approx b$

59. $c = 122$, $B = 65.5°$
   $A = 90° - 65.5° = 24.5°$

$\sin 65.5° = \dfrac{b}{122}$; $\cos 65.5° = \dfrac{a}{122}$; $\tan 65.5° = \dfrac{b}{a}$

$b = 122 \sin 65.5° \approx 111$; $a = 122 \cos 65.5° \approx 51$

67. $b = 51.3$, $c = 111.0$
   $c^2 = a^2 + b^2$; $111^2 = a^2 + 51.3^2$; $a \approx 98.4$

$\sin A = \dfrac{a}{111.0}$; $\cos A = \dfrac{51.3}{111.0}$; $\tan A = \dfrac{51.3}{a}$

Using $\cos A = \dfrac{51.3}{111.0}$, we find $A \approx 62.5°$

$B = 90° - 62.5° \approx 27.5°$

76. Construct a line perpendicular to one side b, as shown. Since $b = 8.25''$, half that is $4.125''$.

Since $\theta = \dfrac{360°}{7}$, $\dfrac{\theta}{2} = \dfrac{1}{2} \cdot \dfrac{360°}{7} = \dfrac{180°}{7}$.

$\sin \dfrac{\theta}{2} = \dfrac{\text{opp}}{\text{hyp}} = \dfrac{4.125}{a}$

$\sin \dfrac{180°}{7} = \dfrac{4.125}{a}$

$a = \dfrac{4.125}{\sin \dfrac{180°}{7}} \approx 9.51$

     4.125 $\boxed{\div}$ $\boxed{(\!(}$ 180 $\boxed{\div}$ 7 $\boxed{)}$ $\boxed{\sin}$ $\boxed{=}$
     Display: $\boxed{9.507155093}$

$\boxed{\text{TI-81}}$ 4.125 $\boxed{\div}$ $\boxed{\text{SIN}}$ $\boxed{(\!(}$ 180 $\boxed{\div}$ 7 $\boxed{)}$
     $\boxed{\text{ENTER}}$

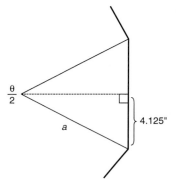

87. $B = 60°$, $b = 8$

$A = 90° - 60° = 30°$

$\sin 60° = \dfrac{8}{c}$, so $c = \dfrac{8}{\sin 60°} = \dfrac{8}{\dfrac{\sqrt{3}}{2}} = \dfrac{8}{1} \cdot \dfrac{2}{\sqrt{3}} = \dfrac{16\sqrt{3}}{3}$

$\tan 60° = \dfrac{8}{a}$, so $a = \dfrac{8}{\tan 60°} = \dfrac{8}{\sqrt{3}} = \dfrac{8\sqrt{3}}{3}$

Exercise 1–4

Answers to odd-numbered problems

1. $\tan \theta \cot \theta$

$\dfrac{1}{\cot \theta} \cot \theta$

1

3. $\cos \theta (1 - \sec \theta)$

$\cos \theta \left(1 - \dfrac{1}{\cos \theta}\right)$

$\cos \theta - \dfrac{\cos \theta}{\cos \theta}$

$\cos \theta - 1$

5. $\sec \theta (\cot \theta + \cos \theta - 1)$

$\sec \theta \cot \theta + \sec \theta \cos \theta - \sec \theta$

$\dfrac{1}{\cos \theta} \dfrac{\cos \theta}{\sin \theta} + \dfrac{1}{\cos \theta} \cos \theta - \sec \theta$

$\dfrac{1}{\sin \theta} + 1 - \sec \theta$

$\csc \theta + 1 - \sec \theta$

7. $\dfrac{\cos \alpha - \sin \alpha}{\cos \alpha}$

$\dfrac{\cos \alpha}{\cos \alpha} - \dfrac{\sin \alpha}{\cos \alpha}$

$1 - \tan \alpha$

9. $1 - \cos^2\theta$

$\sin^2\theta + \cos^2\theta - \cos^2\theta$

$\sin^2\theta$

11. $\cos \beta (\sec \beta - \cos \beta)$

$\cos \beta \sec \beta - \cos^2\beta$

$\cos \beta \dfrac{1}{\cos \beta} - \cos^2\beta$

$1 - \cos^2\beta$

$\sin^2\beta + \cos^2\beta - \cos^2\beta$

$\sin^2\beta$

13. $(\cos \theta + \sin \theta)(\cos \theta - \sin \theta) + 2 \sin^2\theta$

$\cos^2\theta + \cos \theta \sin \theta - \cos \theta \sin \theta - \sin^2\theta + 2 \sin^2\theta$

$\cos^2\theta + \sin^2\theta$

1

15. a. $\sin^2 16°50' + \cos^2 16°50'$

$\sin^2 16.83° + \cos^2 16.83°$

$0.0838 + 0.9162$

1

b. $\sin^2 50° + \cos^2 50°$

$0.5868 + 0.4132$

1

17. $\tan 32°40' \approx 0.6412$

$\dfrac{\sin 32°40'}{\cos 32°40'} \approx \dfrac{0.5398}{0.8418} \approx 0.6412$

19. $\tan x (\cot x + \csc x) = 1 + \sec x$

$\tan x \cdot \cot x + \tan x \cdot \csc x$

$\tan x \cdot \dfrac{1}{\tan x} + \dfrac{\sin x}{\cos x} \cdot \dfrac{1}{\sin x}$

$1 + \dfrac{1}{\cos x}$

$1 + \sec x$

21. $\sin \beta (\cot \beta - \csc \beta + \sin \beta) = \cos \beta - \cos^2\beta$

$\sin \beta \cdot \cot \beta - \sin \beta \cdot \csc \beta + \sin \beta \cdot \sin \beta$

$\sin \beta \cdot \dfrac{\cos \beta}{\sin \beta} - \sin \beta \cdot \dfrac{1}{\sin \beta} + \sin^2\beta$

$\cos \beta - 1 + \sin^2\beta$

$\cos \beta - (\cos^2\beta + \sin^2\beta) + \sin^2\beta$

$\cos \beta - \cos^2\beta$

23. $\cos \alpha (\csc \alpha + \sec \alpha) = \cot \alpha + 1$

$\cos \alpha \cdot \csc \alpha + \cos \alpha \cdot \sec \alpha$

$\cos \alpha \cdot \dfrac{1}{\sin \alpha} + \cos \alpha \cdot \dfrac{1}{\cos \alpha}$

$\dfrac{\cos \alpha}{\sin \alpha} + 1$

$\cot \alpha + 1$

25. 60° **27.** 60° **29.** 11.5° **31.** 77.5° **33.** 33.1°

35. 10° **37.** 30° **39.** 6.5° **41.** 15°

43. 25.3°

45. $\sin B = \dfrac{b}{c}$, $\cos B = \dfrac{a}{c}$, $\tan B = \dfrac{b}{a}$

$\dfrac{b}{a} = \tan B = \dfrac{\sin B}{\cos B} = \dfrac{\dfrac{b}{c}}{\dfrac{a}{c}} = \dfrac{b}{c} \cdot$

$\dfrac{c}{a} = \dfrac{b}{a}$

Solutions to trial exercise problems

8. $\dfrac{\sin \theta + \cos \theta - 2}{\cos \theta} = \dfrac{\sin \theta}{\cos \theta} + \dfrac{\cos \theta}{\cos \theta} - \dfrac{2}{\cos \theta}$

$= \tan \theta + 1 - 2 \sec \theta.$

26. $\sqrt{3} \tan x = 1$

$\tan x = \dfrac{1}{\sqrt{3}}$

$\tan x = \dfrac{\sqrt{3}}{3}$

$x = \tan^{-1} \dfrac{\sqrt{3}}{3}$

$x = 30°$, since $\tan 30° = \dfrac{\sqrt{3}}{3}$

42. $3 \sin 2x = 0.75$

$\sin 2x = 0.25$

$2x = \sin^{-1} 0.25$

$x = \dfrac{\sin^{-1} 0.25}{2}$

$x \approx 7.2°$

0.25 $\boxed{\sin^{-1}}$ $\boxed{\div}$ 2 $\boxed{=}$

Display: $\boxed{7.238756093}$

$\boxed{\text{TI-81}}$ $\boxed{\text{SIN}^{-1}}$ .25 $\boxed{\div}$ 2 $\boxed{\text{ENTER}}$

Chapter 1 review

1. 17.57°, acute **2.** 84.15°, acute

3. 125.62°, obtuse **4.** 39.76°, acute

5. 59°56′52″ **6.** 61.3°

7. $4\sqrt{13} \approx 14.4$ **8.** $\sqrt{595} \approx 24.4$

9. $\sqrt{105} \approx 10.2$ **10.** 52 ft

11. 40.0 ohms **12.** $c = \sqrt{58}$, $\sin A =$

$\dfrac{3\sqrt{58}}{58} \approx 0.3939$, $\cos A = \dfrac{7\sqrt{58}}{58} \approx 0.9191$,

$\tan A = \dfrac{3}{7} \approx 0.4286$, $\csc A = \dfrac{\sqrt{58}}{3}$

≈ 2.5386, $\sec A = \dfrac{\sqrt{58}}{7} \approx 1.0880$,

$\cot A = \dfrac{7}{3} \approx 2.3333$ **13.** $b = 10\sqrt{2}$,

$\cos B = \dfrac{1}{3} \approx 0.333$, $\sin B = \dfrac{2\sqrt{2}}{3} \approx 0.9428$,

$\cot B = \dfrac{\sqrt{2}}{4} \approx 0.3536$, $\sec B = 3$, $\csc B =$

$\dfrac{3\sqrt{2}}{4} \approx 1.0607$, $\tan B = 2\sqrt{2} \approx 2.8284$

14. $c = \sqrt{14}$, $\sin A = \dfrac{\sqrt{14}}{7} \approx 0.5345$, $\cos A$

$= \dfrac{\sqrt{35}}{7} \approx 0.8452$, $\tan A = \dfrac{\sqrt{10}}{5} \approx 0.6325$,

$\csc A = \dfrac{\sqrt{14}}{2} \approx 1.8708$, $\sec A = \dfrac{\sqrt{35}}{5} \approx$

1.1832, $\cot A = \dfrac{\sqrt{10}}{2} \approx 1.5811$

15. $\frac{3}{5}$ **16.** $\frac{5\sqrt{26}}{26}$

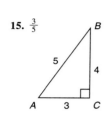
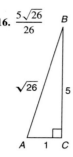

47. csc θ(sin θ − tan θ)

csc θ sin θ − csc θ tan θ

$\frac{1}{\sin θ}\sin θ − \frac{1}{\sin θ}\frac{\sin θ}{\cos θ}$

$1 − \frac{1}{\cos θ}$

$1 − \sec θ$

48. $\frac{\sin θ − 1}{\sin θ}$

$\frac{\sin θ}{\sin θ} − \frac{1}{\sin θ}$

$1 − \csc θ$

49. $\frac{\cos α + 2 − \cot α}{\cos α}$

$\frac{\cos α}{\cos α} + \frac{2}{\cos α} − \frac{\cot α}{\cos α}$

$1 + 2\left(\frac{1}{\cos α}\right) − \frac{\frac{\cos α}{\sin α}}{\cos α}$

$1 + 2\sec α − \frac{1}{\sin α}$

$1 + 2\sec α − \csc α$

50. (1 + sin θ) (1 − sin θ)

1 − sin θ + sin θ − sin²θ

1 − sin²θ

cos²θ + sin²θ − sin²θ

cos²θ

6. 0.4305   **7.** 4.9313   **8.** 1.6107
9. 603.6 watts   **10.** 7.6°   **11.** 76.0°
12. $b ≈ 9.7$, $c ≈ 10.4$, $B = 68.6°$
13. $c ≈ 9.5$, $A ≈ 33.4°$, $B ≈ 56.6°$
14. 15,540 ft
15. cos θ (sec θ − cos θ)   **16.** 15.7°

cos θ sec θ − cos²θ

$\cos θ \frac{1}{\cos θ} − \cos²θ$

$1 − \cos²θ$

$\sin²θ$

Chapter 2

Exercise 2–1

Answers to odd-numbered problems

1. a. yes   **b.** $D = \{3, 4, 6, 7\}$,
$R = \{5, 9, 10\}$ **c.** not one to one
3. a. yes
b. $D = \{−2, 3, 4\}$, $R = \{−2, 3, 4\}$
c. $h^{-1} = \{(−2,−2), (4,3), (3,4)\}$
5. not a function   **7. a.** yes
b. $D = \{1, 2, 3, 4\}$, $R = \{1, 2, 3, 4\}$
c. $f^{-1} = \{(1,1), (2,2), (3,3), (4,4)\}$
9. a. 9   **b.** 19   **c.** 11   **d.** not defined
e. not defined   **11. a.** $(−2,−13)$
b. $(0,−3)$ **c.** $(\sqrt{3},5\sqrt{3} − 3)$
d. $(\frac{1}{2},−\frac{1}{2})$ **e.** $(5,22)$ **13. a.** $(−2,0)$
b. $(0,−6)$ **c.** $(\sqrt{3},−\sqrt{3} − 3)$
d. $\left(\frac{1}{2},\frac{−25}{4}\right)$ **e.** $(5,14)$
15. a. $(−2,1)$ **b.** $(0,−1)$
c. $(\sqrt{3},2 + \sqrt{3})$ **d.** $(\frac{1}{2},−\frac{1}{4})$
e. $(5,29)$ **17. a.** $(−2,46)$ **b.** $(0,2)$
c. $(\sqrt{3},26)$ **d.** $(\frac{1}{2},\frac{31}{16})$ **e.** $(5, 1,852)$
19. a. $(−2,−2)$ **b.** $(0,0)$
c. $\left(\sqrt{3},\frac{\sqrt{3} − 1}{2}\right)$ **d.** $(\frac{1}{2},\frac{1}{7})$ **e.** $(5,\frac{5}{8})$
21. a. $494°$ C   **b.** $476°$ C   **c.** $292°$ C

51. 20.9°

17. $\frac{\sqrt{2}}{4}$ **18.** $\frac{\sqrt{41}}{4}$

19. 0.2672   **20.** 2.6927   **21.** 0.3230
22. 0.6534   **23.** 0.2924   **24.** 1.1098
25. 1.6426   **26.** 13.2347   **27.** 0.6128
28. 1.4617   **29.** 2.0057   **30.** 17.1984
31. a. sin 53.20° ≈ 0.8007, cos 53.20°
≈ 0.5990, tan 53.20° ≈ 1.3367, csc 53.20°
≈ 1.2489, sec 53.20° ≈ 1.6694, cot 53.20°
≈ 0.7481   **b.** sin 53°20′ ≈ 0.8021,
cos 53°20′ ≈ 0.5972, tan 53°20′ ≈ 1.3432,
csc 53°20′ ≈ 1.2467, sec 53°20′ ≈ 1.6746,
cot 53°20′ ≈ 0.7445   **32.** 410.101
33. 39.2°   **34.** 82.1°   **35.** 35.7°
36. 64.8°   **37.** 44.6°   **38.** 9.0°
39. $c ≈ 28.1$, $b ≈ 15.7$, $B ≈ 33.9°$
40. $a ≈ 20.0$, $A ≈ 60.3°$, $B ≈ 29.7°$
41. $c ≈ 9.44$, $A ≈ 25.1°$, $B ≈ 64.9°$
42. $b ≈ 58.9$, $a ≈ 29.9$, $A ≈ 26.9°$
43. 4.39 km   **44.** 36.0 mm
45. sin²45 + cos²45   **46.** cot θ sec θ

$\left(\frac{\sqrt{2}}{2}\right)^2 + \left(\frac{\sqrt{2}}{2}\right)^2$ $\frac{\cos θ}{\sin θ}\left(\frac{1}{\cos θ}\right)$

$\frac{2}{4} + \frac{2}{4} = 1$ $\frac{1}{\sin θ}$

csc θ

Chapter 1 test

1. 26.462°   **2.** 64.21°   **3.** $6\sqrt{3}$
4. 73.8 ft

5. $\frac{3}{4}$

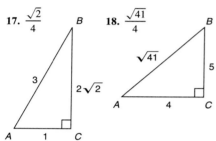

Solutions to trial exercise problems

8. $g = \{(−3,5), (5,8), (8,13), (13,21)\}$
  a. Is a function because no first element repeats.
  b. Domain$_g$ = $\{−3, 5, 8, 13\}$; Range$_g$ = $\{5, 8, 13, 21\}$
  c. Is a one-to-one function because no second element repeats. The inverse is $\{(5,−3),$
  $(8,5), (13,8), (21,13)\}$.

19. $h(x) = \dfrac{x}{x + 3}$

  a. $h(-2) = \dfrac{-2}{-2 + 3} = \dfrac{-2}{1} = -2; \, (-2, -2)$

  b. $h(0) = \dfrac{0}{0 + 3} = \dfrac{0}{3} = 0; \, (0, 0)$

  c. $h(\sqrt{3}) = \dfrac{\sqrt{3}}{\sqrt{3} + 3} = \dfrac{\sqrt{3}}{\sqrt{3} + 3} \cdot \dfrac{\sqrt{3} - 3}{\sqrt{3} - 3} = \dfrac{3 - 3\sqrt{3}}{3 - 9}$

    $= \dfrac{-3(-1 + \sqrt{3})}{-6} = \dfrac{\sqrt{3} - 1}{2}; \, \left(\sqrt{3}, \dfrac{\sqrt{3} - 1}{2}\right)$

  d. $h(\tfrac{1}{2}) = \dfrac{\frac{1}{2}}{\frac{1}{2} + 3} = \dfrac{\frac{1}{2}}{\frac{7}{2}} = \dfrac{1}{2} \cdot \dfrac{2}{7} = \dfrac{1}{7}; \, (\tfrac{1}{2}, \tfrac{1}{7})$

  e. $h(5) = \dfrac{5}{5 + 3} = \dfrac{5}{8}; \, (5, \tfrac{5}{8})$

Exercise 2–2

Answers to odd-numbered problems

1. 60°

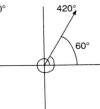

3. 230°

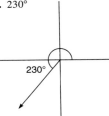

5. 0.6°

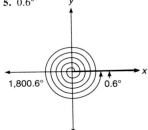

7. 187.9°

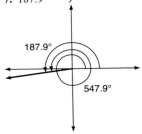

9. 210°

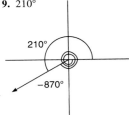

11. 165°

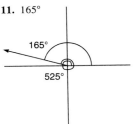

13. 269.7°

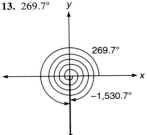

15. 0°

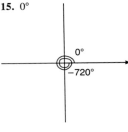

17. 47°

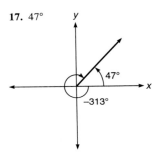

19. 347°   **21.** 353.9°

23. $\sin \theta = \dfrac{2\sqrt{5}}{5}$, $\cos \theta = \dfrac{\sqrt{5}}{5}$, $\tan \theta = 2$, $\csc \theta = \dfrac{\sqrt{5}}{2}$, $\sec \theta = \sqrt{5}$, $\cot \theta = \dfrac{1}{2}$ **25.** $\sin \theta = \dfrac{8\sqrt{89}}{89}$, $\cos \theta = \dfrac{-5\sqrt{89}}{89}$, $\tan \theta = -\dfrac{8}{5}$, $\csc \theta = \dfrac{\sqrt{89}}{8}$, $\sec \theta = -\dfrac{\sqrt{89}}{5}$, $\cot \theta = \dfrac{-5}{8}$

27. $\sin \theta = \dfrac{-\sqrt{2}}{2}$, $\cos \theta = \dfrac{\sqrt{2}}{2}$, $\tan \theta = -1$, $\csc \theta = -\sqrt{2}$, $\sec \theta = \sqrt{2}$, $\cot \theta = -1$ **29.** $\sin \theta = \dfrac{4\sqrt{17}}{17}$, $\cos \theta = -\dfrac{\sqrt{17}}{17}$, $\tan \theta = -4$, $\csc \theta = \dfrac{\sqrt{17}}{4}$, $\sec \theta = -\sqrt{17}$, $\cot \theta = -\dfrac{1}{4}$

31. $\sin \theta = \dfrac{-3\sqrt{13}}{13}$, $\cos \theta = \dfrac{-2\sqrt{13}}{13}$, $\tan \theta = \dfrac{3}{2}$, $\csc \theta = \dfrac{-\sqrt{13}}{3}$, $\sec \theta = \dfrac{-\sqrt{13}}{2}$, $\cot \theta = \dfrac{2}{3}$

33. $\sin \theta = \dfrac{3\sqrt{38}}{19}$, $\cos \theta = \dfrac{-\sqrt{19}}{19}$, $\tan \theta = -3\sqrt{2}$, $\csc \theta = \dfrac{\sqrt{38}}{6}$, $\sec \theta = -\sqrt{19}$, $\cot \theta = \dfrac{-\sqrt{2}}{6}$ **35.** $\sin \theta = -\dfrac{\sqrt{10}}{5}$, $\cos \theta = -\dfrac{\sqrt{15}}{5}$, $\tan \theta = \dfrac{\sqrt{6}}{3}$, $\csc \theta = -\dfrac{\sqrt{10}}{2}$, $\sec \theta = -\dfrac{\sqrt{15}}{3}$, $\cot \theta = \dfrac{\sqrt{6}}{2}$ **37.** $\sin \theta = \dfrac{-\sqrt{10}}{4}$, $\cos \theta = \dfrac{\sqrt{6}}{4}$, $\tan \theta = \dfrac{-\sqrt{15}}{3}$, $\csc \theta = \dfrac{-2\sqrt{10}}{5}$, $\sec \theta = \dfrac{2\sqrt{6}}{3}$, $\cot \theta = \dfrac{-\sqrt{15}}{5}$

39. $\sin \theta = -\dfrac{\sqrt{5}}{5}$, $\cos \theta = \dfrac{2\sqrt{5}}{5}$, $\tan \theta = -\dfrac{1}{2}$,

$\csc \theta = -\sqrt{5}$, $\sec \theta = \dfrac{\sqrt{5}}{2}$, $\cot \theta = -2$ **41.** $\sin \theta = \dfrac{\sqrt{3}}{3}$,

$\cos \theta = \dfrac{\sqrt{6}}{3}$, $\tan \theta = \dfrac{\sqrt{2}}{2}$, $\csc \theta = \sqrt{3}$, $\sec \theta = \dfrac{\sqrt{6}}{2}$, $\cot \theta = \sqrt{2}$

43. $\sin \theta = \dfrac{2\sqrt{5}}{5}$, $\cos \theta = \dfrac{\sqrt{5}}{5}$, $\tan \theta = 2$, $\csc \theta = \dfrac{\sqrt{5}}{2}$,

$\sec \theta = \sqrt{5}$, $\cot \theta = \dfrac{1}{2}$ **45.** $\dfrac{1}{\cos \theta} = \dfrac{1}{\dfrac{x}{r}} = \dfrac{r}{x} = \sec \theta$

47. $\dfrac{\cos \theta}{\sin \theta} = \dfrac{\dfrac{x}{r}}{\dfrac{y}{r}} = \dfrac{x}{y} = \cot \theta$ **49.** $\dfrac{1}{\csc \theta} = \dfrac{1}{\dfrac{r}{y}} = \dfrac{y}{r} = \sin \theta$

51. (x_1, y_1), (x_2, y_2) represent two points with the same
trigonometric functions. The tangent for the point (x_1, y_1) is $\dfrac{y_1}{x_1}$.

The tangent for the point (x_2, y_2) is $\dfrac{y_2}{x_2}$, but $\dfrac{y_1}{x_1} = \dfrac{y_2}{x_2}$, since all

trigonometric functions are the same. Also, $\dfrac{y_1}{x_1}$ is the slope of the

line through $(0,0)$ and (x_1, y_1). Likewise for $\dfrac{y_2}{x_2}$. So $\dfrac{y_1}{x_1} = \dfrac{y_2}{x_2} = m$.

Thus, both (x_1, y_1) and (x_2, y_2) lie on the line $y = mx$. They must be
on the same terminal side, since all the trigonometric functions
have the same sign.

Solutions to trial exercise problems

13. $-1{,}530.3°$
$-1{,}530 \div 360 = -4.25$;
$-1{,}530.3° + 5(360°) =$
$269.7°$
(See the diagram.)

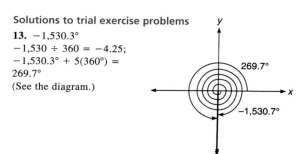

35. $(-\sqrt{3}, -\sqrt{2})$

$r = \sqrt{(-\sqrt{3})^2 + (-\sqrt{2})^2} = \sqrt{3 + 2} = \sqrt{5}$

$\sin \theta = \dfrac{y}{r} = \dfrac{-\sqrt{2}}{\sqrt{5}} \cdot \dfrac{\sqrt{5}}{\sqrt{5}} = -\dfrac{\sqrt{10}}{5}$;

$\csc \theta = \dfrac{r}{y} = \dfrac{\sqrt{5}}{-\sqrt{2}} \cdot \dfrac{\sqrt{2}}{\sqrt{2}} = -\dfrac{\sqrt{10}}{2}$;

$\cos \theta = \dfrac{x}{r} = \dfrac{-\sqrt{3}}{\sqrt{5}} \cdot \dfrac{\sqrt{5}}{\sqrt{5}} = -\dfrac{\sqrt{15}}{5}$;

$\sec \theta = \dfrac{r}{x} = \dfrac{\sqrt{5}}{-\sqrt{3}} \cdot \dfrac{\sqrt{3}}{\sqrt{3}} = -\dfrac{\sqrt{15}}{3}$;

$\tan \theta = \dfrac{y}{x} = \dfrac{-\sqrt{2}}{-\sqrt{3}} \cdot \dfrac{\sqrt{3}}{\sqrt{3}} = \dfrac{\sqrt{6}}{3}$;

$\cot \theta = \dfrac{x}{y} = \dfrac{-\sqrt{3}}{-\sqrt{2}} \cdot \dfrac{\sqrt{2}}{\sqrt{2}} = \dfrac{\sqrt{6}}{2}$

38. $(b, -2b) = (x, y)$
$r = \sqrt{b^2 + (-2b)^2} = \sqrt{5b^2} = \sqrt{5}\sqrt{b^2} = \sqrt{5}b$

$\sin \theta = \dfrac{y}{r} = \dfrac{-2b}{\sqrt{5}b} = -\dfrac{2}{\sqrt{5}} \cdot \dfrac{\sqrt{5}}{\sqrt{5}} = -\dfrac{2\sqrt{5}}{5}$

$\cos \theta = \dfrac{x}{r} = \dfrac{b}{\sqrt{5}b} = \dfrac{1}{\sqrt{5}} \cdot \dfrac{\sqrt{5}}{\sqrt{5}} = \dfrac{\sqrt{5}}{5}$

$\tan \theta = \dfrac{y}{x} = \dfrac{-2b}{b} = -2$

$\csc \theta = \dfrac{1}{\sin \theta} = -\dfrac{\sqrt{5}}{2}$

$\sec \theta = \dfrac{1}{\cos \theta} = \sqrt{5}$

$\cot \theta = \dfrac{1}{\tan \theta} = -\dfrac{1}{2}$

50. As explained in the problem and shown in the figure we have
two points (x_1, mx_1) and (x_2, mx_2) on the terminal side of an angle.
Note that the value m in each case is the same number, since it
is the slope of the line on which both points lie. Using the first
point (x_1, mx_1),

$r_1 = \sqrt{(x_1)^2 + (mx_1)^2} = \sqrt{x_1^2 + m^2 x_1^2}$

$\quad = \sqrt{x_1^2(1 + m^2)} = |x_1|\sqrt{1 + m^2}$

$\sin \theta = \dfrac{y}{r_1} = \dfrac{mx_1}{|x_1|\sqrt{1 + m^2}} = \dfrac{x_1}{|x_1|} \cdot \dfrac{m}{\sqrt{1 + m^2}}$

The value of $\dfrac{x_1}{|x_1|}$ is 1 or -1, depending on the sign of x_1. Thus,

$\sin \theta = \begin{cases} \dfrac{m}{\sqrt{1 + m^2}} & \text{if } x_1 > 0 \\[2ex] -\dfrac{m}{\sqrt{1 + m^2}} & \text{if } x_1 < 0 \end{cases}$

Using the second point (x_2, mx_2),

$r_2 = \sqrt{(x_2)^2 + (mx_2)^2} = \sqrt{x_2^2 + m^2 x_2^2}$

$\quad = \sqrt{x_2^2(1 + m^2)} = |x_2|\sqrt{1 + m^2}$

$\sin \theta = \dfrac{y}{r_2} = \dfrac{mx_2}{|x_2|\sqrt{1 + m^2}} = \dfrac{x_2}{|x_2|} \cdot \dfrac{m}{\sqrt{1 + m^2}}$

As above, the value of $\dfrac{x_2}{|x_2|}$ is 1 or -1, depending on the sign
of x_2. Thus,

$\sin \theta = \begin{cases} \dfrac{m}{\sqrt{1 + m^2}} & \text{if } x_2 > 0 \\[2ex] -\dfrac{m}{\sqrt{1 + m^2}} & \text{if } x_2 < 0 \end{cases}$

Since x_1 and x_2 lie in the same quadrant, they have the same
sign. Therefore, we obtain the same value for $\sin \theta$ using either
point.

Exercise 2-3

Answers to odd-numbered problems

1. II   **3.** I   **5.** IV   **7.** II   **9.** IV
11. III   **13.** 15.8°   **15.** 67.1°
17. 75.3°   **19.** 49.3°   **21.** 1°
23. 80.5°   **25.** 72°   **27.** $\dfrac{\sqrt{2}}{2}$ **29.** $-\dfrac{1}{2}$

31. $-\sqrt{3}$ **33.** $-\dfrac{\sqrt{3}}{2}$ **35.** $\dfrac{1}{2}$

37. $-\dfrac{\sqrt{3}}{3}$ **39.** 0   **41.** 1   **43.** $\dfrac{1}{2}$

45. $-\dfrac{2\sqrt{3}}{3}$ **47.** 0.9178   **49.** 0.6899

51. 0.7813   **53.** 1.0263   **55.** 0.9967
57. -1.0367   **59.** -0.6845
61. 14.5°   **63.** 120°   **65.** -58.0°
67. -36.2°   **69. a.** 110.31 volts
b. 156 volts   **c.** 89.48 volts
d. -65.93 volts   **e.** 132.73 volts
f. 0 volts   **71. a.** 200 lb
b. 181.3 lb   **c.** 128.6 lb

73. $\sin 60° \overset{?}{=} 2\sin 30°$

$\dfrac{\sqrt{3}}{2} \overset{?}{=} 2 \cdot \dfrac{1}{2}$

$\dfrac{\sqrt{3}}{2} \neq 1$; No, it is false.

75. Use the values 30°, 60°, 90° to see if the statement $\sin(\alpha + \beta) = \sin\alpha + \sin\beta$ is true.

$\sin(30° + 60°) \overset{?}{=} \sin 30° + \sin 60°$

$\sin 90° \overset{?}{=} \sin 30° + \sin 60°$

$1 \overset{?}{=} \dfrac{1}{2} + \dfrac{\sqrt{3}}{2}$

$1 \neq \dfrac{1 + \sqrt{3}}{2}$; No, it is false.

Solutions to trial exercise problems

6. $\sec\theta > 0$, $\csc\theta < 0$
If $\sec\theta > 0$, then $\cos\theta > 0$, so θ is in quadrant I or quadrant IV. If $\csc\theta < 0$, then $\sin\theta < 0$, so θ is in quadrant III or quadrant IV. Therefore, θ is in quadrant IV.

19. 130.7°
Since $90° < 130.7° < 180°$, this angle terminates in quadrant II. In quadrant II, $\theta' = 180° - \theta = 180° - 130.7° = 49.3°$

43. $\sin(-690°)$
-690° is coterminal with 30° (add $-690° + 2[360°]$), so $\sin(-690°)$ $= \sin 30° = \dfrac{1}{2}$

52. $\tan 527.2°$
$527.2° - 360° = 167.2°$, so $\tan 527.2°$ $= \tan 167.2°$. Since $167.2°$ terminates in quadrant II, $\theta' = 180° - 167.2°$ $= 12.8°$. The tangent function is negative in quadrant II, so we know that
$\tan 167.2° = -\tan 12.8°$
$= -0.2272$ (to four decimal places).

65. $\tan\theta = -\dfrac{8}{5}$
$\theta = \tan^{-1}(-\dfrac{8}{5}) \approx -58.0°$
Display: $\boxed{-57.99461679}$

Exercise 2-4

Answers to odd-numbered problems

1. 55.6°   **3.** 33.3°   **5.** 200.0°
7. 358.0°   **9.** 22.0°   **11.** 168.7°
13. 224.4°

15. a.

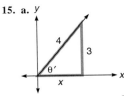

b. $\csc\theta = \dfrac{4}{3}$, $\cos\theta = \dfrac{\sqrt{7}}{4}$,

$\sec\theta = \dfrac{4\sqrt{7}}{7}$, $\tan\theta = \dfrac{3\sqrt{7}}{7}$,

$\cot\theta = \dfrac{\sqrt{7}}{3}$ **c.** $\theta = \theta' \approx 48.6°$

17. a.

b. $\sin\theta = \dfrac{-\sqrt{3}}{2}$, $\csc\theta = \dfrac{-2\sqrt{3}}{3}$,

$\sec\theta = -2$, $\tan\theta = \sqrt{3}$, $\cot\theta = \dfrac{\sqrt{3}}{3}$

c. $\theta' = 60°$, $\theta = 240°$

19. a.

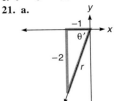

b. $\cos\theta = 0$, $\tan\theta$ undefined, $\cot\theta = 0$, $\csc\theta = 1$, $\sec\theta$ undefined
c. $\theta = \theta' = 90°$

21. a.

b. $\cot\theta = \dfrac{1}{2}$, $\sin\theta = \dfrac{-2\sqrt{5}}{5}$, $\cos\theta$

$= \dfrac{-\sqrt{5}}{5}$, $\csc\theta = \dfrac{-\sqrt{5}}{2}$, $\sec\theta = -\sqrt{5}$
c. $\theta' \approx 63.4°$, $\theta \approx 243.4°$

23. a.

b. $\sin\theta = -\dfrac{1}{5}$, $\cos\theta = \dfrac{-2\sqrt{6}}{5}$,

$\sec\theta = \dfrac{-5\sqrt{6}}{12}$, $\tan\theta = \dfrac{\sqrt{6}}{12}$, $\cot\theta = 2\sqrt{6}$
c. $\theta' \approx 11.5°$, $\theta \approx 191.5°$

25. a.

b. $\sin\theta = -1$, $\cos\theta = 0$, $\sec\theta$ undefined, $\tan\theta$ undefined, $\cot\theta = 0$ **c.** $\theta' = 90°$, $\theta = 270°$

27. a.

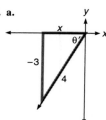

b. $\csc \theta = -\dfrac{4}{3}$, $\cos \theta = \dfrac{-\sqrt{7}}{4}$,

$\sec \theta = \dfrac{-4\sqrt{7}}{7}$, $\tan \theta = \dfrac{3\sqrt{7}}{7}$, $\cot \theta = \dfrac{\sqrt{7}}{3}$

c. $\theta' \approx 48.6°$, $\theta \approx 228.6°$

29. a.

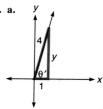

b. $\cos \theta = \dfrac{1}{4}$, $\sin \theta = \dfrac{\sqrt{15}}{4}$, $\csc \theta$

$= \dfrac{4\sqrt{15}}{15}$, $\tan \theta = \sqrt{15}$, $\cot \theta = \dfrac{\sqrt{15}}{15}$

c. $\theta = \theta' \approx 75.5°$

31. a.

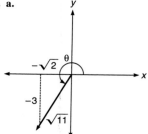

b. $\tan \theta = \dfrac{3\sqrt{2}}{2}$, $\cos \theta = -\dfrac{\sqrt{22}}{11}$, $\sin \theta$

$= -\dfrac{3\sqrt{11}}{11}$, $\csc \theta = -\dfrac{\sqrt{11}}{3}$, $\sec \theta =$

$-\dfrac{\sqrt{22}}{2}$ **c.** $\theta' \approx 64.8°$, $\theta \approx 244.8°$

33. a.

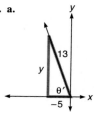

b. $\sec \theta = \dfrac{-13}{5}$, $\sin \theta = \dfrac{12}{13}$, $\csc \theta$

$= \dfrac{13}{12}$, $\tan \theta = \dfrac{-12}{5}$, $\cot \theta = \dfrac{-5}{12}$

c. $\theta' \approx 67.4°$, $\theta \approx 112.6°$

35. a.

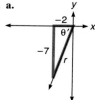

b. $\cot \theta = \dfrac{2}{7}$, $\sin \theta = \dfrac{-7\sqrt{53}}{53}$, $\csc \theta =$

$\dfrac{-\sqrt{53}}{7}$, $\cos \theta = \dfrac{-2\sqrt{53}}{53}$, $\sec \theta = \dfrac{-\sqrt{53}}{2}$

c. $\theta \approx 74.1°$, $\theta \approx 254.1°$

37. a.

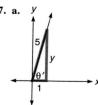

b. $\cos \theta = \dfrac{1}{5}$, $\sin \theta = \dfrac{2\sqrt{6}}{5}$, $\csc \theta$

$= \dfrac{5\sqrt{6}}{12}$, $\tan \theta = 2\sqrt{6}$, $\cot \theta = \dfrac{\sqrt{6}}{12}$

c. $\theta = \theta' \approx 78.5°$

39. a.

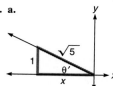

b. $\csc \theta = \sqrt{5}$, $\cos \theta = \dfrac{-2\sqrt{5}}{5}$, $\sec \theta$

$= \dfrac{-\sqrt{5}}{2}$, $\cot \theta = -2$, $\tan \theta = -\dfrac{1}{2}$

c. $\theta' \approx 26.6°$, $\theta \approx 153.4°$

41. a. $\sin \theta = \dfrac{-5\sqrt{29}}{29}$,

$\cos \theta = \dfrac{2\sqrt{29}}{29}$, $\tan \theta = -\dfrac{5}{2}$,

$\sec \theta = \dfrac{\sqrt{29}}{2}$, $\csc \theta = \dfrac{-\sqrt{29}}{5}$, $\cot \theta =$

$-\dfrac{2}{5}$ **b.** 291.8°

43. (−4.85 mm, 4.77 mm)
45. (−5.77 cm, −5.89 cm)
47. 8.8 cm, 60.6°; −8.8 cm, 119.4°; −8.8 cm, 240.6°; 8.8 cm, 299.4°
49. $y \approx -13.5$ in., $x \approx -22.0$ in.
51. $\cot \theta = \dfrac{1}{u}$, $\sin \theta = \dfrac{u}{\sqrt{u^2 + 1}}$,

$\csc \theta = \dfrac{\sqrt{u^2 + 1}}{u}$, $\cos \theta = \dfrac{1}{\sqrt{u^2 + 1}}$,

$\sec \theta = \sqrt{u^2 + 1}$ **53.** $\cot \theta = \dfrac{1}{u}$,

$\sin \theta = \dfrac{-u}{\sqrt{u^2 + 1}}$, $\csc \theta = \dfrac{-\sqrt{u^2 + 1}}{u}$,

$\cos \theta = \dfrac{-1}{\sqrt{u^2 + 1}}$, $\sec \theta = -\sqrt{u^2 + 1}$

55. $\sec \theta = \dfrac{1}{1 - u}$, $\sin \theta = \sqrt{2u - u^2}$,

$\csc \theta = \dfrac{1}{\sqrt{2u - u^2}}$, $\tan \theta = \dfrac{\sqrt{2u - u^2}}{1 - u}$,

$\cot \theta = \dfrac{1 - u}{\sqrt{2u - u^2}}$ **57.** 663.4 ft

Solutions to trial exercise problems
13. $\cos \theta = -\frac{5}{7}$, $\tan \theta > 0$

$\theta' = \cos^{-1}\frac{5}{7} \approx 44.4°$

$\cos \theta < 0$, $\tan \theta > 0$, so θ terminates in quadrant III. Therefore, $\theta = 180° + \theta' \approx 180° + 44.4° \approx 224.4°$.

25. a.

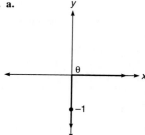

b. $\csc \theta = -1$

$\sin \theta = \dfrac{1}{\csc \theta} = \dfrac{1}{-1} = -1$; $\sin \theta =$

$\dfrac{y}{r} = -1 = \dfrac{-1}{1}$, so we see that $y =$

−1 and $r = 1$ would work. This means

that x must be 0, since $x^2 + y^2 = r^2$. Thus, the point $(0, -1)$ is on the angle, which is shown in the diagram. $\cos \theta = \dfrac{0}{1} = 0$; $\sec \theta = \dfrac{1}{\cos \theta}$, which is not defined in this case. $\tan \theta = \dfrac{y}{x} = \dfrac{-1}{0}$ (not defined); $\cot \theta = \dfrac{x}{y} = \dfrac{0}{-1} = 0$.

c. We can see that $\theta = 270°$ from the diagram.

34. a.

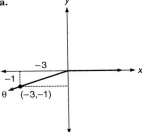

b. $\cos \theta = -\dfrac{3}{\sqrt{10}}$, $\sin \theta < 0$; $x = -3$, $r = \sqrt{10}$.

Computing, $x^2 + y^2 = r^2$
$$9 + y^2 = 10$$
$$y = \pm 1$$

Since $\cos \theta < 0$ and $\sin \theta < 0$, θ terminates in quadrant III, so $y = -1$. (See the diagram.)

$\sin \theta = \dfrac{y}{r} = \dfrac{-1}{\sqrt{10}} \cdot \dfrac{\sqrt{10}}{\sqrt{10}} = \dfrac{-\sqrt{10}}{10}$; $\tan \theta = \dfrac{y}{x} = \dfrac{-1}{-3} = \dfrac{1}{3}$; $\csc \theta = \dfrac{1}{\sin \theta} = -\sqrt{10}$;

$\sec \theta = \dfrac{1}{\cos \theta} = \dfrac{-\sqrt{10}}{3}$; $\cot \theta = \dfrac{1}{\tan \theta} = 3$.

c. $\theta = 180° + \tan^{-1}\dfrac{1}{3} \approx 180° + 18.4° \approx 198.4°$

47. $\sin \theta' = \dfrac{y}{r} = \dfrac{15.5}{17.8}$ (See diagram.)

$\theta' = 60.6°$. The four angles are
$\theta = \theta' = 60.6°$
$= 180° - 60.6° = 119.4°$
$= 180° + 60.6° = 240.6°$
$= 360° - 60.6° = 299.4°$
We know that $r^2 = x^2 + y^2$, so
$17.8^2 = x^2 + 15.5^2$
$17.8^2 - 15.5^2 = x^2$
$76.59 = x^2$, $8.75 = x$. Thus, $x = \pm 8.8$.

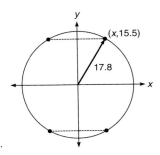

49. 4 ft 3.5 in. $= 51.5$ in.; $r = \dfrac{51.5}{2}$ in. $= 25.75$ in.
$x = r \cos \theta = 25.75 \cos 211.5° = -22.0$ in.
$y = r \sin \theta = 25.75 \sin 211.5° = -13.5$ in.

52. $\cos \theta = u$, and θ terminates in quadrant III. (See the diagram.)

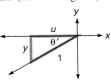

Using the Pythagorean theorem, we find
$y = -\sqrt{1 - u^2}$. $\sin \theta = \dfrac{y}{r} = -\sqrt{1 - u^2}$,

$\tan \theta = \dfrac{y}{x} = \dfrac{-\sqrt{1 - u^2}}{u}$, $\csc \theta = \dfrac{1}{\sin \theta} = \dfrac{-1}{\sqrt{1 - u^2}}$, $\sec \theta = \dfrac{1}{\cos \theta} = \dfrac{1}{u}$,

$\cot \theta = \dfrac{1}{\tan \theta} = -\dfrac{u}{\sqrt{1 - u^2}}$

55. $\cos \theta = 1 - u$, θ in quadrant I. (See the diagram.)

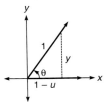

$1^2 = y^2 + (1 - u)^2$
$1 - (1 - 2u + u^2) = y^2$
$2u - u^2 = y^2$
$\sqrt{2u - u^2} = y \ (y > 0)$

$\sec \theta = \dfrac{1}{\cos \theta} = \dfrac{1}{1 - u}$;

$\sin \theta = \dfrac{y}{r} = \sqrt{2u - u^2}$;

$\csc \theta = \dfrac{1}{\sin \theta} = \dfrac{1}{\sqrt{2u - u^2}}$;

$\tan \theta = \dfrac{y}{x} = \dfrac{\sqrt{2u - u^2}}{1 - u}$;

$\cot \theta = \dfrac{1}{\tan \theta} = \dfrac{1 - u}{\sqrt{2u - u^2}}$

57. $AB = 512.4$ feet, $AP = 322.6$ feet, $b = 28.3°$.

$\sin p = \dfrac{AB \sin b}{AP} = \dfrac{512.4(\sin 28.3°)}{322.6}$
≈ 0.7530
$p \approx 48.85°$
$a = 180° - (b + p) \approx 180° - (28.3° + 48.85°) \approx 102.85°$
$BP = \dfrac{AP \sin a}{\sin b} \approx \dfrac{322.6(\sin 102.85°)}{\sin 28.3°} \approx 663.4$ feet

Exercise 2–5

Answers to odd-numbered problems

1. $x^2 + y^2 = 1$ **3.** $\dfrac{\pi}{4}$, 0.79

5. $\dfrac{5\pi}{9}$, 1.75   **7.** $\dfrac{-5\pi}{3}$, -5.24

9. $\dfrac{3\pi}{2}$, 4.71   **11.** $\dfrac{127\pi}{180}$, 2.22

13. $\dfrac{-61\pi}{36}$, -5.32 **15.** 330°

17. 108°   **19.** 40°   **21.** $-510°$

23. $\dfrac{270°}{\pi}$, 85.94°   **25.** $\dfrac{-2,160°}{17\pi}$, $-40.44°$

27. $\dfrac{360°}{\pi}$, 114.59°   **29.** $\dfrac{-900°}{\pi}$, $-286.48°$

31. $\dfrac{\pi}{3}$ **33.** $\dfrac{\pi}{6}$ **35.** $\dfrac{\pi}{3}$ **37.** $\dfrac{\pi}{4}$

39. $\dfrac{\pi}{3}$ **41.** $\dfrac{\pi}{3}$ **43.** $\dfrac{\pi}{6}$

45.

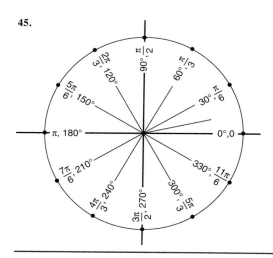

47.

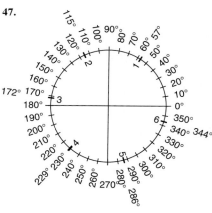

---

49. 2.7 **51.** 6.5 inches **53.** 24 inches
55. 98 in.² **57.** 33.93 cm² **59.** 7.5 in.²
61. 10.60 mm² **63.** 1.24 **65.** 35.5
gallons **67.** 30 mm

Solutions to trial exercise problems

12. $-422°$

$\dfrac{s}{\pi} = \dfrac{\theta°}{180°}$, so $\dfrac{s}{\pi} = \dfrac{-422°}{180°}$, (Cross

multiply.) $s \cdot 180° = \pi(-422°)$,

$s = \dfrac{\pi(-422°)}{180°}$, $s = \dfrac{-211\pi}{90}$ or -7.37

21. $-\dfrac{17\pi}{6}$

$\dfrac{s}{\pi} = \dfrac{\theta°}{180°}$, so $\dfrac{\dfrac{-17\pi}{6}}{\pi} = \dfrac{\theta°}{180°}$, (Cross

multiply.) $\dfrac{-17\pi(180°)}{6} = \pi\theta°$,

$-17\pi(30°) = \pi\theta°$, $\dfrac{-17\pi(30°)}{\pi} = \theta°$,

$-17(30°) = \theta°$, $-510° = \theta°$

29. -5

$\dfrac{s}{\pi} = \dfrac{\theta°}{180°}$, so $\dfrac{-5}{\pi} = \dfrac{\theta°}{180°}$, (Cross

multiply.) $-5(180°) = \pi\theta°$, $\dfrac{-5(180°)}{\pi}$

$= \theta°$, $\dfrac{-900°}{\pi} = \theta°$, $-286.48° = \theta°$

---

43. $-\dfrac{7\pi}{6}$

$-\dfrac{7\pi}{6} + \pi = -\dfrac{7\pi}{6} + \dfrac{1\pi}{6} = \dfrac{5\pi}{6}$

Thus, $\dfrac{5\pi}{6}$ and $-\dfrac{7\pi}{6}$ are coterminal (and

therefore have the same reference

angle). Now find in which quadrant $\dfrac{5\pi}{6}$

terminates.

$0 \quad \dfrac{\pi}{2} \quad \pi$

$0 \quad \dfrac{3\pi}{6} \quad \dfrac{6\pi}{6}$

$\dfrac{3\pi}{6} < \dfrac{5\pi}{6} < \dfrac{6\pi}{6}$, so $\dfrac{\pi}{2} < \dfrac{5\pi}{6} < \pi$, so $\dfrac{5\pi}{6}$

terminates in quadrant II. Therefore, θ'

$= \pi - \theta = \dfrac{6\pi}{6} - \dfrac{5\pi}{6} = \dfrac{\pi}{6}$.

52. $s = \dfrac{L}{r}$; $L = 14.5$ mm, diameter

$= 10.3$ mm. $r = \dfrac{10.3 \text{ mm}}{2} = 5.15$ mm,

$s = \dfrac{14.5 \text{ mm}}{5.15 \text{ mm}} = \dfrac{1,450}{515} = \dfrac{290}{103} \approx 2.8155$

$\dfrac{s}{\pi} = \dfrac{\theta°}{180°}$, so $\dfrac{2.8155}{\pi} \approx \dfrac{\theta°}{180°}$, (Cross

multiply.) $2.8155(180°) \approx \pi\theta°$,

$\dfrac{2.8155(180°)}{\pi} = \theta°$, $161.318° \approx \theta°$

Thus, $\theta° = 161.3°$ or 2.8 (radians).

---

53. Convert 85° to radians.

$\dfrac{85°}{180°} = \dfrac{s}{\pi}$

$s = \dfrac{85\pi}{180} = \dfrac{17\pi}{36}$

The radius of the wheel is $32.4'' \div 2$
$= 16.2''$. The car will move whatever
arc length the angle determines on its
circumference: $L = rs$

$L = 16.2'' \cdot \dfrac{17\pi}{36} = 7.65\pi \approx 24.0$

inches, or 2 feet

61. 15°, 9 mm

15° is $\dfrac{\pi}{12}$ radians

$A = \dfrac{1}{2}sr^2 = \dfrac{1}{2} \cdot \dfrac{\pi}{12} \cdot 9^2 = \dfrac{81\pi}{24} = \dfrac{27\pi}{8}$

≈ 10.60 mm²

Exercise 2–6

Answers to odd-numbered problems

1. $\dfrac{\sqrt{3}}{2}$ **3.** $\dfrac{\sqrt{3}}{2}$ **5.** $-\dfrac{1}{2}$ **7.** $\dfrac{\sqrt{2}}{2}$
9. $-\sqrt{3}$ **11.** $\sqrt{3}$ **13.** $\dfrac{1}{2}$
15. 0.7833 **17.** 0.5463 **19.** 1.5523
21. 0.7457 **23.** 1.4235 **25.** 1.6709
27. $\dfrac{4\pi}{3}$ **29.** $\dfrac{5\pi}{3}$ **31.** $\dfrac{7\pi}{4}$ **33.** $\dfrac{11\pi}{6}$
35. 1.9513 **37.** 3.6259 **39.** 3.4814
41. 0.17 **43.** 1.19 **45.** π
47. $\dfrac{\pi}{18}$ **49.** $\dfrac{\pi}{2}$ or $\dfrac{\pi}{3}$ **51.** $\dfrac{\pi}{3}$ or $\dfrac{\pi}{2}$
53. a. -0.03 **b.** -0.37 **55.** 18.18 cm
57. a. 0.099833417 **b.** 0.479425533
c. 0.841468254 **d.** 0.499999992

Solutions to trial exercise problems

2. $\tan \dfrac{5\pi}{4}$

First we must find the quadrant in which $\dfrac{5\pi}{4}$ terminates.

Remember the following correspondence between values in radians and quadrants, as illustrated in the diagram.

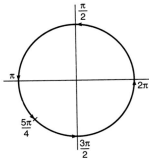

0 to $\frac{1}{2}\pi$: quadrant I; $\frac{1}{2}\pi$ to 1π: quadrant II; 1π to $1\frac{1}{2}\pi$: quadrant III; $1\frac{1}{2}\pi$ to 2π: quadrant IV.

$\dfrac{5\pi}{4} = 1\dfrac{1}{4}\pi$, which, therefore, terminates in quadrant III. For a value that corresponds to an angle that terminates in quadrant III, we form the reference angle by subtracting π:

$1\frac{1}{4}\pi - \pi = \frac{1}{4}\pi = \frac{\pi}{4}$. $\tan\frac{\pi}{4} = \tan 45° = 1$ so $\tan\dfrac{5\pi}{4} = \pm 1$.

Since the corresponding angle terminates in quadrant III, where the tangent function is positive, $\tan \dfrac{5\pi}{4} = 1$.

3. $\cos \dfrac{11\pi}{6}$

$\dfrac{11\pi}{6} = 1\dfrac{5}{6}\pi$, which, therefore, represents an angle that terminates in quadrant IV (see discussion of problem 2). In this quadrant we subtract the value from 2π to obtain the reference angle.

$2\pi - 1\dfrac{5}{6}\pi = \dfrac{1}{6}\pi = \dfrac{\pi}{6}$. $\cos\dfrac{\pi}{6} = \cos 30° = \dfrac{\sqrt{3}}{2}$

Since the cosine function is positive in quadrant IV, we know that our result is positive. Thus, $\cos \dfrac{11\pi}{6} = \dfrac{\sqrt{3}}{2}$.

6. $\sin \dfrac{5\pi}{6}$

$\dfrac{5\pi}{6} = \dfrac{5}{6}\pi$, which corresponds to an angle that terminates in quadrant II. Therefore, the reference angle is $\pi - \frac{5}{6}\pi = \frac{1}{6}\pi$

$= \dfrac{\pi}{6}$. $\sin\dfrac{\pi}{6} = \dfrac{1}{2}$, and $\dfrac{5\pi}{6}$ terminates in quadrant II where the sine function is positive, so $\sin \dfrac{5\pi}{6} = \dfrac{1}{2}$.

24. $\sec 5.2 = \dfrac{1}{\cos 5.2} \approx 2.1344$

5.2 [cos] [1/x]

[TI-81]   [(] [COS] 5.2 [)] [x^{-1}] [ENTER]

Display: [2.134395767]
Make sure calculator is in radian mode.

34. $\sin \theta = -0.5624$
$\theta' = \sin^{-1} 0.5624$
Use the positive value.
$\theta' \approx 0.5973$
$\sin \theta < 0$, $\tan \theta > 0$, so θ terminates in quadrant III. Thus, $\theta = \pi + \theta' \approx 3.74$.

48. $2 \sin \theta - 1 = 0$ or $\sin \theta - 1 = 0$
Zero product property: If $ab = 0$ then $a = 0$ or $b = 0$.
$2 \sin \theta = 1$ or $\sin \theta = 1$
$\sin \theta = \dfrac{1}{2}$

$\theta = \sin^{-1}\dfrac{1}{2} = \dfrac{\pi}{6}$ or $\theta = \sin^{-1}1 = \dfrac{\pi}{2}$

$\theta = \dfrac{\pi}{6}$ or $\dfrac{\pi}{2}$

55. $V = \dfrac{\sqrt{a^2 + b^2 - 2ab \cos \theta}}{\sin \theta}$, $a = 6.2$ cm, $b = 3.5$ cm,

$\theta = 2.6$.

$V = \dfrac{\sqrt{6.2^2 + 3.5^2 - 2(6.2)(3.5) \cos 2.6}}{\sin 2.6} \approx 18.18$ cm

To use a calculator, make sure it is in radian angle mode.

(A)   6.2 [x^2] [+] 3.5 [x^2] [−] 2 [×] 6.2 [×]
    3.5 [×] 2.6 [COS] [=] [$\sqrt{x}$] [÷] 2.6
    [SIN] [=]

(P)   6.2 [x^2] 3.5 [x^2] [+] 2 [ENTER] 6.2 [×] 3.5
    [×]
    2.6 [COS] [×] [−] [$\sqrt{x}$] 2.6 [SIN] [÷]

[TI-81]   [$\sqrt{}$] [(] 6.2 [x^2] [+] 3.5 [x^2] [−] 2
    [×] 6.2 [×] 3.5 [×] [COS] 2.6 [)]
    [÷] [SIN] 2.6 [ENTER]

Display: [18.18497291]

Chapter 2 review

1. a. yes   **b.** $D = \{1, 4, 6, 7\}$,
$R = \{7, 5, 10\}$ **c.** not one to one
2. a. yes
b. $D = \{-2, -1, 1, 2\}$, $R = \{-3, 1, 2, 5\}$
c. $\{(-3,-2), (1,-1), (2,1), (5,2)\}$
3. Not a function   **4. a.** $(-1,6)$
b. $(0,4)$ **c.** $(\sqrt{5},4 - 2\sqrt{5})$ **d.** $(\frac{1}{3}, \frac{10}{3})$
5. a. $(-1,8)$ **b.** $(0,3)$
c. $(\sqrt{5},18 - 2\sqrt{5})$ **d.** $(\frac{1}{3}, \frac{8}{3})$

6. a. $(-1,-4)$ **b.** $(0,-5)$ **c.** $(\sqrt{5},20)$
d. $(\frac{1}{3},-4\frac{80}{81})$ **7. a.** $(-1,\frac{3}{2})$ **b.** $(0,0)$
c. $\left(\sqrt{5},\dfrac{15+3\sqrt{5}}{4}\right)$ **d.** $(\frac{1}{3},-\frac{3}{2})$

8. 105°

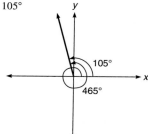

9. 319.75°

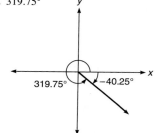

10. 90°

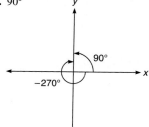

11. 0.6°

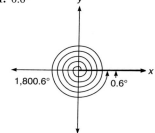

12. 132°18′

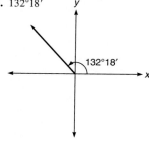

13. 187°26′

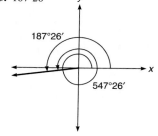

14. 69.3°

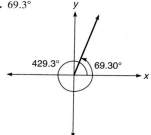

15. 359°45′

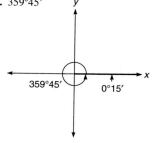

16. $\sin\theta=\frac{-12}{13}$, $\csc\theta=\frac{-13}{12}$, $\cos\theta=\frac{5}{13}$, $\sec\theta=\frac{13}{5}$, $\tan\theta=-\frac{12}{5}$, $\cot\theta=-\frac{5}{12}$

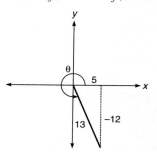

17. $\sin\theta=\dfrac{8\sqrt{89}}{89}$, $\csc\theta=\dfrac{\sqrt{89}}{8}$, $\cos\theta=\dfrac{-5\sqrt{89}}{89}$, $\sec\theta=\dfrac{-\sqrt{89}}{5}$, $\tan\theta=-\dfrac{8}{5}$, $\cot\theta=\dfrac{-5}{8}$

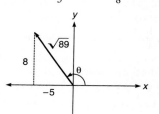

18. $\cos\theta=0$, $\sec\theta$ undefined, $\sin\theta=-1$, $\csc\theta=-1$, $\tan\theta$ undefined, $\cot\theta=0$

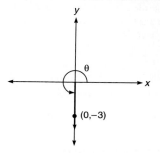

19. $\cos \theta = \frac{2}{3}$, $\sec \theta = \frac{3}{2}$, $\sin \theta = \frac{\sqrt{5}}{3}$,

$\csc \theta = \frac{3\sqrt{5}}{5}$, $\tan \theta = \frac{\sqrt{5}}{2}$, $\cot \theta = \frac{2\sqrt{5}}{5}$

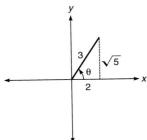

20. $\cos \theta = \frac{-\sqrt{22}}{11}$, $\sec \theta = \frac{-\sqrt{22}}{2}$,

$\sin \theta = \frac{3\sqrt{11}}{11}$, $\csc \theta = \frac{\sqrt{11}}{3}$, $\tan \theta = \frac{-3\sqrt{2}}{2}$, $\cot \theta = \frac{-\sqrt{2}}{3}$

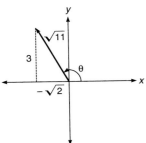

21. $\cos \theta = \frac{\sqrt{7}}{7}$, $\sec \theta = \sqrt{7}$,

$\sin \theta = \frac{-\sqrt{42}}{7}$, $\csc \theta = \frac{-\sqrt{42}}{6}$,

$\tan \theta = -\sqrt{6}$, $\cot \theta = \frac{-\sqrt{6}}{6}$

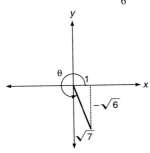

22. $r = \sqrt{a^2 + (-2a)^2} = \sqrt{5a^2} = \sqrt{5}a$

$\sin \theta = \frac{-2a}{\sqrt{5}a} = \frac{-2}{\sqrt{5}} = -\frac{2\sqrt{5}}{5}$,

$\cos \theta = \frac{a}{\sqrt{5}a} = \frac{1}{\sqrt{5}} = \frac{\sqrt{5}}{5}$,

$\tan \theta = \frac{-2a}{a} = -2$, $\csc \theta = -\frac{\sqrt{5}}{2}$, $\sec \theta$

$= \sqrt{5}$, $\cot \theta = -\frac{1}{2}$

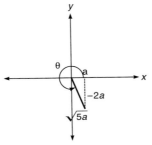

23. III   **24.** III   **25.** IV   **26.** IV
27. II   **28.** II   **29.** III   **30.** IV
31. 46.3°   **32.** 36°44′   **33.** 61°48′
34. 22.7°   **35.** 68.7°   **36.** 74.85°
37. 62.57°   **38.** −0.5505   **39.** $-\frac{1}{2}$
40. 2.1842   **41.** 2   **42.** 1.5818
43. 0.6720   **44.** 2   **45.** −0.6862
46. 0.9159   **47.** 161°   **48.** 141.0°
49. 212.2°   **50.** 294.7°
51. 119.0°   **52.** 193.7°   **53.** 120°
54. 296.6°   **55.** 112.6°
56. $\cos \theta = \frac{3}{5}$, $\sec \theta = \frac{5}{3}$, $\csc \theta = \frac{5}{4}$,
$\tan \theta = \frac{4}{3}$, $\cot \theta = \frac{3}{4}$

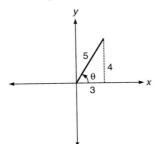

57. $\sec \theta = -2$, $\sin \theta = \frac{-\sqrt{3}}{2}$,

$\csc \theta = \frac{-2\sqrt{3}}{3}$, $\tan \theta = \sqrt{3}$, $\cot \theta = \frac{\sqrt{3}}{3}$

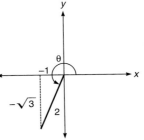

58. $\sec \theta = -\frac{16}{5}$, $\sin \theta = \frac{-\sqrt{231}}{16}$, $\csc \theta$

$= \frac{-16\sqrt{231}}{231}$, $\tan \theta = \frac{\sqrt{231}}{5}$, $\cot \theta =$

$\frac{5\sqrt{231}}{231}$

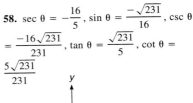

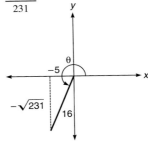

59. $\sec \theta = 4$, $\sin \theta = \frac{-\sqrt{15}}{4}$, $\csc \theta =$

$\frac{-4\sqrt{15}}{15}$, $\tan \theta = -\sqrt{15}$, $\cot \theta = \frac{-\sqrt{15}}{15}$

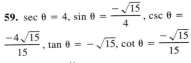

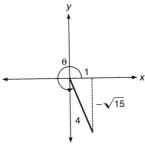

60. $\cot \theta = -\frac{1}{2}$, $\sin \theta = \dfrac{2\sqrt{5}}{5}$, $\csc \theta =$
$\dfrac{\sqrt{5}}{2}$, $\cos \theta = -\dfrac{\sqrt{5}}{5}$, $\sec \theta = -\sqrt{5}$

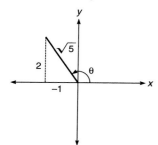

61. $\cos \theta = \dfrac{\sqrt{15}}{4}$, $\sec \theta = \dfrac{4\sqrt{15}}{15}$, $\cot \theta =$
$-\sqrt{15}$, $\tan \theta = \dfrac{-\sqrt{15}}{15}$, $\sin \theta = \dfrac{-1}{4}$

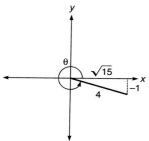

62. $\cos \theta = \dfrac{1}{6}$, $\sin \theta = \dfrac{-\sqrt{35}}{6}$, $\csc \theta =$
$\dfrac{-6\sqrt{35}}{35}$, $\tan \theta = -\sqrt{35}$, $\cot \theta = \dfrac{-\sqrt{35}}{35}$

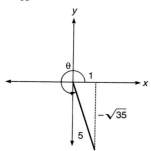

63. $\tan \theta = \frac{1}{2}$, $\sin \theta = \dfrac{-\sqrt{5}}{5}$, $\cos \theta =$
$\dfrac{-2\sqrt{5}}{5}$, $\csc \theta = -\sqrt{5}$, $\sec \theta = \dfrac{-\sqrt{5}}{2}$

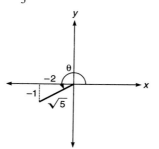

64. $\cot \theta = \frac{2}{7}$, $\sin \theta = \dfrac{-7\sqrt{53}}{53}$, $\cos \theta =$
$\dfrac{-2\sqrt{53}}{53}$, $\csc \theta = \dfrac{-\sqrt{53}}{7}$, $\sec \theta = \dfrac{-\sqrt{53}}{2}$

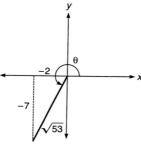

65. $\tan \theta = \frac{7}{2}$, $\sin \theta = \dfrac{-7\sqrt{53}}{53}$, $\cos \theta =$
$\dfrac{-2\sqrt{53}}{53}$, $\csc \theta = \dfrac{-\sqrt{53}}{7}$, $\sec \theta = \dfrac{-\sqrt{53}}{2}$

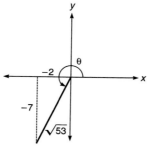

66. $\cot \theta$ undefined, $\sin \theta = 0$, $\cos \theta = 1$,
$\csc \theta$ undefined, $\sec \theta = 1$

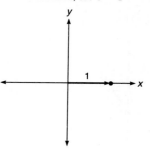

67. $\sin \theta = \frac{1}{4}$, $\cos \theta = \dfrac{-\sqrt{15}}{4}$, $\tan \theta =$
$\dfrac{-\sqrt{15}}{15}$, $\sec \theta = \dfrac{-4\sqrt{15}}{15}$, $\csc \theta = 4$,
$\cot \theta = -\sqrt{15}$

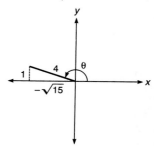

68. $\tan \theta = \dfrac{-z}{\sqrt{1 - z^2}}$

69. $\cos \theta = \dfrac{1}{\sqrt{1 + z^2}}$ **70. a.** 31.06 volts
b. 103.92 volts   **c.** 118.46 volts
d. 10.46 volts   **e.** 0 volts   **f.** -60 volts
71. 337.4 m   **72.** $x \approx -5.2$ mm, $y \approx 7.3$
mm   **73.** $x \approx 7.9$ in., $y \approx 1.4$ in.
74. $x \approx 5.1$ ft, $y \approx -4.6$ ft

75. $\dfrac{2\pi}{3}$, 2.09   **76.** $\dfrac{-43\pi}{36}$, -3.75

77. $\dfrac{43\pi}{18}$, 7.50   **78.** 630°   **79.** 660°

80. $\dfrac{-900°}{7}$, $-128.57°$ **81.** $\dfrac{450°}{\pi}$, 143.24°

82. $\dfrac{-756°}{\pi}$, $-240.64°$ **83.** 12.3 inches

84. 2.3   **85.** $\dfrac{25\pi}{4}$ mm   **86.** 100.8 inches

87. $\dfrac{27\pi}{4}$ in.², 21.21 in.²   **88.** $\dfrac{128\pi}{3}$ mm²,
134.04 mm²   **89.** 16.50 mm²
90. $\dfrac{49\pi}{5}$ in.², 30.79 in.²   **91.** 0.9463

92. -1.3561 **93.** 4.6373 **94.** $\dfrac{-\sqrt{3}}{2}$

95. -1 **96.** $\dfrac{-\sqrt{3}}{2}$ **97.** $\dfrac{\sqrt{3}}{2}$

98. $-\sqrt{3}$ **99.** $-\frac{1}{2}$ **100.** $\sqrt{2}$

101. $\dfrac{11\pi}{6}$ **102.** 2.07 **103.** 0.43

104. 0.5 **105.** $\dfrac{\pi}{3}$ or 0 **106.** 0.1074

Chapter 2 test

1. a. $305°$

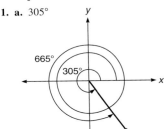

b. $303°$

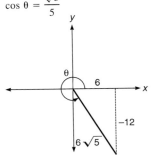

2. $\sin\theta = \dfrac{-2\sqrt{5}}{5}$, $\sec\theta = \sqrt{5}$,

$\tan\theta = -2$, $\csc\theta = \dfrac{-\sqrt{5}}{2}$, $\cot\theta = -\frac{1}{2}$,

$\cos\theta = \dfrac{\sqrt{5}}{5}$

3. $\sin\theta = \dfrac{-3\sqrt{10}}{10}$,

$\csc\theta = \dfrac{-\sqrt{10}}{3}$, $\cos\theta = -\dfrac{\sqrt{10}}{10}$,

$\sec\theta = -\sqrt{10}$, $\tan\theta = 3$,

$\cot\theta = \frac{1}{3}$

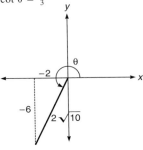

4. $r = \sqrt{(\sqrt{2}a)^2 + a^2} = \sqrt{3a^2} = \sqrt{3}a$

$\sin\theta = \dfrac{a}{\sqrt{3}a} = \dfrac{\sqrt{3}}{3}$, $\cos\theta = \dfrac{\sqrt{2}a}{\sqrt{3}a} = \dfrac{\sqrt{6}}{3}$,

$\tan\theta = \dfrac{a}{\sqrt{2}a} = \dfrac{\sqrt{2}}{2}$, $\csc\theta = \sqrt{3}$,

$\sec\theta = \dfrac{\sqrt{6}}{2}$, $\cot\theta = \sqrt{2}$

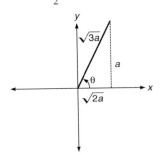

5. a.

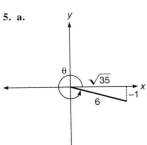

b. $\csc\theta = -6$, $\cos\theta = \dfrac{\sqrt{35}}{6}$,

$\sec\theta = \dfrac{6\sqrt{35}}{35}$, $\tan\theta = \dfrac{-\sqrt{35}}{35}$,

$\cot\theta = -\sqrt{35}$ **c.** $350.4°$

6. a.

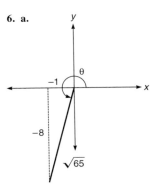

b. $\cot\theta = \dfrac{1}{8}$, $\sin\theta = \dfrac{-8\sqrt{65}}{65}$,

$\cos\theta = \dfrac{-\sqrt{65}}{65}$, $\csc\theta = \dfrac{-\sqrt{65}}{8}$,

$\sec\theta = -\sqrt{65}$ **c.** $262.9°$ **7.** $66.2°$

8. $55.6°$ **9.** 0.8957 **10.** -0.2642

11. 1.1064 **12.** $197.2°$ **13.** $119.0°$

14. 5.1 amperes

15. $x \approx -3.4$ cm, $y \approx -22.3$ cm

16. a. $108.8°$ **b.** 655.1 in.

17. $\dfrac{83\pi}{36}$, 7.24 **18.** $105°$

19. 20.5 inches   **20.** 14.66 cm

21. 1.6709 **22.** $\dfrac{-\sqrt{3}}{2}$

23. 134.04 mm^2 **24. a.** yes   **b.** yes

c. $\{(-3,2), (5,3), (6,5), (12,10)\}$

25. a. $(-4,33)$ **b.** $(\sqrt{2},7 - 3\sqrt{2})$

26. 5.94 **27.** $\dfrac{4\pi}{3}$ **28.** 1.16

29. 0.38 **30.** 0 or $\dfrac{\pi}{6}$ **31.** 0.0589

Chapter 3

Exercise 3–1

Answers to odd-numbered problems

1. a. See figure 3–3.   **b.** See figure 3–6.

c. See figure 3–9.   **3. a.** $\dfrac{\pi}{2} + 2k\pi$

b. $\dfrac{3\pi}{2} + 2k\pi$ **c.** $k\pi$ **5.** $k\pi$ **7. a.** $-\frac{1}{2}$

b. $\dfrac{\sqrt{3}}{2}$ **c.** $\dfrac{-\sqrt{3}}{3}$ **9. a.** $\dfrac{\sqrt{3}}{2}$ **b.** $\frac{1}{2}$

c. $\sqrt{3}$ **11.** odd   **13.** even   **15.** even

17. odd   **19.** even   **21.** even

23. odd   **25.** even

Solutions to trial exercise problems

9. a. $\sin\left(-\dfrac{5\pi}{3}\right) = -\sin\dfrac{5\pi}{3}$

Sine is an odd function.

$\sin\dfrac{5\pi}{3} = -\sin\dfrac{\pi}{3}$

Sine is negative in quadrant IV.

$= -\dfrac{\sqrt{3}}{2},$

so $\sin\left(-\dfrac{5\pi}{3}\right) = -\sin\dfrac{5\pi}{3}$

$= -\left(-\dfrac{\sqrt{3}}{2}\right) = \dfrac{\sqrt{3}}{2}.$

b. $\cos\left(-\dfrac{5\pi}{3}\right) = \cos\dfrac{5\pi}{3}$

Cosine is an even function.

$\cos\dfrac{5\pi}{3} = \cos\dfrac{\pi}{3}$

Cosine is positive in quadrant IV.

$= \dfrac{1}{2},$

so $\cos\left(-\dfrac{5\pi}{3}\right) = \cos\dfrac{5\pi}{3} = \dfrac{1}{2}.$

c. $\tan\left(-\dfrac{5\pi}{3}\right) = -\tan\dfrac{5\pi}{3}$

Tangent is an odd function.

$\tan\dfrac{5\pi}{3} = -\tan\dfrac{\pi}{3}$

Tangent is negative in quadrant IV.

$= -\sqrt{3},$

so $\tan\left(-\dfrac{5\pi}{3}\right) = -\tan\dfrac{5\pi}{3}$

$= -(-\sqrt{3}) = \sqrt{3}.$

17. $f(x) = 3x - 2x^3$

$f(-x) = 3(-x) - 2(-x)^3$

$= -3x + 2x^3$

$-f(x) = -(3x - 2x^3)$

$= -3x + 2x^3$

so $f(-x) = -f(x)$; therefore, f is an odd function.

Exercise 3–2

Answers to odd-numbered problems

1. See figures 3–11, 3–12, and 3–14.

3. $f(x) = \csc(x) = \dfrac{1}{\sin x}$

$f(-x) = \dfrac{1}{\sin(-x)}$

$= \dfrac{1}{-\sin x}$

$= -\dfrac{1}{\sin x}$

$= -\csc(x)$

$= -f(x)$

5. $f(x) = \cot x = \dfrac{1}{\tan x}$

$f(-x) = \cot(-x) = \dfrac{1}{\tan(-x)}$

$= \dfrac{1}{-\tan(x)}$

$= -\dfrac{1}{\tan x}$

$= -\cot x$

$= -f(x)$

Exercise 3–3

Answers to odd-numbered problems

1.

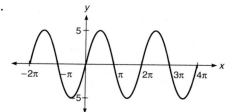

3.

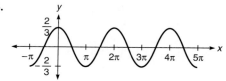

5.

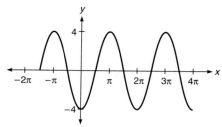

7.

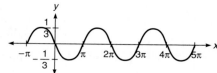

9.

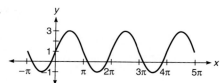

11.

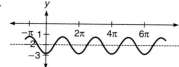

13. amplitude = 2, period = $\dfrac{\pi}{2}$, phase shift = 0

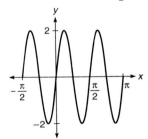

15. amplitude = 1, period = 2π, phase shift = $\dfrac{\pi}{2}$

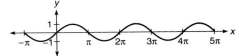

17. amplitude = $\dfrac{2}{3}$, period = $\dfrac{2\pi}{3}$, phase shift = $\dfrac{-\pi}{3}$

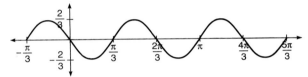

19. amplitude = 1, period = $\dfrac{2\pi}{3}$, phase shift = 0

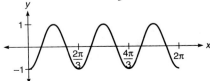

21. amplitude = 1, period = π, phase shift = $\dfrac{-\pi}{4}$

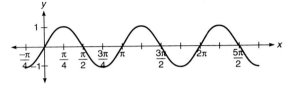

23. amplitude = 1, period = $\dfrac{2\pi}{3}$, phase shift = $\dfrac{-2\pi}{3}$

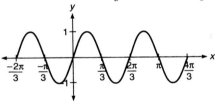

25. amplitude = 1, period = 1, phase shift = 0

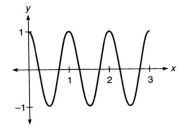

27. amplitude = 2, period = $\dfrac{2\pi}{3}$, phase shift = 0

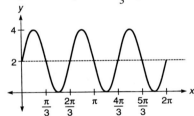

29. amplitude = 3, period = 2π, phase shift = 0

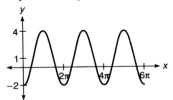

31. amplitude = 2, period = π, phase shift = $\dfrac{\pi}{2}$

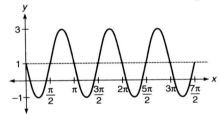

33. amplitude = 1, period = 2, phase shift = 0

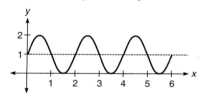

35. $y = -\sin 2x$ **37.** $y = -\cos 3x$ **39.** $y = -\sin(x + 3)$

41. $y = -\sin x - 3$ **43.** $y = -3\cos\left(2x - \dfrac{\pi}{2}\right)$

45. $y = -\sin x$

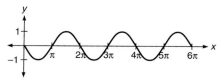

47. $y = \cos\left(x + \dfrac{\pi}{3}\right)$

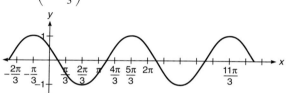

49. $y = \sin(2\pi x - \pi)$

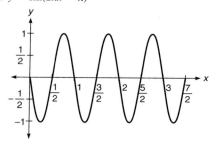

51. $y = -\sin(\pi x - 1)$

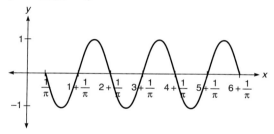

53. $A = 3, B = 4, C = 0, D = 0$ **55.** $A = 2, B = \dfrac{2\pi}{5},$
$C = \dfrac{-2\pi}{5}, D = 0$ **57.** $A = 3, B = 4, C = \dfrac{-\pi}{2}, D = 0$

59. $A = 2, B = \dfrac{2\pi}{5}, C = \dfrac{-9\pi}{10}, D = 0$

61.

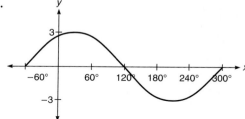

63.

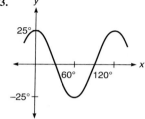

65. $y = 60\sin\left(\dfrac{20x}{3} - 600\right)$

67. $y = 0.5\sin 43x + 23.5$

69.

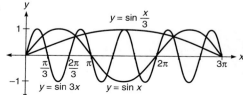

71. Both graphs are the same as figure 3–3, for the sine function.

Solutions to trial exercise problems

11. $y = -\dfrac{3}{4}\cos x - 2$

Period is 2π because the coefficient of the argument is 1. The amplitude is $\frac{3}{4}$, with a reflection about the horizontal axis. There is a vertical shift of 2 units downward. (See the diagram.)

21. $y = -\cos\left(2x + \dfrac{\pi}{2}\right)$

$0 \le 2x + \dfrac{\pi}{2} \le 2\pi$

Subtract $\dfrac{\pi}{2}$.

$-\dfrac{\pi}{2} \le 2x \le \dfrac{3\pi}{2}$

Multiply by $\frac{1}{2}$.

$-\dfrac{\pi}{4} \le x \le \dfrac{3\pi}{4}$

Thus we get one complete cycle of the cosine function, reflected about the horizontal axis (because of the negative coefficient), starting at $-\dfrac{\pi}{4}$ and ending at $\dfrac{3\pi}{4}$. (See the diagram.)

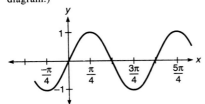

The period is $\dfrac{3\pi}{4} - \left(-\dfrac{\pi}{4}\right) = \dfrac{3\pi}{4} + \dfrac{\pi}{4} = \pi$.

Phase shift is $-\dfrac{\pi}{4}$, and amplitude is 1. We mark the x-axis in increments of one half the period, or $\dfrac{\pi}{2}$, starting at $-\dfrac{\pi}{4}$.

43. $y = -3\cos\left(-2x + \dfrac{\pi}{2}\right)$

Since cosine is an even function, we merely change the sign of the argument. $y = -3\cos\left(2x - \dfrac{\pi}{2}\right)$.

51. $y = \sin(-\pi x + 1)$

Sine is an odd function, so we change both the sign of the coefficient and the sign of the argument. $y = -\sin(\pi x - 1)$.

$0 \le \pi x - 1 \le 2\pi$

Add 1.

$1 \le \pi x \le 2\pi + 1$

Divide by π.

$\dfrac{1}{\pi} \le x \le \dfrac{2\pi + 1}{\pi}$

Phase shift is $\dfrac{1}{\pi}$, period is $\dfrac{2\pi + 1}{\pi} - \dfrac{1}{\pi} = \dfrac{2\pi}{\pi} + \dfrac{1}{\pi} - \dfrac{1}{\pi}$

$= 2$. Amplitude is 1.

We mark the x-axis in increments of one half the period (1), starting at $\dfrac{1}{\pi}$. (We also compute decimal approximations as a

convenience in plotting.) The calculations are as follows:

$\dfrac{1}{\pi} + 1 \approx 1.3$; $\left(\dfrac{1}{\pi} + 1\right) + 1 = \dfrac{1}{\pi} + 2 \approx 2.3$;

$\left(\dfrac{1}{\pi} + 2\right) + 1 = \dfrac{1}{\pi} + 3 \approx 3.3$;

$\dfrac{1}{\pi} + 4 \approx 4.3$; $\dfrac{1}{\pi} + 5 \approx 5.3$; $\left(\dfrac{1}{\pi} + 1\right) - 1 = \dfrac{1}{\pi} \approx 0.3$;

$\dfrac{1}{\pi} - 1 \approx -0.7$.   (See the diagram.)

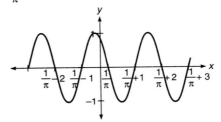

56. Amplitude = 2. We have one cycle between 0 and 3π.

$0 \le x \le 3\pi$

Multiply by $\frac{2}{3}$.

$0 \le \dfrac{2x}{3} \le 2\pi$

Vertical shift = 3, so the equation is $y = 2\sin\left(\dfrac{2x}{3}\right) + 3$.

64. $y = 10\sin(2x - 180°)$ (See the diagram.)

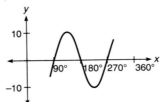

$0° \le 2x - 180° \le 360°$

Add 180°.

$180° \le 2x \le 540°$

Divide by 2.

$90° \le x \le 270°$

67. Amplitude is 0.5; 0° phase shift; period $\left(\dfrac{360}{43}\right)°$; vertical translation 23.5.

$0° \le x \le \dfrac{360°}{43}$

$0° \le 43x \le 360°$

Thus, the argument is $43x$, and we have for

$y = A\sin(Bx + C) + D$,

$A = 0.5$, $B = 43$, $C = 0$, $D = 23.5$, for

$y = 0.5\sin 43x + 23.5$

Exercise 3–4

Answers to odd-numbered problems

1.

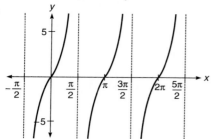

3.

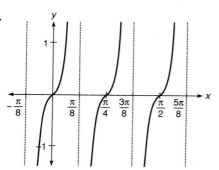

5.

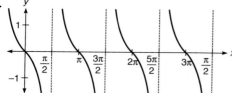

7.

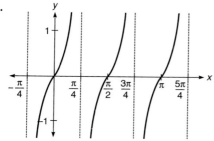

9.

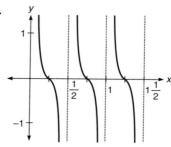

11. $y = -\tan 2x$

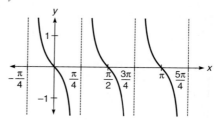

13. $y = \cot \pi x$

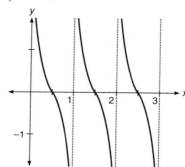

15. $y = -\tan(x + \pi)$

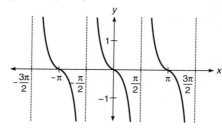

17.

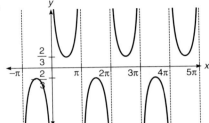

19.

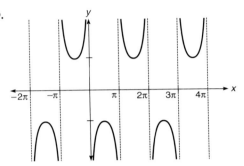

21.

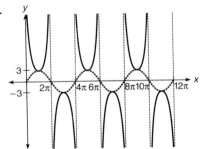

23.

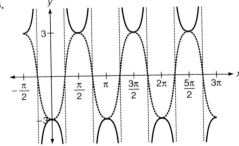

25.

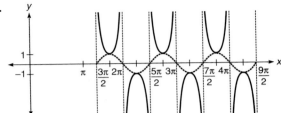

27.

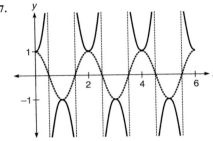

29.

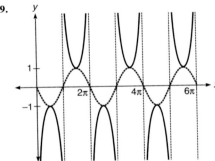

31.

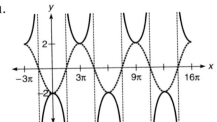

Solutions to trial exercise problems

7. $y = -\cot\left(2x + \dfrac{\pi}{2}\right)$

There is a reversal about the horizontal axis, because of the negative coefficient. To find the beginning and end points for one cycle,

$$0 < 2x + \frac{\pi}{2} < \pi$$

Subtract $\dfrac{\pi}{2}$.

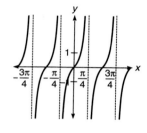

$$-\frac{\pi}{2} < 2x < \frac{\pi}{2}$$

Multiply by $\dfrac{1}{2}$.

$$-\frac{\pi}{4} < x < \frac{\pi}{4}$$

Thus, one complete cycle starts at $\dfrac{-\pi}{4}$ and terminates at $\dfrac{\pi}{4}$, reversed about the horizontal axis. (See the diagram.)

15. $y = \tan(-x - \pi)$

The tangent function is odd, so we change both the sign of the argument and the coefficient of the function.

$y = -\tan(x + \pi)$

We find the beginning and end points.

$$-\frac{\pi}{2} < x + \pi < \frac{\pi}{2}$$

Subtract π.

$-1\tfrac{1}{2}\pi < x < -\tfrac{1}{2}\pi$.

See the diagram.

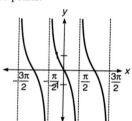

24. $y = \tfrac{2}{3}\sec(3x + \pi)$

We first graph $y = \tfrac{2}{3}\cos(3x + \pi)$.

$0 \le 3x + \pi \le 2\pi$

Subtract π.

$-\pi \le 3x \le \pi$

$$-\frac{\pi}{3} \le x \le \frac{\pi}{3}$$

See the diagram.

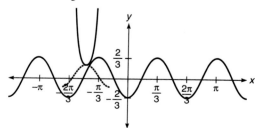

Next we construct the graph of the corresponding secant function. This graph touches the cosine graph at its high and

low values and has vertical asymptotes wherever the cosine graph is 0 (crosses the x-axis). (See the diagram.)

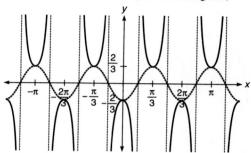

28. $y = \sec(-2x)$

The secant function is even (as is the cosine function), so we simply change the sign of the argument.

$y = \sec 2x$

We graph $y = \cos 2x$ first, then use this to construct the secant graph. (See the diagram.)

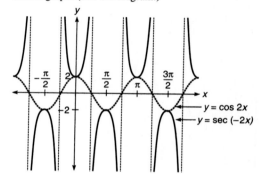

$0 \le 2x \le 2\pi$
$0 \le x \le \pi$

Chapter 3 review

1. See figure 3–3 for the graph; R; $-1 \le y \le 1$; 2π **2.** all multiples of 2π: $2k\pi$, k an integer   **3.** $\dfrac{\sqrt{3}}{2}$ **4.** $-\sqrt{3}$

5. $-\tfrac{1}{2}$ **6.** $\sqrt{2}$ **7.** odd   **8.** even   **9.** odd

10. See figure 3–11.   **11.** domain: $x \ne k\pi$, k an integer; range: R **12.** $f(-x) = \dfrac{-x}{\sec(-x)} = \dfrac{-x}{\sec x} = -f(x)$

13. $f(-x) = \sec(-x) \cdot [\sin(-x)]^2 + (-x)^4 = \sec x \cdot [-\sin x]^2 + x^4 = \sec x \cdot \sin^2 x + x^4 = f(x)$

14. amplitude $= 2$, period $= 2\pi$, phase shift $= 0$

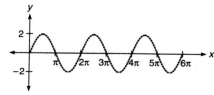

15. amplitude $= \frac{2}{3}$, period $= 2\pi$, phase shift $= 0$

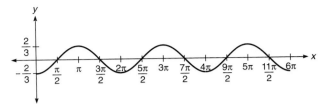

16. amplitude $= 3$, period $= 2\pi$, phase shift $= 0$

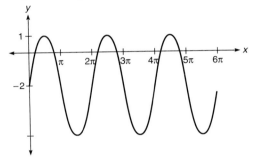

17. amplitude $= 2$, period $= \frac{2\pi}{3}$, phase shift $= 0$

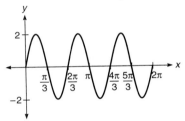

18. amplitude $= 1$, period $= 2\pi$, phase shift $= \frac{-\pi}{3}$

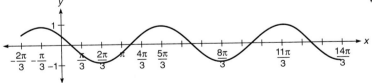

19. amplitude $= 2$, period $= 4\pi$, phase shift $= \frac{-2\pi}{3}$

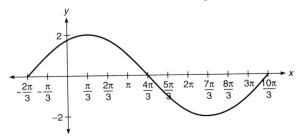

20. amplitude $= 1$, period $= \frac{2}{3}$, phase shift $= 0$

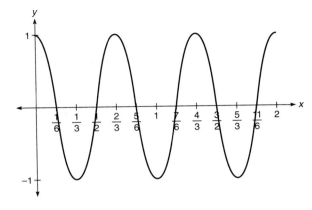

21. amplitude $= 3$, period $= \pi$, phase shift $= 0$

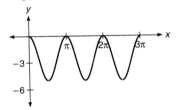

22. $y = \cos\left(2x - \dfrac{\pi}{2}\right)$

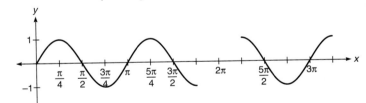

23. $y = -3\sin(x - \pi)$

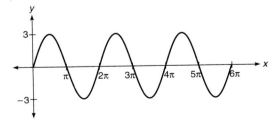

24.

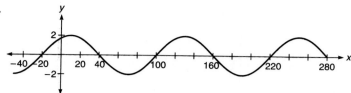

25. amplitude $= 2$, so $A = 2$; $Bx + C = 2x - \dfrac{\pi}{3}$, so $B = 2$,

$C = -\dfrac{\pi}{3}$, and $D = -1$; $y = 2\cos\left(2x - \dfrac{\pi}{3}\right) - 1$

26. $y = \sin\left(\dfrac{2\pi}{23}x + \dfrac{20\pi}{23}\right)$

27.

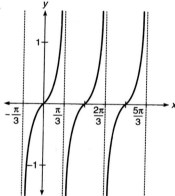

28.

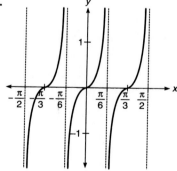

29.

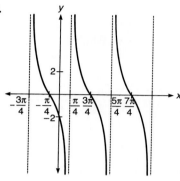

30.

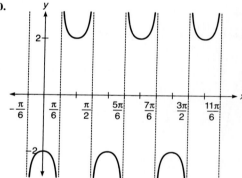

31.

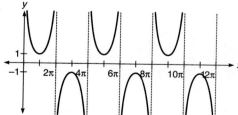

32.

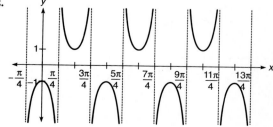

33.

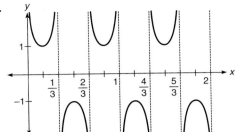

Chapter 3 test

1. $\dfrac{3\pi}{2} + 2k\pi$, k an integer   **2.** $\sqrt{3}$ **3.** odd

4. amplitude $= 2$, period $= 2\pi$, phase shift $= 0$

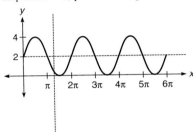

5. amplitude $= 3$, period $= \pi$, phase shift $= 0$

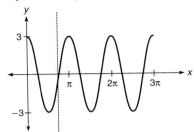

6. amplitude $= 3$, period $= 6\pi$, phase shift $= \dfrac{-3\pi}{2}$

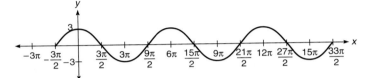

7.

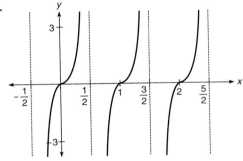

8.

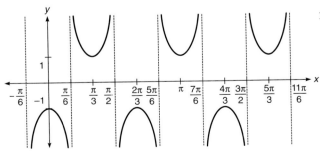

9.

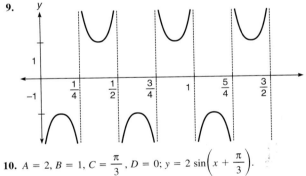

10. $A = 2$, $B = 1$, $C = \dfrac{\pi}{3}$, $D = 0$; $y = 2\sin\left(x + \dfrac{\pi}{3}\right)$.

11.

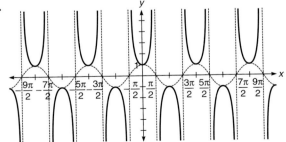

12. $f(-x) = \sec(-x) \cdot \sin(-x) + (-x)^3 = \sec x \cdot (-\sin x) - x^3 = -(\sec x \cdot \sin x + x^3) = -f(x)$

13. $y = \sin\left(\dfrac{\pi}{14}x - \dfrac{5\pi}{14}\right)$

14. $y = 25 \sin\left(\dfrac{12}{5}x + 48°\right) + 10$

Chapter 4

Exercise 4–1

Answers to odd-numbered problems

1. Let $y = f(x) = 2x - 7$. Show $g(y) = x$:
$g(y) = \frac{1}{2}y + 3\frac{1}{2}$
$\quad = \frac{1}{2}(2x - 7) + \frac{7}{2}$
$\quad = x$
Let $y = g(x) = \frac{1}{2}x + \frac{7}{2}$. Show $f(y) = x$:
$f(y) = 2y - 7 = 2(\frac{1}{2}x + \frac{7}{2}) - 7 = x$

3. Let $y = f(x) = \frac{1}{3}x + \frac{8}{3}$. Show $g(y) = x$:
$g(y) = 3y - 8 = 3(\frac{1}{3}x + \frac{8}{3}) - 8 = x$
Let $y = g(x) = 3x - 8$. Show $f(y) = x$:
$f(y) = \frac{1}{3}y + \frac{8}{3} = \frac{1}{3}(3x - 8) + \frac{8}{3} = x$

5. Let $y = f(x) = 2x - 5$. Show $g(y) = x$:
$g(y) = \frac{1}{2}(y + 5) = \frac{1}{2}[(2x - 5) + 5] = x$
Let $y = g(x) = \frac{1}{2}(x + 5)$. Show $f(y) = x$:
$f(y) = 2y - 5 = 2[\frac{1}{2}(x + 5)] - 5 = x$

7. Let $y = f(x) = \dfrac{2}{x - 3}$. Show $g(y) = x$:

$g(y) = \dfrac{2}{y} + 3 = \dfrac{2}{\dfrac{2}{x - 3}} + 3 = (x - 3) + 3 = x$

Let $y = g(x) = \dfrac{2}{x} + 3$. Show $f(y) = x$:

$f(y) = \dfrac{2}{y - 3} = \dfrac{2}{\left(\dfrac{2}{x} + 3\right) - 3} = \dfrac{2}{\dfrac{2}{x}} = x$

9. Let $y = f(x) = 7 - \dfrac{3}{x}$. Show $g(y) = x$:

$g(y) = \dfrac{3}{7 - y} = \dfrac{3}{7 - \left(7 - \dfrac{3}{x}\right)} = \dfrac{3}{\dfrac{3}{x}} = x$

Let $y = g(x) = \dfrac{3}{7 - x}$. Show $f(y) = x$:

$f(y) = 7 - \dfrac{3}{y} = 7 - \dfrac{3}{\dfrac{3}{7 - x}} = 7 - (7 - x) = x$

11. Let $y = f(x) = \dfrac{x}{x - 1}$. Show $g(y) = x$:

$g(y) = \dfrac{y}{y - 1} = \dfrac{\dfrac{x}{x - 1}}{\dfrac{x}{x - 1} - 1}$

$= \dfrac{\dfrac{x}{x - 1}}{\dfrac{x}{x - 1} - 1} \cdot \dfrac{x - 1}{x - 1}$

$= \dfrac{x}{x - (x - 1)} = x$

Let $y = g(x) = \dfrac{x}{x - 1}$. Show $f(y) = x$:

$f(y) = \dfrac{y}{y - 1} = \dfrac{\dfrac{x}{x - 1}}{\dfrac{x}{x - 1} - 1}$

$= \dfrac{\dfrac{x}{x - 1}}{\dfrac{x}{x - 1} - 1} \cdot \dfrac{x - 1}{x - 1}$

$= \dfrac{x}{x - (x - 1)} = x$

13. Let $y = f(x) = x^2 - 9$. Show $g(y) = x$:
$g(y) = \sqrt{y + 9} = \sqrt{(x^2 - 9) + 9}$
$\quad = \sqrt{x^2} = x$ if $x \geq 0$.
Let $y = g(x) = \sqrt{x + 9}$. Show $f(y) = x$:
$f(y) = y^2 - 9 = (\sqrt{x + 9})^2 - 9$
$\quad = (x + 9) - 9 = x$

15. Let $y = f(x) = x^3$ Show $g(y) = x$:
$g(y) = \sqrt[3]{y} = \sqrt[3]{x^3} = x$
Let $y = g(x) = \sqrt[3]{x}$. Show $f(y) = x$:
$f(y) = y^3 = (\sqrt[3]{x})^3 = x$

17. Let $y = f(x) = x^2 - 2x + 3$. Show $g(y) = x$:
$g(y) = \sqrt{y - 2} + 1$
$\quad = \sqrt{(x^2 - 2x + 3) - 2} + 1$
$\quad = \sqrt{x^2 - 2x + 1} + 1$
$\quad = \sqrt{(x - 1)^2} + 1 = x - 1 + 1 = x$
Let $y = g(x) = \sqrt{x - 2} + 1$. Show $f(y) = x$:
$f(y) = y^2 - 2y + 3$
$\quad = (\sqrt{x - 2} + 1)^2 - 2(\sqrt{x - 2} + 1) + 3$
$\quad = [(x - 2) + 2\sqrt{x - 2} + 1] - 2\sqrt{x - 1} - 2 + 3$
$\quad = x$

19. Let $y = f(x) = \dfrac{2x}{x-3}$. Show $g(y) = x$:

$$g(y) = \frac{3y}{y-2} = \frac{3 \cdot \dfrac{2x}{x-3}}{\dfrac{2x}{x-3} - 2}$$

$$= \frac{3 \cdot \dfrac{2x}{x-3}}{\dfrac{2x}{x-3} - 2} \cdot \frac{x-3}{x-3}$$

$$= \frac{3(2x)}{2x - 2(x-3)} = \frac{6x}{6} = x$$

Let $y = g(x) = \dfrac{3x}{x-2}$. Show $f(y) = x$:

$$f(y) = \frac{2y}{y-3} = \frac{2 \cdot \dfrac{3x}{x-2}}{\dfrac{3x}{x-2} - 3}$$

$$= \frac{2 \cdot \dfrac{3x}{x-2}}{\dfrac{3x}{x-2} - 3} \cdot \frac{x-2}{x-2}$$

$$= \frac{6x}{3x - 3(x-2)} = \frac{6x}{6} = x$$

21. function, not one to one
23. not a function

25.

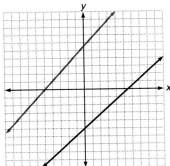

27.

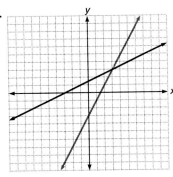

29.

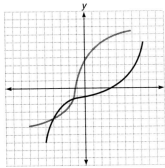

31.

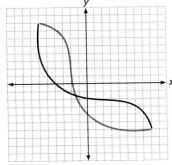

33. $A^{-1}(x) = \dfrac{x}{4} - 4$ **35.** $R^{-1}(x) = \dfrac{20x}{20-x}$

Solutions to trial exercise problems

31. We mark four points on the graph. Any points will do, but the end points and intercepts are good choices.

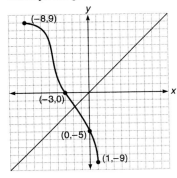

We move these points across the line $y = x$. This is shown in the second figure.

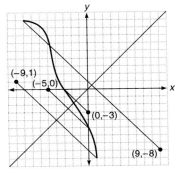

We connect the points and obtain the graph of the inverse function.

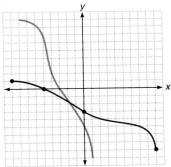

34. $d(t) = 16t^2$

$y = 16t^2$

$t = 16y^2$

$y^2 = \dfrac{t}{16}$

$y = \pm\sqrt{\dfrac{t}{16}}$

$y = \pm\dfrac{\sqrt{t}}{4}$

$y = \dfrac{\sqrt{t}}{4}$ (choose $+$ among $\pm\dfrac{\sqrt{t}}{4}$; to see why, consider that the point $(1,16)$ is in the function d, so the point $(16,1)$ must be in d^{-1}).

$d^{-1}(t) = \dfrac{\sqrt{t}}{4}$

Exercise 4–2

Answers to odd-numbered problems

1. See figure 4–6.   **3.** $-\dfrac{\pi}{6}$, $-30°$

5. $0, 0°$ **7.** $-\dfrac{\pi}{3}$, $-60°$

9. 1.08 rad, 61.9°   **11.** 1.20 rad, 68.8°
13. -1.50 rad, $-86.0°$ **15.** -0.26 rad,
$-14.9°$ **17.** $\dfrac{5\sqrt{39}}{39}$ **19.** $\dfrac{3\sqrt{5}}{5}$

21. $\dfrac{\sqrt{66}}{3}$ **23.** $\dfrac{\sqrt{91}}{10}$ **25.** $\sqrt{1-z^2}$

27. $\dfrac{1+z}{\sqrt{-2z-z^2}}$ **29.** $\dfrac{\sqrt{1-2z}}{1-2z}$ **31.** $\dfrac{\pi}{6}$

33. $-\dfrac{\pi}{6}$ **35.** $\dfrac{\pi}{2}$ **37.** Let f be a
periodic function; then $f(x) = y =$
$f(x + kp) = y$ gives ordered pairs (x,y),
$(x + kp, y)$; second element repeats, so not
one to one.

Solutions to trial exercise problems

7. $\arcsin\left(-\dfrac{\sqrt{3}}{2}\right)$

We want the angle in quadrant I or
quadrant IV whose sine value is $-\dfrac{\sqrt{3}}{2}$.
Since the argument is negative, we
know that we want an angle in
quadrant IV, where the sine function is
negative. Since we have memorized
the fact that $\sin 60° = \dfrac{\sqrt{3}}{2}$, the
reference angle is 60°. Therefore, the
angle is $-60°$, or $-\dfrac{\pi}{3}$ (radians).
(Remember that we use negative
values for the inverse sine function in
quadrant IV.)

13. $\sin^{-1}(-0.9976)$
Calculator:
The keystrokes are the same for radian
and degree mode.
.9976 [+/−] [INV] [SIN]

[TI-81] [SIN⁻¹] [(−)] .9976

[ENTER]
$(= -1.501500431 = -1.50$ to two
decimal places)
$(= -86.02963761° = -86.0°$ to one
decimal place)

21. $\cot\left(\sin^{-1}\dfrac{\sqrt{3}}{5}\right)$

We want the cotangent of a first
quadrant angle whose sine is $\dfrac{\sqrt{3}}{5}$.
Such an angle is shown in the diagram.
The Pythagorean theorem shows that
$x = \sqrt{22}$, so the cotangent of this
angle is $\dfrac{\text{adj}}{\text{opp}} = \dfrac{\sqrt{22}}{\sqrt{3}} = \dfrac{\sqrt{66}}{3}$. (Multiply
numerator and denominator by $\sqrt{3}$.)

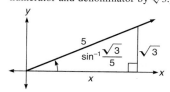

27. $\tan[\sin^{-1}(1 + z)]$, $1 + z < 0$
The argument of the inverse sine
function is negative, so this represents
an angle in quadrant IV. The diagram
shows a reference triangle in quadrant
IV, where the sine of the angle in
standard position is $1 + z$. Now we use
the Pythagorean theorem to find x.
$1^2 = x^2 + (1 + z)^2$
$1 = x^2 + 1 + 2z + z^2$
$-2z - z^2 = x^2$
$\sqrt{-2z - z^2} = x$
Now, the tangent of the angle is
$\dfrac{\text{opp}}{\text{adj}} = \dfrac{1+z}{\sqrt{-2z-z^2}}$
Thus, $\tan[\sin^{-1}(1 + z)]$
$= \dfrac{1+z}{\sqrt{-2z-z^2}}$.

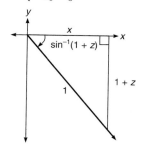

30. $\cot(\sin^{-1}\sqrt{z-1})$
If $\sqrt{z-1} = 0$, we know $\sin^{-1}0 = 0$,
and $\cot 0$ is undefined. Since $\sqrt{z-1}$
< 0 is impossible, we assume $\sqrt{z-1}$
> 0. In this case, we want a first-
quadrant reference triangle. This is
shown in the diagram. We find x.
$x^2 + (\sqrt{z-1})^2 = 1^2$
$x^2 + z - 1 = 1$
$x^2 = 2 - z$
$x = \sqrt{2 - z}$
The cotangent of this angle is
$\dfrac{\text{adj}}{\text{opp}} = \dfrac{\sqrt{2-z}}{\sqrt{z-1}}$.

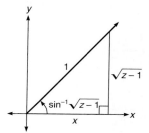

34. $\sin^{-1}\left(\sin\dfrac{11\pi}{6}\right)$

$\sin^{-1}\left(\sin\dfrac{11\pi}{6}\right) = \sin^{-1}\left(-\dfrac{1}{2}\right)$

$= -\dfrac{\pi}{6}$ or $-30°$

Exercise 4–3

Answers to odd-numbered problems

1. a. See figure 4–6.   **b.** See figure 4–8.

c. See figure 4–10.   **3.** $\dfrac{2\pi}{3}$ rad, 120°

5. $\dfrac{\pi}{2}$ rad, 90°   **7.** $\dfrac{\pi}{3}$ rad, 60°

9. $-\dfrac{\pi}{3}$ rad, $-60°$ **11.** $-\dfrac{\pi}{6}$ rad, $-30°$

13. 1.08 rad, 61.9°   **15.** 0.60 rad, 34.4°
17. 0.75 rad, 43.0°   **19.** 0.92 rad, 52.8°
21. -1.50 rad, $-86.0°$ **23.** -0.25 rad,
$-14.3°$ **25.** 3.00 rad, 172°   **27.** $\dfrac{5\sqrt{34}}{34}$

29. $\dfrac{\sqrt{39}}{8}$ **31.** $-\dfrac{\sqrt{5}}{2}$ **33.** $\dfrac{\sqrt{30}}{6}$

35. $\dfrac{10\sqrt{109}}{109}$ **37.** $\sqrt{1-z^2}$

39. $\dfrac{\sqrt{1-z^2}}{z}$ **41.** $\dfrac{1}{\sqrt{1+z^2}}$

43. $\sqrt{1-9z^2}$ **45.** $\sqrt{2+2z+z^2}$

47. $\dfrac{1}{\sqrt{1+2z}}$ **49.** $\dfrac{\pi}{4}$

51. $\dfrac{\pi}{6}$ **53.** 0 **55.** $\sin^{-1}\dfrac{m}{r}$

57. $\tan^{-1}\dfrac{k}{h}$ **59.** $\tan^{-1}\dfrac{2}{x}$

61. $\sin^{-1}\dfrac{3{,}500}{z}$ **63.** $\cos^{-1}(-0.8)$

65. $\tan^{-1}4.1$ **67.** $\tan^{-1}\dfrac{5}{3}$

69. $\tan^{-1}50$ **71.** $\dfrac{\tan^{-1}9}{3}$

73. $\dfrac{2\sin^{-1}(-0.56)}{3}$ **75.** $\dfrac{\sin^{-1}0.75}{4}$

77. $\dfrac{\sin^{-1}\frac{25}{39}}{5}$ **79.** $\dfrac{\tan^{-1}\frac{D}{A}-C}{B}$

81. $\dfrac{\sin^{-1}0.6-3}{2}$

Solutions to trial exercise problems

11. $\tan^{-1}\left(-\dfrac{\sqrt{3}}{3}\right)$

We want the angle in quadrant I or quadrant IV whose tangent is $-\dfrac{\sqrt{3}}{3}$.

We know that $\tan 30°\left(\text{or } \dfrac{\pi}{6}\right)$ is $\dfrac{\sqrt{3}}{3}$.

Thus, the required values are $-30°$ or $-\dfrac{\pi}{6}$.

23. $\arctan(-0.2553)$

Calculator steps are the same in both degree and radian mode.

.2553 ⟦+/−⟧ ⟦INV⟧ ⟦TAN⟧

⟦TI-81⟧ ⟦TAN⁻¹⟧ ⟦(−)⟧ .2553

⟦ENTER⟧

$(=-14.32168996°)$

$(=-0.249960644)$

Thus, rounded, $\arctan(-0.2553)$ $=-14.3°$ or -0.25 (radians).

31. $\tan[\cos^{-1}(-\tfrac{2}{3})]$

$\cos^{-1}(-\tfrac{2}{3})$ is an angle in quadrant II whose cosine is $-\tfrac{2}{3}$. Such an angle is shown in the reference triangle in the diagram. The Pythagorean theorem shows that $y=\sqrt{5}$, and we can then determine that the tangent is $\dfrac{\text{opp}}{\text{adj}}$

$=-\dfrac{\sqrt{5}}{2}$.

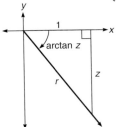

41. $\cos(\arctan z),\ z<0$

$\arctan z$ is an angle in quadrant IV if $z<0$. A reference triangle is shown in the diagram. To find r: $r^2=1^2+z^2$; $r=\sqrt{1+z^2}$ (We know that $r>0$.) Thus, using the reference triangle, $\cos(\arctan z),\ z<0,=\dfrac{1}{\sqrt{1+z^2}}$.

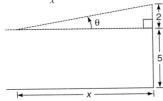

51. $\cos^{-1}\left(\cos\dfrac{11\pi}{6}\right)=\cos^{-1}\left(\dfrac{\sqrt{3}}{2}\right)=\dfrac{\pi}{6}$

59. Refer to the diagram.

$\tan\theta=\dfrac{2}{x}$, so

$\theta=\tan^{-1}\dfrac{2}{x}$.

77. $\dfrac{6\sin 5\theta}{5}=\dfrac{10}{13}$

$\dfrac{6\sin 5\theta}{5}=\dfrac{10}{13}$

Multiply by 5.

$6\sin 5\theta=\dfrac{50}{13}$

Multiply by $\dfrac{1}{6}$.

$\sin 5\theta=\dfrac{50}{78}$

Reduce.

$\sin 5\theta=\dfrac{25}{39}$

$5\theta=\sin^{-1}\dfrac{25}{39}$

Divide by 5.

$\theta=\dfrac{\sin^{-1}\frac{25}{39}}{5}$

81. $\sin(2x+3)=0.6$

$\sin(2x+3)=0.6$

$2x+3=\sin^{-1}0.6$

Subtract 3.

$2x=\sin^{-1}0.6-3$

Divide by 2.

$x=\dfrac{\sin^{-1}0.6-3}{2}$

82. a. The two reference triangles in the first diagram show $\arcsin x$ when $x>0$ and $x<0$. In each case we can see that the tangent of this angle is $\dfrac{x}{\sqrt{1-x^2}}$.

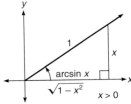

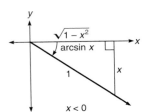

b. In the second diagram we see the reference triangle for arccos x, $x > 0$. It is easy to see that the tangent of the angle arccos x is $\dfrac{\sqrt{1 - x^2}}{x}$.

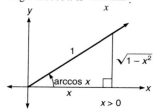

In the third diagram we see both arctan $\dfrac{\sqrt{1 - x^2}}{x}$, $x < 0$, and arccos x, $x < 0$. Note that $\dfrac{\sqrt{1 - x^2}}{x}$, $x < 0 = \dfrac{-\sqrt{1 - x^2}}{|x|}$, $x < 0$. We can see that they differ by π radians.

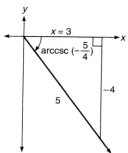

Exercise 4–4

Answers to odd-numbered problems

1. $\dfrac{\pi}{6}$ rad, 30°   3. $\dfrac{\pi}{4}$ rad, 45°

5. $\dfrac{2\pi}{3}$ rad, 120°   7. $\dfrac{\pi}{3}$ rad, 60°

9. $\dfrac{\pi}{2}$ rad, 90°   11. 0.30 rad, 17.3°

13. 1.91, 109.5°   15. 0.19 rad, 10.9°

17. 1.66 rad, 95.2°   19. 0.32 rad, 18.3°

21. $\frac{1}{3}$ 23. $\dfrac{\sqrt{15}}{15}$ 25. $\sqrt{26}$

27. $\frac{3}{5}$ 29. $-\dfrac{\sqrt{11}}{5}$ 31. $\dfrac{1}{z}$

33. $\dfrac{\sqrt{z^2 + 1}}{z}$ 35. $\dfrac{1}{2z}$ 37. $\sqrt{z^2 + 2z}$

39. $\dfrac{3}{z}$

Solutions to trial exercise problems

7. arccsc $\dfrac{2\sqrt{3}}{3}$

By definition, arccsc $\dfrac{2\sqrt{3}}{3}$

$= \arcsin \dfrac{1}{\dfrac{2\sqrt{3}}{3}}$

$= \arcsin\left(\dfrac{3}{2\sqrt{3}} \cdot \dfrac{\sqrt{3}}{\sqrt{3}}\right)$

$= \arcsin \dfrac{3\sqrt{3}}{2 \cdot 3}$

$= \arcsin \dfrac{\sqrt{3}}{2}$

$= 60°$ or $\dfrac{\pi}{3}$

17. $\sec^{-1}(-11.1261)$

$\sec^{-1}(-11.1261) = \cos^{-1}\left(\dfrac{1}{-11.1261}\right)$

by definition.

11.1261 [+/−] [1/x] [INV]

[COS]

[TI-81] [COS⁻¹] [(−)] 11.1261

[x⁻¹] [ENTER]

(= 95.15663191 in degree mode)
(= 1.660796532 in radian mode)
so $\sec^{-1}(-11.1261) = 95.2°$ or 1.66 (radians).

---

27. $\cos[\text{arccsc}(-\frac{5}{4})]$

$\cos[\text{arccsc}(-\frac{5}{4})] = \cos[\arcsin(-\frac{4}{5})]$

by definition.

$\arcsin(-\frac{4}{5})$ is shown in the diagram.

The cosine of this angle is $\frac{3}{5}$. Thus,

$\cos[\text{arccsc}(-\frac{5}{4})] = \frac{3}{5}$.

40. $\sec\left(\cot^{-1}\dfrac{2}{z + 1}\right)$, $z + 1 > 0$

$\cot^{-1}\dfrac{2}{z + 1}$, $z + 1 > 0$, is an angle in quadrant I; a reference triangle is shown in the diagram. We can find r.
$r^2 = 2^2 + (z + 1)^2$
$r^2 = z^2 + 2z + 5$
$r = \sqrt{z^2 + 2z + 5}$
The cosine of the angle is

$\dfrac{2}{\sqrt{z^2 + 2z + 5}}$, and so the secant, which is the reciprocal of the cosine, is $\dfrac{\sqrt{z^2 + 2z + 5}}{2}$.

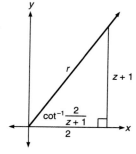

Chapter 4 review

1. Let $y = f(x) = 3x - 5$; show that
$g(y) = x$.

$$g(y) = \frac{y + 5}{3} = \frac{(3x - 5) + 5}{3} = x$$

Let $y = g(x) = \frac{x + 5}{3}$; show that

$f(y) = x$.

$$f(y) = 3y - 5 = 3\left(\frac{x + 5}{3}\right) - 5 = x$$

2. Let $y = f(x) = \frac{3x}{x + 1}$; show that

$g(y) = x$.

$$g(y) = \frac{-y}{y - 3} = \frac{-\dfrac{3x}{x + 1}}{\dfrac{3x}{x + 1} - 3}$$

$$= \frac{-\dfrac{3x}{x + 1}}{\dfrac{3x}{x + 1} - 3} \cdot \frac{x + 1}{x + 1}$$

$$= \frac{-3x}{3x - 3(x + 1)} = x$$

Let $y = g(x) = \frac{-x}{x - 3}$; show that

$f(y) = x$.

$$f(y) = \frac{3y}{y + 1} = \frac{3\dfrac{-x}{x - 3}}{\dfrac{-x}{x - 3} + 1}$$

$$= \frac{3\dfrac{-x}{x - 3}}{\dfrac{-x}{x - 3} + 1} \cdot \frac{x - 3}{x - 3}$$

$$= \frac{-3x}{-x + 1(x - 3)} = x$$

3. no **4.** yes **5.** See figure 4–6.

6. $\text{domain}_{\sin^{-1}}\ 1 \le x \le 1;\ \text{range}_{\sin^{-1}} -\dfrac{\pi}{2} \le$

$y \le \dfrac{\pi}{2}$ **7.** $-\dfrac{\pi}{6}$ rad, $-30°$

8. $\dfrac{\pi}{3}$ rad, $60°$ **9.** $\dfrac{\pi}{6}$ rad, $30°$

10. $\dfrac{-\pi}{4}$ rad, $-45°$ **11.** 0 rad, $0°$

12. $-\dfrac{\pi}{2}$ rad, $-90°$ **13.** 1.34 rad, $76.8°$

14. -0.51 rad, $-29.2°$ **15.** $\dfrac{4}{5}$

16. $\dfrac{\sqrt{15}}{15}$ **17.** $\dfrac{3\sqrt{5}}{5}$ **18.** $\dfrac{z\sqrt{1 - z^2}}{1 - z^2}$

19. $\sqrt{-z^2 - 2z}$ **20.** See figure 4–8.

21. $\text{domain}_{\tan^{-1}}\ R;\ \text{range}_{\tan^{-1}} -\dfrac{\pi}{2} < y < \dfrac{\pi}{2}$

22. $\dfrac{2\pi}{3}$ rad, $120°$

23. $\dfrac{\pi}{6}$ rad, $30°$ **24.** $\dfrac{\pi}{3}$ rad, $60°$

25. $-\dfrac{\pi}{4}$ rad, $-45°$ **26.** $\dfrac{\pi}{3}$ rad, $60°$

27. $-\dfrac{\pi}{4}$ rad, $-45°$ **28.** 1.00 rad, $57.3°$

29. 1.06 rad, $60.8°$ **30.** 1.88 rad, $107.8°$

31. $\dfrac{5\sqrt{34}}{34}$ **32.** 4 **33.** $-\dfrac{\sqrt{5}}{2}$

34. $\dfrac{2\pi}{3}$ rad, $120°$ **35.** $\dfrac{\sqrt{1 - z^2}}{z}$

36. $\dfrac{1}{\sqrt{z^2 + 2z + 2}}$ **37.** $\sin^{-1}\dfrac{j}{k}$

38. $\sin^{-1}\frac{7}{11}$ **39.** $\tan^{-1}\dfrac{35}{x}$

40. $\cos^{-1}0.89$ **41.** $\sin^{-1}(-0.88)$
42. $\sin^{-1}(-0.2)$ **43.** $\tan^{-1}5$

44. $\dfrac{\sin^{-1}0.76}{2}$ **45.** $\dfrac{\cos^{-1}0.7}{3}$

46. $\dfrac{\cos^{-1}(0.6) - 3}{2}$ **47.** $\dfrac{\sin^{-1}0.6}{2}$

48. $\dfrac{\pi}{3}$ rad, $60°$ **49.** $-\dfrac{\pi}{3}$ rad, $-60°$

50. $-\dfrac{\pi}{6}$ rad, $-30°$ **51.** $\dfrac{5\pi}{6}$ rad, $150°$

52. 0.23 rad, $13.2°$ **53.** 0.57 rad, $32.7°$
54. 1.82 rad, $104.3°$ **55.** -0.15 rad,

$-8.6°$ **56.** $\dfrac{\sqrt{2}}{4}$ **57.** $\dfrac{\sqrt{15}}{15}$ **58.** $\dfrac{\sqrt{26}}{26}$

59. $\dfrac{7\sqrt{33}}{33}$ **60.** $\dfrac{\sqrt{z^2 + 1}}{z^2 + 1}$ **61.** $\sqrt{z^2 - 1}$

62. $\sqrt{z^2 + 2z}$ **63.** $\dfrac{1 - z}{\sqrt{-2z + z^2}}$

Chapter 4 test

1. See figure 4–10. **2.** $\text{domain}_{\csc^{-1}}\ |x|$

$\ge 1;\ \text{range}_{\csc^{-1}} \dfrac{-\pi}{2} \le y \le \dfrac{\pi}{2},\ y \ne 0$

3. $\dfrac{2\pi}{3}$ rad, $120°$ **4.** $\dfrac{\pi}{4}$ rad, $45°$

5. $\dfrac{\pi}{6}$ rad, $30°$ **6.** $\dfrac{\pi}{3}$ rad, $60°$

7. 0.97 rad, $55.6°$ **8.** 2.00 rad, $114.6°$
9. 2.31 rad, $132.4°$ **10.** 0.29 rad, $16.6°$

11. $\dfrac{4}{3}$ **12.** $\dfrac{-4\sqrt{17}}{17}$ **13.** $-2\sqrt{2}$

14. $\dfrac{1}{z}$ **15.** $\dfrac{1}{\sqrt{z^2 + 2z + 2}}$

16. $\sqrt{4z^2 - 1}$ **17.** $\dfrac{1 - z}{\sqrt{z^2 - 2z}}$

18. $\sin^{-1}\dfrac{x}{z}$ **19.** $\sin^{-1}\dfrac{52}{x}$

20. $\sec^{-1}2.25$ **21.** $\sin^{-1}(-0.94)$

22. $\dfrac{\sin^{-1}0.75}{3}$ **23.** $\dfrac{3 + \cos^{-1}0.6}{2}$

Chapter 5

Exercise 5–0

Solutions to all problems

1. $\sin \theta(\sin \theta - 1)$
2. $\cos \theta(\cos^2\theta + 3)$
3. $\cos^2\theta(\cos^2\theta - 1)$
  $\cos^2\theta(\cos \theta - 1)(\cos \theta + 1)$
4. $\sin^3\theta(\sin^2\theta - 1)$
  $\sin^3\theta(\sin \theta - 1)(\sin \theta + 1)$
5. $(\cos x - 4)(\cos x + 5)$
6. $(\tan x + 6)(\tan x - 4)$
7. $(2 \sin x - 1)(\sin x - 3)$
8. $3 \cos \theta(3 \cos^2\theta - 5 \cos \theta - 2)$
  $3 \cos \theta(3 \cos \theta + 1)(\cos \theta - 2)$
9. $(2 \csc \theta - 1)(3 \csc \theta - 1)$
10. $\tan \theta(\tan \theta - 1) = 0$
  $\tan \theta = 0$ or $\tan \theta - 1 = 0$
  $\tan \theta = 0$ or $\tan \theta = 1$
11. $\tan^2\theta - \tan \theta - 2 = 0$
  $(\tan \theta - 2)(\tan \theta + 1) = 0$
  $\tan \theta - 2 = 0$ or $\tan \theta + 1 = 0$
  $\tan \theta = 2$ or $\tan \theta = -1$
12. $(2 \sin + 1)(3 \sin \theta + 1) = 0$
  $2 \sin \theta + 1 = 0$ or $3 \sin \theta + 1 = 0$
  $2 \sin \theta = -1$ or $3 \sin \theta = -1$
  $\sin \theta = -\dfrac{1}{2}$ or $\sin \theta = -\dfrac{1}{3}$
13. $(\sec^2\theta - 4)(\sec^2\theta - 1) = 0$
  $(\sec \theta - 2)(\sec \theta + 2)(\sec \theta - 1)$
  $(\sec \theta + 1) = 0$
  $\sec \theta - 2 = 0$ or $\sec \theta + 2 = 0$ or
  $\sec \theta - 1 = 0$ or $\sec \theta + 1 = 0$
  $\sec \theta = \pm 2$ or ± 1
14. $(4 \sin^2\theta - 1)(9 \sin^2\theta - 1) = 0$
  $(2 \sin \theta - 1)(2 \sin \theta + 1)$
  $(3 \sin \theta - 1)(3 \sin \theta + 1) = 0$
  $2 \sin \theta - 1 = 0$ or $2 \sin \theta + 1 = 0$ or
  $3 \sin \theta - 1 = 0$ or $3 \sin \theta + 1 = 0$
  $2 \sin \theta = 1$ or $2 \sin \theta = -1$ or $3 \sin \theta$
  $= 1$ or $3 \sin \theta = -1$
  $\sin \theta = \pm\dfrac{1}{2}$ or $\pm\dfrac{1}{3}$

15. $3 \sin \theta (\frac{2}{3} \sin \theta) + 3 \sin \theta \left(\dfrac{1}{3 \sin \theta}\right)$

$= 1(3 \sin \theta)$

$2 \sin^2\theta + 1 = 3 \sin \theta$

$2 \sin^2\theta - 3 \sin \theta + 1 = 0$

$(\sin \theta - 1)(2 \sin \theta - 1) = 0$

$\sin \theta - 1 = 0$ or $2 \sin \theta - 1 = 0$

$\sin \theta = 1$ or $2 \sin \theta = 1$

$\sin \theta = 1$ or $\frac{1}{2}$

16. $\sin \theta = \dfrac{-(-3) \pm \sqrt{(-3)^2 - 4(1)(-5)}}{2(1)}$

$\sin \theta = \dfrac{3 \pm \sqrt{29}}{2}$

17. $\sec \theta = \dfrac{-3 \pm \sqrt{3^2 - 4(2)(-7)}}{2(2)}$

$\sec \theta = \dfrac{-3 \pm \sqrt{65}}{4}$

18. $u = 2x - 6$

$u^3 - u^2 = 0$

$u^2(u - 1) = 0$

$u^2 = 0$ or $u - 1 = 0$

$u = 0$ or $u = 1$

$2x - 6 = 0$ or $2x - 6 = 1$

$2x = 6$ or $2x = 7$

$x = 3$ or $x = \frac{7}{2}$

19. $u = \dfrac{x}{3} - 1$

$12u^2 - 5u - 2 = 0$

$(3u - 2)(4u + 1) = 0$

$3u - 2 = 0$ or $4u + 1 = 0$

$u = \frac{2}{3}$ or $u = -\frac{1}{4}$

$\dfrac{x}{3} - 1 = \dfrac{2}{3}$ or $\dfrac{x}{3} - 1 = -\dfrac{1}{4}$

$x - 3 = 2$ or $x - 3 = -\frac{3}{4}$

$x = 5$ or $x = 2\frac{1}{4}$

20. $5\left(\dfrac{\pi}{2} - 3\right) + 3\left[\left(\dfrac{\pi}{2} - 3\right) - 7\right]$

$- \left(\dfrac{\pi}{2} - 3\right)$

$u = \dfrac{\pi}{2} - 3$

$5u + 3(u - 7) - u$

$5u + 3u - 21 - u$

$7u - 21$

$7\left(\dfrac{\pi}{2} - 3\right) - 21$

$\dfrac{7\pi}{2} - 21 - 21$

$\dfrac{7\pi}{2} - 42$

21. $u = 3x - \frac{1}{2}$

$\dfrac{2u^2 - 3u + 1}{u^2 - 1}$

$\dfrac{(u - 1)(2u - 1)}{(u - 1)(u + 1)}$

$\dfrac{2u - 1}{u + 1}$

$\dfrac{2(3x - \frac{1}{2}) - 1}{3x - \frac{1}{2} + 1}$

$\dfrac{6x - 1 - 1}{3x + \frac{1}{2}}$

$\dfrac{6x - 2}{3x + \frac{1}{2}} \cdot \dfrac{2}{2}$

$\dfrac{12x - 4}{6x + 1}$

Exercise 5–1

Answers to odd-numbered problems

1. $\dfrac{\sin \theta}{\dfrac{\sin \theta}{\cos \theta}}$

$\dfrac{\sin \theta \cos \theta}{\sin \theta}$

$\cos \theta$

3. $\dfrac{\sin \theta}{\cos \theta} \cdot \dfrac{1}{\sin \theta}$

$\dfrac{1}{\cos \theta}$

$\sec \theta$

5. $\dfrac{\dfrac{\cos^2\theta}{\sin^2\theta}}{\cos^2\theta} \sin^2\theta$

$\cos^2\theta$

7. $\sec^2\theta \cos^2\theta$

$\dfrac{1}{\cos^2\theta} \cos^2\theta$

1

9. $\dfrac{\sec^2\theta - 1}{\sin^2\theta}$

$\dfrac{\tan^2\theta}{\sin^2\theta}$

$\dfrac{\dfrac{\sin^2\theta}{\cos^2\theta}}{\sin^2\theta}$

$\dfrac{1}{\cos^2\theta}$

$\sec^2\theta$

11. $\dfrac{\dfrac{1}{\sin \theta} \sin \theta}{\cot \theta}$

$\dfrac{1}{\cot \theta}$

$\tan \theta$

13. $\cos \theta \sec \theta - \cos^2\theta$

$\cos \theta \dfrac{1}{\cos \theta} - \cos^2\theta$

$1 - \cos^2\theta$

$\sin^2\theta$

15. $\csc^2\theta \sin^2\theta$

$\dfrac{1}{\sin^2\theta} \sin^2\theta$

1

17. $\dfrac{\cos^2\theta}{\sin^2\theta} - \dfrac{1}{\sin^2\theta}$

$\dfrac{\cos^2\theta - 1}{\sin^2\theta}$

$\dfrac{-\sin^2\theta}{\sin^2\theta}$

-1

19. $\tan^2\theta \cot^2\theta + \tan^2\theta$

$\tan^2\theta \cdot \dfrac{1}{\tan^2\theta} + \tan^2\theta$

$1 + \tan^2\theta$

$\sec^2\theta$

21. $\sec^2\theta \cot^2\theta$

$\dfrac{1}{\cos^2\theta} \cdot \dfrac{\cos^2\theta}{\sin^2\theta}$

$\dfrac{1}{\sin^2\theta}$

$\csc^2\theta$

23. $\dfrac{\cos \theta}{\sin \theta} \dfrac{1}{\cos \theta}$

$\dfrac{\dfrac{1}{\sin \theta}}{\dfrac{1}{\sin \theta}}$

$\dfrac{\dfrac{1}{\sin \theta}}{\dfrac{1}{\sin \theta}}$

1

25. $\sin x + \cos x \dfrac{\cos x}{\sin x}$

$\dfrac{\sin^2x + \cos^2x}{\sin x}$

$\dfrac{1}{\sin x}$

$\csc x$

27. $\dfrac{\sin x}{\cos x} \dfrac{1}{\sin x} \cos x$

1

29. $\dfrac{1}{\cos x} - \dfrac{\sin x}{\cos x} \sin x$

$\dfrac{1 - \sin^2x}{\cos x}$

$\dfrac{\cos^2x}{\cos x}$

$\cos x$

31. $\csc x - \csc x \cos x + \cot x - \cot x \cos x$

$\dfrac{1}{\sin x} - \dfrac{1}{\sin x} \cos x + \dfrac{\cos x}{\sin x} - \dfrac{\cos x}{\sin x} \cos x$

$\dfrac{1 - \cos x + \cos x - \cos^2x}{\sin x}$

$\dfrac{1 - \cos^2x}{\sin x}$

$\dfrac{\sin^2x}{\sin x}$

$\sin x$

33. $\csc\theta+\cot\theta$

$\dfrac{1}{\sin\theta}+\dfrac{\cos\theta}{\sin\theta}$

$\dfrac{1+\cos\theta}{\sin\theta}$

35. $\dfrac{\csc\theta}{\sec\theta+\tan\theta}$

$\dfrac{\frac{1}{\sin\theta}}{\frac{1}{\cos\theta}+\frac{\sin\theta}{\cos\theta}}$

$\dfrac{\frac{1}{\sin\theta}}{\frac{1+\sin\theta}{\cos\theta}}$

$\dfrac{\cos\theta}{\sin\theta+\sin^2\theta}$

45. $\dfrac{1}{\sec\theta-\cos\theta}$

$\dfrac{1}{\frac{1}{\cos\theta}-\cos\theta}$

$\dfrac{1}{\frac{1-\cos^2\theta}{\cos\theta}}$

$\dfrac{\cos\theta}{1-\cos^2\theta}$

$\dfrac{\cos\theta}{\sin^2\theta}$

$\dfrac{\cos\theta}{\sin\theta}\,\dfrac{1}{\sin\theta}$

$\cot\theta\csc\theta$

47. $\dfrac{\tan\theta}{\csc\theta}$

$\dfrac{\frac{\sin\theta}{\cos\theta}}{\frac{1}{\sin\theta}}$

$\dfrac{\sin^2\theta}{\cos\theta}$

$\sin\theta\,\dfrac{\sin\theta}{\cos\theta}$

$\sin\theta\tan\theta$

57. $\dfrac{1}{1-\sin x}+\dfrac{1}{1+\sin x}$

$\dfrac{1+\sin x+1-\sin x}{(1-\sin x)(1+\sin x)}$

$\dfrac{2}{1-\sin^2 x}$

$\dfrac{2}{\cos^2 x}$

$2\sec^2 x$

59. $\sin^4 x-\cos^4 x$

$(\sin^2 x+\cos^2 x)(\sin^2 x-\cos^2 x)$

$(1)(1-\cos^2 x-\cos^2 x)$

$1-2\cos^2 x$

37. $\dfrac{1+\csc\theta}{1+\sec\theta}$

$\dfrac{1+\frac{1}{\sin\theta}}{1+\frac{1}{\cos\theta}}$

$\dfrac{1+\frac{1}{\sin\theta}}{1+\frac{1}{\cos\theta}}\cdot\dfrac{\sin\theta\cos\theta}{\sin\theta\cos\theta}$

$\dfrac{\sin\theta\cos\theta+\cos\theta}{\sin\theta\cos\theta+\sin\theta}$

$\dfrac{\cos\theta(\sin\theta+1)}{\sin\theta(\cos\theta+1)}$

$\dfrac{\cos\theta}{\sin\theta}\cdot\dfrac{\sin\theta+1}{\cos\theta+1}$

$\cot\theta\left(\dfrac{1+\sin\theta}{1+\cos\theta}\right)$

39. $\dfrac{\tan^2\theta+\sec^2\theta}{\sec^2\theta}$

$\dfrac{\tan^2\theta}{\sec^2\theta}+\dfrac{\sec^2\theta}{\sec^2\theta}$

$\tan^2\theta\cos^2\theta+1$

$\dfrac{\sin^2\theta}{\cos^2\theta}\cdot\cos^2\theta+1$

$\sin^2\theta+1$

49. $\dfrac{\tan^2\theta}{\sec\theta-1}$

$\dfrac{\sec^2\theta-1}{\sec\theta-1}$

$\dfrac{(\sec\theta+1)(\sec\theta-1)}{(\sec\theta-1)}$

$\sec\theta+1$

51. $\dfrac{\cot x+1}{\cot x-1}$

$\dfrac{\frac{\cos x}{\sin x}+1}{\frac{\cos x}{\sin x}-1}$

$\dfrac{\frac{\cos x+\sin x}{\sin x}}{\frac{\cos x-\sin x}{\sin x}}$

$\dfrac{\cos x+\sin x}{\cos x-\sin x}$

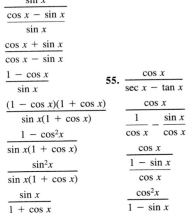

53. $\dfrac{1-\cos x}{\sin x}$

$\dfrac{(1-\cos x)(1+\cos x)}{\sin x(1+\cos x)}$

$\dfrac{1-\cos^2 x}{\sin x(1+\cos x)}$

$\dfrac{\sin^2 x}{\sin x(1+\cos x)}$

$\dfrac{\sin x}{1+\cos x}$

55. $\dfrac{\cos x}{\sec x-\tan x}$

$\dfrac{\cos x}{\frac{1}{\cos x}-\frac{\sin x}{\cos x}}$

$\dfrac{\cos x}{\frac{1-\sin x}{\cos x}}$

$\dfrac{\cos x}{1-\sin x}$

$\dfrac{\cos^2 x}{1-\sin x}$

61. $\cot^2 x\cos^2 x$

$\dfrac{\cos^2 x}{\sin^2 x}(1-\sin^2 x)$

$\dfrac{\cos^2 x}{\sin^2 x}-\cos^2 x$

$\cot^2 x-\cos^2 x$

63. $\dfrac{\tan y-\cot y}{\tan y+\cot y}$

$\dfrac{\tan y-\frac{1}{\tan y}}{\tan y+\frac{1}{\tan y}}$

$\dfrac{\frac{\tan^2 y-1}{\tan y}}{\frac{\tan^2 y+1}{\tan y}}$

$\dfrac{\tan^2 y-1}{\tan^2 y+1}$

$\dfrac{\tan^2 y-1}{\sec^2 y}$

65. $\dfrac{1-\sin x}{1+\sin x}$

$\dfrac{(1-\sin x)(1-\sin x)}{(1+\sin x)(1-\sin x)}$

$\dfrac{1-2\sin x+\sin^2 x}{1-\sin^2 x}$

$\dfrac{1-2\sin x+\sin^2 x}{\cos^2 x}$

$\dfrac{1}{\cos^2 x}-2\left(\dfrac{\sin x}{\cos x}\right)\left(\dfrac{1}{\cos x}\right)+\dfrac{\sin^2 x}{\cos^2 x}$

$\sec^2 x-2\tan x\sec x+\tan^2 x$

$(\tan x-\sec x)^2$

67. $\sec^4 x-\sec^2 x$

$\sec^2 x(\sec^2 x-1)$

$(1+\tan^2 x)(\tan^2 x)$

$\tan^2 x+\tan^4 x$

69. $2\cos^2 y-1$

$\cos^2 y+\cos^2 y-1$

$\cos^2 y-(1-\cos^2 y)$

$\cos^2 y-\sin^2 y$

41. $\sec y-\cos y$

$\dfrac{1}{\cos y}-\cos y$

$\dfrac{1}{\cos y}-\dfrac{\cos^2 y}{\cos y}$

$\dfrac{1-\cos^2 y}{\cos y}$

$\dfrac{\sin^2 y}{\cos y}$

$\dfrac{\sin y}{\cos y}\sin y$

$\tan y\sin y$

43. $\dfrac{1+\cot^2\theta}{\tan^2\theta}$

$\dfrac{1+\frac{\cos^2\theta}{\sin^2\theta}}{\frac{\sin^2\theta}{\cos^2\theta}}$

$\dfrac{\frac{\sin^2\theta+\cos^2\theta}{\sin^2\theta}}{\frac{\sin^2\theta}{\cos^2\theta}}$

$\dfrac{\frac{1}{\sin^2\theta}}{\frac{\sin^2\theta}{\cos^2\theta}}$

$\dfrac{\cos^2\theta}{\sin^4\theta}$

$\dfrac{\cos^2\theta}{\sin^2\theta}\cdot\dfrac{1}{\sin^2\theta}$

$\cot^2\theta\csc^2\theta$

71. Let $\theta = \dfrac{\pi}{6}$:

$$1 - \cos\theta = 1 - \cos\dfrac{\pi}{6}$$

$$= 1 - \dfrac{\sqrt{3}}{2}$$

$$= \dfrac{2 - \sqrt{3}}{2}$$

$$\sin\dfrac{\pi}{6} = \dfrac{1}{2} \neq \dfrac{2 - \sqrt{3}}{2}$$

73. Let $\theta = \dfrac{\pi}{4}$;

$$\sec\dfrac{\pi}{4} \overset{?}{=} \dfrac{1}{\csc\dfrac{\pi}{4}}$$

$$\sqrt{2} \neq \dfrac{1}{\sqrt{2}}$$

75. Let $\theta = \dfrac{\pi}{2}$:

$$\sin^2\theta - 2\cos\theta\sin\theta + \cos^2\theta$$

$$\sin^2\dfrac{\pi}{2} - 2\cos\dfrac{\pi}{2}\sin\dfrac{\pi}{2} + \cos^2\dfrac{\pi}{2}$$

$$1 - 2(0)(1) + 0 = 1$$

$$1 \neq 2$$

77. $\csc\theta + \sec\theta\cot\theta$

$$\csc\dfrac{\pi}{6} + \sec\dfrac{\pi}{6}\cot\dfrac{\pi}{6}$$

$$2 + \left(\dfrac{2\sqrt{3}}{3}\right)\left(\dfrac{3\sqrt{3}}{3}\right)$$

$$2 + 2 = 4$$

$$4 \neq 2$$

79. $\dfrac{1 - \cos\theta}{1 + \cos\theta}$

$$\dfrac{1 - \cos\dfrac{\pi}{4}}{1 + \cos\dfrac{\pi}{4}} = \dfrac{1 - \dfrac{\sqrt{2}}{2}}{1 + \dfrac{\sqrt{2}}{2}} = \dfrac{2 - \sqrt{2}}{2 + \sqrt{2}}$$

$$\sin^2\dfrac{\pi}{4} = \left(\dfrac{\sqrt{2}}{2}\right)^2 = \dfrac{2}{4} = \dfrac{1}{2}$$

$$\dfrac{2 - \sqrt{2}}{2 + \sqrt{2}} \neq \dfrac{1}{2}$$

81. a. $\left(1 - \csc^2\dfrac{\pi}{6}\right)\left(1 - \sec^2\dfrac{\pi}{6}\right)$

$$(1 - 2^2)\left[1 - \left(\dfrac{2}{\sqrt{3}}\right)^2\right]$$

$$(-3)(-\tfrac{1}{3}) = 1$$

b. $\left(1 - \csc^2\dfrac{\pi}{4}\right)\left(1 - \sec^2\dfrac{\pi}{4}\right)$

$$[1 - (\sqrt{2})^2][1 - (\sqrt{2})^2]$$

$$(1 - 2)(1 - 2) = 1$$

c. yes

83. a. $2\sin^2\dfrac{\pi}{6} + \sin\dfrac{\pi}{6}$

$$2\left(\dfrac{1}{2}\right)^2 + \dfrac{1}{2} = 1$$

b. $2\sin^2\dfrac{3\pi}{2} + \sin\dfrac{3\pi}{2}$

$$2(-1)^2 + (-1) = 1$$

c. no; $\theta = \dfrac{\pi}{4}$ is a counterexample

Solutions to trial exercise problems

18. $\tan^2\theta - \sec^2\theta$

$$\dfrac{\sin^2\theta}{\cos^2\theta} - \dfrac{1}{\cos^2\theta}$$

$$\dfrac{\sin^2\theta - 1}{\cos^2\theta}$$

$$\dfrac{-(1 - \sin^2\theta)}{\cos^2\theta}$$

$$\dfrac{-\cos^2\theta}{\cos^2\theta}$$

$$-1$$

32. $\dfrac{\sec^4 y - \tan^4 y}{\sec^2 y + \tan^2 y}$

$$\dfrac{(\sec^2 y + \tan^2 y)(\sec^2 y - \tan^2 y)}{\sec^2 y + \tan^2 y}$$

$$\sec^2 y - \tan^2 y$$

$$(\tan^2 y + 1) - \tan^2 y$$

$$1$$

36. $\dfrac{\sec\theta}{\csc\theta + \cot\theta}$

$$\dfrac{\dfrac{1}{\cos\theta}}{\dfrac{1}{\sin\theta} + \dfrac{\cos\theta}{\sin\theta}}$$

$$\dfrac{\dfrac{1}{\cos\theta}}{\dfrac{1 + \cos\theta}{\sin\theta}}$$

$$\dfrac{1}{\cos\theta} \cdot \dfrac{\sin\theta}{1 + \cos\theta}$$

$$\dfrac{\tan\theta}{1 + \cos\theta}$$

$$\dfrac{\tan\theta}{1 + \cos\theta}$$

52. $\dfrac{\csc y + 1}{\csc y - 1}$

$$\dfrac{\dfrac{1}{\sin y} + 1}{\dfrac{1}{\sin y} - 1}$$

$$\dfrac{\dfrac{1 + \sin y}{\sin y}}{\dfrac{1 - \sin y}{\sin y}}$$

$$\dfrac{1 + \sin y}{\sin y} \cdot \dfrac{\sin y}{1 - \sin y}$$

$$\dfrac{1 + \sin y}{1 - \sin y}$$

84. a. $\tan^4\theta - \tan^2\theta = 6$

$$\theta = \dfrac{\pi}{3}: (\sqrt{3})^4 - (\sqrt{3})^2 = 6$$

$$9 - 3 = 6$$

b. $\theta = \dfrac{4\pi}{3}: (\sqrt{3})^4 - (\sqrt{3})^2 = 6$

$$9 - 3 = 6$$

c. no;

$$\text{let } \theta = 0: 0^4 - 0^2 \neq 6$$

Exercise 5–2

Answers to odd-numbered problems

1. $\cos 72°$ **3.** $\cot 82°$ **5.** $\csc\dfrac{\pi}{6}$

7. $\sin\left(-\dfrac{\pi}{3}\right)$ **9.** $\csc\dfrac{5\pi}{4}$ **11.** 1

13. 1 **15.** 1 **17.** -1 **19.** 1

21. 1 **23.** 1 **25.** 1

27. $\dfrac{\sqrt{6} + \sqrt{2}}{4}$ **29.** $\dfrac{\sqrt{6} + \sqrt{2}}{4}$

31. $\dfrac{\sqrt{6} + \sqrt{2}}{4}$ **33.** $\dfrac{\sqrt{6} - \sqrt{2}}{4}$

35. $\dfrac{\sqrt{2} - \sqrt{6}}{4}$ **37.** $2 + \sqrt{3}$

39. $\dfrac{2\sqrt{14} + 3}{12}$ **41.** $\dfrac{-15 - 12\sqrt{7}}{36 - 5\sqrt{7}}$

43. $\dfrac{13}{85}$ **45.** $\dfrac{-\sqrt{5} - 4\sqrt{2}}{9}$

47. $\dfrac{(8 + \sqrt{5})}{51}\sqrt{17}$ **49.** $-\dfrac{119}{120}$

51. $-\dfrac{\sqrt{5}}{5}$ **53.** $\dfrac{-4\sqrt{6} + \sqrt{5}}{15}$

55. $2 + \sqrt{3}$

57. $\sin(\pi - \theta) = \sin\pi\cos\theta - \cos\pi\sin\theta$
$$= 0\cos\theta - (-1)\sin\theta$$
$$= \sin\theta$$

59. $\cos(\pi - \theta) = \cos\pi\cos\theta + \sin\pi\sin\theta$
$$= (-1)\cos\theta + 0\sin\theta$$
$$= -\cos\theta$$

61. $\tan(\pi - \theta) = \dfrac{\tan\pi - \tan\theta}{1 + \tan\pi\tan\theta}$
$$= \dfrac{0 - \tan\theta}{1 + 0\tan\theta}$$
$$= -\tan\theta$$

63. $\sin(\theta + 2\pi) = \sin\theta\cos 2\pi + \cos\theta\sin 2\pi$
$$= \sin\theta(1) + \cos\theta(0)$$
$$= \sin\theta$$

65. $\tan(\theta + \pi) = \dfrac{\tan\theta + \tan\pi}{1 - \tan\theta\tan\pi}$
$$= \dfrac{\tan\theta + 0}{1 - \tan\theta(0)}$$
$$= \tan\theta$$

67. $\frac{1}{2}[\sin(\alpha + \beta) - \sin(\alpha - \beta)]$
$\frac{1}{2}[\sin \alpha \cos \beta + \cos \alpha \sin \beta - (\sin \alpha \cos \beta - \cos \alpha \sin \beta)]$
$\frac{1}{2}[2 \cos \alpha \sin \beta]$
$\cos \alpha \sin \beta$

69. $\frac{1}{2}[\cos(\alpha - \beta) - \cos(\alpha + \beta)]$
$\frac{1}{2}[\cos \alpha \cos \beta + \sin \alpha \sin \beta - (\cos \alpha \cos \beta - \sin \alpha \sin \beta)]$
$\frac{1}{2}[2 \sin \alpha \sin \beta]$
$\sin \alpha \sin \beta$

71. a. $\frac{11}{29}$ **b.** $3\frac{12}{29}$

73. $\cos(\alpha + \beta) = \cos \alpha \cos \beta - \sin \alpha \sin \beta$
This was shown true in the text.
$\cos(\alpha + (-\beta)) = \cos \alpha \cos(-\beta) - \sin \alpha \sin(-\beta)$
Replace β by $-\beta$. This is valid since the identity is true for all angles and α.
$\cos(\alpha - \beta) = \cos \alpha \cos \beta - \sin \alpha[-\sin \beta]$
$\alpha + (-\beta) = \alpha - \beta; \cos(-\theta) = \cos \theta; \sin(-\theta) = -\sin \theta.$
$\cos(\alpha - \beta) = \cos \alpha \cos \beta + \sin \alpha \sin \beta$
This statement is true since the preceding statements are true.

75. $\cos\left(\dfrac{\pi}{2} - \theta\right) = \sin \theta$
Proved true above.
Let $\alpha = \dfrac{\pi}{2} - \theta$. Then $\theta = \dfrac{\pi}{2} - \alpha$.
$\cos \alpha = \sin\left(\dfrac{\pi}{2} - \alpha\right)$
Substitution of expression (section 5–0).
$\sin\left(\dfrac{\pi}{2} - \theta\right) = \cos \theta$
The variable name α or θ is unimportant.

77. $\sin(\alpha + \beta) = \sin \alpha \cos \beta + \cos \alpha \sin \beta$
Identity [3].
$\sin(\alpha + (-\beta)) = \sin \alpha \cos(-\beta) + \cos \alpha \sin(-\beta)$
$\sin(\alpha - \beta) = \sin \alpha \cos \beta + \cos \alpha[-\sin \beta]$
Cosine is an even function, sine is odd.
$= \sin \alpha \cos \beta - \cos \alpha \sin \beta$
This is identity [4].

79. $\cot\left(\dfrac{\pi}{2} - \theta\right) = \dfrac{1}{\tan\left(\dfrac{\pi}{2} - \theta\right)} = \dfrac{1}{\cot \theta} = \tan \theta.$

81. $\csc\left(\dfrac{\pi}{2} - \theta\right) = \dfrac{1}{\sin\left(\dfrac{\pi}{2} - \theta\right)} = \dfrac{1}{\cos \theta} = \sec \theta.$

Solutions to trial exercise problems

8. $\sin\left(-\dfrac{\pi}{3}\right) = \cos\left(\dfrac{\pi}{2} - \left(-\dfrac{\pi}{3}\right)\right) = \cos \dfrac{5\pi}{6}$

17. $\tan^2 8° - \csc^2 82°$
$\tan^2 8° - \sec^2(90° - 82°)$
$\tan^2 8° - \sec^2 8°$
$-(\sec^2 8° - \tan^2 8°) = -1$

28. $\tan \dfrac{\pi}{12}$
$\tan\left(\dfrac{\pi}{4} - \dfrac{\pi}{6}\right)$
$\dfrac{\tan \dfrac{\pi}{4} - \tan \dfrac{\pi}{6}}{1 + \tan \dfrac{\pi}{4} \tan \dfrac{\pi}{6}}$
$\dfrac{1 - \dfrac{\sqrt{3}}{3}}{1 + 1\left(\dfrac{\sqrt{3}}{3}\right)} \cdot \dfrac{3}{3} = \dfrac{3 - \sqrt{3}}{3 + \sqrt{3}} \cdot \dfrac{3 - \sqrt{3}}{3 - \sqrt{3}}$
$\dfrac{12 - 6\sqrt{3}}{6} = 2 - \sqrt{3}$

40. $\cos \alpha = -\dfrac{12}{13}$, quadrant II; $\sin \beta = \dfrac{1}{2}$, quadrant II.
Find $\cos(\alpha - \beta)$.
$\cos(\alpha - \beta) = \cos \alpha \cos \beta + \sin \alpha \sin \beta$
Find $\cos \alpha$, $\sin \alpha$, $\cos \beta$, $\sin \beta$ from the reference triangles in the figure.
$= -\dfrac{12}{13} \cdot \left(-\dfrac{\sqrt{3}}{2}\right) + \dfrac{5}{13} \cdot \dfrac{1}{2} = \dfrac{12\sqrt{3} + 5}{26}.$

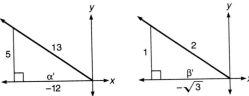

48. $\tan \alpha = \dfrac{3}{4}$, quadrant III; $\sin \beta = -\dfrac{4}{5}$, quadrant III. Find $\cos(\alpha - \beta)$.
$\cos(\alpha - \beta) = \cos \alpha \cos \beta + \sin \alpha \sin \beta$
$= -\dfrac{4}{5}(-\dfrac{3}{5}) + (-\dfrac{3}{5})(-\dfrac{4}{5}) = \dfrac{24}{25}.$

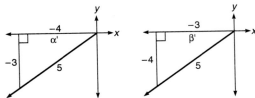

70. For angle α, the hypotenuse is $\sqrt{164} = 2\sqrt{41}$, and for angle β, the hypotenuse is $\sqrt{136} = 2\sqrt{34}$. Thus, $\sin \alpha = \dfrac{8}{2\sqrt{41}}$

$= \dfrac{4}{\sqrt{41}}$; $\cos \alpha = \dfrac{10}{2\sqrt{41}} = \dfrac{5}{\sqrt{41}}$; $\sin \beta = \dfrac{6}{2\sqrt{34}} = \dfrac{3}{\sqrt{34}}$;

$\cos \beta = \dfrac{10}{2\sqrt{34}} = \dfrac{5}{\sqrt{34}}$

Therefore, $\sin(\alpha - \beta) = \sin \alpha \cos \beta - \cos \alpha \sin \beta$

$= \left(\dfrac{4}{\sqrt{41}}\right)\left(\dfrac{5}{\sqrt{34}}\right) - \left(\dfrac{5}{\sqrt{41}}\right)\left(\dfrac{3}{\sqrt{34}}\right)$

$= \dfrac{20}{\sqrt{1{,}394}} - \dfrac{15}{\sqrt{1{,}394}} = \dfrac{5}{\sqrt{1{,}394}}$

$= \dfrac{5\sqrt{1{,}394}}{1{,}394}$

76. $\sin \theta = \cos\left(\dfrac{\pi}{2} - \theta\right)$
We know this is true.
Replace θ by $\alpha + \beta$.

$\sin(\alpha + \beta) = \cos\left[\dfrac{\pi}{2} - (\alpha + \beta)\right]$

$\sin(\alpha + \beta) = \cos\left[\left(\dfrac{\pi}{2} - \alpha\right) - \beta\right]$

Regroup $\dfrac{\pi}{2} - \alpha - \beta$.

$= \cos\left(\dfrac{\pi}{2} - \alpha\right)\cos \beta + \sin\left(\dfrac{\pi}{2} - \alpha\right)\sin \beta$

Use the identity for $\cos(\alpha - \beta)$.
$= \sin \alpha \cos \beta + \cos \alpha \sin \beta$
Use cofunction identities.
Thus, $\sin(\alpha + \beta) = \sin \alpha \cos \beta + \cos \alpha \sin \beta$.

Exercise 5–3

Answers to odd-numbered problems

1. $\sin \dfrac{\pi}{2}$ **3.** $\cos 6\pi$ **5.** $\cos \dfrac{\pi}{5}$

7. $3 \tan 20°$ **9.** $\sin 12\theta$ **11.** $3 \cos 10\theta$

13. $5 \tan 6\theta$ **15.** $2 \cos 14\theta$

17. $3 \cos 6\theta$ **19.** $70°$ **21.** $\dfrac{5\pi}{12}$

23. $35°$ **25.** $20°$ **27.** $\dfrac{\pi}{8}$ **29.** $\dfrac{4\pi}{5}$

31. $\dfrac{24}{25}, \dfrac{7}{25}, \dfrac{24}{7}$ **33.** $-\dfrac{24}{25}, \dfrac{7}{25}, -\dfrac{24}{7}$

35. $\dfrac{5\sqrt{39}}{32}, \dfrac{7}{32}, \dfrac{5\sqrt{39}}{7}$

37. $\dfrac{\sqrt{70}}{10}, -\dfrac{\sqrt{30}}{10}, -\dfrac{\sqrt{21}}{3}$

39. $\dfrac{\sqrt{50 - 20\sqrt{5}}}{10}, -\dfrac{\sqrt{50 + 20\sqrt{5}}}{10}, 2 - \sqrt{5}$

41. $\dfrac{\sqrt{2 - \sqrt{3}}}{2}, \dfrac{\sqrt{2 + \sqrt{3}}}{2}, 2 - \sqrt{3}$

43. $\dfrac{1}{2}\sqrt{2 + \sqrt{3}}, \dfrac{1}{2}\sqrt{2 - \sqrt{3}}, 2 + \sqrt{3}$

45. $\dfrac{\sqrt{4 + \sqrt{6} + 2\sqrt{3} + 2\sqrt{2}} - \sqrt{4 + \sqrt{6} - 2\sqrt{3} - 2\sqrt{2}}}{4}$

47. $\dfrac{\sqrt{2 - \sqrt{2 + \sqrt{3}}}}{2}$

49. $(\sin \theta + \cos \theta)^2$
$\sin^2 + 2 \sin \theta \cos \theta + \cos^2\theta$
$2 \sin \theta \cos \theta + 1$
$\sin 2\theta + 1$

51. $\cos^4\theta - \sin^4\theta$
$(\cos^2\theta + \sin^2\theta)(\cos^2\theta - \sin^2\theta)$
$(1)(\cos 2\theta)$
$\cos 2\theta$

53. $\dfrac{(\cos^2\theta + \sin^2\theta) + (\cos^2\theta - \sin^2\theta)}{(\cos^2\theta + \sin^2\theta) - (\cos^2\theta - \sin^2\theta)}$

$\dfrac{2 \cos^2\theta}{2 \sin^2\theta}$

$\cot^2\theta$

55. $\dfrac{2 \cos 2\theta}{\sin 2\theta}$

$\dfrac{2(\cos^2\theta - \sin^2\theta)}{2 \sin \theta \cos \theta}$

$\dfrac{\cos^2\theta}{\sin \theta \cos \theta} - \dfrac{\sin^2\theta}{\sin \theta \cos \theta}$

$\dfrac{\cos \theta}{\sin \theta} - \dfrac{\sin \theta}{\cos \theta}$

$\cot \theta - \tan \theta$

57. $\sin 2\theta \cos 2\theta$
$2 \sin \theta \cos \theta(\cos^2\theta - \sin^2\theta)$
$2 \sin \theta \cos \theta(\cos^2\theta) - 2 \sin^3\theta \cos \theta$
$2 \sin \theta \cos \theta(1 - \sin^2\theta) - 2 \sin^3\theta \cos \theta$
$2 \sin \theta \cos \theta - 2 \sin^3\theta \cos \theta - 2 \sin^3\theta \cos \theta$
$2 \sin \theta \cos \theta - 4 \sin^3\theta \cos \theta$

59. $\dfrac{2}{1 - \cos 2\theta}$

$\dfrac{2}{1 - (\cos^2\theta - \sin^2\theta)}$

$\dfrac{2}{1 - \cos^2\theta + \sin^2\theta}$

$\dfrac{2}{\sin^2\theta + \sin^2\theta}$

$\dfrac{2}{2 \sin^2\theta}$

$\dfrac{1}{\sin^2\theta}$

$\csc^2\theta$

61. $\dfrac{2(\tan \theta + \tan^3\theta)}{1 - \tan^4\theta}$

$\dfrac{2 \tan \theta(1 + \tan^2\theta)}{(1 - \tan^2\theta)(1 + \tan^2\theta)}$

$\dfrac{2 \tan \theta}{1 - \tan^2\theta}$

$\tan 2\theta$

63. $2 \csc 2\theta \sin \theta \cos \theta$

$2\left(\dfrac{1}{\sin 2\theta}\right)\sin \theta \cos \theta$

$\dfrac{2 \sin \theta \cos \theta}{\sin 2\theta}$

$\dfrac{2 \sin \theta \cos \theta}{2 \sin \theta \cos \theta}$

1

65. $\dfrac{1 - \tan^2\theta}{1 + \tan^2\theta}$

$\dfrac{1 - \dfrac{\sin^2\theta}{\cos^2\theta}}{1 + \dfrac{\sin^2\theta}{\cos^2\theta}}$

$\dfrac{\dfrac{\cos^2\theta - \sin^2\theta}{\cos^2\theta}}{\dfrac{\cos^2\theta + \sin^2\theta}{\cos^2\theta}}$

$\dfrac{\cos^2\theta - \sin^2\theta}{\cos^2\theta + \sin^2\theta}$

$\dfrac{\cos^2\theta - \sin^2\theta}{1}$

$\cos^2\theta - \sin^2\theta$

$\cos 2\theta$

67. $\cos^2 \dfrac{\theta}{2}$

$\left(\pm \sqrt{\dfrac{1 + \cos \theta}{2}} \right)^2$

$\dfrac{1 + \cos \theta}{2}$

$\dfrac{1 + \cos \theta}{2} \cdot \dfrac{1 - \cos \theta}{1 - \cos \theta}$

$\dfrac{1 - \cos^2 \theta}{2 - 2 \cos \theta}$

69. $\cos^2 \dfrac{\theta}{2} \sin^2 \dfrac{\theta}{2}$

$\left(\pm \sqrt{\dfrac{1 + \cos \theta}{2}} \right)^2 \left(\pm \sqrt{\dfrac{1 - \cos \theta}{2}} \right)^2$

$\left(\pm \sqrt{\dfrac{1 - \cos^2 \theta}{4}} \right)^2$

$\dfrac{\sin^2 \theta}{4}$

71. $\tan^2 \dfrac{\theta}{2} + \cos^2 \dfrac{\theta}{2}$

$\left(\pm \sqrt{\dfrac{1 - \cos \theta}{1 + \cos \theta}} \right)^2 + \left(\pm \sqrt{\dfrac{1 + \cos \theta}{2}} \right)^2$

$\dfrac{1 - \cos \theta}{1 + \cos \theta} + \dfrac{1 + \cos \theta}{2}$

$\dfrac{2 - 2 \cos \theta + 1 + 2 \cos \theta + \cos^2 \theta}{2(1 + \cos \theta)}$

$\dfrac{\cos^2 \theta + 3}{2 + 2 \cos \theta}$

73. $\dfrac{\csc \theta - \cot \theta}{2 \csc \theta}$

$\dfrac{\dfrac{1}{\sin \theta} - \dfrac{\cos \theta}{\sin \theta}}{\dfrac{2}{\sin \theta}}$

$\dfrac{\dfrac{1 - \cos \theta}{\sin \theta}}{\dfrac{2}{\sin \theta}}$

$\dfrac{1 - \cos \theta}{2}$

$\left(\pm \sqrt{\dfrac{1 - \cos \theta}{2}} \right)^2$

$\sin^2 \dfrac{\theta}{2}$

75. $\dfrac{1 + \sec \theta}{\sec \theta}$

$\dfrac{1 + \dfrac{1}{\cos \theta}}{\dfrac{1}{\cos \theta}}$

$\dfrac{\dfrac{\cos \theta + 1}{\cos \theta}}{\dfrac{1}{\cos \theta}}$

$\cos \theta + 1$

$2 \left(\dfrac{1 + \cos \theta}{2} \right)$

$2 \left(\pm \sqrt{\dfrac{1 + \cos \theta}{2}} \right)^2$

$2 \cos^2 \dfrac{\theta}{2}$

77. $2 \cos^2 \dfrac{\theta}{2} - \cos \theta$

$2 \left(\pm \sqrt{\dfrac{1 + \cos \theta}{2}} \right)^2 - \cos \theta$

$1 + \cos \theta - \cos \theta$

1

79. $\cos 3\theta = \cos(2\theta + \theta)$

$= \cos(2\theta)\cos \theta - \sin(2\theta)\sin \theta$

$(\cos^2 \theta - \sin^2 \theta)\cos \theta - 2 \sin \theta \cos \theta \sin \theta$

$\cos^3 \theta - \sin^2 \theta \cos \theta - 2 \sin^2 \theta \cos \theta$

$\cos^3 \theta - 3 \sin^2 \theta \cos \theta$

$\cos^2 \theta - 3(1 - \cos^2 \theta)\cos \theta$

$\cos^3 \theta - 3 \cos \theta + 3 \cos^3 \theta$

$4 \cos^3 \theta - 3 \cos \theta$

81. We know that $\sin 4\theta = 4 \cos^3 \theta \sin \theta - 4 \sin^3 \theta \cos \theta$ and $\cos 4\theta = 8 \cos^4 \theta - 8 \cos^2 \theta + 1$ from problem 80.

  a. $\sin 5\theta$

  $= \sin(\theta + 4\theta)$

  $= \sin \theta \cos 4\theta + \cos \theta \sin 4\theta$

  $= \sin \theta (8 \cos^4 \theta - 8 \cos^2 \theta + 1) + \cos \theta (4 \sin \theta \cos \theta$
  $\quad - 8 \sin^3 \theta \cos \theta)$

  $= 4 \sin \theta \cos^2 \theta - 8 \sin^3 \theta \cos^2 \theta + 8 \sin \theta \cos^4 \theta$
  $\quad - 8 \sin \theta \cos^2 \theta + \sin \theta$

  We know $\cos^2 \theta = 1 - \sin^2 \theta$, so that $\cos^4 \theta = (1 - \sin^2 \theta)^2$ $= 1 - 2 \sin^2 \theta + \sin^4 \theta$. Replace $\cos^2 \theta$ and $\cos^4 \theta$ in the equation above:

  $= 4 \sin \theta (1 - \sin^2 \theta) - 8 \sin^3 \theta (1 - \sin^2 \theta)$
  $\quad + 8 \sin \theta (1 - 2 \sin^2 \theta + \sin^4 \theta) - 8 \sin \theta (1 - \sin^2 \theta)$
  $\quad + \sin \theta$

  $= 4 \sin \theta - 4 \sin^3 \theta - 8 \sin^3 \theta + 8 \sin^5 \theta + 8 \sin \theta$
  $\quad - 16 \sin^3 \theta + 8 \sin^5 \theta - 8 \sin \theta + 8 \sin^3 \theta + \sin \theta$

  $= 16 \sin^5 \theta - 20 \sin^3 \theta + 5 \sin \theta$

  b. $\cos 5\theta$

  $= \cos(\theta + 4\theta)$

  $= \cos \theta \cos 4\theta - \sin \theta \sin 4\theta$

  $= \cos \theta (8 \cos^4 \theta - 8 \cos^2 \theta + 1) - \sin \theta (4 \cos^3 \theta \sin \theta$
  $\quad - 4 \sin^3 \theta \cos \theta)$

  $= 8 \cos^5 \theta - 8 \cos^3 \theta + \cos \theta - 4 \cos^3 \theta \sin^2 \theta$
  $\quad + 4 \sin^4 \theta \cos \theta$

  $= 8 \cos^5 \theta - 8 \cos^3 \theta + \cos \theta - 4 \cos^3 \theta (1 - \cos^2 \theta) +$
  $\quad 4(1 - \cos^2 \theta)^2 \cos \theta$

  $= 8 \cos^5 \theta - 8 \cos^3 \theta + \cos \theta - 4 \cos^3 \theta + 4 \cos^5 \theta +$
  $\quad 4 \cos \theta - 8 \cos^3 \theta + 4 \cos^5 \theta$

  $= 16 \cos^5 \theta - 20 \cos^3 \theta + 5 \cos \theta$

83. $\tan \dfrac{\alpha}{2} = \dfrac{1 - \cos \alpha}{\sin \alpha}$; let $\dfrac{\alpha}{2} = \theta$, so $\alpha = 2\theta$.

$$\tan \theta = \frac{1 - \cos 2\theta}{\sin 2\theta}$$

$$= \frac{1 - (1 - 2 \sin^2\theta)}{2 \sin \theta \cos \theta}$$

$$= \frac{2 \sin^2\theta}{2 \sin \theta \cos \theta}$$

$$= \frac{\sin \theta}{\cos \theta}$$

$$= \tan \theta$$

If every instance of θ above were replaced by $\dfrac{\alpha}{2}$, then the statements would still be true, thus proving the identity.

85. a. Problem 41 shows that $\sin 15° = \dfrac{\sqrt{2 - \sqrt{3}}}{2}$.

b. $\sin 15° = \sin(45° - 30°) = \sin 45° \cos 30° - \cos 45° \sin 30°$

$$= \frac{\sqrt{2}}{2} \cdot \frac{\sqrt{3}}{2} - \frac{\sqrt{2}}{2} \cdot \frac{1}{2}$$

$$= \frac{\sqrt{6} - \sqrt{2}}{4}$$

c. $\dfrac{\sqrt{6} - \sqrt{2}}{4} \overset{?}{=} \dfrac{\sqrt{2 - \sqrt{3}}}{2}$

$$\left(\frac{\sqrt{6} - \sqrt{2}}{4}\right)^2 \quad \left(\frac{\sqrt{2 - \sqrt{3}}}{2}\right)^2$$

Square both values.

$$\left(\frac{(\sqrt{6} - \sqrt{2})^2}{16}\right) \quad \frac{2 - \sqrt{3}}{4}$$

$$\frac{6 - 2\sqrt{12} + 2}{16}$$

$$\frac{8 - 4\sqrt{3}}{16}$$

$$\frac{4(2 - \sqrt{3})}{16}$$

$$\frac{2 - \sqrt{3}}{4}$$

87. Identity [5]
$$\cos 2\theta = 2 \cos^2\theta - 1$$
$$\cos 2\theta + 1 = 2 \cos^2\theta$$
$$\cos^2\theta = \frac{1 + \cos 2\theta}{2}$$
$$\cos \theta = \pm\sqrt{\frac{1 + \cos 2\theta}{2}}$$
$$\cos \frac{\alpha}{2} = \pm\sqrt{\frac{1 + \cos \alpha}{2}}$$

Identity [6-a]

$$\tan \frac{\alpha}{2} = \frac{\sin \dfrac{\alpha}{2}}{\cos \dfrac{\alpha}{2}} = \frac{\pm\sqrt{\dfrac{1 - \cos \alpha}{2}}}{\pm\sqrt{\dfrac{1 + \cos \alpha}{2}}}$$

$$= \pm\sqrt{\frac{\dfrac{1 - \cos \alpha}{2}}{\dfrac{1 + \cos \alpha}{2}}}$$

$$= \pm\sqrt{\frac{1 - \cos \alpha}{1 + \cos \alpha}}$$

89. $x = 13\frac{37}{47}$

91. $\sin 2\alpha + \sin 2\beta = 2 \sin(\alpha + \beta) \cdot \cos(\alpha - \beta)$
$2 \sin \alpha \cos \alpha + 2 \sin \beta \cos \beta$
$= 2(\sin \alpha \cos \beta + \cos \alpha \sin \beta)(\cos \alpha \cos \beta + \sin \alpha \sin \beta)$
$= 2(\sin \alpha \cos^2\beta \cos \alpha + \sin^2\alpha \cos \beta \sin \beta$
$\quad + \cos^2\alpha \sin \beta \cos \beta + \cos \alpha \sin^2\beta \sin \alpha)$
$= 2[\sin \alpha \cos^2\beta \cos \alpha + \cos \alpha \sin^2\beta \sin \alpha$
$\quad + \cos^2\alpha \sin \beta \cos \beta + \sin^2\alpha \cos \beta \sin \beta]$
$= 2[\sin \alpha \cos \alpha(\cos^2\beta + \sin^2\beta)$
$\quad + \sin \beta \cos \beta(\cos^2\alpha + \sin^2\alpha)]$
$= 2[\sin \alpha \cos \alpha(1) + \sin \beta \cos \beta(1)]$
$= 2 \sin \alpha \cos \alpha + 2 \sin \beta \cos \beta$

93. $\cos 2\alpha + \cos 2\beta = 2 \cos(\alpha + \beta) \cdot \cos(\alpha - \beta)$
$(2 \cos^2\alpha - 1) + (2 \cos^2\beta - 1)$
$= 2(\cos \alpha \cos \beta - \sin \alpha \sin \beta)(\cos \alpha \cos \beta + \sin \alpha \sin \beta)$
$2 \cos^2\alpha + 2 \cos^2\beta - 2$
$= 2(\cos^2\alpha \cos^2\beta - \sin^2\alpha \sin^2\beta)$
$= 2[\cos^2\alpha \cos^2\beta - (1 - \cos^2\alpha)(1 - \cos^2\beta)]$
$= 2[\cos^2\alpha \cos^2\beta - (1 - \cos^2\beta - \cos^2\alpha + \cos^2\alpha \cos^2\beta)]$
$= 2[-1 + \cos^2\beta + \cos^2\alpha]$
$= 2 \cos^2\alpha + 2 \cos^2\beta - 2$

95. $\cot 2\theta = \dfrac{\cos 2\theta}{\sin 2\theta}$

$$= \frac{\cos^2\theta - \sin^2\theta}{2 \sin \theta \cos \theta}$$

$$= \frac{1}{2} \cdot \frac{\cos^2\theta - \sin^2\theta}{\sin \theta \cos \theta}$$

$$= \frac{1}{2}\left(\frac{\cos^2\theta}{\sin \theta \cos \theta} - \frac{\sin^2\theta}{\sin \theta \cos \theta}\right)$$

$$= \frac{1}{2}\left(\frac{\cos \theta}{\sin \theta} - \frac{\sin \theta}{\cos \theta}\right)$$

$$= \frac{1}{2}(\cot \theta - \tan \theta)$$

$$= \frac{1}{2}\left(\cot \theta - \frac{1}{\cot \theta}\right)$$

Solutions to trial exercise problems

6. $\dfrac{2 \tan \dfrac{\pi}{6}}{1 - \tan^2\dfrac{\pi}{6}}$

$\dfrac{2 \tan \alpha}{1 - \tan^2\alpha} = \tan 2\alpha$; Let $\alpha = \dfrac{\pi}{6}$, so $2\alpha = \dfrac{\pi}{3}$,

and $\tan 2\alpha$ becomes $\tan \dfrac{\pi}{3}$.

8. $8 \cos^2\dfrac{\pi}{2} - 4$

$2 \cos^2\alpha - 1 = \cos 2\alpha$
$8 \cos^2\alpha - 1 = 4 \cos 2\alpha$
  Multiply each member by 4.

Let $\alpha = \dfrac{\pi}{2}$, so $2\alpha = \pi$, and $4 \cos 2\alpha = 4 \cos \pi$.

27. $\cos\theta = \sqrt{\dfrac{1}{2}\left(1 + \cos\dfrac{\pi}{4}\right)}$

$\cos\dfrac{\alpha}{2} = \sqrt{\dfrac{1 + \cos\alpha}{2}}$

$\alpha = \dfrac{\pi}{4}$, so $\dfrac{\alpha}{2} = \dfrac{\pi}{8}$. Thus, θ is $\dfrac{\pi}{8}$, and

$\cos\dfrac{\pi}{8} = \sqrt{\dfrac{1}{2}\left(1 + \cos\dfrac{\pi}{4}\right)}$.

34. $\tan\theta = -\dfrac{3}{4}, \dfrac{3\pi}{2} < \theta < 2\pi$

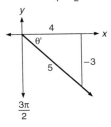

$\sin 2\theta = 2\sin\theta\cos\theta = 2\left(-\dfrac{3}{5}\right)\cdot\dfrac{4}{5} = -\dfrac{24}{25}$

$\cos 2\theta = \cos^2\theta - \sin^2\theta = \left(\dfrac{4}{5}\right)^2 - \left(-\dfrac{3}{5}\right)^2 = \dfrac{7}{25}$

$\tan 2\theta = \dfrac{\sin 2\theta}{\cos 2\theta} = -\dfrac{24}{7}$

38. $\tan\theta = -\sqrt{15}, \dfrac{\pi}{2} < \theta < \pi$: $\cos\theta = -\dfrac{1}{4}$

$\dfrac{\pi}{4} \le \dfrac{\theta}{2} \le \dfrac{\pi}{2}, \left(\dfrac{\theta}{2}\text{ in quadrant I}\right)$ so

$\sin\dfrac{\theta}{2} > 0, \cos\dfrac{\theta}{2} > 0, \tan\dfrac{\theta}{2} > 0.$

$\sin\dfrac{\theta}{2} = \sqrt{\dfrac{1 - \cos\theta}{2}} = \sqrt{\dfrac{1 - \left(-\frac{1}{4}\right)}{2}} = \sqrt{\dfrac{5}{8}}$

$= \dfrac{\sqrt{5}}{2\sqrt{2}} = \dfrac{\sqrt{10}}{4}$

$\cos\dfrac{\theta}{2} = \sqrt{\dfrac{1 + \cos\theta}{2}} = \sqrt{\dfrac{1 + \left(-\frac{1}{4}\right)}{2}} = \sqrt{\dfrac{3}{8}}$

$= \dfrac{\sqrt{3}}{2\sqrt{2}} = \dfrac{\sqrt{6}}{4}$

$\tan\dfrac{\theta}{2} = \sqrt{\dfrac{1 - \cos\theta}{1 + \cos\theta}} = \sqrt{\dfrac{1 - \left(-\frac{1}{4}\right)}{1 + \left(-\frac{1}{4}\right)}}$

$= \sqrt{\dfrac{5}{8} \div \dfrac{3}{8}} = \sqrt{\dfrac{5}{3}} = \dfrac{\sqrt{5}}{\sqrt{3}} = \dfrac{\sqrt{15}}{3}$

42. $22.5°$, or $\dfrac{\pi}{8}$

a. $\sin 22.5° = \sqrt{\dfrac{1 - \cos 45°}{2}} = \sqrt{\dfrac{1}{2}\left(1 - \dfrac{\sqrt{2}}{2}\right)}$

$= \sqrt{\dfrac{2 - \sqrt{2}}{4}} = \dfrac{\sqrt{2 - \sqrt{2}}}{2}$

b. $\cos 22.5° = \sqrt{\dfrac{1 + \cos 45°}{2}} = \sqrt{\dfrac{1}{2}\left(1 + \dfrac{\sqrt{2}}{2}\right)}$

$= \sqrt{\dfrac{2 + \sqrt{2}}{4}} = \dfrac{\sqrt{2 + \sqrt{2}}}{2}$

c. $\tan 22.5° = \sqrt{\dfrac{1 - \cos 45°}{1 + \cos 45°}} = \dfrac{1 - \dfrac{\sqrt{2}}{2}}{\dfrac{\sqrt{2}}{2}} = \dfrac{2 - \sqrt{2}}{\sqrt{2}}$

$= \dfrac{2\sqrt{2} - 2}{2} = \sqrt{2} - 1$

44. $\sin 37.5° = \sin(15° + 22.5°)$

$= \sin 15° \cos 22.5° + \cos 15° \sin 22.5°$

$= \dfrac{\sqrt{2 - \sqrt{3}}}{2} \cdot \dfrac{\sqrt{2 + \sqrt{2}}}{2} + \dfrac{\sqrt{2 + \sqrt{3}}}{2} \cdot \dfrac{\sqrt{2 - \sqrt{2}}}{2}$

$= \dfrac{\sqrt{4 - \sqrt{6} - 2\sqrt{3} + 2\sqrt{2}} + \sqrt{4 - \sqrt{6} + 2\sqrt{3} - 2\sqrt{2}}}{4}$

Note: $\sqrt{2 - \sqrt{3}} \cdot \sqrt{2 + \sqrt{2}} = \sqrt{(2 - \sqrt{3})(2 + \sqrt{2})}$

$= \sqrt{4 + 2\sqrt{2} - 2\sqrt{3} - \sqrt{6}}$

The calculation for $\sqrt{2 + \sqrt{3}} \cdot \sqrt{2 - \sqrt{2}}$ is similar.

80. Find identities for $\sin 4\theta$ in terms of $\sin x$ and $\cos x$, and for $\cos 4\theta$ in terms of $\cos\theta$.

a. $\sin 4\theta = \sin 2(2\theta)$

$= 2\sin 2\theta\cos 2\theta$

$= 2(2\sin\theta\cos\theta)(1 - 2\sin^2\theta)$

$= 4\sin\theta\cos\theta - 8\sin^3\theta\cos\theta$

Depending on how $\cos 2\theta$ is expanded, other possible answers are

$\sin 4\theta = 8\cos^3\theta\sin\theta - 4\cos\theta\sin\theta$

$\sin 4\theta = 4\cos^3\theta\sin\theta - 4\sin^3\theta\cos\theta$

b. $\cos 4\theta = \cos 2(2\theta)$

$= 2\cos^2(2\theta) - 1$

$= 2[\cos 2\theta]^2 - 1$

$= 2[2\cos^2\theta - 1]^2 - 1$

$= 2[4\cos^4\theta - 4\cos^2\theta + 1] - 1$

$= 8\cos^4\theta - 8\cos^2\theta + 1$

89. $\cos \theta_2 = \cos \dfrac{\theta}{2} = \dfrac{8}{9}$; $\cos \theta = \dfrac{8}{x}$

$$\cos \dfrac{\theta}{2} = \sqrt{\dfrac{1 + \cos \theta}{2}}$$

The angles are acute, so we need the positive value.

$$\dfrac{8}{9} = \sqrt{\dfrac{1 + \dfrac{8}{x}}{2}}$$

Substitute values.

$$\dfrac{64}{81} = \dfrac{1 + \dfrac{8}{x}}{2}$$

Square both members.

$$128 = 81\left(1 + \dfrac{8}{x}\right)$$

If $\dfrac{a}{b} = \dfrac{c}{d}$, then $ad = bc$.

$$128 = 81 + \dfrac{648}{x}$$

$$47 = \dfrac{648}{x}$$

$$x = \dfrac{648}{47} = 13\tfrac{37}{47}$$

Exercise 5–4

Answers to odd-numbered problems

1. $\dfrac{3\pi}{4}(135°), \dfrac{7\pi}{4}(315°)$ **3.** $\dfrac{\pi}{3}(60°), \dfrac{5\pi}{3}(300°)$

5. $\dfrac{\pi}{6}(30°), \dfrac{7\pi}{6}(210°)$ **7.** $\dfrac{\pi}{3}(60°), \dfrac{5\pi}{3}(300°)$

9. $\dfrac{\pi}{2}(90°), \dfrac{3\pi}{2}(270°)$ **11.** $0(0°), \pi(180°)$ **13.** $0(0°), \dfrac{3\pi}{2}(270°)$

15. $\dfrac{\pi}{4}(45°), \dfrac{3\pi}{4}(135°), \dfrac{5\pi}{4}(225°), \dfrac{7\pi}{4}(315°)$

17. $0(0°), \pi(180°), \dfrac{\pi}{2}(90°)$ **19.** $0(0°), \pi(180°), \dfrac{\pi}{3}(60°),$

$\dfrac{4\pi}{3}(240°)$ **21.** $\dfrac{3\pi}{2}(270°), \dfrac{\pi}{6}(30°), \dfrac{5\pi}{6}(150°)$

23. $0(0°), \pi(180°), \dfrac{\pi}{4}(45°), \dfrac{3\pi}{4}(135°), \dfrac{5\pi}{4}(225°), \dfrac{7\pi}{4}(315°)$

25. $0(0°), \pi(180°), \dfrac{\pi}{3}(60°), \dfrac{5\pi}{3}(300°)$

27. $\dfrac{5\pi}{6}(150°), \dfrac{11\pi}{6}(330°), \dfrac{\pi}{2}(90°), \dfrac{3\pi}{2}(270°)$

29. $0(0°), \pi(180°), \dfrac{\pi}{2}(90°), \dfrac{3\pi}{2}(270°)$

31. $\dfrac{\pi}{6}(30°), \dfrac{5\pi}{6}(150°), \dfrac{3\pi}{2}(270°)$ **33.** $\dfrac{3\pi}{4}(135°), \dfrac{7\pi}{4}(315°)$

35. $\dfrac{\pi}{3}(60°), \dfrac{5\pi}{3}(300°), \pi(180°)$

37. $\dfrac{\pi}{3}(60°), \dfrac{2\pi}{3}(120°), \dfrac{4\pi}{3}(240°), \dfrac{5\pi}{3}(300°)$

39. $\dfrac{\pi}{4}(45°), \dfrac{3\pi}{4}(135°), \dfrac{5\pi}{4}(225°), \dfrac{7\pi}{4}(315°)$

41. $0(0°), \pi(180°), \dfrac{\pi}{6}(30°), \dfrac{5\pi}{6}(150°)$

43. 0.65, 2.49, 3.42, 6.01 (37.4°, 142.6°, 195.9°, 344.1°)
45. 0.27, 2.08, 3.42, 5.22 (15.7°, 119.3°, 195.7°, 299.3°)
47. 1.26, 2.51, 3.77, 5.03 (72°, 144°, 216°, 288°)
49. 5.08(290.8°), 0.56(32.3°)

51. $\dfrac{\pi}{3} + 2k\pi(60° + k \cdot 360°), \dfrac{5\pi}{3} + 2k\pi(300° + k \cdot 360°)$

53. $\dfrac{5\pi}{6} + k\pi, (150° + k \cdot 180°)$

55. $\dfrac{5\pi}{4} + 2k\pi(225° + k \cdot 360°), \dfrac{7\pi}{4} + 2k\pi(315° + k \cdot 360°)$

57. $\dfrac{\pi}{4} + k\pi(45° + k \cdot 180°)$

59. $\dfrac{\pi}{6} + 2k\pi(30° + k \cdot 360°), \dfrac{5\pi}{6} + 2k\pi(150° + k \cdot 360°)$

61. $\dfrac{2\pi}{3} + 4k\pi(120° + k \cdot 720°), \dfrac{4\pi}{3} + 4k\pi(240° + k \cdot 720°)$

63. $\dfrac{\pi}{3} + \dfrac{2k\pi}{3}(60° + k \cdot 120°)$

65. $\dfrac{\pi}{6} + k\dfrac{\pi}{2}(30° + k \cdot 90°)$

67. $\dfrac{\pi}{6} + k\dfrac{\pi}{2}(30° + k \cdot 90°), \dfrac{\pi}{3} + k\dfrac{\pi}{2}(60° + k \cdot 90°)$

69. $\dfrac{\pi}{3} + k\pi(60° + k \cdot 180°), \dfrac{2\pi}{3} + k\pi(120° + k \cdot 180)$

71. $\dfrac{\pi}{12} + k\dfrac{\pi}{2}(15° + k \cdot 90°)$

73. $\dfrac{\pi}{12} + k\pi(15° + k \cdot 180°), \dfrac{5\pi}{12} + k\pi(75° + k \cdot 180°)$

75. $\dfrac{\pi}{9} + \dfrac{2k\pi}{3}(20° + k \cdot 120°), \dfrac{5\pi}{9} + \dfrac{2k\pi}{3}(100° + k \cdot 120°)$

77. $\dfrac{2\pi}{3} + 4k\pi(120° + k \cdot 720°)$

79. $\dfrac{7\pi}{6}(210°), \dfrac{11\pi}{6}(330°), \dfrac{\pi}{2}(90°)$

81. $0(0°), \pi(180°), \dfrac{2\pi}{3}(120°), \dfrac{4\pi}{3}(240°)$

83. $0(0°), \pi(180°), \dfrac{\pi}{6}(30°), \dfrac{5\pi}{6}(150°)$

85. $0(0°)$ **87.** $\dfrac{\pi}{3}(60°)$ or $\dfrac{5\pi}{3}(300°)$

89. $0(0°), \dfrac{3\pi}{2}(270°)$ **91.** $\dfrac{\pi}{2}(90°), \dfrac{3\pi}{2}(270°), \pi(180°), 0.93(53.1°)$

93. $\dfrac{\pi}{2}$, 1.31   **95.** 0, 0.55, 0.69, 0.72, 0.66

Solutions to trial exercise problems

4. $2 \cos \theta + 1 = 0$

$2 \cos \theta = -1$

$\cos \theta = -\frac{1}{2}$

$\theta' = \cos^{-1} \frac{1}{2} = \frac{\pi}{3}(60°)$

$\cos \theta < 0$ in quadrants II and III, so $\theta = \pi - \theta' =$

$\pi - \frac{\pi}{3} = \frac{2\pi}{3}(180° - 60° = 120°)$ or $\theta = \pi + \theta' =$

$\pi + \frac{\pi}{3} = \frac{4\pi}{3}(180° + 60° = 240°)$.

20. $\cos^2\theta - \frac{1}{2} \cos \theta = 0$

$\cos \theta(\cos \theta - \frac{1}{2}) = 0$

Case 1: $\cos \theta = 0$

$\frac{\pi}{2}(90°)$, $\frac{3\pi}{2}(270°)$

Case 2: $\cos \theta - \frac{1}{2} = 0$

$\cos \theta = \frac{1}{2}$

$\cos \theta > 0$ in quadrants I and IV, so $\theta = \theta' = \frac{\pi}{3}(60°)$

or $2\pi - \theta' = 2\pi - \frac{\pi}{3} = \frac{5\pi}{3}(360° - 60° = 300°)$.

27. $\sqrt{3} \tan \theta \cot \theta + \cot \theta = 0$

$\cot \theta(\sqrt{3} \tan \theta + 1) = 0$

Case 1: $\cot \theta = 0$

$\frac{\cos \theta}{\sin \theta} = 0$

$\cos \theta = 0$

$\frac{\pi}{2}(90°)$ or $\frac{3\pi}{2}(270°)$

Case 2: $\sqrt{3} \tan \theta + 1 = 0$

$\tan \theta = -\frac{\sqrt{3}}{3}$

$\theta' = \tan^{-1} \frac{\sqrt{3}}{3} = \frac{\pi}{6}(30°)$.

$\tan \theta < 0$ in quadrants II and IV, so $\theta = \pi - \theta' =$

$\pi - \frac{\pi}{6} = \frac{5\pi}{6}(180° - 30° = 150°)$ or $2\pi - \theta' =$

$2\pi - \frac{\pi}{6} = \frac{11\pi}{6}(360° - 30° = 330°)$.

33. $\tan x + \cot x = -2$

$\tan x + \frac{1}{\tan x} = -2$

$\tan^2 x + 1 = -2 \tan x$

   Multiply each member by $\tan x$; assume $\tan x \neq 0$.

$\tan^2 x + 2 \tan x + 1 = 0$

$(\tan x + 1)^2 = 0$

$\tan x + 1 = 0$

$\tan x = -1$

$\theta' = \tan^{-1}1 = \frac{\pi}{4}(45°)$

Tangent is negative in quadrants II and IV, so $\theta = \pi - \theta' =$

$\pi - \frac{\pi}{4} = \frac{3\pi}{4}(180° - 45° = 135°)$ or $2\pi - \theta' =$

$2\pi - \frac{\pi}{4} = \frac{7\pi}{4}(360° - 45° = 315°)$.

34. $2 - \sin x - \csc x = 0$

$2 - \sin x - \frac{1}{\sin x} = 0$

$2 \sin x - \sin^2 x - 1 = 0$

$-\sin^2 x + 2 \sin x - 1 = 0$

$\sin^2 x - 2 \sin x + 1 = 0$

$(\sin x - 1)^2 = 0$

$\sin x - 1 = 0$

$\sin x = 1$

$x = \frac{\pi}{2}(90°)$

41. $2 \tan^2 x \sin x = \tan^2 x$

$2 \tan^2 x \sin x - \tan^2 x = 0$

$\tan^2 x(2 \sin x - 1) = 0$

Case 1: $\tan^2 x = 0$

$\tan x = 0$

$\frac{\sin \theta}{\cos \theta} = 0$

$\sin \theta = 0$

$0(0°)$, $\pi(180°)$

Case 2: $2 \sin x - 1 = 0$

$\sin x = \frac{1}{2}$

$\theta' = \sin^{-1}\frac{1}{2} = \frac{\pi}{6}$

$\sin \theta > 0$ in quadrants I and II.

$\theta = \theta' = \frac{\pi}{6}(30°)$ or

$\pi - \frac{\pi}{6} = \frac{5\pi}{6}(150°)$

Recall: If $ax^2 + bx + c = 0$, $c \neq 0$, then

$x = \frac{-b \pm \sqrt{b^2 - 4ac}}{2a}$.

46. $\tan^2 x + 5 \tan x + 2 = 0$

$a = 1, b = 5, c = 2$:

$\tan x = \frac{-5 \pm \sqrt{5^2 - 4(2)}}{2} = \frac{-5 \pm \sqrt{17}}{2}$

Case 1:

$\tan x = \frac{-5 + \sqrt{17}}{2} \approx -0.4384$

$x = \tan^{-1}\left|\frac{-5 + \sqrt{17}}{2}\right| \approx 0.413(23.7°)$

$\tan x < 0$ in quadrants II and IV.

$x = \pi - x' \approx \pi - 0.413 \approx 2.74$

$\quad = 2\pi - x' \approx 2\pi - 0.413 \approx 5.87$

$x = 180° - x' \approx 180° - 23.7° \approx 156.3°$

$\quad = 360° - x' \approx 360° - 23.7° \approx 336.3°$

Case 2:

$$\tan x = \frac{-5 - \sqrt{17}}{2} \approx -4.5616$$

$$x = \tan^{-1}\left|\frac{-5 - \sqrt{17}}{2}\right| \approx 1.355(77.6°)$$

$\tan x < 0$ in quadrants II and IV.

$x = \pi - x' \approx \pi - 1.355 \approx 1.79$

$\quad = 2\pi - x' \approx 2\pi - 1.355 \approx 4.93$

$x = 180° - x' \approx 180° - 77.6° \approx 102.4°$

$\quad = 360° - x' \approx 360° - 77.6° \approx 282.4°$

57. $\tan x = 1$

$$x = \tan^{-1}1 = \frac{\pi}{4}(45°)$$

Primary solutions are in quadrants I and III:

$\frac{\pi}{4}(45°)$ and $\frac{5\pi}{4}(225°)$. These differ by $\pi(180°)$, so we can

write all solutions with one of them: $\frac{\pi}{4} + k\pi(45° + k \cdot 180°)$.

64. $\sec \frac{x}{2} = 1$; $\cos \frac{x}{2} = 1$

Primary solutions: $\frac{x}{2} = \cos^{-1}1 = 0(0°)$

All solutions: $\frac{x}{2} = 0 + 2k\pi(0° + k \cdot 360°)$

$\qquad\qquad x = 4k\pi(k \cdot 720°)$

74. $\sin \frac{\theta}{3} = \frac{\sqrt{3}}{2}$

$\left(\frac{\theta}{3}\right)' = \sin^{-1}\frac{\sqrt{3}}{2} = \frac{\pi}{3}(60°)$

Primary solutions: $\frac{\theta}{3} = \frac{\pi}{3}(60°)$ or $\frac{2\pi}{3}(120°)$

All solutions: $\frac{\theta}{3} = \frac{\pi}{3} + 2k\pi(60° + k \cdot 360°)$ or

$\qquad\qquad \frac{2\pi}{3} + 2k\pi(120° + k \cdot 360°)$

$\theta = \pi + 6k\pi(180° + k \cdot 1{,}080°)$ or

$2\pi + 6k\pi(360° + k \cdot 1{,}080°)$.

81. $\sin 2\theta + \sin \theta = 0$

$2 \sin \theta \cos \theta + \sin \theta = 0$

$\sin \theta(2 \cos \theta + 1) = 0$

Case 1: $\sin \theta = 0$

$\qquad 0(0°), \pi(180°)$

Case 2: $2 \cos \theta + 1 = 0$

$\qquad \cos \theta = -\frac{1}{2}$

$\qquad \frac{2\pi}{3}(120°)$ or $\frac{4\pi}{3}(240°)$

88. $\sin^2\frac{\theta}{2} = \cos \theta$

$\left(\pm\sqrt{\frac{1 - \cos \theta}{2}}\right)^2 = \cos \theta$

$\frac{1 - \cos \theta}{2} = \cos \theta$

$1 - \cos \theta = 2 \cos \theta$

$1 = 3 \cos \theta$

$\frac{1}{3} = \cos \theta$

$\theta' = \cos^{-1}\frac{1}{3}$

$\theta = \cos^{-1}\frac{1}{3}$ or $2\pi - \cos^{-1}\frac{1}{3}$

$\theta = 1.23(70.5°)$ or $5.05(289.5°)$

92. If $A = 0.855$, $B = 1.052$, and $y = 0$, solve for x to the nearest 0.01.

$0 = x \cos 0.855 \cos 1.052 - x^2 \cos 0.855 \sin 1.052$

$\quad - x^3 \sin 0.855$

$0 = 0.32538x - 0.56987x^2 - 0.75457x^3$

$x(0.75457x^2 + 0.56987x - 0.32538) = 0$

$x = 0$ or $0.75457x^2 + 0.56987x - 0.32538 = 0$

$\quad$ Solve the quadratic equation with the quadratic formula.

$x = 0, -1.14, 0.38$

93. If $B = 0.7$, $x = 2$, and $y = -8$, find A to the nearest 0.01.

$-8 = 2 \cos A \cos 0.7 - 4 \cos A \sin 0.7 - 8 \sin A$

$-8 = (2 \cos 0.7)\cos A - (4 \sin 0.7)\cos A - 8 \sin A$

$-8 = 1.5297 \cos A - 2.5769 \cos A - 8 \sin A$

$-8 = -1.0472 \cos A - 8 \sin A$

$8 \sin A - 8 = -1.0472 \cos A$

$\sin A - 1 = -0.1309 \cos A$

$\quad$ Divide each member by 8.

$\sin A = 1 - 0.1309 \cos A$

$(\sin A)^2 = (1 - 0.1309 \cos A)^2$

$\sin^2 A = 1 - 0.2618 \cos A + 0.017134 \cos^2 A$

$1 - \cos^2 A = 1 - 0.2618 \cos A + 0.017134 \cos^2 A$

$0 = 1.0171 \cos^2 A - 0.2618 \cos A$

$0 = \cos A(1.0171 \cos A - 0.2618)$

$\cos A = 0$ or $1.0171 \cos A - 0.2618 = 0$

$A = \cos^{-1}0$ or $1.0171 \cos A = 0.2618$

$A = \frac{\pi}{2}$ or $\cos A = 0.25739$

$A \approx 1.310476103$

Thus, A is $\frac{\pi}{2}$ or 1.31

96. Find θ when $\mathcal{A} = 0.5$ m². Round the answer to the nearest 0.1°.

$\sin \theta \sqrt{1.44 - \sin^2\theta} = 0.5$

$(\sin \theta \sqrt{1.44 - \sin^2\theta})^2 = 0.5^2$

$\sin^2\theta(1.44 - \sin^2\theta) = 0.25$

$1.44 \sin^2\theta - \sin^4\theta = 0.25$

$\sin^4\theta - 1.44 \sin^2\theta + 0.25 = 0$

Let $u = \sin^2\theta$.

$u^2 - 1.44u + 0.25 = 0$

$u \approx 1.2381$	or $u \approx 0.20193$
$\sin^2\theta \approx 1.2381$	or $\sin^2\theta \approx 0.20193$
$\sin \theta \approx \pm\sqrt{1.2381}$	or $\sin \theta \approx \pm\sqrt{0.20193}$
$\sin \theta \approx \pm1.1127$	or $\sin \theta \approx \pm0.44936$
no solution	or $\theta \approx \pm26.7°$

Because $\theta \geq 0$, we choose the positive value for θ.

$\theta \approx 26.7°$

Chapter 5 review

1.
$$\frac{\frac{\cos\theta}{\sin\theta}}{\cos\theta}$$
$$\frac{1}{\sin\theta}$$
$$\csc\theta$$

2. $\sec\theta\dfrac{\sin\theta}{\cos\theta}$
$$\sec\theta\left(\frac{1}{\cos\theta}\right)\sin\theta$$
$$\sec\theta\sec\theta\sin\theta$$
$$\sec^2\theta\sin\theta$$

3. $\dfrac{\tan^2\theta}{\tan^2\theta}$
$$1$$
$$\sin^4\theta\frac{1}{\sin^4\theta}$$
$$\sin^4\theta\csc^4\theta$$

4. $\dfrac{\cot^2\theta}{\tan^2\theta}$
$$\frac{\frac{\cos^2\theta}{\sin^2\theta}}{\frac{\sin^2\theta}{\cos^2\theta}}$$
$$\frac{\cos^4\theta}{\sin^4\theta}$$
$$\cot^4\theta$$

5.
$$\frac{\csc\theta\frac{\sin\theta}{\cos\theta}}{\sin\theta}$$
$$\csc\theta\frac{1}{\cos\theta}$$
$$\csc\theta\sec\theta$$

6. $\sin^2\theta-(1-\sin^2\theta)$
$$\sin^2\theta-1+\sin^2\theta$$
$$2\sin^2\theta-1$$

7. $\dfrac{1}{\sin\theta}-\dfrac{1}{\cos\theta}$
$$\frac{\cos\theta-\sin\theta}{\sin\theta\cos\theta}$$

8. $\dfrac{\sin\theta}{\cos\theta}+\dfrac{\cos\theta}{\sin\theta}$
$$\frac{\sin^2\theta+\cos^2\theta}{\cos\theta\sin\theta}$$
$$\frac{1}{\cos\theta\sin\theta}$$

9.
$$\frac{\frac{1}{\cos\theta}}{\frac{\sin\theta}{\cos\theta}-\frac{\cos\theta}{\sin\theta}}$$
$$\frac{\frac{1}{\cos\theta}}{\frac{\sin^2\theta-\cos^2\theta}{\cos\theta\sin\theta}}$$
$$\frac{\frac{1}{\cos\theta}}{\frac{\sin^2\theta-\cos^2\theta}{\sin\theta}}$$
$$\frac{\sin\theta}{\sin^2\theta-\cos^2\theta}$$

10.
$$\frac{1-\frac{\cos\theta}{\sin\theta}}{\frac{1}{\sin\theta}+1}$$
$$\frac{\frac{\sin\theta-\cos\theta}{\sin\theta}}{\frac{1+\sin\theta}{\sin\theta}}$$
$$\frac{\sin\theta-\cos\theta}{1+\sin\theta}$$

11.
$$\frac{\frac{1}{\cos^2\theta}-1}{\frac{1}{\cos^2\theta}}$$
$$\frac{\frac{1-\cos^2\theta}{\cos^2\theta}}{\frac{1}{\cos^2\theta}}$$
$$\frac{1-\cos^2\theta}{\cos^2\theta}$$
$$\frac{1-\cos^2\theta}{\sin^2\theta}$$

12.
$$\frac{1-\frac{\cos^2\theta}{\sin^2\theta}}{\frac{1}{\sin^2\theta}-1}$$
$$\frac{\frac{\sin^2\theta-\cos^2\theta}{\sin^2\theta}}{\frac{1-\sin^2\theta}{\sin^2\theta}}$$
$$\frac{\sin^2\theta-\cos^2\theta}{1-\sin^2\theta}$$

13. $\csc x-\tan x\cot x$
$$\csc x-\tan x\left(\frac{1}{\tan x}\right)$$
$$\csc x-1$$

14. $\sin^2x+\sin^2x\cot^2x$
$$\sin^2x+\sin^2x\frac{\cos^2x}{\sin^2x}$$
$$\sin^2x+\cos^2x$$
$$1$$

15. $\csc^2x\sec^2x(\cos^2x-\sin^2x)$
$$\left(\frac{1}{\sin^2x}\right)\left(\frac{1}{\cos^2x}\right)(\cos^2x-\sin^2x)$$
$$\frac{1}{\sin^2x}-\frac{1}{\cos^2x}$$
$$\csc^2x-\sec^2x$$

16. $\dfrac{1}{\csc x-\cot x}$
$$\frac{1}{\frac{1}{\sin x}-\frac{\cos x}{\sin x}}$$
$$\frac{1}{\frac{1-\cos x}{\sin x}}$$
$$\frac{\sin x}{1-\cos x}$$

17. $\sec x(\sin x-\cos x)$
$$\frac{1}{\cos x}(\sin x-\cos x)$$
$$\frac{\sin x}{\cos x}-\frac{\cos x}{\cos x}$$
$$\tan x-1$$

18. $\dfrac{\csc^2x-1}{\sin^2x}$
$$\frac{\cot^2x}{\sin^2x}$$
$$\frac{\frac{\cos^2x}{\sin^2x}}{\sin^2x}$$
$$\frac{\cos^2x}{\sin^4x}$$
$$\cos^2x\csc^4x$$

19. $\dfrac{1}{1+\csc x}+\dfrac{1}{1-\csc x}$
$$\frac{1-\csc x+1+\csc x}{1-\csc^2x}$$
$$\frac{2}{1-\csc^2x}$$
$$\frac{2}{-1(\csc^2x-1)}$$
$$\frac{-2}{\cot^2x}$$
$$-2\tan^2x$$

20. $\sin^2x+\sin^2x\cos^2x$
$$\sin^2x(1+\cos^2x)$$
$$(1-\cos^2x)(1+\cos^2x)$$
$$1-\cos^4x$$

21. $\dfrac{\sec^2x}{\cot^2x}$
$$\frac{\tan^2x+1}{\cot^2x}$$
$$\frac{\tan^2x+1}{\frac{1}{\tan^2x}}$$
$$\tan^4x+\tan^2x$$

22. $\dfrac{1-\cot x}{1+\csc x}$
$$\frac{1-\frac{\cos x}{\sin x}}{1+\frac{1}{\sin x}}$$
$$\frac{\frac{\sin x-\cos x}{\sin x}}{\frac{\sin x+1}{\sin x}}$$
$$\frac{\sin x-\cos x}{\sin x+1}$$

23. $\sin\dfrac{\pi}{6}+\cos\dfrac{\pi}{6}$
$$\frac{1}{2}+\frac{\sqrt{3}}{2}$$
$$\frac{1+\sqrt{3}}{2}\neq 1$$

24. $\tan\dfrac{\pi}{4}-\sin\dfrac{\pi}{4}\cos\dfrac{\pi}{4}$
$$1-\left(\frac{\sqrt{2}}{2}\right)\left(\frac{\sqrt{2}}{2}\right)$$
$$1-\frac{1}{2}$$
$$\frac{1}{2}\neq 0$$

25. $\sec\dfrac{\pi}{4}=\sqrt{2}$
$$\frac{1}{\cot\dfrac{\pi}{4}-\csc\dfrac{\pi}{4}}=\frac{1}{1-\sqrt{2}}$$
$$=\frac{1+\sqrt{2}}{-1}=-1-\sqrt{2}\neq\sqrt{2}$$

26. $\dfrac{\sqrt{2} + \sqrt{6}}{4}$ **27.** $\sqrt{3} - 2$

28. $\dfrac{\sqrt{6} + \sqrt{2}}{4}$ **29.** $-2 + \sqrt{3}$

30. a. $\dfrac{-15 + \sqrt{77}}{24}$ **b.** $\dfrac{-15 - \sqrt{77}}{5\sqrt{7} - 3\sqrt{11}}$

31. a. $\dfrac{3\sqrt{5} + 1}{8}$ **b.** $\dfrac{\sqrt{15} + \sqrt{3}}{1 - 3\sqrt{5}}$

32. a. $\dfrac{204}{8\sqrt{119} + 75}$

b. $\dfrac{952 - 75\sqrt{119}}{-40\sqrt{119} - 1{,}785}$

33. $\dfrac{\sin(\alpha + \beta)}{\cos(\alpha - \beta)}$

$\dfrac{\sin \alpha \cos \beta + \cos \alpha \sin \beta}{\cos \alpha \cos \beta + \sin \alpha \sin \beta}$

$\dfrac{\dfrac{\sin \alpha \cos \beta}{\sin \alpha \sin \beta} + \dfrac{\cos \alpha \sin \beta}{\sin \alpha \sin \beta}}{\dfrac{\cos \alpha \cos \beta}{\sin \alpha \sin \beta} + \dfrac{\sin \alpha \sin \beta}{\sin \alpha \sin \beta}}$

$\dfrac{\cot \beta + \cot \alpha}{\cot \alpha \cot \beta + 1}$

34. $\cos\left(\dfrac{3\pi}{2} + \theta\right)$

$\cos \dfrac{3\pi}{2} \cos \theta - \sin \dfrac{3\pi}{2} \sin \theta$

$(0) \cos \theta - (-1) \sin \theta$

$\sin \theta$

35. $\sin\left(\dfrac{\pi}{4} - \theta\right)$

$\sin \dfrac{\pi}{4} \cos \theta - \cos \dfrac{\pi}{4} \sin \theta$

$\dfrac{\sqrt{2}}{2} \cos \theta - \dfrac{\sqrt{2}}{2} \sin \theta$

$\dfrac{\sqrt{2}}{2}(\cos \theta - \sin \theta)$

36. $\dfrac{\cos(\alpha + \beta)}{\sin \alpha \cos \beta}$

$\dfrac{\cos \alpha \cos \beta - \sin \alpha \sin \beta}{\sin \alpha \cos \beta}$

$\dfrac{\cos \alpha \cos \beta}{\sin \alpha \cos \beta} - \dfrac{\sin \alpha \sin \beta}{\sin \alpha \cos \beta}$

$\dfrac{\cos \alpha}{\sin \alpha} - \dfrac{\sin \beta}{\cos \beta}$

$\cot \alpha - \tan \beta$

37. $\cot(\theta + \pi)$

$\dfrac{1}{\tan(\theta + \pi)}$

$\dfrac{1}{\dfrac{\tan \theta + \tan \pi}{1 - \tan \theta \tan \pi}}$

$\dfrac{1}{\dfrac{\tan \theta + (0)}{1 - \tan \theta (0)}}$

$\dfrac{1}{\tan \theta}$

$\cot \theta$

38. $124°$ **39.** 10π **40.** $\dfrac{7\pi}{6}$ **41.** $12°$

42. $3 \sin \theta$ **43.** $2 \tan 8\theta$

44. a. $-\dfrac{5\sqrt{119}}{47}$ **b.** $\dfrac{5\sqrt{119}}{72}$ **45 a.** $-\dfrac{7}{25}$

b. $\dfrac{24}{7}$ **46. a.** $-\dfrac{41}{40}$ **b.** $\dfrac{9}{40}$

47. $\sin 2x - \cos x$

$2 \sin x \cos x - \cos x$

$\cos x(2 \sin x - 1)$

48. $1 + \cos 2x$

$1 + \cos^2 x - \sin^2 x$

$1 + \cos^2 x - (1 - \cos^2 x)$

$1 + \cos^2 x - 1 + \cos^2 x$

$2 \cos^2 x$

49. $\dfrac{\cos 2x}{2 - 4 \sin^2 x}$

$\dfrac{\cos^2 x - \sin^2 x}{2(1 - 2 \sin^2 x)}$

$\dfrac{\cos^2 x - \sin^2 x}{2(\sin^2 x + \cos^2 x - 2 \sin^2 x)}$

$\dfrac{\cos^2 x - \sin^2 x}{2(\cos^2 x - \sin^2 x)}$

$\dfrac{1}{2}$

50. $\dfrac{2 \cot x}{\cot^2 x - 1}$

$\dfrac{\dfrac{2}{\tan x}}{\dfrac{1}{\tan^2 x} - 1}$

$\dfrac{\dfrac{2}{\tan x}}{\dfrac{1 - \tan^2 x}{\tan^2 x}}$

$\dfrac{2 \tan x}{1 - \tan^2 x}$

$\tan 2x$

51. $\sin 2x - \cos 2x$

$2 \sin x \cos x - (\cos^2 x - \sin^2 x)$

$2 \sin x \cos x - \cos^2 x + \sin^2 x$

$2 \sin x \cos x - \cos^2 x + 1 - \cos^2 x$

$2 \sin x \cos x - 2 \cos^2 x + 1$

$2 \cos x(\sin x - \cos x) + 1$

52. $\sqrt{2} - 1$ **53.** $\dfrac{\sqrt{2 + \sqrt{3}}}{2}$

54. $\dfrac{\sqrt{2 + \sqrt{3}}}{2}$ **55.** $\dfrac{\sqrt{2 - \sqrt{2}}}{2}$

56. a. $\dfrac{\sqrt{26}}{26}$ **b.** $\dfrac{1}{5}$ **57. a.** $-\sqrt{\dfrac{6}{3 - \sqrt{5}}}$

b. $\dfrac{-3 + \sqrt{5}}{2}$ **58.** $\dfrac{5}{6}$

59. $\cot \dfrac{\theta}{2}$

$\dfrac{1}{\tan \dfrac{\theta}{2}}$

$\dfrac{1}{\dfrac{\sin \theta}{1 + \cos \theta}}$

$\dfrac{1 + \cos \theta}{\sin \theta}$

60. $\sec^2 \dfrac{\theta}{2} - \tan^2 \dfrac{\theta}{2}$

$\left(1 + \tan^2 \dfrac{\theta}{2}\right) - \tan^2 \dfrac{\theta}{2}$

$1 + \tan^2 \dfrac{\theta}{2} - \tan^2 \dfrac{\theta}{2}$

1

61. $\tan \dfrac{\theta}{2} \csc^2 \dfrac{\theta}{2}$

$\dfrac{\sin \theta}{1 + \cos \theta} \cdot \dfrac{2}{1 - \cos \theta}$

$\dfrac{2 \sin \theta}{1 - \cos^2 \theta}$

$\dfrac{2 \sin \theta}{\sin^2 \theta}$

$\dfrac{2}{\sin \theta}$

62. $\dfrac{\pi}{6}$ **63.** $\dfrac{\pi}{3}$

64. $\dfrac{\pi}{3}, \dfrac{\pi}{2}$ **65.** $\dfrac{\pi}{6}, \dfrac{\pi}{3}$

66. $45°, 90°, 225°, 270°$ **67.** $60°, 120°,$
$240°, 300°$ **68.** $0°, 120°, 240°$ **69.** $30°,$
$150°, 270°$ **70.** $30°, 90°, 150°, 270°$
71. $120°, 180°, 240°$ **72.** $k\pi$

73. $1.31 + k\pi$, $-0.67 + k\pi$

74. $3.52 + 2k\pi$, $5.90 + 2k\pi$

75. $\dfrac{\pi}{3} + 2k\pi$, $\pi + 2k\pi$, $\dfrac{5\pi}{3} + 2k\pi$

76. $\dfrac{\pi}{24}, \dfrac{5\pi}{24}, \dfrac{13\pi}{24}, \dfrac{17\pi}{24}, \dfrac{25\pi}{24}, \dfrac{29\pi}{24},$

$\dfrac{37\pi}{24}, \dfrac{41\pi}{24}$ **77.** $\dfrac{\pi}{3}$ **78.** $\dfrac{\pi}{2}$ **79.** π

80. $12°, 60°, 84°, 132°, 156°, 204°, 228°,$
$276°, 300°, 348°$ **81.** $240°$ **82.** $7.5°,$
$37.5°, 67.5°, 97.5°, 127.5°, 157.5°, 187.5°,$
$217.5°, 247.5°, 277.5°, 307.5°, 337.5°,$
$22.5°, 52.5°, 82.5°, 112.5°, 142.5°, 172.5°,$
$202.5°, 232.5°, 262.5°, 292.5°, 322.5°,$
$352.5°$ **83.** $90°, 210°, 270°, 330°$

84. $\dfrac{\pi}{3} + 2k\pi$, $\pi + 2k\pi$, $\dfrac{5\pi}{3} + 2k\pi$

85. $0.13 + k \cdot \dfrac{\pi}{4}$, $1.22 + k \cdot \dfrac{2\pi}{3}$, $1.92 + k$

$\cdot \dfrac{2\pi}{3}$ **86.** $\dfrac{\pi}{4} + k\pi$, $1.94 + k\pi$, $2.78 + k\pi$

Chapter 5 test

1. $\csc^2 x \sin x \cos x$

$\dfrac{1}{\sin^2 x} \sin x \cos x$

$\dfrac{\cos x}{\sin x}$

$\cot x$

2. $\dfrac{\dfrac{1}{\sin x} - \dfrac{1}{\cos x}}{\dfrac{\sin x}{\cos x} + \dfrac{\cos x}{\sin x}}$

$\dfrac{\dfrac{\cos x - \sin x}{\sin x \cos x}}{\dfrac{\sin^2 x + \cos^2 x}{\sin x \cos x}}$

$\dfrac{\cos x - \sin x}{\sin^2 x + \cos^2 x}$

$\cos x - \sin x$

3. $\cot x - 2 \tan x$

$\cot 45° - 2 \tan 45°$

$1 - 2(1)$

-1

$-1 \neq 1$

4. $\dfrac{8\sqrt{3} - 15}{34}$ **5.** $-\dfrac{240}{289}$

6. 3 **7.** $\dfrac{2}{\sqrt{2 + \sqrt{2}}}$

8. a. $\dfrac{1 + \cot \theta}{\csc \theta}$

$\dfrac{1}{\csc \theta} + \dfrac{\cot \theta}{\csc \theta}$

$\dfrac{1}{\dfrac{1}{\sin \theta}} + \dfrac{\dfrac{\cos \theta}{\sin \theta}}{\dfrac{1}{\sin \theta}}$

$\sin \theta + \cos \theta$

b. $\dfrac{\cos^2 x - 1}{\sin^2 x}$

$\dfrac{-(1 - \cos^2 x)}{\sin^2 x}$

$\dfrac{-\sin^2 x}{\sin^2 x}$

-1

c. $\cos\left(\theta - \dfrac{3\pi}{2}\right)$

$\cos \theta \cos \dfrac{3\pi}{2} + \sin \theta \sin \dfrac{3\pi}{2}$

$\cos \theta(0) + \sin \theta(-1)$

$-\sin \theta$

d. $-1 + 2 \cos x(\cos x - \sin x)$

$-(\sin^2 x + \cos^2 x) + 2 \cos^2 x$

$- 2 \sin x \cos x$

$\cos^2 x - \sin^2 x - 2 \sin x \cos x$

$\cos 2x - \sin 2x$

9. $\dfrac{\pi}{3}, \dfrac{2\pi}{3}, \dfrac{4\pi}{3}, \dfrac{5\pi}{3}$

10. $30°, 120°, 210°, 240°$

11. $0.17 + 2\pi k$, $2.97 + 2\pi k$, $\dfrac{3\pi}{2} + 2\pi k$

12. $18°, 54°, 90°, 126°, 162°, 198°, 234°,$
$270°, 306°, 342°$ **13.** $\pi + 8k\pi,$
$7\pi + 8k\pi, 3\pi + 8k\pi, 5\pi + 8k\pi$ **14.** $\pm m$

Chapter 6

Exercise 6–1

Answers to odd-numbered problems

1. $C = 96°$, $b \approx 16.4$, $c \approx 21.7$
3. $A = 34.4$, $b \approx 0.52$, $c \approx 1.64$
5. $C = 33°$, $c \approx 51.2$, $a \approx 68.7$
7. $B = 20.6°$, $b \approx 0.172$, $c \approx 0.489$
9. $C = 35°$, $a \approx 8.58$, $b \approx 6.16$
11. $A \approx 45.6°$, $C \approx 85.4°$, $c \approx 17.4$
13. $B \approx 18.0°$, $C \approx 30.0°$, $b \approx 1.77$
15. $C \approx 47.4°$, $A \approx 88.9°$, $a \approx 133.9$
    $C \approx 132.6°$, $A \approx 3.7°$, $a \approx 8.7$
17. no solution

19. $B \approx 85.0°$, $A \approx 52.7°$, $a \approx 5.07$
    $B \approx 95.01°$, $A \approx 42.7°$, $a \approx 4.32$
21. $C \approx 26.23°$, $A \approx 108.77°$, $a \approx 10.71$
23. 32.3 miles   **25.** 843,400 miles
27. 15.8 knots   **29.** 25 miles
31. By the definitions of section 2–3,

$\tan A = \dfrac{y}{x}$ in each figure. By the

trigonometric ratios (for a right
triangle) it can be seen in each case

that $\tan C = \dfrac{\text{opposite}}{\text{adjacent}} = \dfrac{y}{b - x}$. (Note

that x is negative in the right figure, so
that $b - x$ is larger than b itself.) Also,
as noted in the problem, $y = h$. Putting
these values in the expression

$\dfrac{b \cdot \tan A \cdot \tan C}{\tan A + \tan C}$ we obtain:

$\dfrac{b \cdot \dfrac{y}{x} \cdot \dfrac{y}{b - x}}{\dfrac{y}{x} + \dfrac{y}{b - x}} = \dfrac{\dfrac{by^2}{x(b - x)}}{\dfrac{yb}{x(b - x)}} = y = h$

33. Let (x, y) be the point at B. It is on the
terminal side of angle A. Then $\cos A =$

$\dfrac{x}{r}$, where r is the length of AB. But

then $r = c$, so $\cos A = \dfrac{x}{c}$, and so c

$\cos A = x$. Using right triangles we see

that in each figure $\cos C = \dfrac{b - x}{a}$, so

that $a \cos C = b - x$. Note that when
A is obtuse (the right-hand figure) x is
negative, so $b - x$ is the length of
$|b| + |x|$. Proceeding with the
information above:

$c \cos A = x$
$\underline{a \cos C = b - x}$
$a \cos C + c \cos A = x + (b - x)$
$a \cos C + c \cos A = b$

Thus, (2) is true.

   (1) can be shown to be true by
putting angle B in standard position
with angle C on the x-axis and
proceeding in the same manner. (2) is
done with angle B in standard position
and angle A on the x-axis. Actually,
this is not really necessary since the
labeling in a triangle is arbitrary, and
thus, for example, we could obtain
(1) by changing the label B to A, C to
B, and A to C, and labeling the sides
appropriately.

35. Consider any triangle ABC; place it as shown in the figure for problem 33, so angle A is in standard position. The figure covers the cases where A is acute, right, or obtuse. Then it can be seen that if h is the height of the triangle, then $h = x$. We know that

$$\sin A = \frac{x}{c} = \frac{h}{c}, \text{ so } h = c \sin A.$$

Then the area is $\frac{1}{2}bh = \frac{1}{2}b(c \sin A) = \frac{1}{2}bc \sin A$.

37. a. It can be seen that the sum of the area of the four triangles shown in the figure is $\frac{1}{2}ab \sin A + \frac{1}{2}cd \sin C + \frac{1}{2}ad \sin D + \frac{1}{2}bc \sin B$. This total is twice as large as the total area of the four-sided figure, so the area of the four-sided figure is $\frac{1}{2}(\frac{1}{2}ab \sin A + \frac{1}{2}cd \sin C + \frac{1}{2}ad \sin D + \frac{1}{2}bc \sin B)$ or $\frac{1}{4}(ab \sin A + ad \sin D + bc \sin B + cd \sin C)$.

b. The difference between the Egyptian formula $\frac{1}{4}(ab + ad + bc + cd)$ and the correct formula $\frac{1}{4}(ab \sin A + ad \sin D + bc \sin B + cd \sin C)$ is the factors $\sin A$, $\sin B$, $\sin C$, and $\sin D$. The value of the sine of each angle is between 0 and 1. Thus,

$$ab \geq ab \sin A$$
$$ad \geq ad \sin D$$
$$bc \geq bc \sin B$$
$$cd \geq cd \sin C$$
$$ab + ad + bc + cd \geq ab \sin A + ad \sin D + bc \sin B + cd \sin C,$$
$$\frac{1}{4}(ab + ad + bc + cd) \geq \frac{1}{2}(ab \sin A + ad \sin D + bc \sin B + cd \sin C)$$

If the figure is a rectangle $A = B = C = D = 90°$, and $\sin A = \sin B = \sin C = \sin D = 1$, so both expressions give the same value.

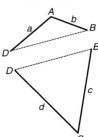

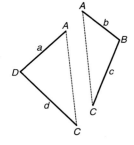

Solutions to trial exercise problems

7. $a = 0.452$, $A = 67.6°$, $C = 91.8°$
$B = 180° - 67.6° - 91.8° = 20.6°$

$$\frac{\sin 67.6°}{0.452} = \frac{\sin 20.6°}{b} = \frac{\sin 91.8°}{c}$$

$$\frac{\sin 67.6°}{0.452} = \frac{\sin 20.6°}{b}$$

$$b = \frac{0.452 \sin 20.6°}{\sin 67.6°}$$

$$b \approx 0.172$$

$$\frac{\sin 67.6°}{0.452} = \frac{\sin 91.8°}{c}$$

$$c = \frac{0.452 \sin 91.8°}{\sin 67.6°}$$

$$c \approx 0.489$$

13. $a = 4.25$, $c = 2.86$, $A = 132°$

$$\frac{\sin 132°}{4.25} = \frac{\sin B}{b} = \frac{\sin C}{2.86}$$

$$\frac{\sin 132°}{4.25} = \frac{\sin C}{2.86} \text{ so } \sin C = \frac{2.86 \sin 132°}{4.25},$$

$$C' = \sin^{-1}\frac{2.86 \sin 132°}{4.25} \approx 30.01°$$

$C \approx 30.01°$ or $180° - 30.01° \approx 149.99°$
Case 1: $C \approx 30.01°$
$B \approx 180° - 132° - 30.01° \approx 17.99°$

$$\frac{\sin 132°}{4.25} \approx \frac{\sin 17.99°}{b}$$

$$b \approx 1.77$$

Thus, the solution is
$B \approx 18.0°$, $C \approx 30.0°$, $b \approx 1.77$.
Case 2: $C \approx 149.99°$
$B = 180° - 132° - 149.99° \approx -101.99$
(No solution.)

15. $b = 92.5$, $c = 98.6$, $B = 43.7°$

$$\frac{\sin A}{a} = \frac{\sin 43.7°}{92.5} = \frac{\sin C}{98.6}$$

$$\frac{\sin 43.7°}{92.5} = \frac{\sin C}{98.6}, \sin C = \frac{98.6 \sin 43.7°}{92.5}$$

$$C' = \sin^{-1}\frac{98.6 \sin 43.7°}{92.5} \approx 47.429°$$

$C \approx 47.429°$ or $180° - 47.429° \approx 132.571°$
Case 1: $C \approx 47.429°$
$A = 180° - 43.7° - 47.429° \approx 88.871$

$$\frac{\sin 88.871°}{a} = \frac{\sin 43.7°}{92.5}$$

$a \approx 133.86$
Solution 1: $C \approx 47.4°$
$A \approx 88.9°$
$a \approx 133.9$
Case 2: $C \approx 132.571°$
$A = 180° - 43.7° - 132.571° \approx 3.729°$

$$\frac{\sin 3.729°}{a} = \frac{\sin 43.7°}{92.5}$$

$a \approx 133.60$
Solution 2: $C \approx 132.6°$
$A \approx 3.7°$
$a \approx 8.7$

27. Angle $A = 90° - 58° = 32°$.

$$\frac{\sin 32°}{8.4} = \frac{\sin B}{12.6}, \sin B = \frac{12.6 \sin 32°}{8.4},$$

so $B' \approx 52.64°$. Thus,
$C = 180° - 32° - 52.64° \approx 95.36°$.

$$\frac{\sin 32°}{8.4} = \frac{\sin 95.36°}{S}; S \approx 15.78.$$

Thus, $S \approx 15.8$ knots.

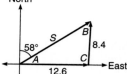

Exercise 6–2

1. $5\sqrt{5}$ **3.** $\sqrt{226}$ **5.** $9\sqrt{2}$
7. $c = 4.0$, $A = 30.7°$, $B = 109.9°$
9. $a = 77.2$, $C = 14.9°$, $B = 41.1°$
11. $b = 38.3$, $C = 25.9°$, $A = 53.8°$
13. $C = 109.0°$, $B = 31.6°$, $A = 39.4°$
15. $C = 105.3°$, $A = 24.4°$, $B = 50.3°$
17. $c = 18.1$, $A = 28.3°$, $B = 12.3°$
19. $a = 28.1$, $C = 40.5°$, $B = 115.0°$
21. $b = 41.8$, $C = 26.3°$, $A = 41.7°$
23. $C = 110.9°$, $B = 30.3°$, $A = 38.3°$
25. $c = 0.28$, $A = 1.12°$, $B = 177.38°$
27. 326.9 feet   **29.** 82.4°   **31.** 125.5°
33. 102.9°   **35.** 40 miles   **37.** 75.0°

39. Yes, the law of cosines can be used because cos 90° is 0:
$$c^2 = a^2 + b^2 - 2ab \cos C$$
$$c^2 = 21.3^2 + 40^2 - 2(21.3)(40)\cos 90°$$
$$c^2 = 21.3^2 + 40^2 - 2(21.3)(40)(0)$$
$$c^2 = 21.3^2 + 40^2$$
$$c \approx 45.3$$
Since cos 90° = 0, the law of cosines is the same as the Pythagorean theorem when the angle used is 90°.

Solutions to trial exercise problems

3. $(-5,-2)$, $(10,-1)$
The distance formula is $d = \sqrt{(x_2 - x_1)^2 + (y_2 - y_1)^2}$. To use it, we must establish the values of x_1, x_2, y_1, and y_2. To find x_1 and y_1, we designate either point as the first point; we will use $(-5,-2)$. Therefore, $x_1 = -5$ and $y_1 = -2$. We now find x_2 and y_2. We use the other point for this: $x_2 = 10$ and $y_2 = -1$. We then fill these values into the formula.
$$d = \sqrt{[10 - (-5)]^2 + [(-1) - (-2)]^2}$$
$$= \sqrt{(10 + 5)^2 + (-1 + 2)^2}$$
$$= \sqrt{(15)^2 + (1)^2}$$
$$= \sqrt{226}$$

9. $b = 61.3$, $c = 23.9$, $A = 124.0°$
$$a^2 = b^2 + c^2 - 2bc \cos A$$
$$a^2 = 61.3^2 + 23.9^2 - 2(61.3)(23.9) \cos 124°$$
$$a = \sqrt{61.3^2 + 23.9^2 - 2(61.3)(23.9)\cos 124°} \approx 77.249$$
Ⓐ 61.3 $\boxed{x^2}$ $\boxed{+}$ 23.9 $\boxed{x^2}$ $\boxed{-}$ 2 $\boxed{\times}$ 61.3 $\boxed{\times}$ 23.9 $\boxed{\times}$ 124 $\boxed{COS}$ $\boxed{=}$ $\boxed{\sqrt{x}}$
Ⓟ 61.3 $\boxed{x^2}$ 23.9 $\boxed{x^2}$ $\boxed{+}$ 2 $\boxed{ENTER}$ 61.3 $\boxed{\times}$ 23.9 $\boxed{\times}$ 124 $\boxed{COS}$ $\boxed{\times}$ $\boxed{-}$ $\boxed{\sqrt{x}}$
$\boxed{\text{TI-81}}$ $\boxed{\sqrt{}}$ $\boxed{(}$ 61.3 $\boxed{x^2}$ $\boxed{+}$ 23.9 $\boxed{x^2}$ $\boxed{-}$ 2 $\boxed{\times}$ 61.3 $\boxed{\times}$ 23.9 $\boxed{COS}$ 124 $\boxed{)}$ $\boxed{ENTER}$
$$\frac{\sin A}{a} = \frac{\sin B}{b} = \frac{\sin C}{c}$$
$$\frac{\sin 124°}{77.249} = \frac{\sin B}{61.3} = \frac{\sin C}{23.9}$$
Find angle C first; it is the smallest and therefore acute.
$$\sin C \approx \frac{23.9 \sin 124°}{77.249}; \quad C \approx 14.9°$$
Ⓐ 23.9 $\boxed{\times}$ 124 $\boxed{\sin}$ $\boxed{\div}$ 77.249 $\boxed{=}$ $\boxed{\sin^{-1}}$
Ⓟ 23.9 $\boxed{ENTER}$ 124 $\boxed{\sin}$ $\boxed{\times}$ 77.249 $\boxed{\div}$ $\boxed{\sin^{-1}}$
$\boxed{\text{TI-81}}$ $\boxed{SIN^{-1}}$ $\boxed{(}$ 23.9 $\boxed{SIN}$ 124 $\boxed{\div}$ 77.249 $\boxed{)}$
$\boxed{ENTER}$
$$B \approx 180° - 14.9° - 124° \approx 41.1°$$
Thus, $a \approx 77.2$, $B \approx 41.1°$, $C \approx 14.9°$.

13. $a = 23.5$, $b = 19.4$, $c = 35.0$
$$c^2 = a^2 + b^2 - 2ab \cos C, \text{ so}$$
$$\cos C = \frac{a^2 + b^2 - c^2}{2ab} = \frac{23.5^2 + 19.4^2 - 35^2}{2(23.5)(19.4)},$$
so $C \approx 108.97° \approx 109.0°$
Ⓐ 23.5 $\boxed{x^2}$ $\boxed{+}$ 19.4 $\boxed{x^2}$ $\boxed{-}$ 35 $\boxed{x^2}$ $\boxed{=}$
$\boxed{\div}$ 2 $\boxed{\div}$ 23.5 $\boxed{\div}$ 19.4 $\boxed{=}$ $\boxed{\cos^{-1}}$
Ⓟ 23.5 $\boxed{x^2}$ 19.4 $\boxed{x^2}$ $\boxed{+}$ 35 $\boxed{x^2}$ $\boxed{-}$ 2
$\boxed{\div}$ 23.5 $\boxed{\div}$ 19.4 $\boxed{\div}$ $\boxed{\cos^{-1}}$

$\boxed{\text{TI-81}}$ $\boxed{COS^{-1}}$ $\boxed{(}$ $\boxed{(}$ 23.5 $\boxed{x^2}$ $\boxed{+}$
19.4 $\boxed{x^2}$ $\boxed{-}$ 35 $\boxed{x^2}$ $\boxed{)}$ $\boxed{\div}$
$\boxed{(}$ 2 $\boxed{\times}$ 23.5 $\boxed{\times}$ 19.4 $\boxed{)}$ $\boxed{)}$ $\boxed{ENTER}$
Since C is the largest angle in the triangle, we know A and B are acute.
$$\frac{\sin A}{a} = \frac{\sin B}{b} = \frac{\sin C}{c}$$
$$\frac{\sin A}{23.5} = \frac{\sin B}{19.4} = \frac{\sin 108.97°}{35}$$
$$\sin A = \frac{\sin 108.97°}{35}(23.5); \; A \approx 39.4°$$
$$B \approx 180° - 39.4° - 109.0° \approx 31.6°$$

31. $A(0,5)$, $B(2,3)$, $C(8,4)$

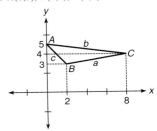

To find the largest angle, we must know which side of the triangle is longest. We find the three lengths.
$$c = \sqrt{(2 - 0)^2 + (3 - 5)^2}$$
$$= \sqrt{8} = 2\sqrt{2}$$
$$b = \sqrt{(8 - 0)^2 + (4 - 5)^2}$$
$$= \sqrt{65}$$
$$a = \sqrt{(8 - 2)^2 + (4 - 3)^2}$$
$$= \sqrt{37}$$
We now see that side b is the longest side; therefore, we need to find the measure of angle B:
$$b^2 = a^2 + c^2 - 2ac \cos B$$
$$\cos B = \frac{a^2 + c^2 - b^2}{2ac}$$
$$= \frac{(\sqrt{37})^2 + (2\sqrt{2})^2 - (\sqrt{65})^2}{2(\sqrt{37})(2\sqrt{2})}$$
$$= \frac{37 + 8 - 65}{4(\sqrt{37})(\sqrt{2})} = -0.581238194$$
$$B = 125.5376778°$$
Ⓐ 37 $\boxed{+}$ 8 $\boxed{-}$ 65 $\boxed{=}$ $\boxed{\div}$ 4 $\boxed{\div}$ 37 $\boxed{\sqrt{x}}$
$\boxed{\div}$ 2 $\boxed{\sqrt{x}}$ $\boxed{=}$ $\boxed{INV}$ $\boxed{COS}$
Ⓟ 37 $\boxed{ENTER}$ 8 $\boxed{+}$ 65 $\boxed{-}$ 4 $\boxed{\div}$ 37 $\boxed{\sqrt{x}}$ $\boxed{\div}$
2 $\boxed{\sqrt{x}}$ $\boxed{\div}$ $\boxed{\cos^{-1}}$
$\boxed{\text{TI-81}}$ $\boxed{COS^{-1}}$ $\boxed{(}$ $\boxed{(}$ 37 $\boxed{+}$ 8 $\boxed{-}$ 65 $\boxed{)}$ $\boxed{\div}$
$\boxed{(}$ 4 $\boxed{\sqrt{}}$ 37 $\boxed{\sqrt{}}$ 2 $\boxed{)}$ $\boxed{)}$ $\boxed{ENTER}$
Thus, to the nearest 0.1°, the measure of B is 125.5°.

Exercise 6–3

Answers to odd-numbered problems

1. $(20\sqrt{3}, 20)$ **3.** $(-53.4, 84.5)$

5. $(-9.4, -3.4)$ **7.** $\left(12\frac{1}{2}, -\frac{25\sqrt{3}}{2}\right)$

9. $(3\sqrt{2}, -3\sqrt{2})$ **11.** $(-0.8, 7.8)$
13. $(5, 53.1°)$ **15.** $(6.0, 120.0°)$
17. $(2.6, -49.1°)$ **19.** $(11.2, -63.4°)$
21. $(7.6, 153.4°)$ **23.** $(3.16, -116.6°)$
25. $(-1, 20)$ **27.** $(8\sqrt{2}, 0)$
29. $(45.2, 31.2°)$ **31.** $(36.5, -122.1°)$
33. $(9.0, -54.2°)$ **35.** $(47.1, 139.7°)$
37. $(6.3, 89.3°)$ **39.** $(20.3, 83.9°)$
41. $(12.9, 21.0°)$ **43.** The aircraft is moving west at 136 knots and north at 63 knots.   **45.** The aircraft is flying east at 193 knots and north at 52 knots.
47. -228 knots = east-west component
      395 knots = north-south component
49. a. 24 nm   **b.** 38 nm   **51.** No; the force vector is $(2,250, 33°)$. The horizontal component f is $2,250 \cos 33° \approx 1,887$ pounds. This is not enough to move the sled.

53.

Force V	Horizontal component V_x	Vertical component V_y
$(1,000, 15°)$	966	259
$(2,000, 15°)$	1,932	518
$(1,000, 30°)$	866	500

Part (a).
Part (b); yes, the components double in value.
Part (c); no, the components do not double.
55. The plane is 40 miles from Orlando, in a direction 59° south of east.
57. $(15.4, -76.8°)$ **59.** $(270.7, 87.5°)$
61. The ship is about 63 knots from its starting position, at an angle of 40° south of west.   **63.** The plane's ground speed is 99 knots, in the direction 47° north of west.
65. The ship is traveling at 26.5 knots in a direction 25.7° north of east.
67. Magnitude is 266 volts at 341°.
69. $(87, 98°)$ The heading of the aircraft is 8° west of north, and its airspeed is 87 knots.   **71.** $(17.7, 76.3°)$ The ships heading is 76.3°, and its speed is 17.7 knots.   **73.** $(320, 130°)$ The tension in the second cable is 320 pounds, and it makes an angle θ of 50° $(180° - 130°)$ with the horizontal.

75. Let $A = (a_1, a_2)$, $B = (b_1, b_2)$, and $C = (c_1, c_2)$ be three vectors in rectangular form. Then,
$(A + B) + C$
$= [(a_1, a_2) + (b_1, b_2)] + (c_1, c_2)$
   The parentheses indicate we add A and B first.
$= (a_1 + b_1, a_2 + b_2) + (c_1, c_2)$
   Two vectors; one is $A + B$, and the other is C.
$= ((a_1 + b_1) + c_1, (a_2 + b_2) + c_2)$
   One vector: $(A + B) + C$.
$= (a_1 + (b_1 + c_1), a_2 + (b_2 + c_2))$
   We can rearrange because real numbers are associative, and the components are real numbers.
$= A + (B + C)$

Solutions to trial exercise problems

3. $(100.0, 122.3°) = (100 \cos 122.3°, 100 \sin 122.3°)$
$\approx (-53.4, 84.5)$
23. $(-\sqrt{2}, -\sqrt{8})$ $|A| = \sqrt{(-\sqrt{2})^2 + (-\sqrt{8})^2} \approx \sqrt{10} \approx 3.16$,
$\theta' \approx 63.43°$; $\theta \approx 63.43° - 180° \approx -116.57°$ $(3.16, -116.6°)$
39. $(15.3, 311°) = (15.3 \cos 311°, 15.3 \sin 311°) = (10.038, -11.547)$
$(20.9, 117°) = (20.9 \cos 117°, 20.9 \sin 117°) = (-9.488, 18.622)$
$(13.2, 83°) = (13.2 \cos 83°, 13.2 \sin 83°) = (1.609, 13.102)$
$= (2.158, 20.177) = (20.3, 83.9°)$

43. $V = (150, 155°)$; $V_x = 150 \cos 155° \approx -136$ (136 knots due west); $V_y = 150 \sin 155° \approx 63$ (63 knots due north). The aircraft is moving west at 136 knots and north at 63 knots.

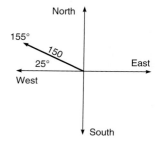

49. 18 knots (18 nautical miles per hour) × 2.5 hours = 45 nm (nautical miles); $V = (45, 32°)$; $V_x = 45 \cos 32° \approx 38$ nm; distance east of the harbor (part b); $V_y = 45 \sin 32° \approx 24$ nm; distance north of the harbor (part a).

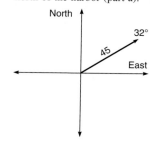

52. $f = 1,700 \cos \theta$. We require $f \geq 1,200$, so $1,200 \geq 1,700 \cos \theta$, or $\frac{12}{17} \geq \cos \theta$. $\cos^{-1}\frac{12}{17} \approx 45.1°$. Thus, $\theta \leq 45.1°$ will move the sled. Note that $\theta \leq 45.1°$ is correct, and not $\theta \geq 45.1°$. This can be seen in the figure. If θ increases, f clearly decreases. Mathematically, the value of $\cos \theta$ increases as θ decreases (for acute angles).

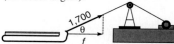

54. At 200 mph, the first leg of the trip is
200 miles. The second is 200 mph ×
0.5 hour = 100 miles. To find d and θ,
we add the vectors (200,0°) and
(100,−60°).

$(200,0°)$ $= (200 \cos 0°, 200 \sin 0°)$ $= (200,0)$
$(100,−60°) = (200 \cos(−60°), 200 \sin(−60°)) \approx (50,−86.60)$
$(250,−86.60) \approx (265,341°)$

Thus, $d \approx 265$ miles, and $\theta \approx 341°$.
The aircraft is 265 miles from
Minneapolis. $360° − 341° = 19°$, so
the aircraft is in a direction 19° south
of east, relative to the city.

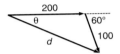

59. $(199,19.0°) = (199 \cos 19°, 199 \sin 19°)$ $\approx (188.15,64.79)$
$(175,131°) = (175 \cos 131°, 175 \sin 131°) \approx (−114.81,132.07)$
$(96,130°)\ \ = (96 \cos 130°, 96 \sin 130°)\ \ \approx (−61.71,73.54)$
$(11.64,270.40) \approx (270.7,87.5°)$

64. $(19.6,170°) = (19.6 \cos 170°, 19.6 \sin 170°) \approx (−19.3,3.4)$
$(7.2,95°)\ \ \ = (7.2 \cos 95°, 7.2 \sin 95°)\ \ \approx (−0.63,7.17)$
$(−19.93,10.58) \approx (22.6,152.0°)$

Thus, its true course is $180° − 152°$
$= 28°$ north of west, at a speed of 22.6
knots.

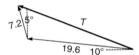

66. $(122,30°) = (122 \cos 30°, 122 \sin 30°) \approx (105.66,61.00)$
$(86,21°)\ \ = (86 \cos 21°, 86 \sin 21°)\ \ \approx (80.29,30.82)$
$(185.94,91.82) \approx (207,26°)$

Magnitude is 207 volts, phase angle
is 26°.

71. We let W represent the water current
vector.

$H + W = T$
$H = T − W$
$\quad = (12.65°) − (6.4,−82°)$
$\quad = (12.65°) + (6.4,−82° + 180°)$
$\quad = (12.65°) + (6.4,98°)$
$\quad = (5.07,10.88) + (−0.89,6.34)$
$\quad = (4.18,17.21) \approx (17.7,76.3°)$

Thus, the ship's heading is 76.3°, and
its speed is 17.7 knots.

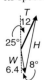

73. The sign is stationary, so the forces
acting on it are balanced (they add to
zero).

$T_1 + T_2 + W = 0$
$T_1 = −T_2 − W$
$\quad = −(456,63°) − (650,270°)$
$\quad = (456,63° + 180°) + (650,270° −$
$\quad\quad 180°)$
$\quad\quad$ To negate a vector, add or
$\quad\quad$ subtract 180° from its direction
$\quad\quad$ angle.
$\quad = (456,243°) + (650,90°)$
$\quad \approx (−207,02,−406.3) + (0,650)$
$\quad\quad$ Convert to rectangular form.
$\quad \approx (−207.02,243.7)$
$\quad\quad$ Convert back to polar form.
$\quad \approx (320,130°)$

Thus, the tension in the second cable is
320 pounds, and it makes an angle θ of
50° $(180° − 130°)$ with the horizontal.

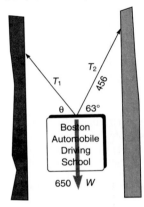

74. Let $A = (a_1,a_2)$ and $B = (b_1,b_2)$ be two
vectors in rectangular form.

Then $A + B = (a_1,a_2) + (b_1,b_2)$
$\quad\quad\quad = (a_1 + b_1,a_2 + b_2)$
$\quad\quad\quad\quad$ Definition of vector
$\quad\quad\quad\quad$ addition.
$\quad\quad\quad = (b_1 + a_1,b_2 + a_2)$
$\quad\quad\quad\quad a_1, a_2, b_1, b_2$ are real
$\quad\quad\quad\quad$ numbers, so their
$\quad\quad\quad\quad$ indicated sum
$\quad\quad\quad\quad$ commutes.
$\quad\quad\quad = B + A$
$\quad\quad\quad\quad$ Definition of vector
$\quad\quad\quad\quad$ addition.

76. The following is for the TI-81:

PRGM EDIT 2   Choose a free location to enter the program. Say 2, by way of example.

A D D V C T R S   Enter these characters as the name of the program.

```
:0→A
:0→B
:Lbl 1
:Input R
:If R=0
:Goto 2
:Input θ
:P▸R(R,θ)
:A+X→A
:B+Y→B
:Goto 1
:Lbl 2
:A→X
:B→Y
:R▸P(X,Y)
:Disp "X,Y"
:Disp X
:Disp Y
:Disp "R,θ"
:Disp R
:Disp θ
```

When running the program one inputs R, then θ, for each vector in polar form. When all vectors have been entered, enter zero (0) for R. The program converts each vector into rectangular form as it is entered, and accumulates the value (x,y) in variables A and B. When all vectors are entered, the accumulated values in A and B are converted to polar form.

Chapter 6 review

1. $C = 121.8°, b = 2.6, c = 12.1$
2. $A = 151°, a = 4.3, c = 0.8$
3. $A = 49°, C = 52°, c = 10.4$
4. $A = 76.5°, B = 70.8°, b = 12.2$; or $A = 103.5°, B = 43.8°, b = 9.0$
5. 48.2 miles   **6.** $c = 3.8, A = 31.9°, B = 118.7°$ **7.** $a = 63.9, C = 18.2°, B = 69.7°$ **8.** $b = 40.2, A = 29.5°, C = 38.5°$ **9.** $A = 106.3°, B = 23.1°, C = 50.5°$ **10.** $C = 135.5°, A = 12.2°, B = 32.3°$ **11.** $c = 2\sqrt{10}, b = 7\sqrt{2}, a = \sqrt{82}, B = 77.9°, C = 38.7°, A = 63.4°$
12. 29.2 km   **13.** (23.8,13.2)

14. (36.3,57.3°)   **15.** $V_x = 370$ knots, $V_y = 256$ knots   **16.** $V_x = 249$ lb, $V_y = 60$ lb   **17.** (47.6,20.6°)
18. (10.8,89.5°)   **19.** (7.2,69.9°)
20. (8.1,187.6°)   **21.** 205 lb, 273°
22. 55 knots, 41° south of east
23. 183 knots, 62° north of west
24. 247 knots, 55° north of west

Chapter 6 test

1. $B = 84.4°, a = 5.3, c = 22.5$
2. $B = 56.3°, A = 61.6°, a = 23.9$
3. $b = 32.8, A = 50.9°, C = 29.1°$
4. $C = 89.1°, A = 39.6°, B = 51.3°$
5. 59 yards   **6.** 53.1°   **7.** $(\sqrt{3},1)$
8. (6.4,51.3°)   **9.** (8.5,84.9°)
10. 584 lb, 65°

Chapter 7

Exercise 7–1

Answers to odd-numbered problems

1. real, 4; imaginary, −5
3. real, −4; imaginary, 1
5. real, 12; imaginary, 0
7. real, −10; imaginary, 2
9. a. $4 + 5i$
   b.

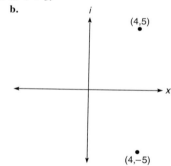

11. a. $-4 - i$
   b.

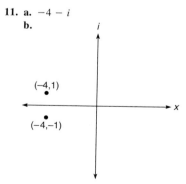

13. a. 12
   b.

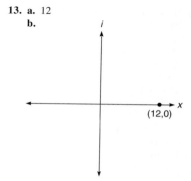

15. a. $-10 - 2i$
   b.

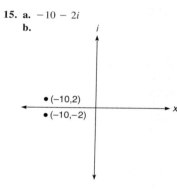

17. $2 + 6i$ **19.** $-9 - 7i$ **21.** $9 - 4i$
23. $-3 + 192i$ **25.** $-20 - 30i$
27. $-46 - 9i$ **29.** $\frac{33}{29} + \frac{10}{29}i$
31. $\frac{-12}{5} - \frac{9}{5}i$ **33.** 5.4 cis (−21.8°)
35. 3.2 cis 108.4°   **37.** 5 cis 126.9°
39. 2 cis 30°   **41.** $3\sqrt{2}$ cis 45°
43. $\sqrt{2}$ cis 225°   **45.** 5 cis 90°
47. $2.9 + 0.8i$ **49.** $3.7 + 2.6i$
51. $1 - i$ **53.** $12.3 - 5.7i$
55. $\dfrac{3}{2} + \dfrac{\sqrt{3}}{2}i$ **57.** $5 - 5\sqrt{3}i$
59. $-\sqrt{10}$ **61.** $2 - 2i$ **63.** 15 cis 75°
65. 10.8 cis(−120°)   **67.** 4 cis 80°
69. $\frac{20}{9}$ cis(−80°)   **71.** 512 cis(−60°)
73. 27 cis(−120°)   **75.** $-8.2 - 0.1i$
77. $2, -1 + \sqrt{3}i, -1 - \sqrt{3}i$
79. $3, 3i, -3, -3i$
81. $-1.1 + 4.9i, -3.7 - 3.4i, 4.8 - 1.5i$
83. 2.5 cis(−20°)   **85.** 50 cis 45°
87. 2.04 cis 6.19°   **89.** $0.75 + 0.86i$
91. Is the following an identity: a cis(−θ) = −a cis θ?
   No. a cis(−θ)
   = $a \cos(-θ) + a \sin(-θ)i$
   = $a \cos θ - a \sin θi$
   but $-a$ cis θ = $-a \cos θ - a \sin θi$.

93. a. $-3 + i$ **b.** $-1 - 3i$
   c. $3 - i$ **d.** $1 + 3i$

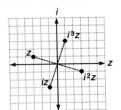

95. a. 6 **b.** $6i$ **c.** -6
   d. $-6i$

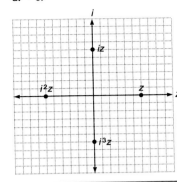

97. a. $-1 - i$ **b.** $1 - i$
   c. $1 + i$ **d.** $-1 + i$

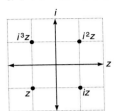

99. a. $\dfrac{\sqrt{3}}{2} + \dfrac{1}{2}i$ **b.** $0.37 + 1.37i$

   c. $0.37 - 1.37i$

101. $r^{\frac{1}{n}} \operatorname{cis}\left(\dfrac{\theta}{n} + \dfrac{k \cdot 360°}{n}\right)$

$$= r^{\frac{1}{n}} \operatorname{cis}\left[\dfrac{\theta}{n} + \dfrac{(an + b) \cdot 360°}{n}\right] \quad \text{Replace } k \text{ by } an + b.$$

$$\dfrac{\theta}{n} + \dfrac{(an + b) \cdot 360°}{n} = \dfrac{\theta}{n} + \dfrac{an \cdot 360°}{n} + \dfrac{b \cdot 360°}{n}$$

$$= \dfrac{\theta}{n} + a \cdot 360° + \dfrac{b \cdot 360°}{n}$$

$$= \left(\dfrac{\theta}{n} + \dfrac{b \cdot 360°}{n}\right) + a \cdot 360°$$

$$= r^{\frac{1}{n}} \operatorname{cis}\left[\left(\dfrac{\theta}{n} + \dfrac{b \cdot 360°}{n}\right) + a \cdot 360°\right]$$

$$= r^{\frac{1}{n}} \cos\left[\left(\dfrac{\theta}{n} + \dfrac{b \cdot 360°}{n}\right) + a \cdot 360°\right] + i r^{\frac{1}{n}} \sin\left[\left(\dfrac{\theta}{n} + \dfrac{b \cdot 360°}{n}\right) + a \cdot 360°\right]$$

$$\cos\left[\left(\dfrac{\theta}{n} + \dfrac{b \cdot 360°}{n}\right) + a \cdot 360°\right] = \cos\left(\dfrac{\theta}{n} + \dfrac{b \cdot 360°}{n}\right)\cos(a \cdot 360°) - \sin\left(\dfrac{\theta}{n} + \dfrac{b \cdot 360°}{n}\right)\sin(a \cdot 360°)$$

$$= \cos\left(\dfrac{\theta}{n} + \dfrac{b \cdot 360°}{n}\right), \text{ because } \cos(a \cdot 360°) = 1 \text{ and } \sin(a \cdot 360°) = 0, \text{ when } a \text{ is an integer.}$$

$$\sin\left[\left(\dfrac{\theta}{n} + \dfrac{b \cdot 360°}{n}\right) + a \cdot 360°\right] = \sin\left(\dfrac{\theta}{n} + \dfrac{b \cdot 360°}{n}\right)\cos(a \cdot 360°) + \cos\left(\dfrac{\theta}{n} + \dfrac{b \cdot 360°}{n}\right)\sin(a \cdot 360°)$$

$$= \sin\left(\dfrac{\theta}{n} + \dfrac{b \cdot 360°}{n}\right), \text{ because } \cos(a \cdot 360°) = 1 \text{ and } \sin(a \cdot 360°) = 0,$$

when a is an integer.

Thus,

$$r^{\frac{1}{n}} \cos\left[\left(\dfrac{\theta}{n} + \dfrac{b \cdot 360°}{n}\right) + a \cdot 360°\right] + i r^{\frac{1}{n}} \sin\left[\left(\dfrac{\theta}{n} + \dfrac{b \cdot 360°}{n}\right) + a \cdot 360°\right]$$

$$= r^{\frac{1}{n}} \cos\left(\dfrac{\theta}{n} + \dfrac{b \cdot 360°}{n}\right) + i r^{\frac{1}{n}} \sin\left(\dfrac{\theta}{n} + \dfrac{b \cdot 360°}{n}\right)$$

$$= r^{\frac{1}{n}} \operatorname{cis}\left(\dfrac{\theta}{n} + \dfrac{b \cdot 360°}{n}\right), \text{ where } b < n.$$

This last expression is one of the previous roots.

Solutions to trial exercise problems

23. $(15 + 4i)(3 + 12i)$
$15(3) + 15(12i) + 4i(3) + 4i(12i)$
$45 + 180i + 12i + 48i^2(i^2 = -1)$
$45 + 192i - 48$
$-3 + 192i$

27. $(2 - 3i)^3$
$(2 - 3i)(2 - 3i)(2 - 3i)$
$[(2 - 3i)(2 - 3i)](2 - 3i)$
$[4 - 12i + 9i^2](2 - 3i)$
$[-5 - 12i](2 - 3i)$
$-10 + 15i - 24i + 36i^2$
$-10 - 36 - 9i$
$-46 - 9i$

31. $\dfrac{3 + 6i}{-2 - i}$

$\dfrac{3 + 6i}{-2 - i} \cdot \dfrac{-2 + i}{-2 + i}$

Multiply by the conjugate of the denominator.

$\dfrac{-6 + 3i - 12i + 6i^2}{4 - 2i + 2i - i^2} = \dfrac{-6 - 9i - 6}{4 + 1}$

$\dfrac{-12 - 9i}{5} = -\dfrac{12}{5} - \dfrac{9}{5}i$

36. $\sqrt{3} - 2i$
$r = \sqrt{(\sqrt{3})^2 + (-2)^2} = \sqrt{7} \approx 2.6.$

$\theta' = \tan^{-1}\dfrac{-2}{\sqrt{3}} \approx -49.1°; a > 0$ to $\theta = \theta'.$

The point is $2.6 \text{ cis}(-49.1°).$

39. $\sqrt{3} + i$
The modulus is $\sqrt{(\sqrt{3})^2 + 1^2} = \sqrt{4} = 2.$

$\tan \theta' = \dfrac{1}{\sqrt{3}}$, so $\theta' = 30°$ (exactly).

$\theta = \theta' = 30°$, since θ is in the first quadrant. Thus, the polar form is $2 \text{ cis } 30°.$

47. $3 \text{ cis } 15°$
$3 \cos 15° + (3 \sin 15°)i = 2.9 + 0.8i$

58. $6 \text{ cis } 135°$
$6(\cos 135° + i \sin 135°)$
$6\left(-\dfrac{\sqrt{2}}{2} + \dfrac{\sqrt{2}}{2}i\right)$
$-3\sqrt{2} + 3\sqrt{2}i$

73. $(3 \text{ cis } 200°)^3 = 3^3 \text{ cis } 3(200)°$
$= 27 \text{ cis } 600°$
$= 27 \text{ cis}(600° - 2 \cdot 360°)$
$= 27 \text{ cis}(-120°)$

76. $(0.8 + 0.6i)^{10}$
We first put the complex number in polar form. The modulus is $\sqrt{0.8^2 + 0.6^2} = \sqrt{1} = 1.$

$\tan \theta' = \dfrac{0.6}{0.8} = \dfrac{3}{4}$, so $\theta' = 36.8699°.$

Since θ terminates in quadrant I, $\theta = 36.8699°$. We now compute:

$(1 \text{ cis } 36.8699)^{10} = 1^{10} \text{ cis}$
$10(36.8699)° = 1 \text{ cis } 368.699° = 1 \text{ cis}$
$8.699°$. Since the original complex number was in its rectangular form, we will put this result in rectangular form.
$1 \text{ cis } 8.699° = \cos 8.699° + i \sin 8.699°$
$= 0.99 + 0.15i = 1.0 + 0.2i$

82. Find the 4 fourth roots of $\sqrt{3} + 3i$ to the nearest tenth.

$\sqrt{3} + 3i = 2\sqrt{3} \text{ cis } 60°$, so
$(\sqrt{3} + 3i)^{1/4} = (2\sqrt{3} \text{ cis } 60°)^{1/4}$
Evaluate $(2\sqrt{3})^{1/4}\text{cis}\left(\dfrac{60°}{4} + \dfrac{k \cdot 360°}{4}\right)$
$\approx 1.364 \text{ cis}(15° + k \cdot 90°)$ for $k = 0, 1, 2, 3.$
$k = 0$: $1.364 \text{ cis}(15°)$
$= 1.364 \cos 15° + 1.364 \sin 15°i$
$\approx 1.3 + 0.4i$
$k = 1$: $1.364 \text{ cis}(15° + 90°)$
$= 1.364 \cos 105° + 1.364 \sin 105°i$
$\approx -0.4 + 1.3i$
$k = 2$: $1.364 \text{ cis}(15° + 180°)$
$= 1.364 \cos 195° + 1.364 \sin 195°i$
$\approx -1.3 - 0.4i$
$k = 3$: $1.364 \text{ cis}(15° + 270°)$
$= 1.364 \cos 285° + 1.364 \sin 285°i$
$\approx 0.4 - 1.3i$

87. $Z_T = \dfrac{Z_1 Z_2}{Z_1 + Z_2} = \dfrac{(2 + i)(3 - 5i)}{(2 + i) + (3 - 5i)}$

$= \dfrac{(2 + i)(3 - 5i)}{5 - 4i} = \dfrac{6 - 7i + 5}{5 - 4i}$

$= \dfrac{11 - 7i}{5 - 4i} = \dfrac{13.038 \text{ cis } 327.529°}{6.403 \text{ cis } 321.340°}$

$= \dfrac{13.038}{6.403} \text{ cis}(327.529° - 321.340°)$

$= 2.04 \text{ cis } 6.19°$

93. a. $-3 + i$

b. $i(-3 + i) = -3i + i^2$
$= -3i - 1$
$= -1 - 3i$

c. $i^2(-3 + i) = -1(-3 + i)$
$= 3 - i$

d. $i^3 z = ii^2 z = i(-1)z$
$= -iz = -i(-3 + i)$
$= 3i - i^2 = 3i - (-1)$
$= 1 + 3i$

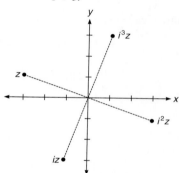

100. $\dfrac{r_1 \text{cis } \theta_1}{r_2 \text{cis } \theta_2} = \dfrac{r_1 \cos \theta_1 + ir_1 \sin \theta_1}{r_2 \cos \theta_2 + ir_2 \sin \theta_2}$

$= \dfrac{r_1(\cos \theta_1 + i \sin \theta_1)}{r_2(\cos \theta_2 + i \sin \theta_2)}$

$= \dfrac{r_1}{r_2} \cdot \dfrac{\cos \theta_1 + i \sin \theta_1}{\cos \theta_2 + i \sin \theta_2}$

$= \dfrac{r_1}{r_2} \cdot \dfrac{\cos \theta_1 + i \sin \theta_1}{\cos \theta_2 + i \sin \theta_2} \cdot \dfrac{\cos \theta_2 - i \sin \theta_2}{\cos \theta_2 - i \sin \theta_2}$

$= \dfrac{r_1}{r_2} \cdot \dfrac{\cos \theta_1 \cos \theta_2 - i \cos \theta_1 \sin \theta_2 + i \sin \theta_1 \cos \theta_2 - i^2 \sin \theta_1 \sin \theta_2}{\cos^2 \theta_2 - i^2 \sin^2 \theta_2}$

$= \dfrac{r_1}{r_2} \cdot \dfrac{\cos \theta_1 \cos \theta_2 + \sin \theta_1 \sin \theta_2 + i(\sin \theta_1 \cos \theta_2 - \cos \theta_1 \sin \theta_2)}{\cos^2 \theta_2 + \sin^2 \theta_2}$

$= \dfrac{r_1}{r_2} \cdot \dfrac{\cos(\theta_1 - \theta_2) + i \sin(\theta_1 - \theta_2)}{1}$

$= \dfrac{r_1}{r_2} \text{ cis}(\theta_1 - \theta_2)$

Exercise 7–2

Answers to odd-numbered problems

The figure shows the answers to odd-numbered problems 1 through 17.

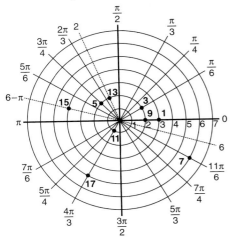

19. $\left(2,\dfrac{13\pi}{6}\right)\left(2,\dfrac{25\pi}{6}\right)\left(-2,\dfrac{7\pi}{6}\right)$

21. $\left(6,\dfrac{23\pi}{6}\right)\left(6,-\dfrac{\pi}{6}\right)\left(-6,\dfrac{5\pi}{6}\right)$

23. $(2,2+2\pi)\ (2,2+4\pi)\ (-2,2+\pi)$

25. $(0,4)$ **27.** $\left(\dfrac{-5\sqrt{3}}{2},\dfrac{5}{2}\right)$

29. $(-2,-2\sqrt{3})$ **31.** $(1.08,1.68)$

33. $(2.05,2.19)$ **35.** $(-2.61,-3.03)$

37. $\left(4,-\dfrac{5\pi}{6}\right)$ **39.** $(2,\pi)$

41. $\left(4\sqrt{2},-\dfrac{3\pi}{4}\right)$ **43.** $(3.61,0.98)$

45. $(4.12,-1.33)$ **47.** $(6.40,0.67)$

49. $\tan\theta=4$ **51.** $r=\dfrac{2}{\sin\theta+3\cos\theta}$

53. $r=\dfrac{b}{\sin\theta-m\cos\theta}$

55. $r^2=\dfrac{5}{\sin^2\theta-2\cos^2\theta}$

57. $r^2=\dfrac{1}{\cos^2\theta+2}$ **59.** $x^2+y^2=y$

61. $x=2$ **63.** $(x^2+y^2)^3=36x^2y^2$

65. $x^4+2x^2y^2+y^4=2xy$

67. $x^3+xy^2=y$

69. $x^2+y^2=4y^2+12y+9$

71. $2(r\cos\theta\ r\sin\theta)=5,\ r^2\sin 2\theta=5,$

$r^2=\dfrac{5}{\sin 2\theta}=5\csc 2\theta$

73. Consider a point $P=(r,\theta)$, where $r<0$. Then $P=(-r,\theta+\pi)$, where $-r>0$. Therefore, since $-r>0,\ y=-r\sin(\theta+\pi)$ is true,

$y=-r\sin(\theta+\pi)$
  A true statement.
$=-r(\sin\theta\cos\pi+\cos\theta\sin\pi)$
  $\sin(\alpha+\beta)=\sin\alpha\cos\beta+\cos\alpha\sin\beta$
$=-r(\sin\theta(-1)+\cos\theta(0))$
$=-r(-\sin\theta)$
$=r\sin\theta$

Thus, $y=r\sin\theta$, even if $r<0$.

75. $(x^2+y^2+2y)^2=x^2+y^2$

77. $(x^2+y^2)^3=(x^2+y^2+4xy)^2$

79. $(x^2+y^2+3x)^2=x^2+y^2$

Solutions to trial exercise problems

15. $(-4,6)$ represents a point with $r=-4$ and $\theta=6$ (radians). We can convert r to a positive value if we add or subtract π from θ. Since $6>\pi$, subtract:

$(-4,6)=(4,6-\pi)$
$\qquad\quad=(4,2.9)$ (approximately).
  (See the diagram.)

To construct an angle of 2.9 radians convert it to $\approx 166°$.

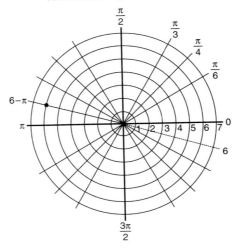

21. $\left(6,\dfrac{11\pi}{6}\right)$

Add 2π to θ:

$\left(6,\dfrac{11\pi}{6}\right)=\left(6,\dfrac{11\pi}{6}+\dfrac{12\pi}{6}\right)$
$\qquad\qquad\;\;=\left(6,\dfrac{23\pi}{6}\right)$

Subtract 2π from θ:

$\left(6,\dfrac{11\pi}{6}\right)=\left(6,\dfrac{11\pi}{6}-\dfrac{12\pi}{6}\right)$
$\qquad\qquad\;\;=\left(6,-\dfrac{\pi}{6}\right)$

To obtain $r<0$, add or subtract an odd multiple of π. We subtract π.

$\left(6,\dfrac{11\pi}{6}\right)=\left(-6,\dfrac{11\pi}{6}-\dfrac{6\pi}{6}\right)$
$\qquad\qquad\;\;=\left(-6,\dfrac{5\pi}{6}\right)$

31. $(2,1)$

$(2,1)=(2\cos 1,2\sin 1)$
$\qquad=(1.08,1.68)$

39. $(-2,0)$ is plotted in the diagram. We can see that $\theta=180°$ or π (radians), and that $r=2$. Thus, $(-2,0)$ (rectangular) $=(2,\pi)$ (polar).

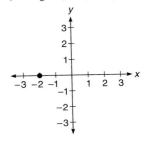

45. $(1,-4)$

$r=\sqrt{1^2+4^2}=\sqrt{17}\approx 4.12$
$\theta'=\tan^{-1}(-4)\approx -1.326$
$x>0$ so $\theta=\theta'$.
$(4.12,-1.33)$

53. $y = mx + b, b \neq 0$

Use $x = r \cos \theta, y = r \sin \theta$.

$y = mx + b$

$r \sin \theta = m(r \cos \theta) + b$

Solve for r when possible.

$r \sin \theta - mr \cos \theta = b$

$r(\sin \theta - m \cos \theta) = b$

$$r = \frac{b}{\sin \theta - m \cos \theta}$$

The quotient is defined when

$\sin \theta - m \cos \theta \neq 0$

$\sin \theta \neq m \cos \theta$

$\dfrac{\sin \theta}{\cos \theta} \neq m, \cos \theta \neq 0$

$\tan \theta \neq m, \cos \theta \neq 0$

$\cos \theta = 0$ implies that θ is an odd

multiple of $\dfrac{\pi}{2}$, representing a vertical

line. However, $y = mx + b$ can only
represent a nonvertical line, so the
condition $\cos \theta \neq 0$ is satisfied.

If $\tan \theta = m$, since $\tan \theta = \dfrac{y}{x}$ if θ is

not an odd multiple of $\dfrac{\pi}{2}$, we have $\dfrac{y}{x}$

$= m$, or $y = mx$. This would be a line
parallel to $y = mx + b$ with $b = 0$, but
the problem specifies that $b \neq 0$. Thus,
we are also guaranteed that $\tan \theta \neq m$.
Therefore, under all conditions for
which $y = mx + b, b \neq 0$ are satisfied,
the polar equation is $r =$

$\dfrac{b}{\sin \theta - m \cos \theta}$.

55. $y^2 - 2x^2 = 5$

$(r \sin \theta)^2 - 2(r \cos \theta)^2 = 5$

$r^2 \sin^2\theta - 2r^2 \cos^2\theta = 5$

$r^2(\sin^2\theta - 2 \cos^2\theta) = 5$

$$r^2 = \frac{5}{\sin^2\theta - 2 \cos^2\theta}$$

63. $r = 3 \sin 2\theta$

$r = 3 \sin 2\theta$

$\sin 2\theta = 2 \sin \theta \cos \theta$

$= 3(2 \sin \theta \cos \theta)$

$= 6\dfrac{y}{r} \cdot \dfrac{x}{r}$

$r^3 = 6xy$

$r = \sqrt{x^2 + y^2} = (x^2 + y^2)^{1/2}$

$[(x^2 + y^2)^{1/2}]^3 = 6xy$

$(x^2 + y^2)^{3/2} = 6xy$, or $(x^2 + y^2)^3 =$

$36x^2y^2$.

69. $r = \dfrac{3}{1 - 2 \sin \theta}$ (Note $r \neq 0$ because

the quotient cannot be 0.)

$$r = \frac{3}{1 - 2\dfrac{y}{r}}$$

$$= \frac{3}{1 - 2\dfrac{y}{r}} \cdot \frac{r}{r} = \frac{3r}{r - 2y}$$

$r(r - 2y) = 3r;$ $r^2 - 2ry = 3r;$

$r^2 = 3r + 2ry$

$r^2 = r(3 + 2y)$

Divide by r, since $r \neq 0$.

$r = 3 + 2y$

$(x^2 + y^2)^{1/2} = 3 + 2y$

$x^2 + y^2 = (3 + 2y)^2$

$x^2 + y^2 = 4y^2 + 12y + 9$

78. Problem 79 in section 5–3 shows that
$\cos 3\theta = 4 \cos^3\theta - 3 \cos \theta$.

$r = 2 \cos 3\theta$

$r = 2(4 \cos^3\theta - 3 \cos \theta)$

$r = 8 \cos^3\theta - 6 \cos \theta$

$r = 8\left(\dfrac{x}{r}\right)^3 - 6\dfrac{x}{r}$

$r = \dfrac{8x^3}{r^3} - \dfrac{6x}{r}$

$r^4 = 8x^3 - 6xr^2$

Multiply each member by r^3.

$(x^2 + y^2)^2 = 8x^3 - 6x(x^2 + y^2)$

$x^4 + 2x^2y^2 + y^4 = 8x^3 - 6x^3 - 6xy^2$

$x^4 - 2x^3 + 2x^2y^2 + 6xy^2 + y^4 = 0$

Exercise 7–3

Answers to odd-numbered problems

1.

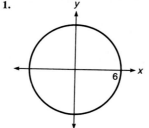

3.

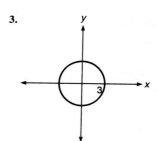

5.

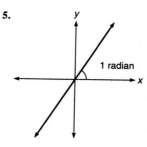

7.

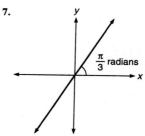

9.

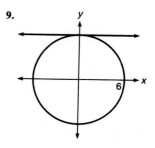

11.

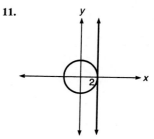

13.

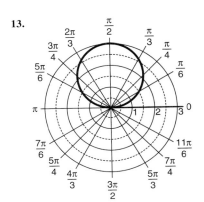

15.

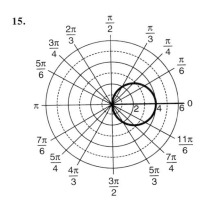

17.

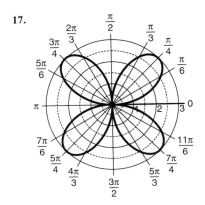

19.

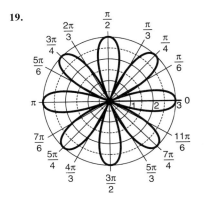

21.

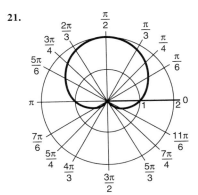

23.

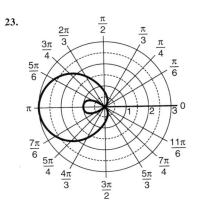

25.

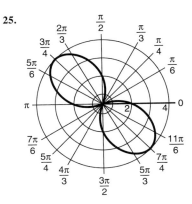

27.

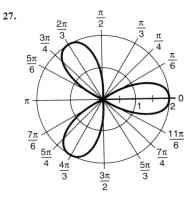

29.

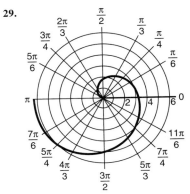

31.

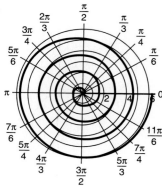

33.

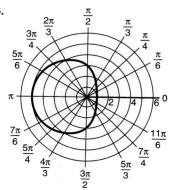

35.

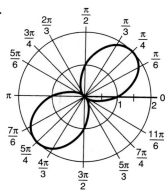

37.

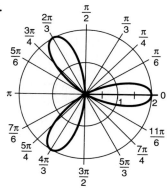

Solutions to trial exercise problems

4. $r = -1$

Since any point $(-1,\theta)$ is equivalent to the point $(1,\theta + \pi)$, and since θ can be any value (since it is not specified), the graph of this equation is equivalent to the graph of $r = 1$, which is a circle with radius 1, centered at the pole.

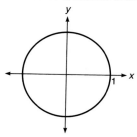

8. $\theta = -1$

The radius r can be any value, but the angle must be -1 (radians). This produces points at all distances from the pole, along the line in which the angle is -1 (radians) or about $-57°$.

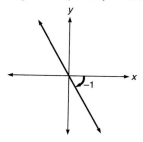

12. $r \sin \theta = -3$
$y = -3$
    Replace $r \sin \theta$ by y.
    This is the horizontal line $y = -3$.

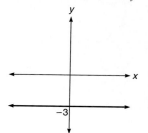

14. $r = 2 \cos \theta$

The following graph shows the rectangular coordinate graph of $r = 2$ cos θ. If we move the "negative lobe" between $\dfrac{\pi}{2}$ and $\dfrac{3\pi}{2}$ by adding π to all x values, it becomes a positive lobe between $\dfrac{3\pi}{2}$ and $\dfrac{5\pi}{2}$. This just repeats the positive lobe that starts at $\dfrac{3\pi}{2}$ in the graph. Thus, we can ignore the negative lobe for finding the polar graph.

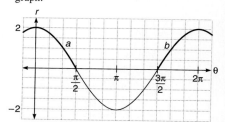

It is easier to imagine what is happening if we move the lobe that starts at 0 to start at 2π. We then see that we have a lobe between $\frac{3\pi}{2}$ and $\frac{5\pi}{2}$, with its maximum value at 2π.

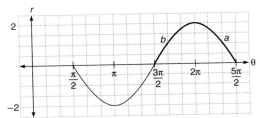

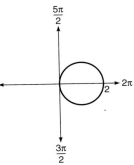

This positive lobe produces a circle between $\frac{3\pi}{2}$ and $\frac{5\pi}{2}$. It takes some experience or a lot of point plotting to know that this lobe is a circle. Remember, however, that graphs of the form $r = k \sin \theta$ or $r \approx k \cos \theta$ produce circles.

26. $r = 1 - \cos 2\theta$

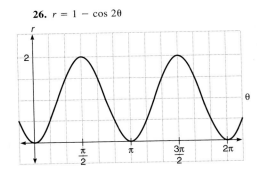

20. $r = \sin 3\theta$

The rectangular coordinate graph of $r = \sin 3\theta$ is shown below. The negative lobes can be ignored because shifting them by π units and flipping them about the θ axis causes them to overlap the positive lobes. We see there are lobes between 0 and $\frac{\pi}{3}$, with

maximum at $\frac{\pi}{6}$, $\frac{2\pi}{3}$, and π, with

maximum at $\frac{5\pi}{6}$, and $\frac{4\pi}{3}$ and $\frac{5\pi}{3}$,

with maximum at $\frac{3\pi}{2}$.

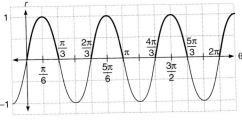

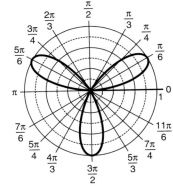

These lobes produce the polar graph shown.

The rectangular graph shows two lobes, one between 0 and π, with maximum at $\frac{\pi}{2}$, and one between π and 2π, with maximum at $\frac{3\pi}{2}$. The two positive lobes produce the polar graph shown. The two lobes are not circles, which would require algebra beyond the scope of this text to show. Of the problems in this text, only those equations categorized in the text as producing circles will in fact produce circles.

32. $r = 1 + \dfrac{\theta}{2}$

This graph is not periodic, and thus an analysis of its rectangular graph is less helpful than in cases where the trigonometric functions are involved. We simply plot points to obtain the graph. It is clear that as the value of θ increases, r increases. This property produces a spiral, which starts at $r = 1$. A table of values and the graph are shown.

θ	r
0	1
$\dfrac{\pi}{2}$	1.8
π	2.6
$\dfrac{3\pi}{2}$	3.4
2π	4.1
$\dfrac{5\pi}{2}$	4.9
3π	5.7

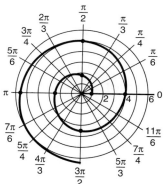

Chapter 7 review

1. real, 3; imaginary, -1 **2.** real, 0; imaginary, 3   **3.** real, 12; imaginary, 0
4. real, 0; imaginary, -1 **5.** $-1 - 2i$
6. $6 + i$ **7.** $63 + 48i$ **8.** $24 + 27i$
9. $12 + 8i$ **10.** $53 - 60i$
11. $\frac{42}{29} - \frac{40}{29}i$ **12.** $\frac{-2}{5} - \frac{3}{10}i$
13. $\frac{3}{7} - \frac{4}{7}i$ **14.** $1 + 4i$
15. $-2 + 4i$ **16.** $\frac{-4}{5} - \frac{7}{5}i$
17. $\frac{-25}{26} + \frac{5}{26}i$

18. a. $-4 - 3i$

b.

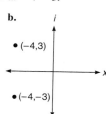

19. a. $-4 - i$

b.

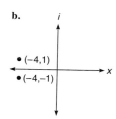

20. a. $-3i$

b.

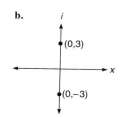

21. a. 17

b.

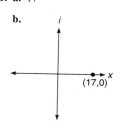

22. $3.6 \text{ cis}(-33.7°)$ **23.** $3.5 \text{ cis } 60°$
24. $2.2 \text{ cis}(-116.6°)$ **25.** $2 \text{ cis}(-30°)$
26. $3\sqrt{2} \text{ cis } 45°$ **27.** $4 \text{ cis}(-90°)$
28. $2.5 + 1.7i$ **29.** $-1.4 - 2.7i$
30. $-\dfrac{3}{2} - \dfrac{3\sqrt{3}}{2}i$ **31.** $5\sqrt{3} - 5i$
32. $6 \text{ cis } 70°$ **33.** $13 \text{ cis } 140°$
34. $8 \text{ cis } 100°$ **35.** $\frac{1}{2} \text{ cis } 36°$
36. $8 \text{ cis } 30°$ **37.** $16 \text{ cis}(-120°)$
38. $0.4 - 0.9i$ **39.** $2, 2i, -2, -2i$

40. $\dfrac{3}{2} + \dfrac{3\sqrt{3}}{2}i, -3, \dfrac{3}{2} - \dfrac{3\sqrt{3}}{2}i$

41. $\frac{13}{3} \text{ cis}(-50°)$

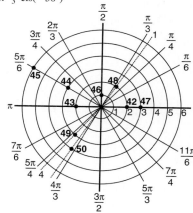

51. $\left(\dfrac{3\sqrt{3}}{2}, \dfrac{-3}{2}\right)$ **52.** $(-2, 2\sqrt{3})$
53. $(-1, \sqrt{3})$ **54.** $(1.08, 1.68)$
55. $(-2.08, 4.55)$ **56.** $(0.88, 0.48)$
57. $(2.24, 0.46)$ **58.** $(5.83, 2.60)$
59. $(4.12, -1.82)$ **60.** $\tan \theta = -3$
61. $r = \dfrac{2}{\sin \theta - 4 \cos \theta}$
62. $r^2 = \dfrac{5}{2 - 3 \cos^2\theta}$ **63.** $r = \dfrac{3 \cos \theta}{\sin^2\theta}$
64. $x^2 + y^2 = y$ **65.** $x = 2$
66. $x^4 + 2x^2y^2 + y^4 = 2xy$
67. $x^3 + xy^2 = y$ **68.** $y = 2$
69. $4x^2 + 3y^2 - 6y - 9 = 0$

70.

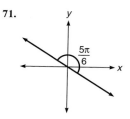

71.

72. $2r \sin \theta = 8$
$r \sin \theta = 4$
$y = 4$

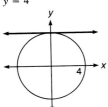

73. $r = 3 \cos \theta$

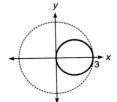

74.

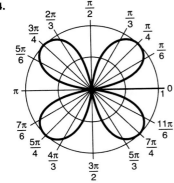

75.

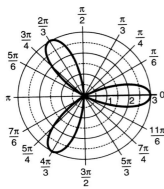

76.

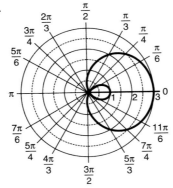

77.

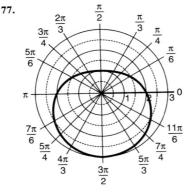

Chapter 7 test

1. $15 - 6i$ **2.** 34 **3.** $\frac{19}{13} - \frac{4}{13}i$
4. $-6 + 8i$ **5.** $6.4 \text{ cis}(-51.3°)$
6. $-1 + \sqrt{3}i$ **7.** $14 \text{ cis } 110°$
8. $3 \text{ cis } 120°$ **9.** $27 \text{ cis } 90°$
10. $2\left(\frac{\sqrt{2}}{2} + \frac{\sqrt{2}}{2}i\right), 2\left(-\frac{\sqrt{2}}{2} + \frac{\sqrt{2}}{2}i\right),$
$2\left(-\frac{\sqrt{2}}{2} - \frac{\sqrt{2}}{2}i\right), 2\left(\frac{\sqrt{2}}{2} - \frac{\sqrt{2}}{2}i\right)$

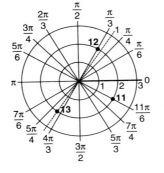

14. $(2.09, 2.15)$ **15.** $(2.08, -4.55)$
16. $\left(2, -\frac{5\pi}{6}\right)$ **17.** $\left(5\sqrt{2}, \frac{3\pi}{4}\right)$
18. $r = \dfrac{5}{\sin \theta + 3 \cos \theta}$
19. $2r^2\sin^2\theta - r \cos \theta = 5$
20. $y = 2$
21. $x^4 + 2x^2y^2 + y^4 = x^2 - y^2$

22.

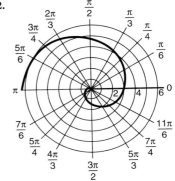

23. $r = 2 \csc \theta$
$r = \dfrac{2}{\sin \theta}$
$r \sin \theta = 2$
$y = 2$

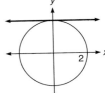

24.

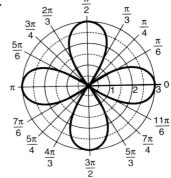

Appendix A

Answers to odd-numbered problems

1.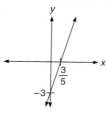

3.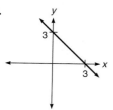

5.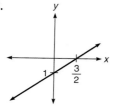

7.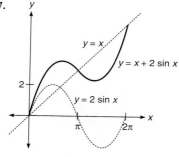

9.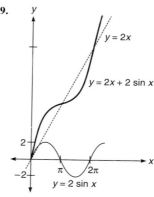

11.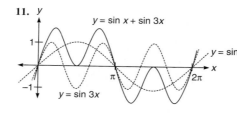

13.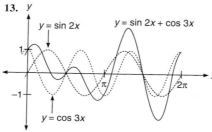

15.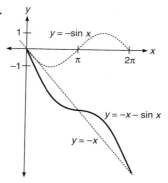

17.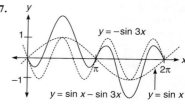

19.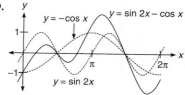

21. a.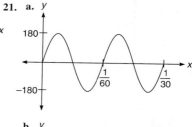

b.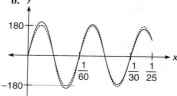

Solutions to trial exercise problems

5. $f(x) = \frac{2}{3}x - 1; y = \frac{2}{3}x - 1$
Let $x = 0$: $y = -1$, so $(0, -1)$ is the
y-intercept.
Let $y = 0$:
$0 = \frac{2}{3}x - 1$
$1 = \frac{2}{3}x$ Multiply by $\frac{3}{2}$.
$\frac{3}{2} = x$, so $(\frac{3}{2}, 0)$ is the x-intercept.
(See the diagram.)

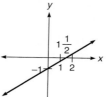

6. $f(x) = -2x;\ y = -2x$

By letting $x = 0$ and then $y = 0$, we find that the x- and y-intercepts are the same point $(0,0)$. Thus, to graph this function we need another point. To get another point, we can let x (or y) be any value but 0, which we have already used. Let $x = 2$; thus, $y = -4$, and $(2,-4)$ is another point to plot. (See the diagram.)

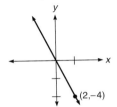

13. $y = \sin 2x + \cos 3x$

First we graph $y = \sin 2x$:

$$0 \le 2x \le 2\pi$$
$$0 \le x \le \pi$$

(shown in short dashed lines in the diagram)

and $y = \cos 3x$:

$$0 \le 3x \le 2\pi$$
$$0 \le x \le \frac{2\pi}{3}$$

(shown in long dashed lines).

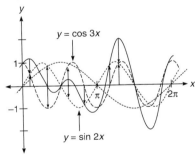

Next we add the ordinates. Remember that wherever one function is zero (crosses the x-axis), the result is the other function. Wherever the functions have equal absolute values but opposite signs, the result is zero. Wherever both functions cross, the result is twice the height of either function. (See the diagram.)

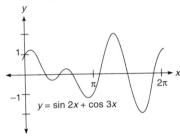

17. $y = \sin x - \sin 3x$

We rewrite the function as $y = \sin x + (-\sin 3x)$. We now graph $y = \sin x$ and $y = -\sin 3x$, and add the ordinates. (See the diagram.)

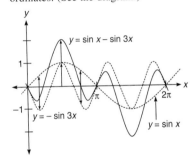

20. $y = 7.5 \sin \frac{\pi}{6}x + 10 \sin \frac{\pi}{3}x$

$0 \le \frac{\pi}{6}x \le 2\pi$. Multiply by $\frac{6}{\pi}$.

$\frac{6}{\pi} \cdot 0 \le \frac{6}{\pi} \cdot \frac{\pi}{6}x \le \frac{6}{\pi} \cdot 2\pi;\ 0 \le x \le 12$.

Similarly,

$0 \le \frac{\pi}{3}x \le 2\pi$. Multiply by $\frac{3}{\pi}$.

$\frac{3}{\pi} \cdot 0 \le \frac{3}{\pi} \cdot \frac{\pi}{3}x \le \frac{3}{\pi} \cdot 2\pi;$

$0 \le 2x \le 12;\ 0 \le x \le 6$.

(See the diagram.)

Appendix B

Answers to odd-numbered problems

1. a.

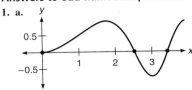

b. 0, 2.5, 3.5   **c.** 0, 2.50662827, 3.54490770

3. a.

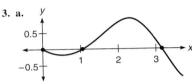

b. 0, 1.1, 3.2   **c.** 0, 1.04719755, 3.14159265 (π)

5. a.

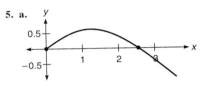

b. 0, 2.5   **c.** 0, 2.47457679

7. a. ± 1.9

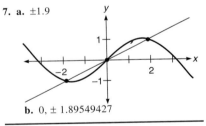

b. 0, $\pm$ 1.89549427

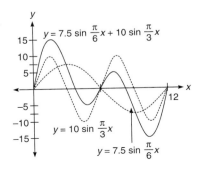

9. a. 1.5

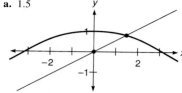

b. 1.47817027

11. The graph of $y = \csc \theta + \cot \theta$, and $y = \dfrac{1 + \cos \theta}{\sin \theta}$ both look like the following.

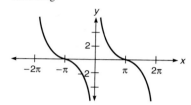

13. The graphs of $y = \dfrac{\csc \theta}{\sec \theta + \tan \theta}$ and of $y = \dfrac{\cos \theta}{\sin \theta + \sin^2 \theta}$ both look like the following.

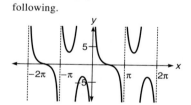

15. The graph of both $y = \dfrac{1}{\sec \theta - \cos \theta}$ and of $y = \cot \theta \csc \theta$ are as follows.

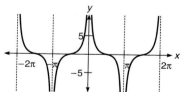

17. See the answers to appendix A.
19. See the answers to appendix A, problem 21.

21. Each graph done with the first 12 terms.

a.

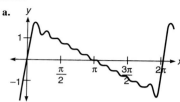

b.

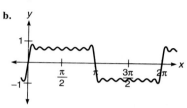

c.

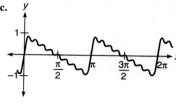

d.

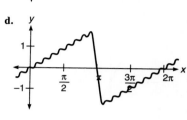

Solutions to trial exercise problems

22. a.

x	$\sin(x)$	$\sin[(4\pi + 1)x]$	$\sin[(8\pi + 1)x]$	$\sin[(12\pi + 1)x]$
0	0.00	0.00	0.00	0.00
0.5	0.48	0.48	0.48	0.48
1	0.84	0.84	0.84	0.84
1.5	1.00	1.00	1.00	1.00
2	0.91	0.91	0.91	0.91
2.5	0.60	0.60	0.60	0.60
3	0.14	0.14	0.14	0.14
3.5	−0.35	−0.35	−0.35	−0.35
4	−0.76	−0.76	−0.76	−0.76
4.5	−0.98	−0.98	−0.98	−0.98
5	−0.96	−0.96	−0.96	−0.96
5.5	−0.71	−0.71	−0.71	−0.71
6	−0.28	−0.28	−0.28	−0.28
6.5	0.22	0.22	0.22	0.22

All functions of the form $y = \sin[(4k\pi + 1)x]$ are equal if x is an integer multiple of $\frac{1}{2}$.

b. The second column of part b of the next table shows the values that these functions produce. They are the same for the four functions. All functions of the form $y = \sin[(8k\pi + 1)x]$ are equal if x is an integer multiple of $\frac{1}{4}$.

c. The second column of part c of the table below shows the values that these functions produce. They are the same for the four functions.

All functions of the form $y = \sin[(20k\pi + 1)x]$ are equal if x is an integer multiple of $\frac{1}{10}$.

Part b			**Part c**	
x	$\sin[(8\pi + 1)x]$		x	$\sin[(20k\pi + 1)x]$
0	0.00		0	0.00
0.25	0.25		0.1	0.10
0.5	0.48		0.2	0.20
0.75	0.68		0.3	0.30
1	0.84		0.4	0.39
1.25	0.95		0.5	0.48
1.5	1.00		0.6	0.56
1.75	0.98		0.7	0.64
2	0.91		0.8	0.72
2.25	0.78		0.9	0.78
2.5	0.60		1	0.84
2.75	0.38		1.1	0.89
3	0.14		1.2	0.93
3.25	−0.11		1.3	0.96

d. In parts a, b, c, we notice that $\frac{1}{2} \cdot 4k\pi = 2k\pi$, $\frac{1}{4} \cdot 8k\pi = 2k\pi$, $\frac{1}{10} \cdot 20k\pi = 2k\pi$, so we know that for $\frac{1}{100}$ we need $\frac{1}{100} \cdot \beta k\pi = 2k\pi$, so $\beta = 200$. Thus, all functions of the form $y = \sin[(200k\pi + 1)x]$ are equal if x is an integer multiple of $\frac{1}{100}$.

e. To see why the generalization of part a is true we consider the following:

If x is an integer multiple of $\frac{1}{2}$ we can describe it as $x = \dfrac{n}{2}$ for some integer n. Then,

$$\sin[(4k\pi + 1)x] = \sin\left[\left(4k\pi + 1\right) \cdot \frac{n}{2}\right] = \sin\left(2nk\pi + \frac{n}{2}\right)$$

$$= \sin 2nk\pi \cos \frac{n}{2} + \cos 2nk\pi \sin \frac{n}{2}$$

$$= 0 \cdot \cos \frac{n}{2} + 1 \cdot \sin \frac{n}{2}$$

$$= \sin \frac{n}{2} = \sin x$$

Thus, as long as x is an integer multiple of $\frac{1}{2}$, $\sin[(4k\pi + 1)x] = \sin x$.

Similar reasoning shows why the generalizations of parts b, c, and d are true.

Index of Applications

Aerodynamics

Mathematical modeling, 25

Aeronautics

Rocket movement, 55, 79

Architecture

Spiral staircase, 28

Astronomy

Sunspot activity, 119

Automotive Engineering

Alternator on engine, 72
ATDC, 47
BTDC, 47
Timing marks on engine, 72

Electronics

Apparent power, 253
Applied voltage in circuit, 79
Average power, 25, 26
Current vs. voltage, 47
Graph of impedance, 243
Impedance diagram, 10, 34
Instantaneous current, 55, 84
Instantaneous voltage, 55, 82
Model AC signal, 116, 117, 119, 132
Ohm's law, 247, 251
Pattern of radiation of antenna, 261
Power in AC circuit, 27
Resistance/impedance in parallel circuit, 140, 251
Total circuit impedance, 7, 26

Engineering

Shape of cam on sewing machine, 261

General

Angle determined by picture at observer's eye, 156
Angle of depression from aircraft, 156
Angle of elevation of rocket, 156

Area of sector at airport terminal, 72
Biorhythms, 132
Centigrade/Fahrenheit temperature conversion, 140
Distance to building, 224
Distance to object, 27, 35, 153, 214, 215, 238
Flagpole, 7, 10, 34, 164
Height of building, 164
Height of ladder, 24
Ladder on fire truck, 10
Locate lost aircraft, 237
Movement of hang glider, 213
Path of amusement park ride, 272
Sheet metal work, 221
Weight of steel bar, 37
Wheel on automobile, 71, 83
Wheel on ski lift cable, 71

Geology

Model earth's ice ages, 119

History

Ancient Egyptian formula for area of quadrilateral, 216

Machining

Distance across flats of hexagonal stock, 26
Length of part, 35
Numerically controlled machine, 58, 61, 83, 237
Saw cut along diagonal, 10
Tip of threading tool, 27

Manufacturing

Industrial robot, 84
Laser device to cut cloth, 61, 83
Numerically controlled machine, 223, 252
Path of industrial robot, 261
Piece of wood being mass produced, 27

Medicine

Interpreting electrocardiogram, 79
Scanning diagnostic device, 61

Military Science

Relative strength of troops, 11

Index

A

"A Chaotic Search for *i*," 192
Acute angle, 3
Adjacent side in triangle, 4
A History of π, 62
Ambiguous case of law of sines, 210, 236
Amplitude of sine or cosine function, 102
Angle, 2
    acute, 3
    obtuse, 3
    reference, 49, 80
    right, 3
    straight, 3
    vertex of, 2
Angle in standard position, 42, 80
Angle measurement, 2
Angle of depression, 27
Angle of elevation, 27
Angles, quadrantal, 49, 80
Arc, 1
Arccos (inverse cosine function), 148, 162
Arccosecant (inverse cosecant function), 159, 162
Arccot (inverse cotangent function), 157, 162
Arc length, 63
Arcsecant (inverse secant function), 159, 162
Arcsin (inverse sine function), 142, 162
Arctan (inverse tangent function), 151, 162
Area of sector of a circle, 69, 81
Argand diagram, 243
Argument of a function, 105
ASTC rule, 48, 49, 80
Asymptotes, 93
ATDC, 47

B

Basic cosine cycle, 105, 129
Basic sine cycle, 105, 129
Beckmann, Petr, 62
BTDC, 47

C

Calculator, electronic, 2
Cardioid (graph of polar equation), 271
Celestial sphere, 1
Chaotic behavior in iterative systems, 192
Chord, 1
Chudnovsky, G. V. and D. V., 62
Circumference of a circle, 62
Cofunction identities, 178, 203
Columbia University, 62

Complementary angles, 179
Complex conjugate, 240, 272
Complex number
    graph of, 243
    polar form, 244, 272
    rectangular form, 240, 272
Complex numbers
    addition and subtraction, 241, 276
    division, 242, 246, 272
    equality of, 241, 272
    multiplication, 241, 246, 272
Conditional equation, 28, 31, 167
Conjugate of a binomial, 171
Coordinate plane, 41
Coordinates of ordered pair, 41
Cosecant function, 43
Cosecant function, graph of, 95, 123, 130
Cosecant trigonometric ratio, 13, 14
Cosine function, 43
Cosine function, graph, 90, 129
Cosine trigonometric ratio, 11
Cotangent function, 43, 98
Cotangent function, graph of, 119, 130
Cotangent trigonometric ratio, 13, 14
Coterminal angles (degrees), 42
Coterminal angles (radian measure), 66
CT (computed tomography) scanner, 41

D

Decimal degree system, 3
Degree mode of calculator, 21
Degrees, 2, 33
De Moivre's theorem, 247
De Moivre's theorem for roots, 248
Descartes, René, 239
Direction of vector, 225
Distance formula, 216
DMS (degree, minute, second) system, 3
Domain of function, 37
Double-angle identities, 184, 203

E

Elements, 3
Equation, 166
    conditional, 28, 31, 167
    identity, 28, 167
    linear, 167
Equivalent equations using substitution, 168
Euclid, 3
Euclidean geometry, 3
Even function, 90

The Primary Trigonometric Ratios

If θ is either of the two acute angles in a right triangle, then

$$\sin \theta = \frac{\text{length of side opposite } \theta}{\text{length of hypotenuse}},$$

$$\cos \theta = \frac{\text{length of side adjacent to } \theta}{\text{length of hypotenuse}},$$

$$\tan \theta = \frac{\text{length of side opposite to } \theta}{\text{length of side adjacent to } \theta}.$$

The Trigonometric Functions

Let θ be an angle in standard position, and (x, y) be any point on the terminal side of angle θ, except $(0,0)$. Let $r = \sqrt{x^2 + y^2}$ be the distance from the origin to the point. Then

$$\sin \theta = \frac{y}{r}, \ \cos \theta = \frac{x}{r}, \ \tan \theta = \frac{y}{x},$$

$$\csc \theta = \frac{r}{y}, \ \sec \theta = \frac{r}{x}, \ \cot \theta = \frac{x}{y}.$$

Radian Measure

Let θ be an angle in standard position with degree measure $\theta°$ and radian measure s. Then $\dfrac{s}{\pi} = \dfrac{\theta°}{180°}$.

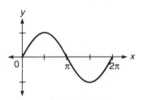

Basic sine cycle

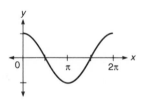

Basic cosine cycle

Inverse Trigonometric Functions

$y = \sin^{-1}x$ means (1) $\sin y = x$

                  (2) $-\dfrac{\pi}{2} \le y \le \dfrac{\pi}{2}$

                  (3) $-1 \le x \le 1$

$y = \cos^{-1}x$ means (1) $\cos y = x$

                  (2) $0 \le y \le \pi$

                  (3) $-1 \le x \le 1$

$y = \tan^{-1}x$ means (1) $\tan y = x$

                  (2) $-\dfrac{\pi}{2} < y < \dfrac{\pi}{2}$

$y = \cot^{-1}x$ means (1) $\cot y = x$

                  (2) $0 < y < \pi$

$$\sec^{-1}x = \cos^{-1}\frac{1}{x} \text{ if } |x| \ge 1.$$

$$\csc^{-1}x = \sin^{-1}\frac{1}{x} \text{ if } |x| \ge 1.$$

$$\cot^{-1}x = \frac{\pi}{2} - \tan^{-1}x$$

Reciprocal Identities

$$\csc \theta = \frac{1}{\sin \theta}, \ \sec \theta = \frac{1}{\cos \theta}, \ \cot \theta = \frac{1}{\tan \theta}$$

Tangent, Cotangent Identities

$$\tan \theta = \frac{\sin \theta}{\cos \theta}, \ \cot \theta = \frac{\cos \theta}{\sin \theta}$$

Pythagorean Identities

$$\sin^2\theta + \cos^2\theta = 1$$
$$\sec^2\theta = \tan^2\theta + 1$$
$$\csc^2\theta = \cot^2\theta + 1$$

Sum and Difference Identities

$$\sin (\alpha + \beta) = \sin \alpha \cos \beta + \cos \alpha \sin \beta$$
$$\sin (\alpha - \beta) = \sin \alpha \cos \beta - \cos \alpha \sin \beta$$
$$\cos (\alpha + \beta) = \cos \alpha \cos \beta - \sin \alpha \sin \beta$$
$$\cos (\alpha - \beta) = \cos \alpha \cos \beta + \sin \alpha \sin \beta$$
$$\tan (\alpha + \beta) = \frac{\tan \alpha + \tan \beta}{1 - \tan \alpha \tan \beta}$$
$$\tan (\alpha - \beta) = \frac{\tan \alpha - \tan \beta}{1 + \tan \alpha \tan \beta}$$

Cofunction Identities

$$\sin\left(\frac{\pi}{2} - \theta\right) = \cos \theta, \ \tan\left(\frac{\pi}{2} - \theta\right) = \cot \theta,$$
$$\sec\left(\frac{\pi}{2} - \theta\right) = \csc \theta$$

Double-Angle Identities

$$\sin 2\alpha = 2 \sin \alpha \cos \alpha$$
$$\cos 2\alpha = \cos^2\alpha - \sin^2\alpha$$
$$= 1 - 2 \sin^2\alpha$$
$$= 2 \cos^2\alpha - 1$$
$$\tan 2\alpha = \frac{2 \tan \alpha}{1 - \tan^2\alpha}$$